American Heart Association Recommendations for the Prevention of Bacterial Endocarditis

Table 1. Cardiac Conditions Associated With Endocarditis

ENDOCARDITIS PROPHYLAXIS RECOMMENDED	ENDOCARDITIS PROPHYLAXIS NOT RECOMMENDED
High-Risk Category	**Negligible-Risk Category (no greater risk than the general population)**
Prosthetic cardiac valves, including bioprosthetic and homograft valves	Isolated _____ ' septal defect
Previous bacterial endocarditis	Surgic_____ ' defect,
Complex cyanotic congenital heart disease (e.g., single ventricle states, transposition of the great arteries, tetralogy of Fallot)	ver_____ atent ductus ? _____ beyond 6 mo)
Surgically constructed systemic pulmonary shunts or conduits	_____ /pass graft surgery _____ .nout valvar
Moderate-Risk Category	_____ .ial, or innocent heart
Most other congenital cardiac malformations (other than above an_ below)	_____ aki disease without valvar
Acquired valvar dysfunction (e.g., rheumatic heart disease)	_____ eumatic fever without valvar .ion
Hypertrophic cardiomyopathy	Ca____ _ pacemakers (intravascular and epicardial) and implanted defibrillators
Mitral valve prolapse with valvar regurgitation and/or thickened leaflets	

Table 2. Prophylactic Regimens for Dental, Oral, Respiratory Tract, or Esophageal Procedures

SITUATION	AGENT	REGIMEN*
Standard general prophylaxis	Amoxicillin	Adults: 2.0 g; children: 50 mg/kg orally 1 h before procedure
Unable to take oral medications	Ampicillin	Adults: 2.0 g IM or IV; children: 50 mg/kg IM or IV within 30 min before procedure
Allergic to penicillin	Clindamycin *or*	Adults: 600 mg; children: 20 mg/kg orally 1 h before procedure
	Cephalexin[†] *or* cefadroxil[†] *or*	Adults: 2.0 g; children; 50 mg/kg orally 1 h before procedure
	Azithromycin *or* clarithromycin	Adults: 500 mg; children: 15 mg/kg orally 1 h before procedure
Allergic to penicillin and unable to take oral medications	Clindamycin *or*	Adults: 600 mg; children: 20 mg/kg IV within 30 min before procedure
	Cefazolin[†]	Adults: 1.0 g; children: 25 mg/kg IM or IV within 30 min before procedure

IM, intramuscularly; IV, intravenously.

* Total children's dose should not exceed adult dose.

[†] Cephalosporins should not be used in individuals with immediate-type hypersensitivity reaction (urticaria, angioedema, or anaphylaxis) to penicillins.

Adapted with permission from Dajani AS, Taubert KA, Wilson W, Bolger AF, Bayer A, Ferrieri P, et al. Prevention of bacterial endocarditis: Recommendations by the American Heart Association. Circulation. 1997;96(1):358–366. Tables 1 and 4.

Antibiotic Prophylaxis for Dental Patients with Total Joint Replacement
Joint advisory statement of the American Dental Association and the American Academy of Orthopaedic Surgeons.

Table 1. Patients at Potential Increased Risk of Hematogenous Total Joint Infection*

PATIENT TYPE	CONDITION PLACING PATIENT AT RISK
All patients during first two years following joint replacement	Not applicable
Immunocompromised/immunosuppressed patients	Rheumatoid arthritis Systemic lupus erythematosus Drug or radiation-induced immunosuppression
Patients with comorbidities†	Previous prosthetic joint infections Malnourishment Hemophilia HIV infection Type 1 (insulin-dependent) diabetes Malignancy

*Based on Ching and colleagues,[1] Brause,[2] Murray and colleagues,[3] Poss and colleagues,[4] Jacobson and colleagues,[5] Johnson and Bannister,[6] Jacobson and colleagues[7] and Berbari and colleagues.[8]
†Conditions shown for patients in this category are examples only; there may be additional conditions that place such patients at risk of experiencing hematogenous total joint infection.

Table 2. Incidence Stratification of Bacteremic Dental Procedures*

INCIDENCE	DENTAL PROCEDURE
Higher Incidence†	Tooth extraction Periodontal procedures (surgery, subgingival placement of fibers/strips, scaling, probing, recall maintenance) Implant placement and replantation of avulsed teeth Endodontic (root canal) instrumentation or surgery only beyond the apex Initial placement of orthodontic bands (not brackets) Intraligamentary and intraosseous local anesthetic injection Prophylactic cleaning of teeth or implants where bleeding is anticipated
Lower Incidence‡§	Restorative dentistry# (operative and prosthodontic) with or without retraction cord Local anesthetic injections (nonintraligamentary and nonintraosseous) Intracanal endodontic treatment; post placement, buildup Rubber dam placement Postoperative suture removal Placement of removable prosthodontic/orthodontic appliances Taking of impressions Fluoride treatment Taking radiographs Adjustment of orthodontic appliances

*Adapted with permission of the publisher from Dajani AS, Taubert KA, Wilson W, et al.[9]
†Prophylaxis should be considered for patients with total joint replacement who meet the criteria in Table 1. No other patients with orthopedic implants should be considered for antibiotic prophylaxis prior to dental treatment/procedures.
‡Antibiotic prophylaxis not indicated.
§Clinical judgment may indicate antibiotic prophylaxis in selected circumstances involving significant bleeding.
#Includes restoration of carious (decayed) or missing teeth.

Table 3. Suggested Antibiotic Prophylaxis Regimens

PATIENT TYPE	SUGGESTED DRUG	REGIMEN
Patients not allergic to penicillin	Cephalexin, cephradrine, or amoxicillin	2 g orally 1 hr prior to the dental procedure
Patients not allergic to penicillin and unable to take oral medications	Cefazolin or ampicillin	Cefazolin 1 g or ampicillin 2 g IM or IV 1 hr prior to the dental procedure
Patients allergic to penicillin	Clindamycin	600 mg orally 1 hr prior to the dental procedure
Patients allergic to penicillin and unable to take oral medication	Clindamycin	600 mg IV 1 hr prior to the dental procedure

Advisory Statement from ADA and AAOS: Antibiotic prophylaxis for dental patients with total joint replacements, JADA 2003;134(7):895–899. Tables 1, 2, and 3. Reprinted by permission of ADA Publishing.

1. Ching DW, Gould IM, Rennie JA, Gibson PI. Prevention of late haematogenous infection in major prosthetic joints. J Antimicrob Chemother 1989;23:676–80. 2. Brause BD. Infections associated with prosthetic joints. Clin Rheum Dis 1986;12:523–35. 3. Murray RP, Bourne MH, Fitzgerald RH Jr. Metachronous infection in patients who have had more than one total joint arthroplasty. J Bone Joint Surg Am 1991;73(10):1469–74. 4. Poss R, Thornhill TS, Ewald FC, Thomas WH, Batte NJ, Sledge CB. Factors influencing the incidence and outcome of infection following total joint arthroplasty. Clin Orthop 1984;182:117–26. 5. Jacobson JJ, Millard HD, Plezia R, Blankenship JR. Dental treatment and late prosthetic joint infections. Oral Surg Oral Med Oral Pathol 1986;61:413–7. 6. Johnson DP, Bannister GG. The outcome of infected arthroplasty of the knee. J Bone Joint Surg Br 1986;68(2):289–91. 7. Jacobson JJ, Patel B, Asher G, Wooliscroft JO, Schaberg D. Oral Staphylococcus in elderly subjects with rheumatoid arthritis. J Am Geriatr Soc 1997;45:1–5. 8. Berbari EF, Hanssen AD, Duffy MC, Ilstrup DM, Harmsen WS, Osmon DR. Risk factors for prosthetic joint infection: case–control study. Clin Infect Dis 1998;27:1247–54. 9. Dajani AS, Taubert KA, Wilson W, et al. Prevention of bacterial endocarditis: recommendations by the American Heart Association. From the Committee on Rheumatic Fever, Endocarditis and Kawasaki Disease, Council on Cardiovascular Disease in the Young. JAMA 1997;277:1794–801.

Lippincott Williams & Wilkins'
Dental Drug Reference
with Clinical Implications

Frieda Atherton Pickett, RDH, MS
Géza T. Terézhalmy, DDS, MA

Lippincott Williams & Wilkins'
Dental Drug Reference
with Clinical Implications

Frieda Atherton Pickett, RDH, MS
Adjunct Associate Professor
Dental Hygiene Program
East Tennessee State University
Johnson City, TN
Former Associate Professor and Clinical Coordinator
Caruth School of Dental Hygiene
Baylor College of Dentistry
Dallas, TX

Géza T. Terézhalmy, DDS, MA
Endowed Professor in Clinical Dentistry
Dental School
Professor, Department of Pharmacology
Graduate School of Biomedical Sciences
The University of Texas Health Science Center at San Antonio
San Antonio, TX

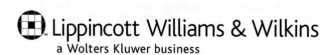 Lippincott Williams & Wilkins
a Wolters Kluwer business

Executive Editor: John Goucher
Senior Publisher: Julie K. Stegman
Managing Editor: Heather A. Rybacki
Marketing Manager: Hilary Henderson
Manager, Software Development: David Horne
Copy Editors: Sue E. Flint, Alison T. Kelley, Jenifer F. Walker, MA
Proofreaders: Kristi Lukens, Raymond Lukens
Manufacturing Coordinator: Dana Jackson
Cover Designer: Jason Delaney
Internal Designer: Karen Savage
Typesetter: Maryland Composition
Printer & Binder: Malloy Litho, Inc.

Library of Congress Cataloging-in-Publication Data

Pickett, Frieda Atherton.
  Lippincott Williams & Wilkins' dental drug reference with clinical implications / Frieda A. Pickett, Geza T. Terezhalmy.
      p. ; cm.
  ISBN 0-7817-7762-3
  1. Dental pharmacology—Handbooks, manuals, etc. I. Terezhalmy, G. T. (Geza T.) II. Title. III. Title: Dental drug reference with clinical implications. IV. Title: Lippincott Williams and Wilkins' dental drug reference with clinical implications.
  [DNLM: 1. Pharmaceutical Preparations—Handbooks. 2. Dentistry—Handbooks. QV 39 P597L 2006]
  RK701.P63 2006
  615'.10246176—dc22

                        2005030521

To purchase additional copies of this book, call our customer service department at **(800) 638-3030** or fax orders to **(301) 824-7390**. For other book services, including chapter reprints and large quantity sales, ask for the Special Sales department.

For all other calls originating outside of the United States, please call **(301) 714-2324**.

Visit Lippincott Williams & Wilkins on the Internet: **http://www.lww.com**. Lippincott Williams & Wilkins customer service representatives are available from 8:30 am to 4:30 pm, EST, Monday through Friday, for telephone access.

05 06 07 08 09 10 11
1 2 3 4 5 6 7 8 9 10

Preface

Lippincott Williams and Wilkins' Dental Drug Reference with Clinical Implications is designed as a quick and concise resource for dental professionals. This unique reference delivers clinically relevant information to be used chairside during the review of a patient's medical history. In addition to providing data on the drugs encountered and used in dentistry, *LWW's Dental Drug Reference with Clinical Implications* also serves as an up-to-date reference for the pharmacological management of orodental pain, oral infections, and common mucocutaneous conditions, and also presents a practical approach to relevant adverse drug events.

The text begins with a discussion of general principles of pharmacology and adverse drug events, an understanding of which is essential for the rational use of drugs in the prevention, diagnosis, and treatment of disease. Subsequent chapters provide insightful information related to the risk stratification and dental management of the patient taking medication for a variety of systemic diseases, and a common sense approach to the potential medical emergencies one may encounter in the oral health care setting. Prescription examples can be found in the section on the medical management of selected oral conditions.

The attached CD-ROM contains expanded but concise information relevant to the management of odontogenic pain and infection, plus full-color clinical photographs of common mucocutaneous conditions and oral manifestations of adverse drug effects.

Readers may receive continuing education credits for the personal study of the Clinical Medicine and Therapeutics chapters in Section 1. Refer to the inside front cover for additional details.

The A to Z Listing of Drugs provides information relevant to dentistry on over 3,500 formulations. We have made every effort to include current, up-to-date information as it was available at the time of manuscript preparation. However, the user should be cautioned that therapeutic recommendations change as new drugs and new drug information becomes available. Information on all drugs listed in the text can be printed from the CD-ROM and placed in patient charts.

The appendices present information that is not readily available in other reference sources but which may be helpful to the oral health care provider. This includes a Spanish-English translation guide, a list of herbal and nutritional supplements and how they may effect dental care, and product-specific information such as toothpastes that do not contain sodium laurel sulfate.

Our goal in writing *LWW's Dental Drug Reference with Clinical Implications* was to provide relevant, concise information in a conveniently-sized book that can be stored in the dental operatory. Our focus was to include drugs likely to be reported on the health history and drugs that the dental professional would be likely to use. For that reason, not all drugs are included. If the user encounters a drug that has not been included, but should be, you are asked to notify LWW via e-mail to DDR@LWW.com.

Frieda Atherton Pickett, RDH, MS
Géza T. Terézhalmy, DDS, MA

How to Use This Book

Lippincott Williams and Wilkins' Dental Drug Reference with Clinical Implications is divided into three sections.

Section 1: Clinical Medicine and Therapeutics may be read at one's convenience or may be referred to during the clinical decision-making process. The chapters on General Principles of Pharmacology and Adverse Drug Events (the latter of which includes corresponding clinical photographs on the CD-ROM) provide crucial information on prescribing or using drugs in the clinical setting, and on how other drugs the patient may be taking will affect their oral care. Current recommendations for Medical Management of Pain and Medical Management of Odontogenic Infections can be found on the CD-ROM; the Table of Contents for both of these chapters are listed in this book for your reference. The chapter on the Medical Management of Selected Oral Conditions includes sample prescriptions and corresponding clinical images that can be viewed on the CD-ROM. The first section of the book is rounded out with a chapter on Clinical Medicine, with recommendations for the dental management of patients with selected systemic diseases, and a chapter outlining a stepwise approach to the Management of Medical Emergencies in the Oral Health Care Setting. The University of Texas Health Science Center at San Antonio, Dental School, is offering Continuing Education credits based on these seven chapters. Instructions on how to obtain CE credits can be found on the inside front cover.

Section 2: A to Z Listing of Drugs includes concise therapeutic information for individual drugs likely to be reported on the health history, along with expanded information on drugs prescribed by the dentist. Drugs are listed alphabetically by generic name, brand names, and synonyms, with brand name and synonym listings directing you to the appropriate generic drug name. The *concise drug monographs* present information relevant to the oral health care treatment plan. *Drugs likely to be prescribed or used by the dental professional* are identified by a tooth icon (🦷) next to the generic name and contain expanded information to include dosages for the various forms of the product (topical, oral, injectable), pharmacokinetics of the drug, and the pregnancy risk category of the drug.

The following outlines the elements that are included in each drug monograph. Points of information that appear only for drugs prescribed or used by the dental professional are indicated by the tooth icon (🦷).

GENERAL INFORMATION

Drug Name	The generic drug name is listed at the top of each drug monograph, followed by the phonetic pronunciation in parentheses. The pronunciations are based on the USAN Council officially designated pronunciations. If there are alternate generic names used for a particular drug, they will appear in small black font after the written pronunciation, enclosed in parentheses. Common synonyms are preceded by the title "Synonyms."
Trade Name	U.S. trade names for each drug are listed in bold black font. If the drug is administered or prescribed by a dental care provider, the available dosage forms and dosages follow the trade drug name. Common Canadian trade names are indicated by the Canadian flag icon (🇨🇦). Common Mexican trade names are preceded by the Mexican

flag icon (██◐██). If a trade name is available in both the U.S. and Canada or Mexico, it will appear in the U.S. list only.

Drug Class The drug class indicates the drug's classification or therapeutic category.

DEA Schedule If a drug is a controlled substance, the U.S. Drug Enforcement Administration schedule is listed.

PHARMACOLOGY

Action Action describes how the drug works.

Uses Uses list all approved indications for the drug.

Unlabeled Uses Unlabeled uses (indications for which the drug is frequently used but for which it is not approved) are given when applicable.

Contraindications Contraindications are listed when appropriate. Hypersensitivity to a given drug is always a contraindication and, therefore, this fact is assumed and has not been repeated for every monograph. *Standard Considerations* appears when there are no specific contraindications other than hypersensitivity.

⟨ Usual Dosage The route of administration and typical dosages are provided. Where applicable, dosages are organized by age group and/or condition.

⟨ Pharmacokinetics The Pharmacokinetics section details the absorption (ASORP), distribution (DIST), metabolism (METAB), excretion rate (EXCRET), onset, peak, and duration of the drug, along with useful information on how pharmacokinetic factors differ in certain populations (SPECIAL POP).

Drug Interactions Drug interaction information indicates the drug category or specific dental drug likely to interact with the subject drug, the likely mechanism of the interaction, and the clinical dental recommendation for the interaction. For *concise drug monographs*, only drug interactions that are relevant to dental treatment are listed, under the heading Drug Interactions Related to Dental Therapeutics. For *drugs that are likely to be used or prescribed by a dental professional*, a more comprehensive listing of interactions is provided.

Drug interaction information included throughout the drug monographs is based primarily on clinical reports, with some theoretical interactions. Since new drug interactions are being reported daily, it is important to note that the absence of information does not always imply safety.

Adverse Effects Common or life-threatening adverse reactions for the drug are listed according to the following body systems: oral, central nervous system (CNS), cardiovascular system (CVS), gastrointestinal system (GI), and respiratory system (RESP). Other applicable adverse reactions are listed after the miscellaneous (MISC) heading.

CLINICAL IMPLICATIONS

General
The General section addresses the implications of the drug effects or of the medical condition for which the drug is prescribed. The information provided here may reflect potential changes to the treatment plan and should be reviewed thoroughly prior to initiation of treatment.

Pregnancy Risk Category
Indicates the FDA pregnancy risk category for the drug.

Oral Health Education
The section on Oral Health Education lists information that should be shared with the patient or caregiver, including information on the drug's administration, potential side effects, and safety precautions.

Section 3: Appendices provide clinically useful information in an easy-to-use format. Drugs Listed by Therapeutic Category or Condition can be referenced when the patient cannot recall the name of a drug being taken. Locate the category the agent would most likely fall under, such as "antihypertensive agents," and have the patient look through the list of drug names to identify the drug being used. The Abbreviations appendix defines the abbreviations and acronyms used throughout the drug monographs. Herbal and Nutritional Supplements of Interest to Dentistry lists dentally-relevant information for supplements likely to be consumed. This list is not all-inclusive, and suggestions for updates or additions can be submitted to LWW via e-mail to DDR@LWW.com. Spanish/English Dental Communication Guidelines covers common phrases to assist the dental professional when communicating with a Spanish-speaking patient. The appendix on In-Office Preventive Products is comprised of specific information on products in various categories, including: fluoride varnishes; toothpastes without sodium laurel sulfate, cinnamon or methylparaben; products with therapeutic levels of xylitol; and oral rinses without alcohol. The Laboratory Values for Normal Limits appendix, found on the CD-ROM, addresses normal values as well as safe limit values for the most common laboratory tests the dental professional would consider when completing a medical consultation.

The full text of this handbook is included on the CD-ROM in an easy-to-use, searchable format. Drug information can be printed from the CD and placed into a patient's record for quick reference.

The last and first pages of the text summarize recommendations for antibiotic prophylaxis prior to dental procedures likely to result in significant bleeding. The American Heart Association recommendations to prevent bacterial endocarditis following specific oral procedures can be found at the front of the book; the American Dental Association/American Academy of Orthopedic Society recommendations for total joint replacement (TJR) situations are printed at the back of the book.

Acknowledgments

The authors wish to express their sincere gratitude for the contributions made by the Editorial Review Board, who were selected on the basis of their extensive experience and knowledge.

This book would not have been possible without the assistance and cooperation of my colleague, Géza T. Terézhalmy, DDS, MA. He is a wonderful coauthor, pleasant to work with, and encouraging in his demeanor. This text represents a true collaboration between dentistry and dental hygiene science. My appreciation for the support and encouragement of my husband, Russell Pickett, should be mentioned. His philosophy is: "Whatever you need, you should have." I rather like that idea.

Frieda A. Pickett, RDH, MS

This book is dedicated to my mentor, colleague, and friend, the late Dr. William K. Bottomley, who instilled in me an academic discipline essential for lifelong learning; to Frieda A. Pickett, RDH, MS, who conceived the idea of this book; and to my wife, Rebecca, without whose encouragement and support implementation of a project of this magnitude would not have been possible.

Géza T. Terézhalmy, DDS, MA

Editorial Review Board Members and Contributors

Jacquelyn W. Johnson, RDH, MS
Associate Professor of Dental Hygiene
Tarrant County College
Hurst, TX

Kristy H. Lucas, PharmD
Assistant Professor
Departments of Clinical Pharmacy and Internal Medicine
Schools of Pharmacy and Medicine
West Virginia University-Charleston
Charleston, WV

Steven Wayne Mifflin, PhD
Professor of Pharmacology
Department of Pharmacology
Graduate School of Biomedical Sciences
The University of Texas Health Science Center at San Antonio
San Antonio, TX

Stephen B. Milam, DDS, PhD
Professor and Chair
Hugh B. Tilson Endowed Chair
Department of Oral and Maxillofacial Surgery, Dental School
The University of Texas Health Science Center at San Antonio
San Antonio, TX

Karen Ridley, RDH, MS
Assistant Professor of Dental Hygiene
Department of Periodontics and Oral Medicine
University of Michigan School of Dentistry
Ann Arbor, MI

Jean Tyner, RDH, BS
Instructor of Dental Hygiene
Florence Darlington Technical College
Florence, SC

Laura J. Webb, CDA, RDH, MS
Independent Consultant
LJW Education Services
www.ljweduserv.com
Fallon, NV

Table of Contents

Clinical Medicine and Therapeutics

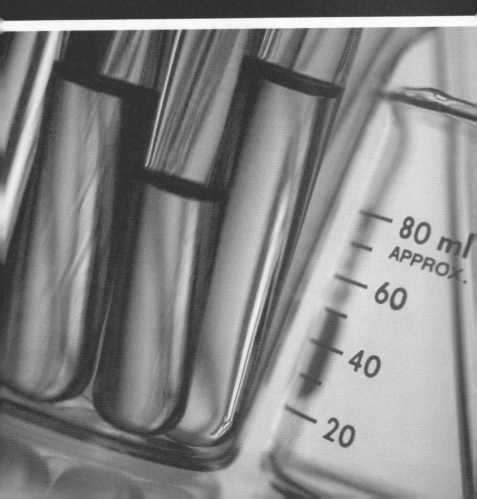

1 General Principles of Pharmacology

Table of Contents

INTRODUCTION

The science of pharmacology is the study of drugs. Historically, the clinician was responsible for information about the sources, physical and chemical properties, and compounding and dispensing of drugs. These activities are now delegated to pharmacologists and pharmacists. Today, the practitioner's responsibility requires the clinical application of this knowledge. Understanding how chemicals affect physiological homeostasis at the molecular level forms the basis for developing sound therapeutic strategies. Consequently, rational clinical use of therapeutic agents for prevention, diagnosis, and treatment of disease requires an understanding of basic pharmacological principles. These principles apply to all therapeutic agents (including vitamins, herbals, and nutritional supplements) and pertain to pharmacodynamic, pharmacokinetic, and pharmacotherapeutic variables.

PHARMACODYNAMICS

Pharmacodynamics is the study of molecular interactions between drugs and body constituents. It relates to the biochemical and physiological actions of drugs. Drugs circulating in the vascular compartment are carried to tissues. The first step in initiating a drug-induced effect is the formation of a complex between the drug and a cell component generally known as the **drug receptor**. The **receptor site** where a drug acts to initiate a series of biochemical and physiological effects is the **site of action** of that drug. The molecular events that follow drug-receptor interactions are called the **mechanisms of action** of drugs. However, it should be understood that not all drugs produce their effects by interacting with specific receptors. A number of drugs form chemical bonds with small molecules, chelating agents, or metallic cations. A practical example of this type of drug-receptor interaction is the therapeutic neutralization of gastric acid by antacids. Many other drugs act by physiochemical mechanisms that are not yet understood.

RECEPTORS

Drug receptors are cellular macromolecules (Figure 1-1). They may be metabolic or regulatory enzymes or coenzymes; proteins or glycoproteins associated with transport mechanisms; or structural and functional components of lipid membranes or nucleic acids. A single cell may have hundreds of receptor sites. Drugs attach to or interact with these receptor sites by covalent, ionic, hydrogen, hydrophobic, or Van der Waals binding and produce a definable pharmacological response. Hydrogen binding and ionic binding are the most common. These interactions require little energy and may be easily broken. The affinity of a drug for a particular receptor and the type of binding is intimately related to the drug's chemical structure. Affinity is expressed by its **dissociation constant** (K_D), the concentration of a drug required in solution to achieve 50% occupancy of its receptors. It is generally accepted that the law of mass action, which states that

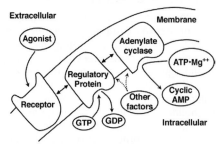

Figure 1-1. Drug receptors are cellular macromolecules.

chemicals go across semipermeable biological membranes from high concentration to low concentration to reach equilibrium, governs most drug-receptor interactions.

AGONISTS

Drugs that have a direct stimulatory effect on a receptor are called **agonists**. The ability of a drug to interact with a receptor and initiate a response is the function of its **intrinsic activity**, which is related to the chemical structure of the drug. The measured response in an agonist-receptor system may be the end result of several successive "events" initiated by the agonist-receptor interaction. A **strong agonist** produces a significant physiological response when only a relatively small number of receptors are occupied. A small dose of the drug will produce the desired effect, i.e., the drug has good affinity and good intrinsic activity. A weak agonist must be bound to many more receptors to produce the same effect. A much larger dose of the drug will be required to produce the desired effect, i.e., the drug has weak affinity and low intrinsic activity. A **partial agonist** has good affinity but very low intrinsic activity; it will never produce the same effect as a strong agonist or a weak agonist even when all receptors are occupied.

ANTAGONISTS

A drug that interferes with the activities of an agonist may be classified as either competitive or noncompetitive. A **competitive antagonist** blocks the agonist-binding domain of the receptor. It forms a reversible drug-receptor complex, which can be overcome by increasing the concentration of the agonist and, consequently, the inhibition is surmountable. An **irreversible antagonist** also competes with the agonist for the agonist-binding domain but it forms a permanent drug-receptor complex, which is insurmountable.

A **noncompetitive antagonist** binds to a receptor site other than the agonist-binding domain; this type of antagonist produces a conformational change and irreversibly prevents an agonist-receptor interaction. An increase in agonist concentration in the presence of a noncompetitive antagonist will not produce the response expected for that agonist and is consequently also insurmountable.

Mixed agonist-antagonists are drugs that have both agonistic and antagonistic properties. When used alone, such a drug behaves as an agonist. However, when another drug that competes for the same receptor site is administered concurrently, the agonist-antagonist will also act as an antagonist.

RECEPTOR CLASSIFICATION

Receptors are classified according to the type of drug that they interact with or according to the specific physiological response produced by the drug-receptor complex. By evaluating the effects of different agonists in the presence of a given antagonist, receptor sites may also be subclassified. For example, cholinergic receptors can be activated either by muscarine or nicotine. However, only the response to muscarine is antagonized by atropine, whereas curare will only antagonize the response to nicotine. This evidence suggests that acetylcholine can bind to or activate at least two different receptor sites, which are either muscarinic or nicotinic. Similarly, receptors and receptor subtypes exist for many other agents. The number of any given receptor type or subtype on a cell may also vary. Certain disease states or drugs taken long term and/or in large doses may increase (up-regulate) or decrease (down-regulate) the number of receptors and provide a degree of adaptability in the face of changing physiological events.

EFFICACY

Efficacy is the magnitude of response obtained from optimal receptor site occupancy by a drug. As seen with the affinity of drugs for a particular receptor, the efficacy of a drug is also related to its chemical structure. This concept is referred to as the *structural activity* (or intrinsic activity) *relationship (SAR).* The graded dose-response relationship is the quantification of a specific response elicited by a drug over a range of dosages. This relationship is expressed visually and mathematically with a dose-response curve. The curve is established by placing the logarithmic value for dosage (or *log dose*) on the x-axis and the quantified response on the y-axis (Figure 1-2). The upper plateau of the dose-effect curve represents the efficacy or the maximal effect of a drug associated with a specific dose. The maximum dose of a drug associated with optimal response is called the *ceiling dose* of that drug.

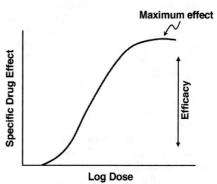

Figure 1-2. The efficacy or the maximum effect of a drug is represented by the upper plateau of the dose-response curve.

POTENCY

Potency relates two or more drugs by comparing the doses required to produce a given effect. Potency is related to the affinity of a drug to its receptor, whereas efficacy is related to the intrinsic activity of that drug once a drug receptor complex is formed. It is determined by the relative position of the dose-response curve along the dose axis (Figure 1-3). Note that for any given effect, the dose of drug A is always smaller than that required for drug B. The maximal effect of drug A (A_1) is reached at a lower dose than the same maximal effect of drug B (B_1). Drug A is considered more potent than drug B yet they have the same efficacy. An understanding of the concept of potency is important in determining drug dosage; however, high or low potency is significant only if the administration of an effective dose becomes impractical.

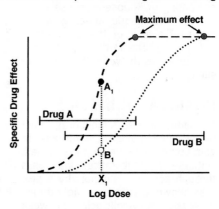

Figure 1-3. Potency relates to two or more drugs by comparing the doses required to produce a given effect.

TOXICITY

Any drug at a high enough concentration can produce a toxic effect. In the context of this discussion, **toxicity** refers to the undesirable effects associated with the given therapeutic use of a drug. These adverse effects may be exaggerations of direct effects seen at higher dosages or multiple concurrent "side" effects occurring at therapeutic dosage levels. For example, barbiturates may produce sedation and drowsiness at therapeutic levels but death at increased dosage levels. This is an extension of the intended therapeutic effect of central nervous system depression. An antihistamine, which is intended to antagonize histamine action, may also bind to receptors in the central nervous system (CNS) and cause drowsiness. In this case, the drowsiness is a concurrent side effect, not an extended response.

The dose of a drug required to produce a response of specific intensity in 50% of the individuals within the same population is the **median effective dose** (ED50) (Figure 1-4). If death is the measured end point, the median effective dose is expressed as the **median lethal dose** (LD50). A steep dose-response curve indicates a narrow dosage range between minimal and maximal effects. Consequently, the risk for toxic or even lethal dosage levels can be greater because of the narrower dosage range. The margin of safety of a drug may be expressed by its **therapeutic index,** the actual ratio of LD50 and ED50. The margin of safety may also be established by comparing 99% dose-response curve for the therapeutic effect with the curve for a toxic or the lethal effect (Figure 1-5). The farther apart these two curves lie, the wider the margin of safety.

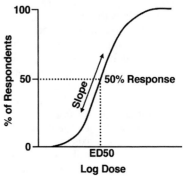

Figure 1-4. The dose of a drug required to produce a response of specific intensity in 50% of the individuals within the same population is the median effective dose (ED50).

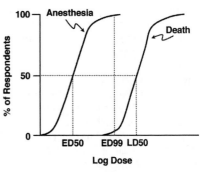

Figure 1-5. The margin of safety of a drug may be expressed by its therapeutic index, the actual ratio of LD50 and ED50, or by comparing the 99% dose-response curve for the therapeutic effect with the curve for the toxic effect.

PHARMACOKINETICS

To produce an effect, most drugs must pass through biological membranes to gain access to their receptor(s). Small, water-soluble substances may pass through aqueous channels by a process known as **filtration**. Most drugs, however, are weak acids or weak bases too large to pass through aqueous channels. The passage of these drug molecules across cell membranes is achieved by *passive diffusion* along a concentration gradient. The concept of *facilitated diffusion* assumes that the drug forms a complex with a component of the cell membrane on one side. The complex is then carried through the membrane, the drug is released, and the carrier returns to the original surface to repeat the process. Facilitated transport does not require energy and does not proceed against a concentration gradient. *Active transport* is characterized by selectivity, competitive inhibition, requirement for energy, saturability, and movement against an electrochemical gradient. Some water-insoluble substances are engulfed by the cell membrane and are released unchanged in the cytoplasm by the process known as *pinocytosis*.

ABSORPTION

Most drugs are weak acids or weak bases that diffuse through the lipid component of the cell membrane as a function of the drug's molecular weight, lipid solubility coefficient, pK_a (the pH at which a drug is 50% ionized and 50% un-ionized), and concentration. In general, drugs with a small molecular weight will cross biological membranes more readily than drugs with a large molecular weight. The nonpolar, un-ionized form of a drug will diffuse across biological membranes more readily than its ionized, polar fraction. Drugs administered in high concentration are more readily absorbed than low concentrations of the same drug. A drug's formulation and its route of administration further influence absorption.

Routes of drug administration

Enteral. The oral route is the most common, convenient, and economical method of drug administration. It is also the most unpredictable. When a drug is administered enterally, its rate of absorption into the systemic circulation is influenced by the inherent characteristics of the drug, the pH of the gastrointestinal tract, the presence of food in the stomach, gastric motility, splanchnic blood flow, and importantly, patient compliance with the prescribed drug regimen. In addition, the anatomical relationship between the liver and the gastrointestinal tract and the blood supply of these organs has important implications on drug absorption. Because the liver is situated between enteric sites of absorption and the systemic circulation, it can profoundly influence the bioavailability of a drug given orally—an action that has been described as the *first-pass effect*. *Bioavailability* is defined as the fraction of the dose of a drug that enters the systemic circulation. A drug given orally that is efficiently removed from the bloodstream by the liver will have a low bioavailability.

Parenteral. Intravenous (IV) administration provides for accurate and immediate deposition of drugs into the bloodstream unaffected by hepatic first-pass metabolism. The dose can be adjusted to patient response; however, once a drug is injected there is no recall. Sterile formulations of soluble substances and an aseptic technique are required. Local irritation and thromboembolic complications may occur with some drugs.

Following subcutaneous (SC) injection, a drug's rate of absorption into the bloodstream is slow and sufficiently constant to provide a sustained effect. The incorporation of a vasoconstrictor into a drug formulation may further retard the rate of absorption. Local tissue irritation characterized by sloughing, necrosis, and severe pain may occur.

Intramuscular (IM) injections allow for rapid absorption of aqueous solutions into the bloodstream. Oily or other nonaqueous vehicles may provide slow, constant absorption. Substances considered too irritating by the IV and SC routes may, in some instances, be given intramuscularly.

Topical. Absorption of drugs through skin and mucosa by passive diffusion is proportional to their concentration and lipid solubility. Because venous drainage from the mouth is via the superior vena cava, sublingual administration of certain drugs is effective owing to the large area of vascular flow. This direct absorption also has an advantage over enteric administration because it circumvents the metabolic first-pass breakdown in the liver. The large pulmonary absorptive surface allows for rapid access of gaseous, volatile agents to the circulation. Drugs administered by inhalation may act locally or cross the alveoli; they then travel in the systemic blood flow and act at the appropriate receptor site. Concentration is controlled at the alveolar level, since most of these drugs are exhaled immediately. The rectal route of drug administration may be useful in young children and for unconscious or vomiting patients; however, absorption is unpredictable.

DISTRIBUTION

Following absorption into the circulation, drugs are distributed both into the extracellular and intracellular environments. Diffusion into the extracellular space occurs rapidly. However, many drugs are bound to plasma proteins, which limit their ability to leave the vascular compartment and affect their concentration in tissues and at their sites of action. Plasma protein binding is a nonselective process. Many drugs compete with each other and with endogenous substances for these binding sites. Once a drug leaves the vascular compartment, it may accumulate in tissues in higher than expected concentrations as a result of the pK_a of the drug and the pH of the environment. Highly perfused organs such as the heart, liver, kidney, and brain will receive most of the drug within minutes of absorption. Muscle, most viscera, skin, and fat may require a much longer amount of time before equilibrium is achieved. The distribution of drugs to the CNS and cerebrospinal fluid is further restricted by the blood-brain barrier. However, the only limiting factor associated with highly lipid-soluble uncharged drugs is cerebral blood flow. Redistribution may affect the duration of a drug effect when a compound of high lipid solubility acts on the brain or cardiovascular system after administration and then is redistributed to other tissues.

METABOLISM

Lipid-soluble weak acids and bases are not readily eliminated from the body. Metabolism fosters drug excretion by biotransforming them into more polar, water-soluble fractions, although many drug metabolites maintain a degree of pharmacological activity. If drug metabolites are active, termination of drug action takes place by further biotransformation or by excretion of the active metabolites. The chemical reactions associated with biotransformation may be nonsynthetic (Phase I) or synthetic (Phase II). In a Phase I reaction, a drug is oxidized or reduced to a more polar compound. In a Phase II reaction, an endogenous macromolecule is conjugated to the drug. Drugs undergoing conjugation reactions (Phase II) may have already undergone Phase I biotransformation. The hepatic microsomal enzyme (cytochrome P450) system is responsible for the biotransformation (oxidation/reduction) of most drugs. However, enzymes in plasma and renal, pulmonary, and gastrointestinal metabolism make notable contributions. The cytochrome P450 enzyme system can be "induced" to increase or reduce the rate of a drug's metabolism and is responsible for many adverse drug effects. Nonmicrosomal enzyme activity also contributes to the process of biotransformation. However, nonmicrosomal enzymes involved in drug biotransformation are not usually inducible.

EXCRETION

Drugs are excreted from the body either unchanged or as metabolites. Polar compounds are excreted more readily than nonpolar compounds. Consequently, lipid-soluble substances have to be metabolized to more polar fractions before they can be excreted. The kidney is the most important organ responsible for the elimination of drugs and their metabolites from the body. Renal excretion may involve three processes: glomerular filtration, which depends on fractional plasma protein binding and filtration rate; active tubular excretion, a nonselective carrier system for organic ions; and passive tubular reabsorption of un-ionized drugs, which results in net passive reabsorption. Many metabolites formed in the liver are excreted via the bile into the intestinal tract. If these metabolites are subsequently hydrolyzed and reabsorbed from the gut (enterohepatic recirculation), drug action is prolonged. Pulmonary excretion is important mainly for the elimination of anesthetic gases and vapors. Drugs excreted in milk are potential sources of unwanted pharmacological effects in nursing infants. Other routes, such as saliva, sweat, and tears, are quantitatively unimportant.

The removal of most drugs from the body follows exponential or *first-order kinetics*. Assuming a relatively uniform distribution of a drug within the body (considered to be a single compartment), first-order kinetics implies that a constant fraction of the drug is eliminated per unit time. The rate of exponential kinetics may be expressed by its *constant* (k), the fractional change per unit time, or its *half-life* ($t_{1/2}$), the time required for the plasma concentration of a drug to decrease by 50%. The *distribution half-life* represents the rapid decline in plasma drug concentration as 50% of the drug is distributed throughout the body. The *elimination half-life* reflects the time required to metabolize and excrete 50% of the drug from the system. Multiple dosage intervals, which are shorter than the drug's half-life, will lead to a plateau level of accumulation of the drug over four half-lives. This plateau, known as the *steady-state concentration*, represents a rate of administration that is equal to the rate of elimination. Fluctuations in the plasma concentrations will occur as a function of the dosage interval and the drug's elimination half-life (Figure 1-6). Assuming first-order kinetics, it takes approximately four half-lives to eliminate a drug from the body. The elimination of some drugs (such as alcohol) may follow *zero-order kinetics*, implying that a constant amount of the drug is eliminated per unit time.

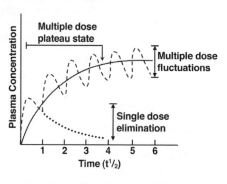

Figure 1-6. The effect of dosing on plasma concentrations.

PHARMACOTHERAPEUTICS

Pharmacotherapeutic principles relate to the use of drugs in the diagnosis, prevention, and treatment of disease. The dosing regimen, which takes into account the route, amount, and frequency of drug administration, influences the onset and duration of drug action. If the desired full effect of a drug must be achieved promptly, a *loading dose*, which is larger than the maintenance dose, must be employed. Following the administration of maintenance doses, a drug's concentration in plasma is characterized by the time course of accumulation, the maximal amount accumulated, and the fluctuations associated with the dose interval and the half-life of the drug. Dosage intervals are predicated on the fluctuation in drug concentration that can be tolerated without toxicity or loss of efficacy. However, different patients show significant variations in response to the same dosage regimen. Optimal pharmacotherapy depends on the clinician's awareness of the sources of such variations, which include both disease-related and patient-related factors.

Pharmacogenetic Factors

Genetic determinants may affect both pharmacokinetic and pharmacodynamic factors and contribute to the normal variability of drug effects. The dose of a drug required to produce a specific response in an individual is referred to as the *individual effective dose*. If a drug produces its usual effect on a patient at an unexpectedly high dose, the patient is said to be *hyporeactive*. A patient is said to be *hyperreactive* when a drug produces its effect at an unexpectedly low dose. Decreased response to a drug as a result of prior exposure to the drug is described as *tolerance*. When this occurs, cross-tolerance may develop to the effects of other, structurally related drugs. In the case of tolerance, drug dosage must be increased to maintain an acceptable therapeutic response. When tolerance develops rapidly, subsequent to the administration of only a few doses of a drug, the response is described as *tachyphylaxis*. An unusual reaction of any intensity, irrespective of drug dosage, observed in a small percentage of the patients is referred to as *idiosyncrasy* or an *idiosyncratic reaction*.

Weight of the Patient

Optimal therapeutic doses intended to produce a specific effect are generally determined in terms of the amount of drug per kilogram of body weight of the patient. Although there are many rules and formulas to calculate dosages, doses based on manufacturers' recommendations or the prescriber's experience provide the most reasonable approach to dosing.

The Pregnant Patient

Fetal abnormalities occur in 3% to 6% of pregnancies in the United States; drugs are considered to be responsible for 1% to 5% of these malformations. The physiochemical properties of the drug and the genetic determinants of both the mother and the fetus will influence the extent to which an agent will affect the developing fetus. Such genetically determined factors affect the rate of absorption, metabolism, and elimination of a drug by the mother, the drug's rate of placental transfer, or the way a drug interacts with the cells and tissues of the embryo or fetus. Each drug has a threshold concentration above which fetal abnormalities can occur and below which no effects are discernible. Whether a drug reaches the threshold concentration in the fetus depends on the chemical nature of the agent (molecular weight, protein binding, lipid solubility, pK_a); interacting drugs, herbals, and dietary supplements consumed by the patient; and maternal pharmacokinetic factors.

During pregnancy the maternal plasma volume increases (by 20% at midgestation and 50% at term), total plasma protein concentrations decrease, total body fat increases, and, therefore, the apparent volume of distribution for many drugs increases. At the same time, drugs excreted by the kidneys may have increased rates of clearance as a result of increased cardiac output, increased renal blood flow, and increased glomerular filtration rate. Consequently, in-

Table 1-1.	FDA Risk Stratification of Drugs
Category A:	Controlled studies in women fail to demonstrate a risk to the fetus in the first trimester; possibility of fetal harm appears remote.
Category B:	Either animal studies do not indicate a risk to the fetus and there are no controlled studies in women, or animal studies have shown an adverse effect but controlled studies in women failed to demonstrate risk.
Category C:	Either animal studies do not indicate fetal risk and there are no controlled studies in women, or studies in women and animals are not available.
Category D:	There is positive evidence of fetal risk, but the benefits may be acceptable despite the risk.
Category X:	There is definite fetal risk based on studies in animals or humans, or based on human experience, and the risk clearly outweighs any possible benefit.

Briggs GG, Freeman RK, Yaffe SJ. A Reference Guide to Fetal and Neonatal Risk—Drugs in Pregnancy and Lactation. 5th ed. Philadelphia: Lippincott Williams & Wilkins; 1998.

creased dosage of a drug may have to be administered to the mother during critical periods of pregnancy. Most drugs in the maternal bloodstream cross the placenta by simple diffusion along the concentration gradient. During early pregnancy the placental membrane is relatively thick, which tends to reduce permeability. The thickness decreases and the surface area of the placenta increases in the later trimesters, increasing the passage of drugs.

Human teratogenicity is not predictable. Major malformations are usually the result of exposure to drugs during the critical period of organogenesis (first trimester). Exposure during the second and third trimesters primarily affects organ function. Any drug in the fetal system at the time of birth must rely on the infant's own metabolic and excretory capabilities, which have not yet fully developed. Consequently, drugs given near term, especially those with long half-lives, may have a prolonged effect on the newborn. Finally, drugs that cause maternal addiction are also known to cause fetal addiction and the fetus may undergo withdrawal following delivery. To assist practitioners in prescribing drugs for the pregnant patient, the U.S. Food and Drug Administration (FDA) has established a code for categorizing drugs according to their potential to cause fetal injury (Table 1-1). In certain clinical situations, drug administration to resolve an emerging dental problem may be unavoidable in a pregnant woman and may require the use of local anesthetics, analgesics, antibiotics, and anxiolytic agents.

THE NURSING PATIENT

With the increasing recognition of the advantages of breast-feeding, clinicians must often weigh the risks versus benefits of drug therapy in lactating women. The rate of passage of a drug from plasma to milk depends on the characteristics of the drug, such as the drug's molecular weight, lipid solubility, pK_a, and degree of plasma protein binding. Small water-soluble nonelectrolytes pass into milk by simple diffusion through aqueous channels in the mammary epithelial membrane that separates plasma from milk; equilibrium is reached rapidly and the drug's concentration in milk approximates plasma levels. With larger molecules, only lipid-soluble drugs can pass through the membrane. The pK_a of weak electrolytes is an important determinant of drug concentration in milk because the pH of milk is generally lower (more acidic) than that of plasma and milk can act as an "ion trap" for weak bases. At equilibrium, basic drugs may become more concentrated in milk. Conversely, acidic drugs are limited in their ability to enter milk because the concentration of the nonionized free form in milk is higher than it is in plasma, causing a net transfer of the drug from milk to plasma.

The ratio of drug concentration in breast milk to drug concentration in maternal plasma is called the *milk-to-plasma drug-concentration ratio*. Most drugs for which data are available have a milk-to-plasma ratio of 1 or less; about 25% have ratios of more than 1; and about 15% have ratios of more than 2. If the precise concentration of a drug in breast milk over time is known, one can estimate the dose the infant will ingest per unit of time by assuming intake of a specific amount of milk (e.g., 150 mL per kilogram of body weight per day). This estimated dose is then expressed as a percentage of the therapeutic (or equivalent) dose for the infant. For most drugs, the dose below which there is no clinical effect in infants is unknown. This uncertainty led to arbitrarily defining as "safe" a value of no more than 10% of the therapeutic dose for infants.

Factors that determine the advisability of using a particular drug in a nursing mother include the potential for acute or long-term dose-related and non–dose-related toxicity, dosage and duration of therapy, age of the infant, quantity of milk consumed by the infant, and the drug's effect on lactation. To minimize the infant's exposure to medications in milk, clinicians should consider the following strategies: withhold drug therapy; delay drug therapy temporarily; choose a drug that passes poorly into milk; use alternative routes of drug administration (i.e., topical, inhalation); advise the mother to avoid nursing at peak plasma concentrations of the drug; administer the drug to the mother before the infant's longest sleep period; and/or withhold breast-feeding temporarily.

THE PEDIATRIC PATIENT

Pediatric drug therapy presents a unique challenge to clinicians. Often there is a paucity of pediatric-specific data in the literature from which to derive appropriate dosage regimens. Dosage forms are usually designed with the adult population in mind, and the dosage cannot easily be individualized for children. Even when appropriate dosage forms for children are available, palatability, resistance to taking medications, and compliance issues may hinder optimal therapy. Finally, children often do not react the same way adults do to certain medications (i.e., paradoxical hyperactivity, which may be observed in children taking chloral derivatives or barbiturates). Clinicians must, therefore, use medications for which data are extrapolated on the basis of limited pharmacodynamic and pharmacokinetic knowledge. Conservative dosage, especially initially, with close monitoring for dose-related effects is imperative. Information on specific drugs administered or prescribed by dentists can be found in the pediatric dosage section of individual drug monographs.

Pharmacodynamics

Pharmacodynamic factors are poorly studied in the pediatric population. Responses to specific drug concentrations may be different from responses in the adult population. Medications tolerated by adult patients, such as acetylsalicylic acid (aspirin) for fever, may be inappropriate for pediatric patients (may result in Reye syndrome).

Pharmacokinetics

At birth, the gastric pH is neutral but falls to values of 1 to 3 in the first day of life. Subsequently, the pH returns toward neutrality, because gastric acid secretion is low in the first several months of life. Adult values are usually achieved by the age of 2 years or by the time an oral health care provider would see a child for the first time. Generally, drug distribution approaches adult values (in L/kg) by the first year of life. In the pediatric patient, hepatic activity may greatly exceed that observed in adult patients on a weight-adjusted basis. A decrease in hepatic activity (relative to body weight) begins after a child weighs approximately 30 kg (66 lb). Drug dosages typically begin to approach adult values in adolescence. The kidneys are functionally immature at birth, but glomerular filtration and tubular secretion reach adult values by the first year of life.

THE ELDERLY PATIENT

Geriatric drug therapy is another important area of therapeutics because of the growing elderly population, their disproportionately high use of medications, and their increased risk of adverse drug events. Optimization of drug therapy in the elderly requires an understanding of how aging and concomitant disease affect the pharmacodynamics and pharmacokinetics of drugs, an appreciation for the wide physiological variability in the elderly population, and acknowledgment of the elderly patient's expectations about therapy. The results of drug studies using young adult subjects cannot be extrapolated accurately to the elderly. Conservative dosage, especially initially, with close monitoring for dose-related effects is imperative. Information on specific drugs administered or prescribed by dentists can be found in the geriatric dosage section of individual drug monographs.

Pharmacodynamics

The number and sensitivity of drug receptors can change with age and concomitant disease states and produce altered, often exaggerated, drug responses. Whereas it appears that there are age-related decreases in the number and/or affinity of some receptor subtypes, increased receptor sensitivity to certain drugs with aging might contribute to the higher frequency of adverse drug events.

Pharmacokinetics

Absorption. With aging there is some decrease in gastric secretions, acidity, emptying, peristalsis, absorptive surface area, and splanchnic blood flow. These changes predict an altered extent and/or rate of absorption for orally administered drugs. However, some of these factors counterbalance each other (i.e., gastric acidity and emptying, decreased absorptive surface, and decreased peristalsis) and produce no clinically appreciable difference in bioavailability.

Distribution. Total body water and lean body mass decrease while body fat increases in proportion to total body weight with age. These factors alter the volume of distribution (V_d). The V_d relates the amount of drug in the body to the concentration of drug in the blood. The V_d for lipophilic drugs is increased and for hydrophilic drugs is decreased. Although cardiac output does not appear to decrease with age, some chronic diseases affecting the elderly do contribute to a decrease in cardiac output and regional blood flow; blood may be preferentially shunted away from the liver and kidneys to the brain, heart, and muscles, explaining the slowed excretion of some drugs and an increased sensitivity to others. Although plasma albumin is not decreased by age alone, it does decrease with frailty, catabolic disease states, and immobility seen in many elderly. A decrease in plasma albumin can increase the percentage of free drug available for pharmacological effect, metabolism, and excretion. Fluctuations in plasma albumin concentrations are more important with highly protein-bound (>90%) weak acids, such as acetylsalicylic acid.

Metabolism. Liver size and hepatic blood flow decrease with age, especially with concomitant hepatic disease. Liver size decreases by 28% in elderly men and by 44% in elderly women, and hepatic blood flow decreases by 35% when compared with young adults. Such changes can limit the first-pass effect on drugs with high extraction and markedly reduce their metabolism.

Renal elimination. Renal blood flow, glomerular filtration, and tubular secretion all decrease with age. Creatinine clearance (Cl_{cr}) decreases approximately 1% per year after age 40. Volume depletion, congestive heart failure, and renal disease can further decrease renal function and reduce drug excretion.

THE PATIENT WITH HEPATIC DYSFUNCTION

The spectrum of liver disease is extremely wide. Most of the underlying pathophysiological mechanisms are accounted for by autoimmune disease, viral infection, and toxic insult, which lead to hepatitis and cirrhosis. Patients with acute hepatitis usually experience transient reduction in liver function. Patients with chronic hepatitis and cirrhosis demonstrate permanent loss of functional hepatocytes. Liver dysfunction is one of the most common causes of morbidity in patients receiving pharmacotherapeutic agents. Most adverse drug reactions in the presence of liver disease are related to altered pharmacokinetics.

Pharmacokinetics

Metabolism. Enteric medications must pass through the liver before undergoing systemic distribution. In the presence of liver disease, one can expect decreased hepatic blood flow, portal vein hypertension, and shunting of blood around the liver. This leads to a reduced hepatic first-pass effect. A decrease in hepatic first-pass effect can result in large increases in steady-state concentrations of drugs within the blood circulation.

Distribution. The liver also produces albumin, which binds weak acids in the blood. In patients with hepatic dysfunction, the production of these proteins declines. When this is the case, the fraction of free drug in blood increases because of reduced protein binding. In addition, high concentrations of endogenous substances in blood that are normally eliminated by the liver, such as bilirubin, further displace drugs from their plasma protein binding sites. A higher free fraction of the drug in the blood increases the volume of distribution, leads to a longer half-life, and further increases its pharmacological effects.

Excretion. Lipid-soluble drugs are biotransformed to some degree by the liver for subsequent excretion, primarily by the kidney. Hepatic abnormalities lead to a reduced capacity to metabolize drugs and to reduced hepatobiliary and/or renal clearance, factors that increase the elimination half-life of drugs and contribute to toxicity.

Unfortunately, there is no single laboratory test that can be used to assess liver function. The most widely accepted predictor of liver disease to estimate the ability of the liver to metabolize drugs is to determine the Child-Pugh score (Table 1-2). The Child-Pugh score consists of five laboratory tests or clinical symptoms: total bilirubin, serum albumin, prothrombin time, ascites, and hepatic encephalopathy. Each of these areas is given a score of 1 (normal) to 3 (severely abnormal) and the scores for the five areas are totaled. The Child-Pugh score for a patient with normal liver function is 5, whereas the score for

Table 1-2.	Child-Pugh Scores for Patients With Liver Disease		
TEST/SYMPTOMS	SCORE 1 POINT EACH	SCORE 2 POINTS EACH	SCORE 3 POINTS EACH
Total bilirubin (mg/dL)	< 2.0	2.0–3.0	> 3.0
Serum albumin (g/dL)	> 3.5	2.8–3.5	< 2.8
Prothrombin time (seconds prolonged over control)	< 4	4–6	> 6
Ascites	Absent	Slight	Moderate
Hepatic encephalopathy	None	Moderate	Severe

Pugh RNH, Murray-Lyon IM, Dawson JL, Pietroni MC, Williams R. Transection of the oesophagus for bleeding oesophageal varices. Br J Surg 1973;60:646–649.

a patient with grossly abnormal serum albumin, total bilirubin, and prothrombin time values, in addition to severe ascites and hepatic encephalopathy, is 15. For drugs that are metabolized primarily by the liver, a Child-Pugh score of 8 to 9 is grounds for a moderate decrease (~25%) in initial daily dose for drugs, while a score of 10 or greater indicates that a significant decrease (~50%) in initial daily dose is required.

THE PATIENT WITH RENAL DYSFUNCTION

Renal failure is said to occur when the kidneys are no longer able to carry out their normal excretory functions. The condition may be either acute or chronic. In acute failure, there is a sudden marked reduction in urine flow associated with an episode of infection, trauma, severe burns, blood transfusion, or the administration of a nephrotoxic drug. Chronic renal failure frequently follows glomerulonephritis, pyelonephritis, and nephritic syndrome. Most patients with chronic renal failure may also have other medical problems that either contributed to the development of renal dysfunction or are a complication of chronic renal failure. Many of these conditions respond to pharmacotherapy. Consequently, patients with renal failure are at increased risk for adverse drug events because of the number of drugs they are taking, concurrent medical problems, and impaired renal function. Drug-related complications, however, can be minimized by the rational use of drugs based on an understanding of pharmacokinetic changes associated with renal failure.

Pharmacokinetics

Absorption. The absorption of enteric drugs may be altered in renal failure because of associated gastrointestinal disturbances characterized by nausea, vomiting, and diarrhea. Weak acids may have diminished absorption because of an increased gastric pH secondary to increased salivary urea levels. In addition, many patients with decreased renal function routinely take aluminum or calcium antacids (for calcium/phosphorous abnormalities), which may also alter pH-dependent drug absorption.

Distribution. The V_d of drugs may be increased, decreased, or unchanged in patients with renal failure. An example of a drug with an increased V_d is naproxen. This may be secondary to hypoalbuminemia or competitive displacement from its protein-binding sites caused by the accumulation of acidic by-

products in uremia. Most organic acids, such as the salicylates, exhibit decreased plasma protein binding. Weak organic bases have either decreased (diazepam) or unchanged (lidocaine) plasma protein binding in uremia.
Metabolism. Many drugs are biotransformed before being excreted. These processes occur predominantly in the liver and result in the formation of water-soluble, usually less toxic, polar compounds, which are readily excreted. Obviously, advanced liver disease significantly affects the metabolism of many drugs, but there is also evidence that renal failure can lead to abnormalities in hepatic biotransformation. Mixed-function oxidation systems, conjugation, reduction, and hydrolysis reactions may be slowed in uremia. Drugs metabolized to active or toxic compounds (even if metabolized at a slow rate) that are excreted by the kidney may accumulate to toxic levels in renal failure patients.
Renal elimination. The degree to which renal failure impairs drug elimination depends largely on the percentage of drug excreted by the kidneys. For many drugs, linear correlates have been established between the elimination half-life of the drug and creatinine clearance (Cl_{cr}). Consequently, when presented with a patient with impaired renal function for whom drug dosage regimen decisions are to be made, one should look to the Cl_{cr} as an index of renal function. Mathematically:

$$Cl_{cr} = 140 - age \times body\ weight/serum\ creatinine \times 72$$

where body weight is in kg and serum creatinine is in mg/dL. Adjustment of drug dosage in renal disease may be necessary only when Cl_{cr} is below 30 to 40 mL/min. For a drug excreted entirely by the kidney, adjustment is simple. A 50% decline in renal function necessitates either halving the dose or doubling the usual dosage interval. The variable interval method leads to more extreme peak-through levels and is best for drugs with long half-lives.

THE PATIENT ON HEMODIALYSIS

Drug prescribing is further complicated when patients with renal failure are put on hemodialysis because they may lose therapeutic levels of some drugs in the dialysis bath. Many factors contribute to the rate of drug removal, such as the type of dialyzer equipment (conventional vs. high-flux), dialysis membrane characteristics (cuprophane vs. polysulfone), dialysate flow rate (most conventional hemodialysis runs are 4 hours whereas high-flux dialysis procedures last 2 to 2.5 hours), and specific properties of the drug in question (molecular weight, lipid solubility, volume of distribution, plasma protein binding). Drugs with a small molecular weight (<500 daltons) cross conventional cuprophane dialysis membranes readily. Large molecular weight drugs are not effectively removed by conventional dialysis. The polysulfone membranes used in high-flux dialysis systems, however, readily remove large molecular weight compounds. Drugs with high water solubility are more easily removed to the aqueous dialysate than more lipid-soluble compounds. Lipid-soluble compounds also have a larger volume of distribution and are not accessible for removal. Plasma protein binding of a drug further determines how effectively it can be dialyzed. Drugs with a high degree of protein binding are poorly removed by dialysis because the drug-protein complex is too large to cross most dialysis membranes. Drug dialysis data are not readily available for many drugs. A sensible rule to follow for drugs that may be substantially removed by dialysis is to administer maintenance doses at the conclusion of dialysis treatment.

COMPLIANCE

A *compliant patient* is one who follows the therapeutic regimen recommended by the clinician. In contrast, a patient is considered noncompliant if the patient fails to follow a regimen to the extent that therapeutic goals are not achieved. There are several determinants of compliance that take into consideration the disease, the patient, the practitioner, the treatment regimen, economic factors, and the interaction of each of these factors. Patient trust in the clinician and treatment as established during the office visit is important. A patient tends to be more compliant if he or she has a good understanding of the illness and the therapy. Therefore, good communication between the clinician and patient is a major aid to compliance. A positive office visit and attitude, along with individualization of regimens and good follow-up on the clinician's part, improve compliance.

The nature of the illness itself has an important influence on the patient. The more serious or disabling an illness is, the more likely the patient will follow the regimen. The patient's perception of the severity of the illness is the major factor influencing compliance. The longer the duration of treatment, the less will be the compliance as time goes on. This is especially true if symptoms are relieved before drug therapy is to be discontinued. The regimen itself may be discouraging or confusing to the patient because of multiple drug use, scheduling of dosages, side effects, cost, and access to or dispensing of the drug.

Noncompliance in the pediatric patient is complicated by a parent-guardian factor. The major reason for noncompliance in children is a dislike for the taste or smell of the medication. If it is frustrating to the parent-guardian to give the medication, they are more likely to skip doses or discontinue the medication when symptoms disappear. One must also consider the possibility of a negative parent-guardian attitude transferring to the child. If the child is attending school, the regimen should have a convenient schedule for doses coordinated with the school schedule. Consider recommending specific times rather than generalizing.

Noncompliance in the geriatric patient is not uncommon. They may fail to fill prescriptions because of transportation problems, expense, or lack of trust in the doctor or therapy. Poor comprehension of the therapy and concurrent multiple drug therapies are common reasons for omission of doses. Difficulty in opening packages or swallowing pills, poor memory, and visual or hearing impairment may also contribute to confusion in compliance. A good understanding of the patient's needs and fears will help the clinician to individualize drug therapy for better compliance. Repetition of directions with written instructions and clear labeling is helpful.

PRESCRIPTION WRITING

The essence of prescription writing is to ensure that the pharmacist knows exactly which drug formulation and dosage to dispense, and the patient has explicit written instructions for self-administration of the prescribed drug. It is practical to consider the prescription to consist of three components: a heading, a body, and a closing. The heading identifies the prescriber (name, phone number, and address), exhibits the date of the prescription, and lists the patient information (name, age, and address). The body tells the pharmacist the specific drug, dosage unit or concentration, and amount to be dispensed. It also provides directions to the patient (transcribed by the pharmacist to the packaged drug), which states precisely how the patient is to self-administer the drug. The closing exhibits the signature of the prescriber, the prescriber's U.S. Drug Enforcement Administration (DEA) number (if applicable), instructions to the pharmacist about product selection (generic versus brand name), and other items.

Table 1-3.	Metric and Household Measures
Weight	
kilogram = kg	1 kg = 1000 g
gram = g	1 g = 1000 mg
milligram = mg	1 mg = 1/1000 g
pound = lb	1 kg = 2.2 lb
grain = gr	1 gr = 65 mg
Volume	
liter = L	1 L = 1000 mL
milliliter = mL	1 mL = 1/1000 L
teaspoonful = tsp	1 tsp = 5 mL
tablespoonful = tbs	1 tbs = 15 mL
drop = gt (drops = gtt)	1 mL = 15 gtt
fluid ounce = fl oz	1 fl oz = 30 mL

METRIC AND HOUSEHOLD MEASURES

The metric system is the language of scientific measurement and should always be used in prescription writing (Table 1-3). Solid drugs are dispensed by weight (mg) and liquid drugs by volume (mL). Although the clinician will direct the pharmacist to dispense a liquid preparation in milliliters, it is generally necessary to convert this to a convenient household measurement in directions to the patient (Table 1-3). When greater accuracy is required, the patient may need to use a graduated cylinder or a calibrated dropper.

ABBREVIATIONS

Abbreviations are used in prescription writing to save time and to make alteration of a prescription by the patient more difficult (Table 1-4). However, unless a practitioner writes a large number of prescriptions daily, he or she saves little time using abbreviations. Since abbreviations are more likely to be misinterpreted by the pharmacist than are instructions written in full, the practitioner should ensure the clarity of the information.

REGULATIONS

The U.S. Food and Drugs Act of 1906 was the first federal law to regulate interstate commerce in drugs. It was rewritten and reenacted to become the Federal Food, Drug, and Cosmetic Act of 1938. This law and its subsequent amendments, enforced by the FDA of the U.S. Department of Health and Human Services, prohibit interstate commerce in drugs that have not been shown to be safe and effective. They further regulate labeling and packaging and establish

Table 1-4.	Commonly Used Abbreviations		
dispense = disp		as needed = prn	
number = no		every hour = qh	
capsule = cap		every day = qd	
tablet = tab		twice a day = bid	
label = sig		3 times a day = tid	
by mouth = po		4 times a day = qid	
at once = stat		discontinue = d/c	

standards for strength and purity. Over the years, Congress has enacted more than 50 pieces of legislation related to drug control. The Controlled Substances Act of 1970 collects and conforms most of these diverse laws into one piece of legislation. The law is designed to improve the administration and regulation of manufacturing, distribution, and dispensing of drugs, and to provide a "closed" system for the legitimate handlers of controlled substances. Individual states or local governments may legislate additional requirements concerning controlled substances. Whenever state and federal laws differ, the more stringent law must be followed.

Every practitioner who administers, prescribes, or dispenses controlled substances must be registered with the Drug Enforcement Administration, Registration Unit, P.O. Box 28083, Central Station, Washington, DC 20005. The 1984 Diversion Control Amendments, a part of the Comprehensive Crime Control Act, give the attorney general authority to deny an application for registration if it is determined that the issuance of such registration would be inconsistent with the public interest. In determining the public interest, the following factors are considered: the recommendation of the appropriate state licensing board or professional disciplinary authority, the applicant's experience in dispensing or conducting research with respect to controlled substances, and the applicant's conviction record under federal or state laws relating to the manufacture, distribution, or dispensing of controlled substances.

Controlled substances

The drugs that come under the jurisdiction of the Controlled Substances Act of 1970 are divided into five schedules (Table 1-5). All prescription orders for controlled substances must be written in ink or typewritten; must bear the full name and address of the patient; must list the full name, address, and DEA registration number of the practitioner; must be dated; and must be manually signed by the practitioner. When prescribing a controlled substance, the clinician must write out the actual amount in addition to giving an Arabic number or Roman numeral to discourage alterations in written prescription orders. To avoid misprescribing, overprescribing, or inappropriate prescribing, clinicians must also be aware of gimmicks and techniques used by drug abusers to obtain controlled substances, be cautious of patients who self-diagnose and self-prescribe, and be alert to a series of "new" patients all complaining of similar symptoms.

CONCLUSION

It should be emphasized that drugs seldom exert their beneficial effects without also causing adverse side effects. The inevitability of this therapeutic dilemma lends credence to the statement that there are no "absolutely" safe biologically active agents. In dealing with this certainty, the clinician familiar with the molecular mechanisms of drug action, principles of disposition, and therapeutic and toxic effects of drugs has the advantage. By reviewing a patient's medical history, the clinician can identify the medically or pharmacologically compromised patient and avoid prescribing drugs that may produce potential drug-drug, drug-disease, or drug-food interactions, or cause drug-induced illness. It cannot be overemphasized that patients may fail to report the intake of over-the-counter preparations and herbal and other dietary supplements, as well as illicit drugs, and, therefore, a patient's health and drug profile must also reflect an adequate social history. Furthermore, clinicians should avoid misprescribing, overprescribing, or inappropriate prescribing and be aware of gimmicks and techniques used by drug seekers to obtain controlled substances.

Table 1-5.	Drug Schedules	
	DESCRIPTION	**EXAMPLE(S)**
SCHEDULE I (C-I)	C-I drugs have no legal medical use in the United States and have a high abuse potential. They may be used for research purposes and must be obtained from governmental agencies.	• hallucinogens • marijuana • selected opiates (heroin, opium derivatives)
SCHEDULE II (C-II)	C-II drugs have legal medical uses in the United States, but they have a high abuse potential, which may lead to severe psychological and/or physical dependence. A written prescription order is required for C-II drugs. The refilling of C-II prescription orders is prohibited. In the case of a bona fide emergency, a practitioner may telephone a prescription order to a pharmacist. In such a case, the drug prescribed must be limited to the amount needed to treat the patient during the emergency period. Such oral orders must be followed up by a written order within 72 hours.	• amphetamines • selected opiates (morphine and congeners, codeine congeners, methadone) • some barbiturates
SCHEDULE III (C-III)	C-III drugs have legal medical uses in the United States and a moderate abuse potential, which may lead to moderate psychological and/or physical dependence. A prescription order for C-III drugs may be issued either orally or in writing to the pharmacist and may be refilled up to five times within six months after the date of issue, if so authorized on the prescription. After five refills or after six months, a new oral or written prescription is required.	• anabolic steroids • selected opiates (acetaminophen [APAP] w/ codeine)

(continues)

Table 1-5.	Drug Schedules *(continued)*	
	DESCRIPTION	**EXAMPLE(S)**
SCHEDULE IV (C-IV)	C-IV drugs have legal medical uses in the United States and a low abuse potential, which may lead to moderate psychological and/or physical dependence. A prescription order for C-IV drugs may be issued either orally or in writing to the pharmacist and may be refilled up to five times within six months after the date of issue, if so authorized on the prescription. After five refills or after six months, a new oral or written prescription is required.	• benzodiazepines • selected opiates (propoxyphene) • some barbiturates
SCHEDULE V (C-V)	C-V drugs have legal medical uses in the United States and a low abuse potential, which may lead to moderate psychological and/or physical dependence. A prescription order for C-V may be issued either orally or in writing to the pharmacist and may be refilled if so authorized on the prescription.	• selected opiates (cough and diarrhea preparations)

BIBLIOGRAPHY

1. American Academy of Pediatrics, Committee on Drugs. The transfer of drugs and other chemicals into human milk. Pediatrics 1994;93:137–150.

2. Anand AC, Chawala YK. Prescribing drugs for patients with liver disease. Natl Med J India 1999;12(5):217–224.

3. Anderson PO. Drug use during breast-feeding. Clin Pharm 1991;10:594–624.

4. Andrade SE, Gurwitz JH, Davis RL, et al. Prescription drug use in pregnancy. Am J Obstet Gynecl 2004;191:398–407.

5. Benet LZ, Zia-Amirhosseini P. Basic principles of pharmacokinetics. Toxicol Pathol 1995;23(2):115–23.

6. Breckenridge A. Science, medicine and clinical pharmacology. The Lilly lecture 1994. Br J Clin Pharmacol 1995;40(1): 1–9.

7. Doering PL, Boothby LA, Cheok M. Review of pregnancy labeling of prescription drugs: is the current system adequate to inform of risk? Am J Obstet Gynecol 2002;187:333–339.

8. Epstein JB. Understanding placebos in dentistry. J Am Dent Assoc 1984;109:71–74.

9. Gleiter CH, Gundert-Remy U. Gender differences in pharmacokinetics. Eur J Drug Metab Pharmacokinet 1996;21(2): 123–128.

10. Goldman P. Rate-controlled drug delivery. N Engl J Med 1982;307:286–290.

11. Greenblatt DJ, Sellers EM, Shader RI. Drug disposition in old age. N Engl J Med 1982;306:1081–1088.

12. Harris RZ, Benet LZ, Schwartz JB. Gender effects in pharmacokinetics and pharmacodynamics. Drugs 1995;50(2): 222–239.

13. Howard CR, Lawrence RA. Breast-feeding and drug exposure. Obstet Gynecol Clin North Am 1998;25:195–217.

14. Inaba T, Nebert DW, Burchell B, et al. Pharmacogenetics in clinical pharmacology and toxicology. Can J Physiol Pharmacol 1995;73(3):331–338.

15. Ito S. Drug therapy for breast-feeding women. N Engl J Med 2000;343:118–126.

16. Kacew S. Adverse effects of drugs and chemicals in breast milk on the nursing infant. J Clin Pharmacol 1993;33: 213–221.

17. Kinirons MT, Crome P. Clinical pharmacokinetic considerations in the elderly. An update. Clin Pharmacokinet 1997; 33(4):302–312.

18. Koch-Weser J. Drug administration in hepatic disease. N Engl J Med 1983;309:1616–1622.

19. Koch-Weser J. Rate-controlled drug delivery. N Engl J Med 1982;307:286–290.

20. Loebstein R, Lalkin A, Koren G. Pharmacokinetic changes during pregnancy and their clinical relevance. Clin Pharmacokinet 1997; 33(5):328–343.

21. Morgan DJ, McLean A. Clinical pharmacokinetic and pharmacodynamic considerations in patients with liver disease. Clin Pharmacokinet 1995;29(5):370–391.

22. Niederhauser VP. Prescribing for children: issues in pediatric pharmacology. Nurse Pract 1997;22(3):16–18, 23, 26–28.

23. Pfeifer S. Pharmacokinetic drug interactions. Part 1: Drugs A-C. Pharmazie 1995;50(3):163–179.

24. Phillips KA, Veenstra DL, Oren E, Lee JK, Sadee W. Potential role of pharmacogenomics in reducing adverse drug reactions. JAMA 2001;286:2270–2279.

25. Pugh RNH, Murray-Lyon IM, Dawson JL, Pietroni MC, Williams R. Transection of the oesophagus for bleeding oesophageal varices. Br J Surg 1973;60:646–649.

26. Reichen J. Prescribing in liver disease. J Hepatol 1997;(26)1:36–40.

27. Rescigno A. Fundamental concepts in pharmacokinetics. Pharmacol Res 1997;35(5):363–390.

28. Rescigno A. Pharmacokinetics, science or fiction? Pharmacol Res 1996;33(4–5):227–233.

29. Rudd P, Lenert L. Pharmacokinetics as an aid to optimising compliance with medications. Clin Pharmacokinet 1995; 28(1):1–6.

30. Trocóniz IF. Population-based approach to the assessment of pharmacokinetic-pharmacodynamic data. Methods Find Exp Clin Pharmacol 1996;18(Suppl C):51–52.

31. Vesell ES. Genetic host factors: determinants of drug response. N Engl J Med 1985;313:261–262.

32. Vestal RD. Aging and pharmacology. Cancer 1997;80(7):1302–1310.

33. Ward RM. Pharmacological treatment of the fetus. Clinical pharmacokinetic considerations. Clin Pharmacokinet 1995; 28(5):343–350.

34. Welling PG. Differences between pharmacokinetics and toxicokinetics. Toxicol Pathol 1995;23(2):143–147.

35. Williams RL. Drug administration in hepatic disease. N Engl J Med 1983;390:1616–1622.

2 Adverse Drug Events

Table of Contents

INTRODUCTION

Clinicians and patients both acknowledge the major role played by drugs in modern health care. As we observe changing demographic and disease trends, despite the availability of more than a thousand active ingredients in several thousand different formulations, it can be anticipated that new and better drugs are still needed. Understanding how chemicals affect body homeostasis at the molecular level serves as the foundation for developing new drugs and provides the basis for rational pharmacotherapy.

Drugs, including herbal remedies and various dietary supplements, seldom exert their beneficial effects without also causing adverse events. The inevitability of this therapeutic dilemma lends credence to the statement that there are no "absolutely" safe biologically active agents. When selecting a drug necessary to obtain a desired therapeutic effect, prescribers must take into consideration the diagnosis, individual variations in physiological homeostatic mechanisms, variations in disease states, and drug-related pharmacodynamic and pharmacokinetic variables. Oral health care providers, like other health care professionals, should be aware of the spectrum of drug-induced events and should be actively involved in monitoring for and reporting adverse drug events (ADEs).

ETIOLOGY AND EPIDEMIOLOGY

It is estimated that as many as 75% of office visits to general medical practitioners and internists are associated with the initiation or continuation of pharmacotherapy. Pharmacotherapy of this magnitude predisposes patients to ADEs. The frequency of clinically important ADEs is difficult to estimate, but it has been reported that between 3% and 11% of hospital admissions could be attributed to ADEs. The incidence of ADEs during hospitalization ranges from 0.3% to 44%, depending on the type of hospital, definition of an ADE, and study methodology. Although the U.S. Food and Drug Administration (FDA) has one of the most rigorous approval requirements in the world to authorize the marketing of new drugs (Table 2-1), clinical trials cannot and should not be expected to uncover every potential ADE.

Premarketing study groups generally include only 3,000 to 4,000 subjects. From a statistical perspective, a population of 30,000 would have to be exposed to the drug to have a 95% chance of detecting an ADE with an incidence of 1 in 10,000 subjects. Therefore, ADEs that occur at a low frequency can be easily missed. In addition, premarketing clinical trials are of relatively short duration. ADEs that develop with chronic use or those that have a long latency period may also escape detection. Study groups often exclude children, women, and the elderly, and they are seldom representative of the population exposed to the drug after FDA approval. Finally, the efficacy of a drug is evaluated for only a narrow set of indications and does not extend to the actual evolving use of a drug. Consequently, premarketing clinical trials detect only the most common ADEs. Those occurring more frequently than 1 in 1,000 subjects will be observed and subsequently listed in the product's official labeling at the time of approval.

ADEs may be classified as Type A or Type B (Table 2-2). They can range from mild to severe reactions and can lead to hospitalization, permanent disability, or death. **Type A ADEs**, with the exception of drug overdose, are associated with the administration of therapeutic dosages of a drug, are usually predictable and avoidable, and are responsible for most ADEs. **Type B ADEs** are generally independent of the dose and are rarely predictable or avoidable. While they are uncommon, type B reactions are often among the most serious and poten-

Table 2-1.	The Chronology of Testing and Introducing New Drugs	
PRECLINICAL TESTING (3.5 YEARS)	**CLINICAL TRIALS (8.5 YEARS)**	**POSTMARKETING SURVEILLANCE**
Laboratory studies • Isolation or synthesis of a new chemical Animal studies • Assess safety and biological activity Pharmaceutical company files an Investigational New Drug (IND) application with the FDA • FDA approval IND reviewed and approved by the Institutional Review Board where the studies will be conducted • Progress reports on clinical trials submitted to FDA annually	Phase I (1 year): • 20 to 80 healthy volunteers • Dosage range • Safety profile Phase II (2 years): • 100 to 300 volunteers with a specific disease • Short-term effectiveness • Adverse drug events Phase III (3 years): • 1,000 to 3,000 volunteers with a specific disease • Long-term effectiveness • Adverse drug events Pharmaceutical company files a New Drug Application (NDA) with the FDA • FDA approval	Monitoring for safety during postmarketing clinical use to determine the true risk-benefit profile of the new drug • Pharmaceutical company must continue to submit periodic reports to the FDA • Case reports of adverse drug reactions • Quality control records • FDA may require additional clinical trials (Phase IV studies)
5,000 potential drugs evaluated	5 drugs are approved for clinical trials	1 drug approved for marketing

tially life threatening of all ADEs and they are the major cause of important drug-induced illness. These reactions seem to affect certain organ systems, most commonly the liver, the hematopoietic system, or the skin and mucosa. With the exception of immediate hypersensitivity reactions, e.g., anaphylaxis (which can develop in seconds to minutes), Type B events require up to 12 weeks of drug exposure. Some ADEs may be delayed even further and appear a long time after drug therapy has been discontinued.

Table 2-2.	Classification of Adverse Drug Events
TYPE A REACTIONS	**TYPE B REACTIONS**
Predictable	Unpredictable
• Overdose	• Idiosyncratic reactions
• Cytotoxic reactions	• Immunologic/Allergic reactions
• Drug-drug interactions	• Pseudoallergic reactions
• Drug-food interactions	• Teratogenic effects
• Drug-disease interactions	• Oncogenic effects

MECHANISMS ASSOCIATED WITH TYPE A REACTIONS

Cytotoxic reactions

Most **cytotoxic reactions** involve the formation of unstable or reactive metabolites and are related to some abnormality that interferes with the normal metabolism and/or excretion of therapeutic dosages of a drug; cytotoxic reactions can also result from a drug overdose. These events lead to the saturation of hepatic enzyme systems. Two main mechanisms underlie the formation of these intermediate compounds during biotransformation: an oxidative pathway, which leads to the formation of electrophilic compounds capable of binding covalently with cellular macromolecules; and a reductive pathway, which gives rise to intermediate compounds with an excess of electrons (free radicals, anionic radicals). These substances react with oxygen and produce reactive metabolites, which overwhelm antioxidant defense systems (superoxide dismutase, glutathione peroxidase). Covalent binding to proteins and the oxidation of biological macromolecules both lead to direct cytotoxic effects.

Drug-drug interactions

Two or more drugs administered in therapeutic dosages at the same time or in close sequence may (1) act independently, (2) interact to increase or diminish the magnitude or duration of action of one or more drugs, or (3) interact to cause an unintended reaction. Drug-drug interactions may be complex and even unexplained, but they all seem to have either a pharmacodynamic or a pharmacokinetic basis because the same pharmacological mechanisms that account for a drug's efficacy also account for many of its adverse effects.

Pharmacodynamic drug-drug interactions. In *pharmacodynamic interactions*, the intended or expected effect produced by a given plasma level of a drug in the presence of a second drug is altered. These types of interactions may be characterized as (1) pharmacological interactions, (2) physiological interactions, (3) chemical interactions, or (4) drug-related receptor alterations (Table 2-3).

Pharmacokinetic drug-drug interactions. The duration and intensity of a drug's action is a function of the plasma level of the drug, which is directly related to the drug's rate of absorption, distribution, metabolism, and excretion. One or more of these rates may be altered by concomitant drug therapy resulting in unexpected differences in the plasma levels of a drug (Table 2-4).

Drug-food interactions

An awareness of significant drug-food interactions can help the clinician to identify the nutrients that may interact with certain medications. This information can be used to educate patients and optimize pharmacotherapy.

Table 2-3.	Pharmacodynamic Drug-drug Interactions	
TYPE	**MECHANISMS**	**EXAMPLE(S)**
Pharmacological	Drug A and drug B compete for the same receptor site and as a function of their respective concentrations either produce (an agonist) or prevent (an antagonist) an effect	• Opioids vs. naloxone • Acetylcholine vs. atropine • Epinephrine vs. adrenergic receptor blocking agents
Physiological	Drug A and drug B interact with different receptor sites and either enhance each other's action or produce an opposing effect via different cellular mechanisms	• Cholinergic agents enhance the action of diazepam • Epinephrine opposes the action of histamine • Epinephrine opposes the action of lidocaine
Chemical	Drug A interacts with drug B and prevents drug B from interacting with its intended receptor	• Protamine sulfate inhibits heparin
Receptor alterations	Drug A, when administered long term, may either increase or decrease the number of its own receptors or alter the adaptability of receptors to physiological events	• α_1-adrenergic receptor agonists down-regulate their own receptors • β_1-adrenergic receptor antagonists up-regulate their own receptors

Interactions affecting absorption. Nutrients may protect the gastric mucosa from irritants, but they may also act as a mechanical barrier that prevents drug access to mucosal surfaces and reduces or slows the absorption of some drugs. Conversely, a meal with high fatty acid content will actually increase the absorption of lipid-soluble drugs. Chemical interactions, chelating reactions with food components, can produce inactive complexes. The interaction of tetracycline with calcium in milk and other dairy products is an example of a chelating reaction. Similarly, ferrous or ferric salts can bind with tetracyclines and fluoroquinolones, preventing their absorption. An interaction between zinc and fluoroquinolones may also result in the formation of inactive complexes and decreased absorption.

Interactions affecting metabolism. Components in grapefruit juice inhibit the CYP450 3A4 isoenzyme and can greatly increase (up to threefold) the bio-

Table 2-4.	Pharmacokinetic Drug-drug Interactions	
TYPE	**MECHANISMS**	**EXAMPLE(S)**
Interactions affecting absorption	Drug A, by causing vaso-constriction, interferes with the systemic absorption of drug B	Epinephrine vs. li-docaine (or other local anesthetic agents)
	Drug A, by forming a complex with drug B, interferes with the systemic absorption of drug B	Calcium vs. tetracycline
	Drug A, by delaying gastric emptying, delays the systemic absorption of drug B, which is absorbed primarily in the intestine	Opioids vs. acetaminophen
	Drug A, by elevating gastric pH, prevents the absorption of drug B (a weak acid)	Antacids vs. acetylsalicylic acid
Interactions affecting distribution	Drug A (a weak acid), by competing for plasma protein binding with drug B, increases the plasma level of drug B	Acetylsalicylic acid vs. sulfonylureas and many other drugs
Interactions affecting metabolism	Drug A, by increasing or decreasing hepatic microsomal enzyme activity responsible for the metabolism of drug B, increases or decreases the plasma level of drug B respectively	Macrolides, azole antifungals, and ethanol (long-term use) increase the plasma level of many drugs; H_2-receptor antagonists decrease the plasma level of many drugs
	Drug A, by decreasing hepatic nonmicrosomal enzyme activity responsible for the metabolism of drug B, increases the plasma level of drug B	MAO-inhibitors increase the plasma level of benzodiazepines
	Drug A, by inhibiting the enzyme acetaldehyde dehydrogenase, interferes with the further metabolism of intermediate metabolites (oxidation product) of drug B	Disulfiram and metronidazole inhibit the metabolism of intermediate metabolites of ethanol

(continues)

Table 2-4.	Pharmacokinetic Drug-drug Interactions *(continued)*	
TYPE	**MECHANISMS**	**EXAMPLE(S)**
Interactions affecting renal excretion	Drug A, which competes with drug B for the same excretory transport mechanisms in the proximal tubules, increases the plasma level of drug B	Acetylsalicylic acid and probenecid increase the plasma level of penicillin and other weak acids
	Drug A, by alkalizing the urine, decreases the plasma level of drug B	Sodium bicarbonate decreases the plasma level of weak acids
	Drug A, by acidifying the urine, decreases the plasma level of drug B	Ammonium chloride decreases the plasma level of weak bases
Interactions affecting biliary excretion	Drug A, by increasing bile flow and the synthesis of proteins, which function in biliary conjugation mechanisms, decreases the plasma level of drug B	Phenobarbital decreases the plasma level of many drugs
	Drug A binds drug B, which would undergo extensive enterohepatic recirculation, and decreases the plasma level of drug B	Activated charcoal and cholestyramine decreases the plasma level of many drugs

MAO, monoamine oxidase.

availability of numerous drugs, such as some calcium channel-blocking agents, benzodiazepines, and warfarin.

Interactions affecting excretion. Changes in the pH of kidney fluids can inhibit excretion of some drugs. For example, large doses of vitamin C (ascorbic acid) may cause acidic drugs to be reabsorbed, delaying excretion and increasing plasma levels of a drug.

Drug-disease interactions

A drug prescribed for the treatment of one disease may have an adverse effect on a different condition that has been generally well controlled. Additionally, certain disease states can interfere with the metabolism and/or excretion of drugs in general.

Pharmacodynamic interactions. Nonselective beta$_1$-adrenergic receptor antagonists, such as propranolol, prescribed for the treatment of chronic stable angina, hypertension, or cardiac arrhythmia, can induce an asthma attack in susceptible individuals by blocking beta$_2$-adrenergic receptors and increasing airway resistance. Beta$_1$-adrenergic receptor antagonists and calcium channel-blocking agents, which can be used for the management of hypertension, chronic stable angina, and certain cardiac arrhythmias, can in some instances precipitate cardiac complications secondary to negative inotropism (decreased contractility), peripheral vasodilatation, and decreased nodal conductance. Beta$_1$-adrenergic receptor antagonists can also adversely affect carbohydrate metabolism and inhibit endogenous epinephrine-mediated hyperglycemic response to excessive insulin levels, thus placing the diabetic patient at risk for hypoglycemia. Cyclooxygenase (COX)-1 inhibitors, especially acetylsalicylic acid (ASA), can lead to gastrointestinal bleeding in patients with preexisting peptic ulcer disease. COX-1, COX-2, and COX-3 inhibitors and amoxicillin may induce renal toxicity in patients with preexisting renal dysfunction. Uncontrolled hypothyroidism increases the sensitivity of patients to sedative/anxiolytic agents and opioids, whereas uncontrolled hyperthyroidism predisposes to epinephrine-induced hypertension and cardiac arrhythmias.

Pharmacokinetic interactions. Hepatic dysfunction can affect drug metabolism and biliary excretion. Renal insufficiency can be expected to impair renal drug elimination. Cardiac disease can often result in reduced metabolic activity in general because of poor oxygenation and organ perfusion. All of these conditions can lead to elevated plasma concentration of drugs and associated adverse drug effects. Patients with congestive heart failure may become symptomatic while receiving beta$_1$-adrenergic receptor blocking agents because these drugs decrease cardiac output and reduce glomerular filtration and sodium excretion, increasing the risk of edema. In patients with liver disease, drugs metabolized primarily by the liver (such as acetaminophen) may induce further hepatic dysfunction, even at therapeutic levels, when taken on a long-term basis.

MECHANISMS ASSOCIATED WITH TYPE B REACTIONS

Idiosyncratic reactions

Drug metabolism is largely dominated by oxidation reactions catalyzed by the CYP450 enzyme system. There are ten isoforms of the CYP450 enzyme system and this genetic polymorphism may lead to significant differences in the efficacy and toxicity of drugs. The effect of genetic polymorphism on catalytic activity is most prominent for five isoforms (CYP1A2, CYP2C9, CYP2C19, CYP2D6, and CYP3A4). CYP3A4 alone is involved in the metabolism of about half of all drugs currently prescribed (Table 2-5). Drugs that are substrates of the same CYP isoenzyme (i.e., metabolized by the same isoenzyme) may competitively inhibit each other. Other drugs may inhibit or induce CYP isoen-

Table 2-5.	Important Relationships Between Drugs Prescribed by Oral Health Care Providers and CYP Enzymes		
CYP ISOENZYMES	**SUBSTRATES**	**INHIBITORS**	**INDUCERS**
CYP2C9	Ibuprofen	Fluconazole	
CYP2C19	Diazepam		
CYP2D6	Codeine Hydrocodone		
CYP3A4	Erythromycin Clarithromycin Alprazolam Midazolam Triazolam	Erythromycin Clarithromycin Fluconazole Ketoconazole Itraconazole	Carbamazepine

zyme activity without being substrates. The therapeutic consequences of this genetic polymorphism will depend on the intrinsic character of the drug, on the importance of the deficient metabolic pathway in the overall metabolism of the drug, and on the possible existence of alternative metabolic pathways.

Allergic/immunological reactions

A familial predisposition to drug allergy has been reported, and it is suggested that specific human leukocyte antigen (HLA) genes are involved in the reaction to at least some drugs. In susceptible patients, alkylation and/or oxidation of cellular macromolecules by drug metabolites may lead to the production of antigens. The production of antigens is patient dependent, clearly not related to the dose administered, and is unpredictable. Allergic reactions to drugs are characterized by specificity to a given agent, transferability by antibodies or lymphocytes, and recurrence when reexposure to the offending drug occurs. Most allergic reactions to drugs tend to occur in young or middle-aged adults; drug allergy is observed twice as frequently in women as men.

Type I (immediate) hypersensitivity reactions. Exposure to an allergen results in antigen-specific antibody production dominated by the immunoglobulin E (IgE) isotype. IgE antibodies bind to mast cells, basophils, and eosinophils associated with mucosal and epithelial tissues. The simultaneous binding of an antigen to adjacent IgE molecules fixed to Fc receptors triggers degranulation of mast cells and basophils, resulting in the production and release of histamine, leukotrienes, prostaglandins, chemokines, enzymes, and cytokines (Figure 2-1). Histamine produces peripheral vasodilatation and increased capillary permeability. Leukotrienes and prostaglandins promote smooth muscle contraction, increased vascular permeability, and increased mucus secretion. Chemokines attract eukocytes, enzymes break down tissue matrix proteins, and the cytokines promote inflammatory activities in target tissues.

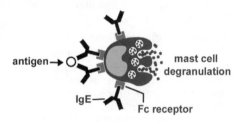

Figure 2-1. Type I (immediate) hypersensitivity reaction.

Type II (cytotoxic) hypersensitivity reactions. IgG antibodies mediate the basic cytotoxic immune reaction. The antibodies bind to antigen-coated host cells, followed by complement activation and cell lysis induced by the active byproducts of the complement cascade (Figure 2-2).

Type III (immune-complex) hypersensitivity reactions. Immune-complex reactions are also mediated by IgG antibodies and result in the formation of large,

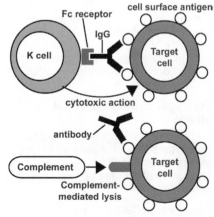

Figure 2-2. Type II (cytotoxic) hypersensitivity reaction.

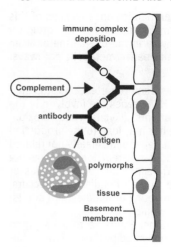

Figure 2-3. Type III (immune-complex) hypersensitivity reaction.

insoluble anti-gen-antibody com-plexes (Figure 2-3). These immune complexes adhere to target tissues, initiate intense complement activa-tion, aggregate leukocytes and plate-lets to form thrombi and occlude arte-rioles, and produce either localized or systemic complications.

Type IV (delayed) hypersensitiv-ity reactions. Delayed reactions are closely related to cellular immunity in that specifically sensitized CD4+ T-lymphocytes initiate the reaction (Fig-ure 2-4). Initial sensitization occurs slowly, over a 10-day to 14-day period. Small molecular weight drugs bind co-valently to host cell membrane pro-teins or *hapten-carrier conjugates*. A subsequent exposure causes the im-munologically committed lymphocytes to react with the allergen (antigens) and release cytokines (lymphokines), which activate macrophages and amplify the inflammatory response.

Pseudoallergic reactions

Pseudoallergic reactions cannot be explained on an immunological basis. These ADEs occur in patients who had no prior exposure to the drug. Penicillin, codeine, morphine, and vancomycin directly activate mast cells through non-IgE receptor pathways and initiate the release of histamine and other bioactive media-tors. Angiotensin-converting enzyme (ACE) inhibitors block the degrada-tion of vasoactive substances such as bradykinin and prostaglandin. COX-1 inhibitors, by inhibiting the ac-tivity of cyclooxygenase, increase the production of leukotriene-related metabolic products.

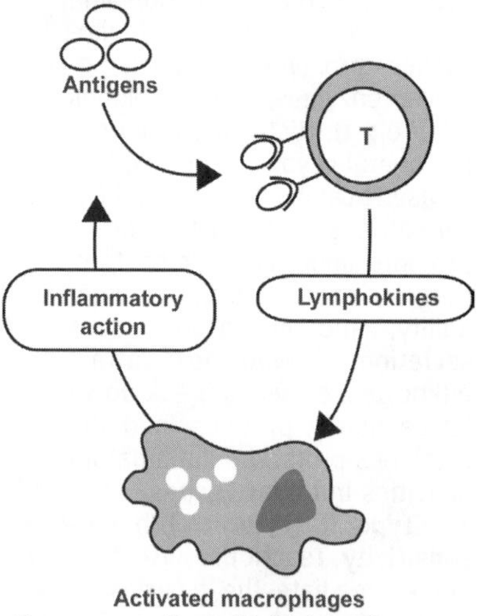

Teratogenic/developmental effects

Figure 2-4. Type IV (delayed) hypersensitivity reaction.

Teratogens are substances capable of causing physical or functional disor-ders in the fetus in the absence of toxic effects on the mother. Direct teratogenic effects depend on the achievement of drug or metabolite concentrations in the fetus at a critical time period, especially from the third to the twelfth week of gestation.

Oncogenic effects

Oncogenic effects associated with drug therapy may be primary or second-ary. *Primary oncogenic effects* may be produced by certain procarcinogenic drugs, which are converted into carcinogens by polymorphic oxidation reactions. Covalent binding of these reactive metabolites to DNA leads to mutagenic and carcinogenic effects. *Secondary oncogenic effects* are associated with therapeutic immunosuppression, leading to the reactivation of latent infection with oncogenic viruses (i.e., hepatitis B virus [HBV], hepatitis C virus [HCV], cytomegalovirus [CMV], herpes simplex virus [HSV], human papillomavirus [HPV], and the Epstein-Barr virus [EBV]). The pattern of cancer incidence from secondary effects is distinctly different from that in the general population, with a marked excess in the occurrence of (1) carcinoma of the skin and lips, (2) non-Hodgkin lymphoma, (3) Kaposi sarcoma (KS), (4) carcinoma of the uterus, (5) hepatobiliary carcinoma, (6) carcinoma of the vulva and perineum, (7) renal carcinoma, and (8) sarcomas (other than KS). The prevalence of de novo malignancies associated with therapeutic immunosuppression ranges from 4% to 18%. The malignancies occur in a relatively young group of patients (average age at the time of transplantation is 42 years), at a fairly predictable time interval, and within a relatively short period of time after transplantation.

CLINICAL MANIFESTATIONS OF ADVERSE DRUG EVENTS

The clinical manifestations of ADEs may reflect primary (direct) or secondary (indirect) adverse effects. Primary or secondary adverse effects associated with Type A reactions are those dose-dependent effects that are not desired for the given therapeutic use of a drug. These adverse effects account for most of the ADEs and may be exaggerations of direct effects or multiple concurrent "side" effects. Similarly, the clinical manifestations of ADEs associated with Type B reactions are either primary or secondary, but they may or may not be dose dependent.

TYPE A REACTIONS

Cytotoxic effects

Hepatocellular toxicity. Drug-induced liver injury is a potential complication of nearly every medication that is prescribed. One such drug, acetaminophen (APAP), is metabolized primarily by conjugation into inactive metabolites. When the capacity of conjugation reactions is exceeded, the CYP2E1 enzyme is activated and a highly reactive intermediate metabolite is synthesized. While it can be detoxified through glutathione-mediated conjugation, depletion of glutathione (excessive doses of APAP [>5 therapeutic doses in a 24-hour period], malnutrition, and ethanol abuse) allows the reactive metabolite to accumulate and bind covalently to cellular macromolecules and disrupt hepatic cell function. Clinical signs and symptoms of APAP overdose include nausea, vomiting, anorexia, and abdominal pain. A few days later, elevated bilirubin presents as jaundice (see Figure 2-5 ✿ and Figure 2-6 ✿ on CD-ROM).

Cytotoxic mucositis. Cancer chemotherapeutic agents produce extensive injury to certain cancer cells, but they are not selectively tumoricidal and may arrest the growth and maturation of normal cells. The degree of toxicity usually depends on the specific agent, dosage, schedule and route of administration, and patient-related predisposing factors. Mucositis appears clinically as erythematous or diffuse ulcerative lesions. Certain chemotherapeutic agents are more stomatotoxic than others, and chemotherapy-related mucositis may contribute to systemic infection by odontopathic, periodontopathic, and transient oral microorganisms. Other drugs may also produce cytotoxic reactions that affect oral soft tissues (see Figure 2-7 🦷, Figure 2-8 🦷, Figure 2-9 🦷, Figure 2-10 🦷, and Figure 2-11 🦷 on CD-ROM).

Gastrointestinal disturbances

Nausea and vomiting. The physiological purpose of nausea is to prevent food intake; that of vomiting is to expel food or other toxic substances present in the upper part of the gastrointestinal tract. The vomiting center, located in the brain, is the origin of the final common pathway along which different impulses induce emesis. The second important medullary site is the chemoreceptor trigger zone. The chemoreceptor trigger zone is outside the blood-brain barrier and, thus, it is accessible to drugs circulating either in the blood or in the cerebrospinal fluid. The vomiting center, activated by impulses that originate in the chemoreceptor trigger zone, induces nausea and vomiting. Protracted vomiting may cause electrolyte imbalance, dehydration, and malnutrition syndrome, and it may result in mucosal laceration and esophageal hemorrhage.

Opioid analgesics can either induce or block emesis. Both the emetic and antiemetic action can be blocked by naloxone (an opioid antagonist), which suggests that both effects are mediated by opiate receptors. Studies using selective opiate-receptor agonists suggest that the delta and/or kappa receptors are the emetic receptors and the mu receptors mediate an antiemetic effect. In addition, dopamine (D_2), histamine (H_1), muscarinic, and serotonin (5-HT_3) receptor agonists have been implicated in causing nausea and vomiting.

Constipation. Constipation may be defined as the passage of excessively dry stool, infrequent stool, or stool of insufficient size. It involves the subjective sensations of incomplete emptying of the rectum, bloating, passage of flatus, lower abdominal discomfort, anorexia, malaise, headache, weakness, and giddiness. Constipation may be of brief duration (e.g., when one's living habits and diet change abruptly), or it may be a lifelong problem. The administration of many drugs (anticholinergic drugs found in many over-the-counter medications, antiparkinsonian drugs with anticholinergic properties, antihistamines, neuroleptics, antidepressants, anticonvulsants, opioid analgesics, and antacids) may lead to constipation.

Diarrhea. Diarrhea and associated fecal urgency and incontinence may be defined as passage of liquefied stool with increased frequency. Chronic diarrhea may be due to lactose intolerance, inflammatory bowel disease, malabsorption syndromes, endocrine disorders, irritable bowel syndrome, and the abuse of laxatives and antacids. Infection (viral or bacterial), toxins, or drugs such as antibacterial agents are the usual causes of acute diarrhea.

Urinary incontinence

Urinary incontinence caused by medications can be attributed to a number of mechanisms. Diuretics cause incontinence by increasing urinary flow. Other drugs cause this problem as a result of overflow, stemming from urinary retention. Drugs acting in this manner include anticholinergic agents and adrenergic agonists, such as ephedrine and theophylline. Other agents affecting incontinence are sedative-hypnotics, anxiolytics, neuroleptics, opioids, and sialagogues.

Mood alterations

Several agents have been implicated in causing depression in susceptible patients. Depression is a frequent consequence of treatment with antihypertensive agents, beta-adrenergic antagonists, cardiac glycosides, benzodiazepines, barbiturates, levodopa, indomethacin, phenothiazines, and steroids. Delirium (acute confusional states) in some cases may also be attributed to drug therapy.

The primary offending agents include anticholinergic agents, psychotropics, cardiac glycosides, opioids, and sedative-hypnotic agents.

Cardiovascular dysfunction

Several drugs can have adverse effects on cardiovascular function. Orthostatic hypotension occurs when there is a positionally related drop in the blood pressure, putting the patient at risk for syncope. Drugs known to produce orthostatic hypotension include antihypertensive agents, antidepressants and other psychotropic agents, alcohol, and levodopa. Digoxin, a drug used to treat congestive heart failure and atrial arrhythmias, is also associated with causing cardiac arrhythmias. Macrolide antibiotics are also known to cause cardiac arrhythmias (QT interval prolongation) and this cardiac effect is amplified in combination with some calcium channel blockers, azole antifungal agents, and protease inhibitors because of CYP3A4 isoenzyme inhibition. The serious consequence of this interaction is the torsade de pointes ventricular arrhythmia.

Equilibrium problems

Patients at increased risk for falls include those with impaired vision, impaired mobility and cognition, postural hypotension, and peripheral neuropathy. The administration of certain drugs to an individual so predisposed may contribute to falls. Drugs commonly implicated in falls include benzodiazepines, antidepressants, neuroleptics, barbiturates, phenytoin, antiarrhythmic agents, and alcohol.

Xerostomia

Qualitative and quantitative changes in saliva lead to reduced lubrication; antibacterial, antiviral, and antifungal activity; loss of mucosal integrity; loss of buffering capacity; reduced lavage and cleansing of oral tissues; interference with normal remineralization of teeth; and altered digestion, taste, and speech. The major classes of drugs causing xerostomia include anticholinergic agents, antidepressants, antihypertensive agents, antipsychotics, diuretics, antihistamines, central nervous system stimulants, systemic bronchodilators, and a small number of cancer chemotherapeutic agents. The consequence of long-term salivary gland hypofunction is an increased risk for periodontal disease and root surface caries. Altered salivary flow and composition may be important predisposing factors to oral candidiasis, and reduced salivary amylase and IgA levels may be associated with an increased incidence of oral infections with opportunistic bacterial pathogens (see Figure 2-12 ✺, Figure 2-13 ✺, Figure 2-14 ✺, and Figure 2-15 ✺ on CD-ROM).

Bleeding diatheses

ASA acetylates cyclooxygenase, which results in the inhibition of platelet thromboxane A_2 biosynthesis. This reduces the ability of platelets to stick or clump together and form a clot. Because platelets lack the ability to synthesize new proteins, the defect induced by ASA cannot be repaired during their life span. Therefore, after treatment with ASA is stopped, cyclooxygenase activity recovers slowly (4 to 7 days) as a function of platelet turnover. Clopidogrel, a thienopyridine, inhibits adenosine diphosphate receptor-mediated platelet activity. Clopidogrel added to ASA can further increase the potential for bleeding.

The oral anticoagulant warfarin reduces clot formation by inhibiting the formation of vitamin K–dependent clotting factors, primarily Factor VII. The parenteral anticoagulant heparin interferes with the activities of Factors II and X. The most common side effect of both warfarin and heparin is hemorrhage. Hemorrhages may present clinically as gingival bleeding or submucosal bleeding with hematoma formation. Cancer chemotherapeutic agents may secondarily induce profound thrombocytopenia (<20,000 mm^3). Hemorrhage may occur anywhere in the mouth and may be spontaneous or precipitated by trauma or existing disease (see Figure 2-16 ✸, Figure 2-17 ✸, Figure 2-18 ✸, Figure 2-19 ✸, and Figure 2-20 ✸ on CD-ROM).

Bacterial infections

If a patient complains of diarrhea with lower abdominal cramping and is currently taking, or has taken in the recent past, clindamycin or a broader spectrum penicillin or cephalosporin, the clinician must consider the possibility of a bacterial superinfection. The worst finding of a bacterial superinfection is pseudomembranous colitis associated with an overgrowth of *Clostridium difficile* in the gastrointestinal tract. Bacterial infections often contribute to morbidity and mortality in association with therapeutic immunosuppression. A wide range of bacteria, including odontopathic, periodontopathic, and transient pathogens of the oral flora, may manifest as ulcerative lesions. The normal signs of infection are not always obvious, with pain, fever, and the presence of a lesion observed most consistently (see Figure 2-21 ✸ on CD-ROM).

Fungal infections

Antibacterial chemotherapy and therapeutic immunosuppression, including inhaled corticosteroids, are often complicated by infection with *Candida albicans* and other fungal organisms. Oral candidiasis may appear as white, raised, or cottage cheese—like growths that can be scraped off, leaving a red and sometimes hemorrhagic base. Candidiasis may also appear as an erythematous lesion under dental prostheses. Once pathogenic, *C. albicans* may spread to the esophagus or lungs via deglutition or droplet aspiration, or through the hematological route. Eventually, all organ systems may be affected (see Figure 2-22 ✸ and Figure 2-23 ✸ on CD-ROM).

Viral infections

Herpes simplex virus infections. Clinical manifestations of recurrent HSV infections in patients undergoing therapeutic immunosuppression may be observed on the lips and intraorally on all tissues. The ulcerations are quite painful. The optimal period of observation for the detection of recurrent HSV infections is during the 7- to 14-day period following the administration of chemotherapy. Primary HSV infections appear to account for fewer than 2% of infections in these patients (see Figure 2-24 ✸ on CD-ROM).

Varicella zoster virus infection. Recurrent infection with the varicella zoster virus, known as herpes zoster, is a painful, unilateral vesiculation that may follow the distribution of a branch of the trigeminal nerve. The lesions coalesce into large ulcerations and may linger for weeks before remission occurs (see Figure 2-25 ✸ and Figure 2-26 ✸ on CD-ROM).

Epstein-Barr virus infection. Infection with the EBV has been associated with a wide range of syndromes in solid organ transplant recipients. In the oral cavity, the EBV has been causally related to hairy leukoplakia, characteristically found on the lateral border of the tongue in patients with therapeutic immunosuppression (see Figure 2-27 ✸ on CD-ROM).

Gingival hyperplasia

Gingival hyperplasia (GH) in patients taking phenytoin has long been recognized. GH also occurs in patients treated with cyclosporine (an immunosuppressive agent) and calcium channel-blocking agents. The mechanisms responsible for GH are unknown, but they may be related to calcium metabolism and the inflammatory changes resulting from poor oral hygiene. Gingival enlargement is usually noted within 1 to 2 months after the initiation of therapy and appears to affect primarily the labial/facial interdental papillae. Although the enlarged tissue may be firm and painless, it is often associated with erythematous and edematous chronic inflammation. The patient may report pain, gingival bleeding, and difficulty with mastication as a result of the hyperplastic tissue. (See Figure 2-28 ✿, Figure 2-29 ✿, and Figure 2-30 ✿ on CD-ROM.)

Neurological complications

Oral pain. Oral pain may be secondary to drug-induced mucositis. During therapeutic immunosuppression, acute exacerbations of chronic periodontal or apical infections can also precipitate pain. Finally, pain or paresthesia may be associated with the administration of certain cytotoxic chemotherapeutic agents (i.e., the plant alkaloids, vinblastine, and vincristine).

Tardive dyskinesia. Tardive dyskinesia (TD) is an example of an adverse drug effect produced by certain psychotropic drugs. It is characterized by uncontrolled, repetitive movements of the lips, tongue, and mouth, which may occur after several months on the drug. It is irreversible and can impair the ability of a patient to wear dental prostheses and complicate the delivery of routine dental care.

Taste alterations. Many drugs, including ACE inhibitors, griseofulvin, phenindione, D-penicillamine, metronidazole, benzodiazepines, methamphetamines, levodopa, chlorhexidine, methocarbamol, dimethyl sulfoxide, gold salts, and lithium have been implicated in dysgeusia. The mechanism of action in taste alteration is poorly understood but may be associated with drug effect on trace metals.

Inadequate nutrition

Drug therapy may compromise the nutrition and caloric intake of the patient by inducing nausea and anorexia. Excessive nutrients may be lost to vomiting and diarrhea. Enteritis, malabsorption, and impaired liver function further interfere with the nutritional status of the patient. The cytotoxic effects of chemotherapeutic agents on the oral mucosa also predispose the patient to pain, difficulty in mastication, and dysphagia. Altered or reduced taste associated with many drugs further contributes to inadequate intake of food.

TYPE B REACTIONS

Idiosyncratic reactions

An unusual reaction of any intensity observed in a small percentage of the patients is referred to as *idiosyncrasy*. If a drug produces its usual effect on a patient at an unexpectedly high dose, the patient is said to be *hyporeactive*. A patient is said to be *hyperreactive* when a drug produces its effect at an unexpectedly low dosage. Some of this diversity in rates of response can be attributed to differences in the rate of drug metabolism. Among the various CYP450 enzymes, CYP2D6 has been studied the most extensively and various phenotypes have been identified. Patients who lack CYP2D6 activity will exhibit poor metabolism of certain drugs; patients who have normal enzyme activity will exhibit normal metabolism; those with reduced activity will exhibit intermediate metabolism; and those with markedly enhanced enzyme activity will exhibit ultrarapid metabolism. If the consequence is reduced drug metabolism, it leads to excessive therapeutic effects and associated adverse reactions. If the consequence is accelerated metabolism, it results in insufficient therapeutic response.

The CYP2D6 enzyme is involved in the metabolism of more than 100 drugs. In most cases, this results in deactivation of the drug; however, in the case of codeine, this metabolic pathway leads to the conversion of the prodrug (codeine) into its active metabolite. The CYP2D6 enzyme converts codeine to morphine, a crucial step in bioactivation, since the affinity of codeine for the mu-opioid receptor is only 1/200th to 1/3000th that of morphine. The analgesic, respiratory, psychomotor, and miotic effects of codeine are markedly attenuated in people with poor metabolism by the CYP2D6 enzyme. Conversely, for people with ultrarapid metabolism, the greater amount of morphine being produced will result in exaggerated pharmacological effects and may lead to life-threatening opioid intoxication. The frequency of the phenotype associated with poor metabolism is 5% to 10% of the white population. Similarly, the frequency of the phenotype associated with ultrarapid metabolism is also 5% to 10%.

Allergic/immunological reactions

In general, topical drug administration is more likely to sensitize than parenteral administration; in turn, parenteral administration is more likely to sensitize than oral administration. The dose, duration, and frequency of administration can also influence drug allergy, and single doses tend to produce less sensitization than prolonged treatment. The preferential sites for cellular injury in allergic reactions involve the vascular endothelium, conjunctivae, mucosa of the upper respiratory tract, bronchial mucosa, and epithelial cells of the skin. *Immediate hypersensitivity reactions* occur during the first hour after drug exposure. *Delayed hypersensitivity reactions* may occur during the first 3 days after drug exposure. *Late reactions*, often of the mucocutaneous or hematological type, occur more than 3 days after drug intake.

Type I (immediate) hypersensitivity reactions. The IgE-mediated reaction is experienced within minutes of exposure to a specific drug. Histamine produces peripheral vasodilatation and increased capillary permeability. Leukotrienes and prostaglandins promote smooth muscle contraction, increased vascular permeability, and increased mucous secretion. Chemokines attract leukocytes, enzymes break down tissue matrix proteins, and the cytokines promote inflammatory activities in target tissues. Local intracutaneous exposure to a drug can lead to a wheal-and-flare reaction. Ingestion of a drug can cause cramping, vomiting, and diarrhea as a result of smooth muscle contraction. If the drug is disseminated to the skin, urticaria can occur. Involvement of the nasopharynx and upper airway results in allergic rhinitis. Involvement of the oropharyngeal area can lead to angioedema. Activation of mast cells in the submucosa of the lower airways results in allergic asthma. Hypotension, a result of vasodilation, may be the first sign of anaphylaxis as a result of exposure to significant systemic doses of the drug, which is followed by respiratory collapse and shock. Rapid detection of signs and symptoms with immediate intervention is necessary to prevent serious complication and death (see Figure 2-31 ✸, Figure 2-32 ✸, and Figure 2-33 ✸ on CD-ROM).

Type II (cytotoxic) hypersensitivity reactions. Antibody titer may take 7 to 12 days to rise after exposure to the antigen before a significant fever, urticaria, swelling of the face and feet, lymphadenopathy, and arthralgia occur. These effects may be transient and insignificant, and the patient is usually able to tolerate the reaction without necessity for allergy therapy. A clinical example of this type of allergic reaction is drug-induced hemolytic anemia.

Type III (immune-complex) hypersensitivity reactions. Immune complexes adsorb to host tissue, initiate intense complement activation, and produce either localized (Arthus reaction) or systemic complications (serum sickness). Leukocytes and platelets aggregate to form thrombi, occlude the arterioles, and lead to redness, edema, hemorrhage, and ischemic necrosis of tissues. Deposition of immune complexes can be observed in biopsy specimens, which demonstrate an irregular (lumpy-bumpy) layer of antibody/complement-coated host tissue (see Figure 2-34 🟢 and Figure 2-35 🟢 on CD-ROM).

Type IV (delayed) hypersensitivity reactions. Sensitization occurs at the time of initial exposure to a drug. A subsequent exposure causes the immunologically committed lymphocytes to react with the drug and release lymphokines, which initiate an inflammatory response. Within 24 to 28 hours, the patient develops symptoms such as fever, malaise, erythema, and edema in target tissues. With repeated exposure to the antigenic challenge, the response becomes more profound (see Figure 2-36 🟢, Figure 2-37 🟢, Figure 2-38 🟢, and Figure 2-39 🟢 on CD-ROM).

Pseudoallergic reactions

The clinical manifestations of pseudoallergic reactions are similar to those associated with allergic reactions. A classic example of such reactions is the patient who gets hives after being administered penicillin, codeine, morphine, or vancomycin. ACE inhibitors block kinin degradation and induce angioedema, and COX-1 inhibitors can cause asthma and hives by inhibiting the activity of cyclooxygenase and increasing the production of leukotriene-related metabolic products (see Figure 2-40 🟢 and Figure 2-41 🟢 on CD-ROM).

Lichenoid stomatitis

The clinical appearance of lichenoid stomatitis is indistinguishable from oral lichen planus (LP). Like oral LP, these lesions most often affect the buccal mucosa, gingivae, and lateral borders of the tongue and may be reticular, erythematous, or atrophic. Various drugs including diuretics (thiazides, furosemide, spironolactone), beta$_1$-adrenergic receptor blocking agents (labetalol, propranolol), ACE-inhibitors (captopril), and COX-1 inhibitors have been implicated as etiologic agents in the development of lichenoid lesions. It is believed such agents act as haptens and alter the antigenicity of epithelial self-antigens. The diagnosis is confirmed when the condition resolves after the offending drug is discontinued (see Figure 2-42 🟢 and Figure 2-43 🟢 on CD-ROM).

Erythema multiforme and Stevens-Johnson syndrome

Erythema multiforme (EM) is an acute, frequently recurrent mucocutaneous vesiculobullous erosive disorder. Typically a self-limiting process, severity varies from mild (EM minor) to moderate (EM major) to potentially fatal (Stevens-Johnson syndrome [SJS] and toxic epidermal necrolysis [TEN]). The etiology of EM has not been clearly established, although it likely represents a genetically predisposed immunologic host response to antigenic challenge. Most cases of EM minor and EM major are related to an infectious agent (typically HSV), whereas most cases of SJS and TEN are related to pharmacological agents (most frequently sulfonamides, anticonvulsive drugs, and COX-1 inhibitors).

Cutaneous lesions usually begin as erythematous papules that progress to form the more characteristic iris or target lesions. In the vast majority of cases, mucosal lesions tend to appear abruptly and manifest as painful vesiculobullous ulcerations and erosions. The oral mucosa is most frequently involved; ocular and genital involvement is seen in more severe forms. Although any oral site may be involved, lesions on the unattached mucosal tissues predominate and hemorrhagic crusting of the lips is highly characteristic and virtually pathognomonic. Ocular involvement manifests as conjunctivitis, periorbital edema, and photophobia. Most mucocutaneous lesions tend to heal completely in 2 to 6 weeks. In severe cases, scarring and permanent visual impairment may ensue. Fatal forms are rare (<1%) (see Figure 2-44 🎄, Figure 2-45 🎄, Figure 2-46 🎄, Figure 2-47 🎄, Figure 2-48 🎄, and Figure 2-49 🎄 on CD-ROM).

Teratogenic/developmental effects

Drug-related developmental toxicity may produce altered growth (terata), growth retardation, functional deficits or impairments, and death of the fetus. Behavioral teratogens disrupt normal behavioral development after prenatal exposure. Fetal abnormalities in the United States occur in 3% to 6% of pregnancies; drugs are considered to be responsible for 1% to 5% of these malformations.

Oncogenic effects

Malignancies of the skin and lips. Skin and lip malignancies are the most frequent ADEs to develop following therapeutic immunosuppression. The reported incidence of lip cancer in organ transplant patients varies from 7% to 8.1% (versus 0.3% in the general population). The average age of patients is 42 years and the mean latency from transplantation to malignancy is 5.3 years. Most squamous cell carcinomas (SCCs) are low grade but a significant percentage behaves aggressively, with lymph node metastasis in 5.8% of the cases, leading directly to the death of 4.9% of all transplant patients (versus 1% to 2% in the general population). (See Figure 2-50 🎄 on CD-ROM.)

Kaposi sarcoma. The incidence of KS following therapeutic immunosuppression in organ transplant recipients is 5.6% (compared with 0.02% to 0.07% in the general population). Sixty percent of the patients have KS confined to skin, conjunctiva, or oropharyngeal mucosa. In addition, 24% of patients with visceral KS have no skin involvement but 3% have oral involvement (see Figure 2-51 🎄 on CD-ROM).

Lymphoproliferative disease, Hodgkin and non-Hodgkin lymphoma, leiomyoma, leiomyosarcoma, and spindle-cell sarcoma. Lymphoproliferative disease, Hodgkin and non-Hodgkin lymphoma, leiomyoma, leiomyosarcoma, and spindle-cell sarcoma have been associated with therapeutic immunosuppression in solid organ transplant recipients. Lymphoproliferative disease is the most severe and can be life threatening. (See Figure 2-52 🎄, Figure 2-53 🎄, Figure 2-54 🎄, and Figure 2-55 🎄 on CD-ROM.)

PREVENTING ADVERSE DRUG EVENTS

Preventing ADEs is a critical part of clinical practice. Oral health care providers must have an awareness of and have access to information related to ADEs. To minimize such events, they must develop a rational approach to the use of pharmacotherapeutic agents in the management of oral/odontogenic problems.

ACCURATE DIAGNOSIS

Diagnosis is the bridge between the study of disease and the treatment of illness. Unfortunately, the establishment of an accurate diagnosis before the initiation of therapy is not always possible. Patients often have vague and multiple somatic symptoms that may be misinterpreted and lead to inappropriate therapeutic intervention. Meticulous documentation of the patient's medical history and an appropriate physical examination are fundamental to establishing the correct diagnosis.

CRITICAL ASSESSMENT OF THE NEED FOR PHARMACOTHERAPY

In the management of most oral/odontogenic conditions, nonpharmacological intervention (primary dental care) is a more appropriate and safer alternative to pharmacotherapy. Practitioners must avoid "rationalized activism." The rational activist assumes that it is better to overtreat than not to treat at all. Even though the risk may be small, the subsequent benefits may not justify prescribing a drug with the potential to cause a serious ADE.

BENEFITS VERSUS RISKS OF DRUG THERAPY

Practitioners must avoid "symptomatic reflex prescribing." The reflex prescriber, the agent of brief encounters, is typically concerned with the patient's symptoms and caters to the patient's demands, disregarding the therapeutic balance. Benefits should always outweigh the risks when a drug is prescribed. If clinicians were to observe this basic principle routinely, then the number of unnecessary or inappropriate prescriptions would be reduced, thus minimizing the number of patients at risk.

INDIVIDUALIZATION OF DRUG THERAPY

Individualization of drug therapy involves the consideration of both drug-related and patient-related variables. Drug-related factors, in addition to the choice and dosage of a drug, should include consideration of the route of administration, formulation, and other drugs the patient may be taking. A review of patient-related variables must include genetic factors, age, sex, race, weight, occupation, lifestyle, and systemic disease. Errors in medications, which may lead to ADEs, are related to such factors as progressing age, multiple illnesses, living alone, and poor coping ability of ambulatory patients with their environment.

PATIENT EDUCATION

Take time to explain the role of drugs in the treatment of a disease. Pay special attention to impaired intellect, poor vision, and diminished hearing. Simple and clear instructions on how and when to take drugs should be given both by the clinician and the pharmacist, reinforced by clear labeling of containers, and written on the patient's own drug report card. Special labels are available for blind or visually impaired patients.

CONTINUOUS REASSESSMENT OF THERAPY

Assess the patient's response frequently for efficacy, ADEs, and compliance. Adjust dosages as may be required and discontinue unnecessary medications. When new signs and symptoms are reported, rule out drug-induced etiology. Mild and chronic disorders that require prophylactic therapy, disorders in which the consequences of stopping therapy may be delayed, complex regimens, and frequent dosing lend themselves to noncompliance. A by-product of poor compliance is hoarding of drugs. This phenomenon can further contribute to noncompliance and ADEs because patients may confuse new bottles with old ones, take medications that have deteriorated with age, or use hoarded drugs for the wrong purpose.

DIAGNOSING ADVERSE DRUG EVENTS

The diagnosis of ADEs is highly subjective and imprecise. Symptomatic complaints that may be assumed to be drug-induced, such as fatigue, inability to concentrate, and excessive sleepiness, have been reported by healthy individuals not taking any medications. In another study, investigators found that 58% of the patients receiving a placebo complained of one or more ADEs. However, drugs as disease-producing and symptom-producing agents should always be

Table 2-6.	A Stepwise Process to the Diagnosis of ADEs
Step 1	Identify the drug(s) taken by the patient.
Step 2	Verify that the onset of signs and symptoms was after the initiation of pharmacological intervention.
Step 3	Determine the time interval between the initiation of drug therapy and the onset of ADEs.
Step 4	Stop drug therapy and monitor the patient's status.
Step 5	If appropriate, restart drug therapy and monitor for recurrence of ADEs.

considered in the formulation of a differential diagnosis, and a stepwise process can be helpful in assessing possible drug-related adverse events (Table 2-6).

REPORTING ADVERSE DRUG EVENTS

The FDA has the regulatory responsibility for ensuring the safety of all marketed drugs. Drug manufacturers are required by federal regulations to notify the FDA of adverse events of which they are aware. Hospitals must also maintain an ADE surveillance program to fulfill accreditation requirements by the Joint Commission on Accreditation of Healthcare Organizations (JCAHO). However, the success of any surveillance program is dependent on active participation by individual clinicians. In an effort to increase awareness to the extent of drug-induced adverse events, the Commissioner of the Food and Drug Administration launched MEDWatch, an initiative designed to educate health care professionals about the critical importance of being aware of, monitoring for, and reporting ADEs. It is not necessary to prove causality; a suspected association constitutes sufficient reason to report.

The FDA is not interested in ADEs that are resolved by stopping drug therapy or changing the dosage, or those that have responded to prescription medications. The FDA considers an ADE serious, and consequently reportable, if it required hospitalization, if medical or surgical intervention was required to prevent permanent damage, if it resulted in disability, if it produced a congenital abnormality, or if the outcome was death. Reports may be sent directly to the FDA by several different mechanisms (Table 2-7). The FDA holds the identity of the patient in strict confidence. The reporter's identity may be shared with the manufacturer of the product unless otherwise indicated on the reporting form. Based on these reports, the FDA may send out letters to health care

Table 2-7.	Reporting Serious ADEs
FDA FORM 3500	
Web site	Go to: http://www.fda.gov/medwatch/report/hcp.htm • Complete and submit Form 3500 ONLINE, or • Download a copy of Form 3500 and FAX the completed form to 1-800-FDA-0178, or • Download a copy of Form 3500 and MAIL back the completed form using the postage-paid, addressed envelope form
Phone	Call 1-800-FDA-1088 to report by telephone

professionals notifying them of the ADE; require warning labels or changes to the drug name or packaging; require further epidemiological investigations and/or manufacturer-sponsored postmarketing studies; conduct inspections of manufacturers' facilities and/or records; or require that the drug be withdrawn from the market.

CONCLUSION

ADEs evolve through the same physiological and pathological pathways as normal disease and are difficult to distinguish. Prerequisites to considering ADEs in the differential diagnosis of a patient's disease or clinical symptoms include an awareness that an ever-increasing number of patients are taking more and more medications (polypharmacy); recognition that many drugs will remain in the body for weeks after therapy is discontinued; clinical experience; and familiarity with relevant literature about ADEs. It is equally important to recognize that some ADEs occur rarely, and detection based on clinical experience or reports in the medical literature is impossible at times. However, timely reporting of ADEs can save lives, reduce morbidity, and decrease the cost of health care.

BIBLIOGRAPHY

1. Al-Khatib SM, LaPointe NM, Kramer JM, Califf RM. What clinicians should know about the QT interval. JAMA 2003;289: 2120–2127.
2. Andrade SE, Gurwitz JH, Davis RL, et al. Prescription drug use in pregnancy. Am J Obstet Gynecol 2004;191:398–407.
3. Beard K. Adverse reactions as a cause of hospital admissions in the aged. Drugs Aging 1992;2:356–357.
4. Bhatt AD, Sane SP, Vaidya AB. Understanding the mechanisms of adverse drug reactions. J Assoc Physicians India 1994;42(2):132–134, 139–141.
5. Caraco Y. Genes and the response to drugs. N Engl J Med 2004;351:2867–2869.
6. Chan H-L, Stern RS, Arndt KA, et al. The incidence of erythema multiforme, Stevens-Johnson syndrome, and toxic epidermal necrolysis: a population-based study with particular reference to reactions caused by drugs among outpatients. Arch Dermatol 1990;126:43–47.
7. Ciancio SG. Medications' impact on oral health. J Am Dent Assoc 2004;135:1440–1448.
8. Edwards IR, Aronson JK. Adverse drug reactions: definitions, diagnosis, and management. Lancet 2000;356: 1255–1259.
9. Gasche Y, Daali Y, Fathi M, et al. Codeine intoxication associated with ultrarapid CYP2D6 metabolism. N Engl J Med 2004;351:2827–2831.
10. Green DM. Pre-existing conditions, placebo reactions, and "side effects."Ann Intern Med 1964;60:255–265.
11. Hersh EV, Moore PA. Drug interactions in dentistry. The importance of knowing your CYPs. J Am Dent Assoc 2004;135: 298–311.
12. Irey NS. Tissue reactions to drugs. Am J Pathol 1976;82:617–647.
13. Johnson JM, Barash D. A review of postmarketing adverse drug experience reporting requirements. Food Drug Cosmetic Law J 1991;46:6654–6672.
14. Juurlink DN, Mamdani M, Kopp A, Laupacis A, Redelmeier DA. Drug-drug interactions among elderly patients hospitalized for drug toxicity. JAMA 2003;289:1652–1658.
15. Karch FE, Lasagna L. Adverse drug reactions: a critical review. JAMA 1975;234:1236–1241.
16. Karch FE, Smith CL, Kerzner B, Mazzullo JM, Weintraub M, Lasagna L. Adverse drug reactions—a matter of opinion. Clin Pharmacol Ther 1976;19:489–492.
17. Kessler DA. Introducing MEDWatch: a new approach to reporting medication and device adverse effects and product problems. JAMA 1993;269:2765–2768.
18. Knowles SR, Uetrecht J, Shear NH. Idiosyncratic drug reactions: the reactive metabolite syndromes. Lancet 2000;356: 1587–1591.
19. Lakshmanan MC, Hershey CO, Breslan D. Hospital admissions caused by iatrogenic disease. Arch Intern Med 1986;146: 1931–1934.
20. Lazarou J, Pomeranz BH, Corey PN. Incidence of adverse drug reactions in hospitalized patients. JAMA 1998;279: 1200–1205.
21. Lee WM. Drug-induced hepatotoxicity. N Engl J Med 1995;333(17):1118–1127.
22. Lewis JA. Post-marketing surveillance: how many patients? Trends Pharmacol Sci 1981;2:93–94.
23. Maskalyk J. Grapefruit juice: potential drug interactions. CMAJ 2002;167:279–280.
24. Meyer UA. Pharmacogenetics and adverse drug reactions. Lancet 2000;356:1667–1671.

25. Moore PA, Gage TW, Hersh EV, Yagiela JA, Haas DA. Adverse drug interactions in dental practice. Professional and educational implications. J Am Dent Assoc 1999;130:47–54.

26. Neugut AI, Ghatak AT, Miller RL. Anaphylaxis in the United States. Arch Intern Med 2001;161:15–21.

27. Nolan L, O'Malley K. Prescribing for the elderly. Part I: Sensitivity of the elderly to adverse drug reactions. J Am Geriatr Soc 1988;36:142–149.

28. Park BK, Pirmohamed M, Kitteringham NR. Idiosyncratic drug reactions: a mechanistic evaluation of risk factors. Br J Clin Pharmacol 1992;34:377–395.

29. Phillips KA, Veenstra DL, Oren E, Lee JK, Sadee W. Potential role of pharmacogenomics in reducing adverse drug reactions. JAMA 2001;286:2270–2279.

30. Reidenberg MM, Lowenthal DT. Adverse nondrug reactions. N Engl J Med 1968;279:678–679.

31. Ti TY. The role of the doctor in drug safety. Ann Acad Med Singapore 1993;22(1):54–56.

32. Torpet LA, Kragelund C, Reibel J, Nautofte B. Oral adverse drug reactions to cardiovascular drugs. Crit Rev Oral Biol Med 2004;15:28–46.

33. Vincent PC. Drug-induced aplastic anemia and agranulocytosis: incidence and mechanisms. Drugs 1986;31:52–63.

34. Waller PC. Dealing with variability: the role of pharmacovigilance. J Pharm Pharmacol 1994;46(Suppl 1):445–449.

3 Medical Management of Acute Odontogenic Pain

The full text for this chapter can be found on the *LWW's Dental Drug Reference with Clinical Implications* CD-ROM ❁. The Table of Contents is included here for your reference.

Table of Contents

Lidocaine hydrochloride
Mepivacaine hydrochloride
Prilocaine hydrochloride
Articaine hydrochloride
Secondary line of treatment
Bupivacaine hydrochloride
Tertiary line of treatment
Procaine hydrochloride
Adverse Drug Events
Toxic reactions
Local toxicity
Systemic toxic reactions
Methemoglobinemia
Sympathetic reactions
Allergic reactions
Psychomotor reactions
Vasopressor syncope
Hyperventilation
Local anesthetic agents, epinephrine, and pregnancy

ANALGESICS

Pharmacodynamic Considerations
Cyclooxygenase inhibitors
Opioid-receptor agonists
Pharmacokinetic Considerations
Cyclooxygenase inhibitors
Opioid-receptor agonists
Pharmacotherapeutic Considerations
Primary line of treatment
Acetylsalicylic acid
Acetaminophen
Secondary line of treatment
Cyclooxygenase-1 inhibitors
Cyclooxygenase-inhibitor/opioid combinations
Tramadol
Tertiary line of treatment

Adverse Drug Events
  Cyclooxygenase inhibitors
    Intolerance
    Gastropathy
    Antithrombotic effects
    Pregnancy-related events
    Local and systemic salicylate toxicity
    Hepatic toxicity
    Renal toxicity
  Opioid-receptor agonists
    Gastropathy
    Intolerance
    Cardiovascular effects
    Respiratory effects
    CNS effects
    Pregnant and nursing women
    Geriatric patients
    Tolerance
    Dependence
    Overdose

The Medical Management of Chronic (Neuropathic) Pain

Conclusion

Bibliography

4 Medical Management of Odontogenic Infections

The full text for this chapter can be found on the *LWW's Dental Drug Reference with Clinical Implications* CD-ROM ✸. The Table of Contents is included here for your reference.

Table of Contents

Medical
5 Management of Selected Oral Conditions

Table of Contents

INTRODUCTION

Although most oral conditions are self-limiting, they often produce enough discomfort, concern, or embarrassment to prompt the patient to seek some form of therapy. In addition, the epidemiological association of some of these conditions with neoplasia has placed health care professionals under increased pressure to treat such lesions to reduce not only the discomfort, but also the potential risk of neoplastic changes. In some instances, treatment is also required to minimize the likelihood that the patient will transmit an infection to others. As the scope of oral medicine continues to expand, the dental professional is confronted with ever-increasing advertising and promotion of prescription drugs, paralleled by excessive public faith in the efficacy of such drugs. The intent of this chapter is to discuss the diagnosis of common orally related primary and secondary conditions, and their established management protocols.

ACUTE ODONTOGENIC PAIN

The most common complaint causing a person to seek the services of an oral health care provider is pain. Consequently, the primary obligation and ultimate responsibility of every clinician is not only to restore function but also to relieve pain. Pain is an unpleasant sensory and emotional experience, associated with actual or potential tissue damage. Stimuli that provoke pain receptors may be mechanical, thermal, or chemical. Chemical agents that occur naturally in the environment of pain receptors following acute tissue damage include adenosine, adenosine triphosphate, serotonin, histamine, bradykinin, cytokines, prostaglandins, and other neuroactive substances, which initiate the release of substance P, calcitonin-gene-related peptide (CGRP), and glutamate from nerve terminals. Whereas substance P and CGRP are considered to be neuromodulators involved in evoking neurogenic inflammation, glutamate is now thought to be the primary pain neurotransmitter. It activates nociceptive receptors, which generate impulses that are transmitted along peripheral fibers to the central nervous system (CNS).

DIAGNOSIS

Complaints of anguish, postural displays, groaning, wincing, and grimacing are all equated with pain, along with limitation of normal activity (function), excessive rest, social withdrawal, and medication demand or intake. Patients in pain tend to behave in ways appropriate to their cultural heritage. This perspective recognizes that pain can be altered and shaped by the social consequences of its expression or display. Refer to Chapter 3: *Medical Management of Acute Odontogenic Pain* on CD-ROM ✿.

MANAGEMENT

Proper management of pain requires an understanding of its complexity, an appreciation for the factors that determine its expression in the clinical setting, and the implementation of sound clinical and pharmacological strategies. Ultimately, the choice of a therapeutic intervention for acute odontogenic pain is determined largely by the nature of the patient's problem, the resources available, the comparative complexity of the procedure to eliminate the underlying cause, and the cost to the patient. Most patients can attain satisfactory relief of acute odontogenic pain through an approach that incorporates primary dental care in conjunction with local anesthesia and the administration of analgesics.

Topical anesthetic agents

The ideal topical anesthetic agent should have rapid onset of action, a duration of action appropriate for the clinical situation, and minimal systemic absorption. Most available topical anesthetic agents produce the desirable effect in about 1 to 3 minutes. Benzocaine, 20%, is an effective topical anesthetic agent when used before the injection of local anesthetics. It has a relatively rapid onset and short duration of action and its systemic absorption through mucous membranes is limited. Lidocaine is available in 2% viscous, 5% ointment and liquid, and 10% spray formulations. Toxicity related to these agents has largely been attributed to the use of large doses with excessive systemic absorption. The ability of topical anesthetic agents to interfere with the pharyngeal phase of swallowing and cause aspiration has been documented.

Local anesthetic agents

Local anesthetic agents produce loss of sensation in a circumscribed area of the body without loss of consciousness or central control of vital functions. The choice of the agent and the technique used for its administration are important determinants of activity (Table 5-1). Local anesthetic agents currently available may conveniently be divided into three categories based on their relative duration of anesthetic action. Procaine (medical formulation only) has a relatively short duration of action. Lidocaine, mepivacaine, articaine, and prilocaine represent agents of intermediate duration, and bupivacaine will produce anesthesia of long duration. When indicated, local anesthesia may be supplemented with an oral benzodiazepine, nitrous oxide, or intravenous sedation.

Analgesics

Three types of analgesics are available for the management of acute odontogenic pain: cyclooxygenase (COX)-inhibitors, opioid analgesics, and adjuvant drugs. An adjuvant may either enhance the efficacy of an analgesic or it may have an analgesic activity of its own. Caffeine in doses of 65 to 200 mg enhances the analgesic effect of acetylsalicylic acid (ASA), acetaminophen (APAP), and ibuprofen in dental and other acute pain syndromes. Hydroxyzine, an antihistamine, in doses of 25 to 50 mg enhances the analgesic effect of opioids in postoperative pain and significantly reduces the incidence of opioid-induced nausea and vomiting. Corticosteroids, through their anti-inflammatory and phospholipase-inhibitory effects, can produce analgesia in some patients with pain of inflammatory origin.

Primary line of therapy. ASA is the standard for the comparison and evaluation of orally effective analgesics. APAP is as effective as ASA with similar potency and time-effect curve. ASA, 650 mg, and APAP, 650 mg, are equianalgesic to 200 mg of ibuprofen; 200 mg of ibuprofen is equianalgesic to 275 mg of naproxen sodium. So:

$$\text{APAP 650 mg} \leftrightarrow \text{ASA 650 mg} \leftrightarrow \text{ibuprofen 200 mg}$$
$$\leftrightarrow \text{naproxen sodium 275 mg}$$

Consequently, over-the-counter (OTC) formulations of ASA, APAP, ibuprofen, or naproxen sodium are the drugs of choice for the management of mild odontogenic pain.

Table 5-1. Formulations and Other Characteristics of Selected Local Anesthetic Agents

DRUGS AND FORMULATIONS	PKA	% FREE BASE AT PH 7.4	FDA RISK STATUS	MG/ML	TOXIC DOSE MG/KG (MAXIMUM RECOMMENDED DOSE)
Procaine (Novocaine)					
2% plain (medical formulation)	8.9	3	C	20	6.0 (300)
Lidocaine (Xylocaine, others)					
2% plain	7.9	24	B	20	4.5 (300)
2% w/epinephrine 1:50,000	7.9	24	B	20	7.0 (200)
2% w/epinephrine 1:100,000	7.9	24	B	20	7.0 (500)
2% w/epinephrine 1:200,000	7.9	24	B	20	7.0 (500)
Mepivacaine (Carbocaine, others)					
3% plain	7.6	39	C	30	6.6 (400)
2% w/levonordefrin 1:20,000	7.6	39	C	20	6.6 (550)
Articaine (Septocaine)					
4% w/epinephrine 1:100,000	7.8	25	C	40	7.0 (500)
Prilocaine (Citanest)					
4% plain	7.9	24	B	40	8.0 (600)
4% w/epinephrine 1:200,000	7.9	24	B	40	8.0 (600)
Bupivacaine (Marcaine)					
0.5% w/epinephrine 1:200,000	8.1	17	C	5	2.0 (90)

OTC

ASA, 500-mg tablets, take 2 tablets four times a day, maximum daily dose 4000 mg

Ibuprofen (Advil), 200-mg tablets, take 2 tablets four times a day, maximum daily dose 2400 mg

Naproxen (Aleve), 200-mg tablets, take 2 tablets four times a day, maximum daily dose 1375 mg

APAP, 500-mg tablets, take 2 tablets four times a day, maximum daily dose 4000 mg

Secondary line of therapy. In the management of acute moderate-to-severe odontogenic pain, full doses of COX-1 inhibitors are as effective as or more effective than full doses of ASA or APAP. Some have also been shown to be as effective as or more effective than oral codeine, hydrocodone, propoxyphene, and pentazocine in combination with ASA or APAP. Propoxyphene and pentazocine, even in combination with ASA or APAP, offer no clinically relevant advantage over codeine or hydrocodone combinations.

Ibuprofen, 800-mg tablets

Disp: 10 tablets

Sig: Take 1 tablet three times a day until all tablets are taken.

Naproxen sodium, 275-mg tablets

Disp: 10 tablets

Sig: Take 2 tablets stat, then 1 tablet three times a day until all tablets are taken.

Hydrocodone w/ibuprofen, 7.5-mg/200-mg tablets

Disp: 24 tablets

Sig: Take 2 tablets four times a day until all tablets are taken.

Hydrocodone w/APAP, 5-mg/500-mg tablets

Disp: 24 tablets

Sig: Take 2 tablets four times a day until all tablets are taken.

Tramadol w/APAP, 37.5-mg/325-mg tablets

Disp: 24 tablets

Sig: Take 2 tablets four times a day until all tablets are taken.

Tertiary line of therapy. Morphine, hydromorphone, methadone, levorphanol, and oxycodone are all effective in the management of severe pain. These drugs can relieve practically all forms of pain, including visceral. Of these, oxycodone in combination with a COX-1 (ASA or ibuprofen) or a COX-3 (APAP) inhibitor is the drug of choice for the management of severe odontogenic pain. Oxycodone, 10 mg, in oral doses is equianalgesic with 90 mg of codeine. A single dose of oxycodone, 5 mg, with ibuprofen, 400 mg, has been shown to be more effective than oxycodone, 5 mg, or ibuprofen, 400 mg, or a placebo in the management of acute odontogenic pain following extractions.

 Oxycodone w/ibuprofen, 5-mg/400-mg tablets

Disp: 24 tablets

Sig: Take 2 tablets four times a day until all tablets are taken.

 Oxycodone w/APAP, 7.5-mg/500-mg tablets

Disp: 24 tablets

Sig: Take 2 tablets four times a day until all tablets are taken.

ODONTOGENIC INFECTIONS

The oral environment harbors more than 300 bacterial species. These include both gram-positive and gram-negative organisms, which may be aerobic, anaerobic, or facultative. The number of isolated strains in most odontogenic infections ranges from 1 to 10 with an average number of approximately 4 isolates per infection. The most common organisms responsible for odontogenic infections are viridans streptococci (*S. oralis, S. sanguis,* and *S. mitis), Peptostreptococcus, Fusobacterium,* pigmented and nonpigmented *Prevotella, Gemella, Porphyromonas,* and *Bacteroides* species. Refer to Chapter 4: *Medical Management of Odontogenic Infections* on CD-ROM ✹.

DIAGNOSIS

Oral bacterial infections primarily affect the teeth (caries) and pulpal, periodontal, or pericoronal tissues. Patients commonly present with pain, erythema, and edema, and report difficulty chewing. Patients presenting with a serious infection typically exhibit fever, chills, trismus, lymphadenopathy, and swelling. Rapid respiration and hypotension are more ominous signs of a life-threatening condition with cardiorespiratory compromise.

Management

Most odontogenic infections can be resolved satisfactorily with timely débridement (primary dental care). Odontogenic infections that fail to respond to débridement may spread into anatomical spaces contiguous with fascial planes and lead to serious, even life-threatening situations. This is especially true in immunocompromised patients. In addition, when patients present with malaise, fever, chills, trismus, rapid respiration, lymphadenopathy, swelling, and hypotension or when transient bacteremia may adversely affect the general health of the patient, appropriate antibacterial chemotherapy is indicated. Patients who initially present with signs of impending airway compromise, marked trismus (<25 mm), or dehydration (e.g., marked malaise, disorientation, tachycardia) should be admitted to the hospital for urgent or emergency care.

Primary line of therapy

Unless the patient has an allergy to the penicillin, the appropriate empirical drug of choice for the treatment of an uncomplicated odontogenic infection is penicillin VK. It has good activity against most oral facultative gram-positive cocci and gram-negative anaerobes. Most odontogenic infections will require 5 days of antibacterial chemotherapy. Begin with a loading dose, followed by maintenance doses for the remainder of the time. The patient should be instructed to notify the clinician if symptoms do not significantly improve in 2 to 3 days. In such circumstances, it is prudent to reevaluate the patient because this may indicate noncompliance or, possibly, bacterial drug resistance and the need to modify the therapeutic regimen, and/or the need for a culture and susceptibility test.

Some gram-positive (*S. oralis, S. sanguis,* and *S. mitis*) and gram-negative organisms exhibit resistance related to structural changes in penicillin-binding proteins. In addition, staphylococci and many gram-negative bacteria can synthesize beta-lactamase enzymes, which hydrolyze beta-lactam antibiotics. A therapeutic strategy to counter such resistance is to administer a broad-spectrum penicillin, such as amoxicillin in combination with clavulanic acid, a beta-lactamase inhibitor. Unfortunately, amoxicillin is also beta-lactamase susceptible and certain beta-lactamases produced by gram-negative bacteria now confer resistance to clavulanic acid as well. Consequently, the administration of a broad-spectrum penicillin offers little therapeutic advantage over penicillin VK in the management of odontogenic infections.

 Penicillin VK, 500-mg tablets

Disp: 21 tablets

Sig: Take 2 tablets stat, then 1 tablet four times a day until all tablets are taken.

If significant improvement is not noted with penicillin VK in 48 to 72 hours, the empirical addition (for 7 days) of metronidazole to penicillin VK is reasonable because it is beta-lactamase resistant. Although certain oral microorganisms such as *Streptococcus* species, *Actinomyces* species, and *Actinobacillus actinomycetemcomitans* exhibit natural or intrinsic resistance to metronidazole (they lack the enzyme nitroreductase necessary to convert metronidazole to its active metabolites), metronidazole in combination with penicillin VK provides excellent coverage for mixed odontogenic infections dominated by obligate anaerobes.

Metronidazole, 250-mg tablets

Disp: 29 tablets

Sig: Take 2 tablets stat, then 1 tablet four times a day until all tablets are taken.

Secondary line of therapy

Erythromycin, a member of the macrolide class of antibiotics, has been suggested as the empirical drug of choice for the treatment of odontogenic infections in patients who are allergic to beta-lactam antibiotics. However, many oral gram-negative anaerobes have natural or intrinsic resistance to erythromycin because the structure of the outer bacterial cell membrane restricts entry of the drug. Resistance to erythromycin has also been related to the ability of certain microorganisms to block ribosomal erythromycin-receptor sites. Unfortunately, this mechanism contributes not only to erythromycin resistance, but also because of microsomal receptor overlap, these microorganisms will be resistant to clindamycin. Finally, certain bacteria have developed resistance to erythromycin by activating efflux pumps, which act to remove intracellular erythromycin, and these efflux pumps can also affect the intracellular concentration of beta-lactam antibiotics and beta-lactamase inhibitors.

Although there is a paucity of data demonstrating the efficacy of clarithromycin and azithromycin in the treatment of odontogenic infections, these newer macrolide antibacterial agents may be better alternatives to erythromycin because of their extended spectrum against facultative and some obligate anaerobes, more favorable tissue distribution, fewer side effects, and a once a day (azithromycin) or twice a day (clarithromycin) dosage schedule. However, their substantially higher cost and the association of sudden death from cardiac causes following the oral administration of macrolides (with the exception of azithromycin) are compelling reasons to recommend clindamycin as a more appropriate alternative for patients allergic to beta-lactam antibacterial agents.

Azithromycin, 250-mg tablets

Disp: 8 tablets

Sig: Take 2 tablets stat, then 1 tablet every day until all tablets are taken.

Tertiary line of therapy

Beta-lactam antibiotic use in the recent past increases the likelihood for the emergence of beta-lactamase–producing bacteria. When a patient presents with an unresolved odontogenic infection following treatment with a beta-lactam antibacterial agent, the administration of a beta-lactamase–stable antibacterial drug, such as clindamycin, should be considered. Similarly, the initial empirical drug of choice for the treatment of a complicated odontogenic infection is also clindamycin. It is not only beta-lactamase resistant but it has excellent activity against gram-positive cocci and most oral gram-negative anaer-obes. Some authorities also point to clindamycin as an increasingly attractive choice in the treatment of all odontogenic infections, but concerns about associ-ated gastric side effects (i.e., pseudomembranous colitis), higher cost, and, importantly, the potential for drug-resistance to clindamycin should prompt caution in using it as a primary line of treatment.

R
Clindamycin, 300-mg tablets

Disp: 29 tablets

Sig: Take 2 tablets stat, then 1 tablet four times a day until all tablets are taken.

ACTINIC CHEILOSIS

Actinic cheilosis is the labial equivalent of actinic keratosis and, as such, repre-sents the early clinical manifestation of a continuum, which may ultimately progress to squamous cell carcinoma. The cause of actinic cheilosis is chronic exposure to sunlight, especially from an early age. Although ultraviolet-B (UV-B) radiation is principally responsible, ultraviolet-A (UV-A) radiation adds to the risk. Other risk factors include a fair complexion, outdoor occupations, and immunosuppression. Men are affected more often than women, and although most cases occur in men after the age of 40, the condition is increasingly being diagnosed in younger men.

DIAGNOSIS

The diagnosis is based on history and clinical findings. The lip appears dry, mottled, and opalescent, with white or gray plaques that are slightly ele-vated and cannot be stripped off (Figure 5-1 ❀ on CD-ROM). Isolated areas of hyperkeratosis may also be evident. Lip pliability or elasticity may be decreased and the normally distinct definition of the vermilion-cutaneous border may be lost. Other clinical signs include erythematous or hemorrhagic areas, parallel marked folds, and an unobtrusive "chapped lip" appearance.

MANAGEMENT

The potentially progressive nature of actinic cheilosis to squamous cell carcinoma emphasizes the need for early recognition and implementation of preventive and therapeutic strategies. Any time a lesion exhibits induration, ulceration, bleeding, rapid growth, or pain, an immediate biopsy is indicated.

Prevention

The American Cancer Society recommends avoiding sun exposure when UV rays are strongest (10 AM to 4 PM); covering up exposed skin; wearing a hat that shades the neck, face, and ears; wearing sunglasses; and using a sunscreen. The patient should consistently use a broad-spectrum sunscreen product with an SPF of 30 or higher. Ideally, the product chosen should block both UV-B and UV-A (formulations containing zinc oxide, avobenzone, or Mex-oryl) and be specifically formulated for use on the lip. Sunscreen should be applied liberally 15 to 30 minutes before anticipated exposure and reapplied liberally after any vigorous activity that may wash or rub the sunscreen away.

Broad-spectrum sunscreens

Blistex Clear Advantage [OTC]
Disp: 1 tube
Sig: Apply to lip 30 minutes prior to sun exposure and every hour thereafter while in the sun.

Burnout SPF 32 [OTC] *(multiple flavors)*
Disp: 1 tube
Sig: Apply to lip 30 minutes prior to sun exposure and every hour thereafter while in the sun.

Zinc Stick SPF 30+ [OTC] *(multiple flavors)*
Disp: 1 stick
Sig: Apply to lip 30 minutes prior to sun exposure and every hour thereafter while in the sun.

HERPETIC INFECTIONS

Herpetic infections are caused by either herpes simplex virus type-1 (HSV-1) or herpes simplex virus type-2 (HSV-2). A unique feature of these viruses is their ability to establish latency following primary infection and thus create the potential for recurrence. An estimated 500,000 cases of primary infection and 100,000,000 cases of recurrent infection occur annually in the United States.

DIAGNOSIS

The diagnosis of herpetic infections is based on history and clinical findings. Laboratory tests such as Tzanck smear, serology, and culturing are rarely necessary, but assist in the diagnosis of equivocal cases.

Most PRIMARY HERPETIC INFECTIONS are asymptomatic or mildly symptomatic and typically occur between 2 to 3 years of age. Symptomatic primary infection usually presents as herpetic gingivostomatitis. Nonspecific prodromal signs and symptoms of fever, malaise, irritability, headache, and cervical lymphadenopathy typically occur 1 to 3 days before the development of painful oral lesions characterized by widespread vesicular eruptions and gingival inflammation (Figures 5-2 ❋ and 5-3 ❋ on CD-ROM). All oral soft tissues may be affected. Within a few days, the vesicles coalesce, rupture, and form large, irregularly shaped erosions or ulcerations. The lesions heal without scarring in 1 to 2 weeks. In some cases the pain may be intense and interfere with eating and drinking, placing the patient at risk for dehydration and malnutrition. Conditions that predispose to systemic dissemination include immunological immaturity, malignancy, malnutrition, pregnancy, and therapeutic or acquired immunosuppression.

After primary infection, an estimated 15% to 40% of the patients experience a RECURRENT HERPETIC INFECTION, most commonly recurrent herpes labialis

(RHL). Patients usually relate prodromal sensations of tingling, itching, burning, or pain before the eruption of the characteristic focal vesicular lesions affecting the lip vermilion (Figure 5-4 ❀ on CD-ROM) or other perioral sites such as the skin or ala of the nose. The vesicles rapidly rupture and crust, with ultimate uneventful healing occurring within 2 weeks. Viral shedding precedes the prodromal period and continues into convalescence; when this occurs, the patient should be considered infectious. This can lead both to autoinoculation and cross-infection. Less frequently observed are intraoral recurrent herpetic eruptions (Figure 5-5 ❀ on CD-ROM). Small clusters of lesions are usually restricted to the keratinized mucosa. Numerous trigger factors such as ultraviolet radiation, trauma, menstruation, fever, and immunosuppression have been implicated. In immunocompromised patients the lesions are usually more severe and recovery is protracted.

MANAGEMENT

There exists no cure for HSV and its establishment of latency. Therapy is tailored to the individual patient, taking into account the severity of the infection and the patient's overall health.

Primary line of therapy for primary herpetic infection

Strategies are targeted to ensure adequate hydration and nutrition and provide palliation. A topical anesthetic agent such as diphenhydramine hydrochloride or lidocaine viscous and, if necessary, a systemic analgesic should be prescribed. When topical anesthetics are used, the patient or guardian should be warned that these agents may increase the risk of self-induced trauma, may interfere with the pharyngeal phase of swallowing, and may lead to aspiration. Systemic analgesics such as APAP or, in rare instances, an APAP/codeine formulation may have to be prescribed. ASA should be avoided for children younger than 18 years of age because of the risk of Reye syndrome.

Nutritional supplements

Ensure Plus [OTC]
Disp: 25 cans
Sig: Three to 5 cans in divided doses throughout the day. Serve cold.

Carnation Instant Breakfast [OTC] *(various flavors)*
Disp: 1 package
Sig: Three to 5 servings daily. Prepare as indicated on label.

Topical anesthetic agents

Diphenhydramine (Children's Benadryl) elixir 12.5 mg/5 mL [OTC]
Disp: 8 ounces
Sig: Rinse with 1 teaspoonful every 2 hours and spit out.

Diphenhydramine (Children's Benadryl) elixir 12.5 mg/5 mL [OTC] 4 ounces mixed with Kaopectate or Maalox [OTC] 4 ounces (50% mixture by volume)

Disp: 8 ounces

Sig: Rinse with 1 teaspoonful every 2 hours and spit out.

Lidocaine (Xylocaine) viscous 2%

Disp: 100 mL

Sig: Rinse with 1 teaspoonful for 1 minute and expectorate, before meals and at bedtime.

Systemic analgesics

Acetaminophen (Tylenol), 325-mg tablets

Disp: 50 tablets

Sig: Take 2 tablets every 4 to 6 hours for pain and fever. Do not exceed 4 grams per 24-hour period.

Acetaminophen 300 mg with codeine 30 mg (Tylenol With Codeine) tablets

Disp: 24 tablets

Sig: Take 1 to 2 tablets four times a day for pain.

Secondary line of therapy for primary herpetic infection

Patients with a primary herpetic infection who are immunocompromised, manifest immunologic immaturity, or present with evidence of systemic dissemination should be promptly referred for medical evaluation and management. Possible signs and symptoms of dissemination include the presence of extraoral lesions, conjunctivitis, ocular pain, visual impairment, lethargy, dysphagia, hemiparesis, or seizure.

Primary line of therapy for recurrent herpes infection

RHL, while often painful and at times unsightly, is self-limiting and often requires no treatment. All patients should be advised to avoid touching the lesion and practice good hygiene to reduce the risk of autoinoculation. Several OTC topical agents are marketed to provide palliation and promote the healing of RHL. However, docosanol (Abreva) is the only OTC formulation specifically approved by the U.S. Food and Drug Administration (FDA) for the treatment of RHL. For patients who manifest frequent recurrent episodes or who otherwise desire antiviral therapy, the FDA has approved three prescription antiviral agents. Regardless of the agent chosen, therapy is most effective when initiated during prodrome. Finally, prescribing a lip balm with an SPF of 15 or greater may prevent future RHL.

Antiviral agents

Docosanol (Abreva) cream [OTC]

Disp: 2-gram tube

Sig: Apply to affected area 5 times per day during waking hours for 4 days. Initiate therapy promptly at prodrome.

Penciclovir (Denavir), 1% cream

Disp: 2-gram tube

Sig: Apply to affected area every 2 hours while awake for 4 days. Initiate therapy promptly at prodrome.

Acyclovir (Zovirax), 5% cream

Disp: 2-gram tube

Sig: Apply to affected area 5 times per day. Initiate therapy promptly at prodrome.

Valacyclovir (Valtrex), 1000-mg tablets

Disp: 4 tablets

Sig: Take 2 tablets twice a day for 1 day.

Sunscreen for prevention

Blistex Clear Advantage [OTC]

Disp: 1 tube

Sig: Apply to lip 30 minutes prior to sun exposure and every hour thereafter while in the sun.

Recurrent intraoral herpetic lesions typically occur as an isolated event associated with an antecedent traumatic event, such as may occur with dental manipulation. Such cases only require recognition, reassurance, and, if necessary, palliation with the application of a topical anesthetic.

Secondary line of therapy for recurrent herpetic infection

For the immunocompromised patient, antiviral therapy has been shown to be of benefit in reducing pain and accelerating healing. To improve patient compliance, oral famciclovir may be a better alternative to topical acyclovir ointment. For all cases, therapy is most effective when initiated during prodrome.

Famciclovir (Famvir), 125-mg tablets

Disp: 10 tablets

Sig: Take 1 tablet twice a day.

R̶x Acyclovir (Zovirax), 5% ointment
Disp: 3-gram tube
Sig: Apply to affected area every 3 hours (6 times per day) for 7 days. Initiate therapy promptly at prodrome.

Tertiary line of therapy for recurrent herpetic infection

Patients with a recurrent herpetic infection who are nonresponsive to the above therapies or who present with evidence of possible dissemination should be promptly referred for medical evaluation and management.

CANDIDIASIS

Candidiasis is the most frequently occurring opportunistic fungal infection to affect humans. Whereas most cases are caused by *Candida albicans*, other species have been implicated, especially in immunosuppressed patients. *C. albicans* is ubiquitous as evidenced by its ability to exist in a commensal state in such areas as the skin and the gastrointestinal and genitourinary tracts. In the oral cavity, carriage rates of up to 75% have been reported. The shift from a state of commensalism to a pathogenic infection is almost always associated with an underlying predisposing factor. Established predisposing factors include immunosuppression, immunological immaturity, certain medications, salivary changes, malignancies, numerous endocrinopathies, epithelial alterations, nutritional deficiencies, high-carbohydrate diet, poor oral hygiene, dental prostheses, advanced age, and smoking.

Diagnosis

In the majority of cases, the diagnosis of oral candidiasis is based on clinical signs and symptoms. For equivocal cases, exfoliative cytology, culture, or biopsy may be necessary. Because many patients carry *C. albicans* in a commensal state, the presence of hyphae is usually required to confirm infection when using cytology. Patients with oral candidiasis may be asymptomatic or complain of a burning sensation, dysgeusia, or dysphagia. Oral candidiasis may manifest a variety of clinical presentations.

Pseudomembranous candidiasis is characterized by the presence of creamy, white, curdled milk-like papules or plaques on the mucosal tissues, most commonly affecting buccal and labial mucosa, palate, tongue, and oropharynx (Figure 5-6 🌑 on CD-ROM). These lesions may be wiped away to expose an underlying erythematous base.

Erythematous candidiasis (atrophic) manifests as red patches, most commonly noted on the tongue dorsum or palate (Figure 5-7 🌑 on CD-ROM). A burning sensation is often related by the patient. Erythematous candidiasis may occur in a patient wearing a dental prosthesis, in which case the erythema is usually limited to the denture-bearing surface.

Chronic hyperplastic candidiasis presents as white papules or plaques, most commonly affecting the buccal mucosa or tongue (Figure 5-8 🌑 on CD-ROM). This variant cannot be easily wiped off and represents the least commonly observed form.

Angular cheilitis presents as a discomforting cracking or fissuring of the lip commissures (Figure 5-9 🌑 on CD-ROM) and frequently occurs in conjunction with other variants of oral candidiasis. Concurrent involvement of staphylococci and streptococci is the rule.

MEDIAN RHOMBOID GLOSSITIS is a unique form of candidiasis that appears as an erythematous area of papillary loss confined to the dorsal aspect of the tongue, just anterior to the circumvallate papillae (Figure 5-10 ❀ on CD-ROM). Median rhomboid glossitis is frequently asymptomatic.

MANAGEMENT

Essential to any management strategy is a thorough review of the patient's medical and dental histories to identify predisposing factors. Acute cases attributed to short-term antibiotic therapy are usually easily managed, whereas chronic or recurrent cases attributed to a poorly controlled systemic disease may be more problematic and require medical referral. In all cases, the goals of therapy are to remove any predisposing factors when possible, to prevent further spread or dissemination, to provide symptomatic relief, and, when appropriate, to provide patient education to reduce the risk of recurrence.

Primary line of therapy

For mild localized lesions, the use of a topical antifungal agent such as nystatin, clotrimazole, or ketoconazole is usually effective. Improvement should be noted within a week, at which time the topical therapy should be continued for another 3 to 5 days. The efficacy of topical formulations is largely dependent on prolonged contact time with the affected tissues. Thus, patients must be instructed on the appropriate use of topical therapies. Both nystatin solution and clotrimazole troches contain sucrose, which may limit their use in patients with diabetes and/or who are at high risk for caries. Topical fluoride agents should be used during prolonged therapy to reduce caries risk. In cases of candidiasis associated with a dental prosthesis, it is important to also treat the prosthesis. Specifically, the prosthesis should not be worn during sleep but should be soaked in an antifungal solution. Most commercial denture solutions exhibit antifungal properties, as does nystatin solution, chlorhexidine gluconate, and sodium hypochlorite.

 Nystatin (Mycostatin) lozenges, 200,000 units/lozenge
Disp: 70 lozenges
Sig: Let 1 lozenge slowly dissolve in mouth 5 times per day.

 Nystatin suspension, 100,000 units/mL
Disp: 240 mL
Sig: Rinse with 1 teaspoonful for 2 minutes and swallow 4 times per day.

 Clotrimazole (Mycelex), 10-mg troches
Disp: 70 troches
Sig: Let 1 troche slowly dissolve in mouth 5 times per day.

Ketoconazole (Nizoral), 2% cream

Disp: 15-gram tube

Sig: Apply thin coating to affected areas after meals and at bedtime.

Secondary line of therapy

For patients nonresponsive to topical therapy or noncompliant or intolerant with its use, a systemic oral antifungal agent is often effective. Available drugs include ketoconazole, fluconazole, and itraconazole. Fluconazole is usually the drug of choice because it is readily absorbed and exhibits a better safety profile than ketoconazole. Itraconazole is usually reserved for treating candidiasis resistant to fluconazole.

Fluconazole (Diflucan), 100-mg tablets

Disp: 15 tablets

Sig: Take 2 tablets stat, then take 1 tablet daily until gone.

Tertiary line of therapy

Patients at continual risk of candidiasis, such as may occur with HIV infection or other immunosuppressive disorders, are often placed on long-term systemic antifungal therapy. In such cases, long-term fluconazole therapy may prove effective, but the risk of developing resistance is high. Tertiary therapies fall under the purview of the patient's physician.

XEROSTOMIA

Dry mouth or xerostomia is not a specific disease entity, but it may occur in conjunction with a number of significant local and systemic factors (Table 5-2). It is quite common for the patient to manifest more than one factor contributing to his or her xerostomia.

DIAGNOSIS

The diagnosis of xerostomia is usually readily made by clinical examination. Characteristic clinical findings include a noticeable lack of wetness to the mucosal tissues and teeth; saliva that is thick and ropey; absence of saliva pooling in the floor of the mouth; red, dry, and atrophic mucosa; an atrophic and fissured tongue (Figure 5-11 ● on CD-ROM); incisal and smooth surface caries; and candidiasis. When used as a retractor, the dental mirror will often stick to the xerostomic patient's buccal mucosa. Once the clinical diagnosis of a dry mouth is made, a careful and exhaustive review of the patient's medical history must be obtained to identify any predisposing factors.

MANAGEMENT

Depending on the etiology, treatment strategies for xerostomia may be either targeted or palliative and supportive, or both.

Primary line of therapy

Efforts to remove or reduce identified predisposing factors should be undertaken whenever possible. Underlying systemic disorders that predispose to xerostomia should be medically addressed. A consultation with the patient's

Table 5-2.	Causes of Xerostomia
Local factors	• Reduction in salivary flow as a result of heavy smoking and alcohol intake, altered psychic states, and/or idiopathic conditions • Congenital absence or aplasia of one or more of the major salivary glands or ducts (rare) • Glandular hyperplasia associated with mumps, sialolithiasis, and sialoadenitis • Neoplasms, which usually affect an isolated gland (although there may be infiltration of multiple glands in leukemia and lymphoma)
Systemic conditions	• Uncontrolled diabetes mellitus • Sjögren syndrome, a relatively common condition that typically affects women between the ages of 40 to 60 and is characterized clinically by parotid enlargement and histologically by lymphocytic infiltration of the salivary glands • Collagen vascular or connective tissue disorders such as systemic lupus erythematosus, scleroderma, mixed connective tissue disease, and polydermatomyositis
Specific drug classes	• Anticholinergics • Antidepressants • Antihypertensives • Antipsychotics • Diuretics • Gastrointestinals • Antihistamines • CNS stimulants • Systemic bronchodilators • Antineoplastics—the most problematic and profound form of xerostomia is seen secondary to external irradiation of the head and neck

physician is warranted to attempt to discontinue, reduce, or change any medications that predispose to xerostomia. Patient education to reduce exposure to OTC medications that predispose to xerostomia should be provided. Patients should be advised to maintain hydration throughout the day; practice thorough and meticulous oral hygiene (specifically, use a fluoride dentifrice twice a day, 0.05% sodium fluoride rinses daily, and remove and clean prostheses at night); avoid products that irritate the mucosa (alcohol, tobacco, acidic or spicy food, and fruits and vegetables with high acid content); reduce their sugar intake; use xylitol-containing or sugar-free gums or candies to stimulate salivation; and use a humidifier at night. Alcohol-containing mouthrinses should be avoided because they have an additive drying effect on the mucosa.

Secondary line of therapy

Regardless of the etiology, the secondary line of therapy is added to the primary line of therapy and is focused on palliation, reducing oral disease progression, and improving the patient's quality of life.

Salivary substitute

Various salivary substitutes are available. However, these agents represent poor imitators of natural saliva and patient acceptance is notoriously poor.

 Sodium carboxymethyl cellulose 0.5% aqueous solution [OTC]

Disp: 8 ounces

Sig: Use as a rinse as needed throughout day.

 Commercial saliva substitute [OTC] (i.e., Entertainer's Secret, Breathtech, Moist Plus, Optimoist, OralBalance, Salivart, others)

Disp: One bottle

Sig: Use as a rinse as needed throughout day.

Sialogogues

For patients with residual salivary function, a sialagogue may prove beneficial. Pilocarpine (Salagen) is approved for the treatment of xerostomia associated with head and neck radiotherapy and Sjögren syndrome; cevimeline (Evoxac) is approved for the treatment of xerostomia associated with Sjögren syndrome. Either drug may be prescribed on a trial basis to improve salivary flow in all patients with xerostomia. They should be used with caution in patients with significant cardiovascular disease, asthma, chronic bronchitis, chronic obstructive pulmonary disease (COPD), cholelithiasis, biliary tract disease, and nephrolithiasis. Common side effects include sweating, headache, nausea, gastrointestinal upset, urinary frequency, rhinitis, and flushing. Either drug may be titrated to attempt to maximize effect while minimizing side effects.

 Pilocarpine HCl (Salagen), 5-mg tablets

Disp: 21 tablets

Sig: Take 1 tablet three times a day 1/2 hour prior to meals. Dose may be titrated to 2 tablets three times a day.

 Cevimeline (Evoxac), 30-mg capsules

Disp: 21 capsules

Sig: Take 1 capsule three times a day 1/2 hour prior to meals. Dose may be titrated to minimize side effects.

Chlorhexidine gluconate and supplemental fluoride for caries control

An alcohol-free formulation of chlorhexidine gluconate rinse and supplemental topical fluoride should be prescribed to reduce caries development. The additional application of a fluoride varnish on a regular basis may be beneficial. An antifungal agent is often necessary to address the near ubiquitous occurrence of candidiasis (see section on candidiasis, p. 70). Because of the lack of salivary flow in the patient with xerostomia, the use of a systemic antifungal agent is typically more tolerable and effective than topical formulations. Last, patients with xerostomia should be placed on an accelerated recall schedule, typically every 3 months.

℞ Chlorhexidine gluconate (alcohol-free formulation), 0.12% rinse

Disp: 16-ounce bottle

Sig: 1/2-ounce rinse for 1 minute, twice a day, every day, for 2 weeks, followed by 1/2-ounce rinse for 1 minute, twice a day, 1 to 2 days per week (*for maintenance*).

℞ Commercial neutral fluoride (Acclean, Karigel-N, PreviDent 5000 Plus, Topex, Thera-Flur-N, others), 1.1% gel

Disp: One bottle

Sig: Apply to teeth 5 to 10 minutes daily in custom tray (*preferred method*) OR use as a dentifrice once daily.

℞ Commercial stannous fluoride (Acclean Home Care gel, Gel-Tin, Omnii Gel, Plak Smacker, Stop, Take Home Care, others), 0.4% gel

Disp: One bottle

Sig: Apply to teeth 5 to 10 minutes daily in custom tray (*preferred method*) OR use as a dentifrice once daily.

℞ Commercial fluoride varnish (Duraflor, Duraphat, CavityShield)

Sig: Apply to teeth after professional cleaning

RECURRENT APHTHOUS STOMATITIS

Recurrent aphthous stomatitis (RAS) is recognized as the most commonly observed oral mucosal disease to affect humans. For most, RAS proves to be a localized self-limiting episodic annoyance. For others, RAS may be so severe as to interfere with eating and drinking and/or be associated with an underlying, often serious, systemic condition. The specific etiology of RAS is unknown but likely involves an alteration in the cell-mediated immune system. Possible causes include local factors (trauma, toothpaste allergy or sensitivity), nutritional deficiencies (iron, folic acid, zinc, B_1, B_2, B_6, B_{12}), absorptive disorders (gluten-sensitive enteropathy, celiac sprue), food allergies, and other systemic conditions (Behçet disease, Crohn disease, systemic lupus erythematosus [SLE], cyclic neutropenia, HIV, Reiter syndrome).

DIAGNOSIS

There are three distinct forms of RAS: minor, major, and herpetiform. The lesions typically are confined to the nonkeratinized oral mucosa. The diagnosis of RAS is usually easily established after obtaining a thorough history and noting the characteristic clinical presentation. Biopsy is rarely required but may prove useful to rule out other conditions in the differential, such as lichen planus, mucous membrane pemphigoid, and pemphigus.

MINOR RAS is by far the most common form and presents as recurrent, round, clearly defined, shallow ulcerations less than 1 cm in diameter (Figure 5-12 ✿ on CD-ROM). The presence of an intense erythematous halo around the ulceration is characteristic. The patient may relate a prodrome of a localized altered sensation. The patient is afebrile but may present with discrete submandibular lymphadenopathy. Complete resolution without scarring occurs in 7 to 14 days.

MAJOR RAS is similar in appearance to minor RAS, but the lesions are larger than 1 cm in diameter (Figure 5-13 ✿ on CD-ROM). The ulcerations are deeper, often persist for weeks to months, and may heal with scarring. Their presence may indicate the presence of a more serious underlying condition.

HERPETIFORM RAS is characterized by the clustering of numerous small (2- to 3-mm) shallow ulcerations on nonkeratinized mucosa (Figure 5-14 ✿ on CD-ROM). The lesions may coalesce to form a more diffuse ulceration. Healing may take 1 to 4 weeks and scarring is possible.

MANAGEMENT

A primary goal in the management of RAS is to identify and eliminate or manage any contributory factors or conditions associated with the RAS. Appropriate medical consultation and/or referral is warranted for RAS associated with systemic conditions such as nutritional deficiencies, Behçet disease, and HIV. Targeted lesion therapy is aimed at palliation, promoting healing, and reducing recurrence.

Primary line of therapy

There are numerous prescription and OTC topical gels, creams, ointments, and rinses marketed for the treatment of RAS. Commonly found ingredients include corticosteroids, covering agents, antiseptics, oxygenating agents, anti-inflammatory agents, cauterizing agents, and topical anesthetics. No validated studies exist to demonstrate the clinical superiority of any formulation over another. Problems related to the consistent application and retention of these agents often limit their effectiveness. Topical steroid ointments may be compounded with a mucosal adherent (i.e., Orabase) to improve and prolong retention. A rinse formulation may be more effective to treat widespread or hard-to-reach lesions. Topical corticosteroids predispose to oral candidiasis and prolonged use may lead to mucosal atrophy.

Fluocinonide (Lidex), 0.05% ointment

Disp: 15-gram tube

Sig: Apply thin layer to lesions after each meal and at bedtime.

Dexamethasone (Decadron) elixir, 0.05 mg/5 mL

Disp: 100 mL

Sig: Rinse with 1 teaspoon for 2 minutes 4 times a day and expectorate.

Amlexanox (Aphthasol), 5% oral paste

Disp: 5-gram tube

Sig: Dab on lesion 4 times a day.

Orabase Soothe-N-Seal Protective Barrier [OTC]

Disp: 1 package

Sig: Apply as per manufacturer's directions every 6 hours as needed.

Secondary line of therapy

The secondary line of therapy entails the use of a systemic corticosteroid and is indicated for patients whose symptoms are not relieved by primary therapy or for patients whose initial presentation warrants a more aggressive treatment approach. Prednisone, prescribed at 1 mg/kg per day as a single morning dose for 1 to 2 weeks, is the most commonly chosen systemic corticosteroid for use. The development of secondary candidiasis is predictable, thus concurrent antifungal therapy is indicated. Although short-term corticosteroid regimens are generally safe, the patient may experience insomnia, nervousness, indigestion, increased appetite, and weight gain. Relative contraindications include gastrointestinal ulcerations, diabetes, glaucoma, psychoses, renal disorders, osteoporosis, seizures, heart failure, and hypertension. The therapeutic response of RAS is usually rapid and dramatic. However, recurrence is likely. For some, when the lesions recur, the prompt application of a topical agent will be all that is necessary to manage their RAS. Others will require occasional repeat, high-dose, short-term corticosteroids to control acute exacerbations.

Prednisone (Deltasone), 10-mg tablets

Disp: 70 (*for a 70-kg patient*) tablets

Sig: Take 7 tablets by mouth each morning with food or milk.

Tertiary line of therapy

A more aggressive therapeutic protocol is indicated for patients whose RAS is recalcitrant to secondary lines of therapy. Tertiary lines of therapy include chronic systemic corticosteroid regimens, chronic systemic corticosteroid regimens with steroid-sparing agents, or thalidomide. All of these protocols are associated with potentially serious side effects and should only be undertaken in close cooperation with the patient's physician.

ORAL LICHEN PLANUS

The exact etiology of lichen planus is not known but it is believed to be an autoimmune disease with a genetic predisposition. It is the most common dermatologic disease with oral manifestations. An estimated 65% of patients with dermal lichen planus experience oral lichen planus (OLP), with the buccal mucosa the most commonly affected site. Trauma, viral and bacterial infections, emotional stress, and drug therapy have all been implicated as precipitating factors. A possible association between OLP and oral squamous cell carcinoma mandates all cases of OLP be followed closely.

DIAGNOSIS

Dermal lesions appear characteristically on the flexor surfaces of the arms and legs, but they may also involve other areas of the skin. They typically present as purple, polygonal, pruritic papules. Oral lesions may be present before, during, or after dermal eruptions, or they may represent the sole manifestation of the disease. Other common sites of occurrence include the tongue, lips, floor of mouth, palate, and gingiva. A simple classification system recognizes three forms of OLP: reticular, atrophic, and erosive.

RETICULAR OLP, the most frequently occurring form of OLP, is characterized by mucosal keratotic lines, plaques, or papules that often create a lacy or reticular pattern (Wickham striae) (Figure 5-15 ❀ on CD-ROM). The patient may be unaware of this form of OLP because it is typically asymptomatic.

ATROPHIC (erythematous) and EROSIVE (ulcerated) areas may occur in reticular OLP (Figure 5-16 ❀ on CD-ROM), frequently causing sufficient discomfort to induce the patient to seek treatment. Affected areas may range in size from a few millimeters to several centimeters.

All three forms may occur simultaneously and vary in predominance over time in a given patient. The observation of the characteristic Wickham striae, especially with the presence of characteristic dermal lesions, usually makes for a straightforward diagnosis. However, a biopsy is recommended because the characteristic lacy keratotic component of OLP is often lacking and many other disorders may clinically mimic OLP.

MANAGEMENT

There is no cure for OLP, and oral lesions tend to be more persistent and recalcitrant to therapy than concurrent dermal lesions. Strategies are aimed at relieving symptoms and reducing exacerbations and progression. Asymptomatic reticular cases only require routine follow-up for change, whereas symptomatic cases usually require some form of drug therapy.

Primary line of therapy

For patients with mild to moderately symptomatic OLP, a topical corticosteroid is usually prescribed. Therapy is empirical and the agent chosen depends largely on the lesion presentation, patient preference, and practitioner experience. Ointments or gels work well for localized lesions, whereas elixirs are better suited for more widespread presentations. Ointments may also be mixed with an oral paste such as Orabase to improve adhesion. When effective, improvement should be apparent within 2 weeks. Once improvement is noted, the dosing is titrated down to the lowest dose required to maintain patient comfort. Measures to reduce the predictable risk of developing secondary candidiasis should be undertaken.

Intermediate-potency topical steroid

Triamcinolone acetonide (Kenalog), 0.1% cream

Disp: 15-gram tube

Sig: Apply thin coating to affected areas after meals and at bedtime. Do not eat or drink for 30 minutes.

Betamethasone valerate (Betatrex), 0.1% ointment

Disp: 15-gram tube

Sig: Apply thin coating to affected areas after meals and at bedtime. Do not eat or drink for 30 minutes.

High-potency topical steroid

Fluocinonide (Lidex), 0.05% ointment

Disp: 15-gram tube

Sig: Apply thin coating to affected areas after meals and at bedtime. Do not eat or drink for 30 minutes.

Dexamethasone (Decadron) elixir, 0.5 mg/5 mL

Disp: 100 mL

Sig: Rinse with 1 teaspoonful for 2 minutes 4 times a day and spit out.

Ultra-potent topical steroid

Clobetasol propionate (Temovate), 0.05% ointment

Disp: 15-gram tube

Sig: Apply thin coating to affected areas after meals and at bedtime. Do not eat or drink for 30 minutes.

Secondary line of therapy

For moderate to severe OLP or for cases unresponsive to topical corticosteroids, a systemic steroid should be used. Localized lesions may respond favorably to the local injection of an agent such as triamcinolone acetonide. The most commonly used systemic corticosteroid is prednisone. The approach is to prescribe a high-dose (40 to 80 mg/day), short-course (no more than 10 days) regimen to maximize the therapeutic effect while minimizing long-term side effects such as hypothalamic-pituitary-adrenal axis suppression. However, other possible adverse effects such as insomnia, mood swings, nervousness, diarrhea, fluid retention, muscle weakness, and hypertension may occur. Consultation with a physician is recommended before prescribing systemic corticosteroids for patients with hypothyroidism, heart failure, peptic ulcer disease, ulcerative colitis, cirrhosis, and thromboembolic disorders. Patients who respond favorably to a short-course systemic regimen should be placed on a topical agent with the goal of reducing acute exacerbations.

For local injection

$\mathbf{R}_\chi$ Triamcinolone acetonide (Kenalog) suspension, 10 g/mL

Disp: 5 mL

Sig: Inject 0.2 to 0.4 mL into base of lesion

For systemic oral course

$\mathbf{R}_\chi$ Prednisone (Deltasone), 10-mg tablets

Disp: 70 tablets (*for a 70-kg patient*)

Sig: Take 7 tablets by mouth each morning until lesions resolve, then decrease by 1 tablet each successive day.

Tertiary line of therapy

For patients nonresponsive to the secondary line of therapy or for those who quickly relapse after cessation of short-term steroid therapy, a more aggressive approach is necessary. Long-term corticosteroid regimens with or without additional agents such as immunosuppressants or immunomodulators may be beneficial for such patients. However, the side-effect liability is such that these medications should only be prescribed by or in close collaboration with the patient's physician.

ERYTHEMA MULTIFORME

Erythema multiforme (EM) is the global term applied to a spectrum of acute mucocutaneous vesiculobullous erosive disorders. Typically a self-limiting process, the severity of EM varies from mild (EM minor and oral EM) to moderate (EM major) to potentially fatal (Stevens-Johnson syndrome [SJS] and toxic epidermal necrolysis [TEN]). The pathophysiology of EM has not been clearly established, although it likely represents a genetically predisposed allergic host response to antigenic challenge. In susceptible patients, an immunological attack against keratinocytes expressing nonself antigens results in apoptosis and subsequent necrolysis. Most cases of oral EM, EM minor, and EM major are related to an infectious agent, usually the herpes simplex virus. Other organisms implicated include β-hemolytic streptococci, coccidiomycosis, Coxsackie virus, diphtheria, Epstein-Barr virus, herpes zoster, influenza virus type-A, measles, mumps, *Mycoplasma pneumoniae*, and vaccinia. In contrast, most cases of SJS and TEN are related to pharmacological agents, most frequently sulfonamides, anticonvulsive drugs, and nonsteroidal anti-inflammatory drugs (NSAIDs). In addition, EM has been reported to develop following immunizations or radiotherapy, whereas other reports associate it with Crohn disease, Addison disease, lupus erythematosus, pregnancy, sarcoidosis, and malignancies such as

Hodgkin disease, multiple myeloma, and others. Still, in many cases a causative agent is not identified.

DIAGNOSIS

EM may occur at any age, however it has its greatest propensity in young adults. The onset of the eruption is rapid (12 to 24 hours) and at times it is associated with fever, symptoms of respiratory tract infection, and muscular aches. Table 5-3 summarizes the spectrum of EM. The typical abrupt onset combined with the presence of characteristic mucocutaneous lesions (i.e., target lesions, vesiculobullous erosive oral lesions, serohemorrhagic crusting of the lips [Figures 5-17 ✿ and 5-18 ✿ on CD-ROM]) makes for a straightforward diagnosis. Historical evidence of prior occurrence and/or exposure to a possible causative drug or infectious agent reinforces the diagnosis.

MANAGEMENT

Most cases of EM are self-limiting with resolution occurring in 1 to 6 weeks. For such cases, treatment is generally palliative and symptomatic. The withdrawal of any suspected causative medications should be undertaken and a careful history obtained to identify any other possible underlying causes.

Primary line of therapy

Topical anesthetic

Anesthetic mouth rinses such as diphenhydramine or viscous lidocaine may be prescribed for oral pain. Such agents may be mixed with Kaopectate or Maalox to improve local retention.

Diphenhydramine (Children's Benadryl) elixir, 12.5 mg/5 mL [OTC]

Disp: 8 ounces

Sig: Rinse with 1 teaspoonful every 2 hours and spit out.

Diphenhydramine (Children's Benadryl) elixir, 12.5 mg/5 mL [OTC] 4 ounces mixed with Kaopectate or Maalox [OTC] 4 ounces (50% mixture by volume)

Disp: 8 ounces

Sig: Rinse with 1 teaspoonful every 2 hours and spit out.

Nutritional supplement

Adequate hydration and nutrition are mandatory. Nutritional supplements may be prescribed to ensure the maintenance of adequate nutritional intake.

Ensure Plus [OTC]

Disp: 25 cans

Sig: Three to 5 cans in divided doses throughout the day. Serve cold.

Table 5-3.   Spectrum of Erythema Multiforme

SPECTRUM	CUTANEOUS INVOLVEMENT	MUCOSAL INVOLVEMENT	OUTCOME
EM minor	Target lesion, acral distribution, negative Nikolsky sign	Often absent	Recovery; possible recurrence
EM major	As above	Prominent oral involvement; vesiculoerosive erosions with fibrinous pseudomembrane; characteristic hemorrhagic lip involvement	Recovery; possible recurrence; rare mortality
SJS	Widespread small blisters, macules, atypical target lesions predominate on torso; epidermal detachment in <10% body surface area; positive Nikolsky sign	As above, possibly more extensive; ocular and genital involvement common	Fatal in 5% to 10% of cases; possible scarring; possible recurrence
TEN	Widespread small blisters, macules, atypical target lesions predominate on torso; epidermal detachment in >30% body surface area; positive Nikolsky sign	As above	Fatal in up to 35% of cases; possible scarring; possible recurrence
Oral EM	Typical target lesions frequently absent	Oral lesions predominate clinical picture	Recovery; possible recurrent and chronic forms

EM, erythema multiforme; SJS, Stevens-Johnson syndrome; TEN, toxic epidermal necrolysis.

> ℞ Meritene Food Supplement [OTC]
>
> *Disp*: 1-pound can (various flavors)
>
> *Sig*: Three servings daily. Prepare as indicated on label. Serve cold.

Corticosteroids

The use of systemic corticosteroids for the treatment of EM, particularly the more severe forms, remains controversial and has not been validated in clinical trials. Any potential value of corticosteroid therapy is likely predicated on its prompt administration to a patient who presents at the earliest onset of the EM.

> ℞ Prednisone (Deltasone), 10-mg tablets
>
> *Disp*: 70 tablets (*for a 70-kg patient*)
>
> *Sig*: Take 7 tablets by mouth each morning until lesions resolve, and then decrease by 1 tablet each successive day.

Secondary line of therapy

Referral to a physician is warranted for all cases of EM nonresponsive to primary therapy or any suspected case of SJS or TEN. These cases often require a multidiscipline approach to management, in a manner similar to that of a patient with extensive burns.

Prevention

For cases of EM associated with herpes simplex infection, prophylactic antiviral therapy often proves beneficial. For cases of EM attributed to a specific drug, strict avoidance of the suspect drug and all drugs with cross-reactive potential is mandatory to preclude recurrence. For cases in which the cause is unknown, patient education concerning the possibility of recurrence and the necessity to ensure prompt medical intervention is recommended.

For herpes-associated erythema multiforme (HAEM)

> ℞ Acyclovir (Zovirax), 400-mg capsules
>
> *Disp*: 90 capsules
>
> *Sig*: Take 1 capsule 3 times daily until all capsules are taken.

> ℞ Valacyclovir (Valtrex), 500-mg capsules
>
> *Disp*: 30 capsules
>
> *Sig*: Take 1 capsule daily until all capsules are taken.

CICATRICIAL PEMPHIGOID

Cicatricial pemphigoid (CP), also known as mucous membrane pemphigoid, is a rare chronic mucocutaneous bullous condition. It is a heterogeneous autoimmune disease, characterized by the production of autoantibodies against basement membrane zone (BMZ) antigens. The mean age of onset of CP is 62 years and it appears to have a 2:1 predilection for women, without racial or geographical bias.

Diagnosis

The most common sites affected by CP are the oral tissues, conjunctiva, and skin. These are followed in prevalence by genital, pharyngeal, laryngeal, nasal, and esophageal involvement. Oral CP is most commonly found on the buccal and labial aspects of the attached gingiva, followed by the buccal or labial mucosa, palate, tongue, and pharynx (Figures 5-19 ✿ and 5-20 ✿ on CD-ROM). Gingival lesions may be characterized as desquamative (positive Nikolsky sign), erythematous, painful, and, at times, hemorrhagic. The primary oral mucosal lesions of CP are vesiculobullous and tend to rupture within hours, resulting in painful erosions or ulcerations with smooth borders. Although oral mucosal lesions usually heal slowly without scarring, scarring as a result of submucosal fibrosis is a key feature of disease progression in other sites such as the conjunctiva and larynx.

The diagnosis is confirmed by histological, immunopathological, and serological studies. Histological specimens are often nonspecific, but typically demonstrate subepithelial blistering and the presence of a dense submucosal inflammatory infiltrate. Direct immunofluorescence of perilesional tissue reveals a characteristic linear deposition of immunoglobulin G (IgG) and complement 3 (C3) along the BMZ. Indirect immunofluorescence examination using salt-split skin as the substrate may demonstrate several anti-BMZ antibodies associated with CP.

Management

The extent of the dentist's involvement in managing CP depends on the presentation. For cases of CP restricted to the oral cavity, the dentist should be prepared to deliver initial therapeutic interventions. However, cases of CP manifesting extraoral involvement require a multidisciplinary approach to therapy, usually coordinated by a dermatologist. In all cases, the dentist should be familiar with immunopharmacological strategies intended to minimize morbidity or induce remission; participate in monitoring the patient's response to therapy; and anticipate, recognize, and report treatment-related adverse drug events to the primary caregiver.

Primary line of therapy

For mild cases of CP limited to the oral cavity, a regularly applied topical high-potency or ultra-potency corticosteroid ointment or gel may be all that is necessary to successfully manage the illness. Ointments may also be mixed with an oral paste such as Orabase to improve adhesion. For lesions restricted to the gingiva, custom trays may be fabricated to improve the delivery of steroids to the affected tissues. The frequency of application should be titrated down to the minimum required to maintain lesion control and patient comfort. Measures to reduce the predictable risk of developing secondary candidiasis should be undertaken. In addition, the patient should be educated to reduce the risk of trauma and to maintain excellent oral hygiene. All teeth and restorations should be smooth and free of jagged edges.

High-potency topical steroid

Fluocinonide (Lidex), 0.05% ointment

Disp: 15-gram tube

Sig: Apply a thin layer to affected areas after each meal and at bedtime. Do not eat or drink for 30 minutes.

Ultra-potent topical steroid

> R̸
> Clobetasol propionate (Temovate), 0.05% ointment
> *Disp*: 15-gram tube
> *Sig*: Apply a thin coating to affected areas after meals and at bedtime. Do not eat or drink for 30 minutes.

Secondary line of therapy

In the management of recalcitrant cases, a regimen of dapsone may be added to the first line of therapy. Dapsone, a sulfone antimicrobial agent, is a competitive antagonist of para-aminobenzoic acid (PABA) and prevents the normal use of PABA in the synthesis of folic acid. It also inhibits the chemotaxis of polymorphonuclear leukocytes, reduces their accumulation in the upper dermis, and directly diminishes tissue inflammation. Dapsone is associated with several potentially serious side effects such as headache, hemolytic anemia, methemoglobinemia, bone marrow suppression, and liver toxicity. Its use is contraindicated in patients with glucose-6-phophate dehydrogenase deficiency. The complete blood count, with white blood cell differential, should be established at baseline and monitored every 2 weeks during therapy. The development of agranulocytosis warrants immediate drug cessation and prompt medical evaluation. To reduce the risk of side effects, a small initial dose is prescribed with future doses gradually tapered up to reach therapeutic levels. Once control is obtained, the dosage is gradually reduced to the minimum required for maintenance. Partial or complete remission may be observed after 2 to 12 weeks of treatment with 75 to 150 mg of dapsone daily.

> R̸
> Dapsone, 25-mg tablets
> *Disp*: 60 tablets
> *Sig*: Take 1 tablet once a day for 3 days, then take 2 tablets once a day for 3 days, then take 3 tablets once a day for 3 days, then take 4 tablets once a day for 3 days, then take 6 tablets once a day for 4 days.

Tertiary line of therapy

For cases of oral CP not controlled by topical steroids and dapsone and for cases of CP manifesting extraoral involvement, more aggressive therapeutic measures are prescribed. Initially, a regimen of long-term systemic corticosteroid and dapsone may induce disease remission. However, severe nonresponsive cases of CP often require still more aggressive immunosuppressive therapies with agents such as azathioprine, methotrexate, mycophenolate mofetil, cyclophosphamide, tacrolimus, or mitomycin C. The side effect liability of all tertiary lines of therapy is such that they should only be prescribed by or in close collaboration with the patient's physician.

PERICORONITIS

Pericoronitis, seen most commonly in young adults, is a localized gingivitis associated with a partially erupted tooth. Although it may be associated with any deciduous or succedaneous tooth, it most often affects the permanent third molars. Bacterial plaque and food debris accumulate beneath the operculum, providing an ideal milieu for rapid bacterial growth. The ensuing bacterial infection consists of a predominately anaerobic flora mainly consisting of alpha-hemolytic streptococci, *Veillonella*, *Prevotella*, *Bacteroides*, *Capnocytophaga*, *Campylobacter*, and *Actinomyces* species. Contributing factors include lowered systemic resistance, decreased flow of saliva, poor eating habits, lack of sleep, and inadequate oral hygiene.

DIAGNOSIS

The diagnosis of pericoronitis is usually straightforward. Mild or early cases present with pain or discomfort associated with gingival inflammation around the offending tooth. Frequently, occlusal trauma from an opposing, often su-praerupted tooth acts to aggravate or occasionally initiate the process. Palpation of inflamed gingival tissue will usually elicit a purulent exudate. More advanced cases may manifest malaise; fever; lymphadenopathy; foul taste; pain in the ear, throat, and floor of the mouth; peritonsillar and pharyngeal inflammation; cellulitis; and loss of masticatory function. Severe cases may involve the buccal, submental, submandibular, vestibular, and pterygoid spaces. Rarely, cases caused by virulent pathogens may spread rapidly to the brain, throat, and mediastinum.

MANAGEMENT

The extent of treatment depends on the severity of pericoronitis, the presence of systemic complications, and the feasibility of retaining the involved tooth.

Primary line of therapy

Mild cases of pericoronitis usually respond promptly to therapies that establish drainage, remove sources of trauma, improve oral hygiene, and relieve pain. Drainage can often be established by simply inserting a periodontal probe under the operculum. The area should be thoroughly irrigated with saline or an antiseptic rinse such as 0.8% povidone iodine, 3% hydrogen peroxide diluted to half-strength with saline, or 0.12% chlorhexidine gluconate. A wick of iodoform gauze may be temporarily inserted under the operculum to allow for continuous drainage. The patient is further instructed to rinse with warm salt water for 2 minutes every waking hour.

For cases in which the opposing tooth is traumatizing the operculum, the opposing tooth should either be extracted or undergo an odontoplasty to reduce the traumatic insult. Patients should be advised to rest; avoid drinking alcoholic beverages and smoking cigarettes; maintain hydration; and eat a soft, balanced diet. The importance of oral hygiene must be stressed and its relationship to pericoronitis discussed. For patients with mild-to-moderate pain, an NSAID or an opioid combination may be prescribed.

Ibuprofen (Motrin), 400-mg tablets
Disp: 20 tablets
Sig: Take 1 tablet every 4 to 6 hours.

Secondary line of therapy

For patients manifesting systemic signs of infection (fever, lymphadenopathy, and malaise), an antimicrobial regimen should be prescribed and added to the aforementioned primary therapeutic measures. Penicillin remains the initial drug of choice. However, there is growing concern that the use of a beta-lactam antibiotic may select for beta-lactamase-producing bacteria, resulting in clinical failure. For such cases, or for patients unable to take penicillin, metronidazole is a better choice.

R̸ Penicillin VK, 500-mg tablets

Disp: 20 tablets

Sig: Take 2 tablets stat then 1 tablet four times a day until all tablets are taken.

R̸ Metronidazole (Flagyl), 500-mg tablets

Disp: 20 tablets

Sig: Take 1 tablet four times a day until all tablets are taken.

Tertiary line of therapy

Any patient nonresponsive to conservative therapy or who initially presents with severe signs of infection such as severe trismus, cellulitis, dehydration, or pending respiratory embarrassment should be immediately referred to an oral and maxillofacial surgeon or an emergency care facility.

Prevention

Many cases of pericoronitis may be prevented by the timely extraction of teeth that are either malposed or have insufficient room to fully erupt. The extraction of third molars in the presence of pericoronitis is controversial. Some experts caution that extracting teeth in the presence of pericoronitis increases the risk of developing septicemia, cavernous sinus thrombosis, or mediastinal abscess. They recommend extraction of the offending tooth once the pericoronitis has been appropriately managed.

ALVEOLAR OSTEITIS

Alveolar osteitis (AO), or dry socket, is a relatively common postextraction complication that affects mandibular third-molar sites ten times more frequently than other sites. It is postulated that surgical trauma or the presence of existing inflammation leads to the release of bioactive substances from the alveolar bone or adjacent tissues that convert plasminogen in the clot to the fibrinolytic agent plasmin. Plasmin acts to dissolve the clot, which leads to the release of kinins. Numerous predisposing factors have been associated with AO including smoking, oral contraceptive use, gender, surgical trauma, practitioner inexperience, preexisting infections, inadequate infection control, increased patient age, and insufficient irrigation during surgery. AO is a transient phenomenon that will resolve itself in about 7 to 10 days, albeit with significant discomfort.

DIAGNOSIS

The diagnosis of AO is usually easily made and is based on the presence of an empty extraction site 2 to 3 days postprocedure, severe pain in and around the extraction site that often radiates, and halitosis. AO is unlikely to occur within the first 24 hours postextraction. Occasionally, fever, trismus, and lymphadenopathy may be present, but such findings may also indicate the presence of infection. Other conditions to consider in the differential include retained tooth or bony fragments, foreign debris, or fracture.

MANAGEMENT

Unfortunately, no universally accepted or validated protocols exist to prevent or manage AO. Indeed, some protocols that have been shown to prolong and/or worsen AO continue to be practiced by some clinicians. Almost all proposed protocols incur additional office visits, substantial extra costs, and may induce an adverse reaction. If an adverse reaction were to occur, defending the use of an unproven product may prove difficult. However, in spite of all the apparent contradictions in the literature, some prudent recommendations can be offered.

Prevention

Prudent measures to prevent AO should be undertaken for all patients undergoing an extraction. Whenever possible, plaque levels and associated inflammation should be reduced. For patients taking oral contraceptives, the surgery should be scheduled during days 23 to 28 of the menstrual cycle. A chlorhexidine rinse should be administered immediately before surgery and for 1 week postoperatively. An atraumatic surgical technique should be used with attention to irrigate the extraction site with saline; ensure the removal of any bone or tooth fragments; and verify the formation of a viable clot. Verbal and written postoperative instructions should be provided to emphasize the need to avoid smoking, sucking through a straw, drinking carbonated beverages, and vigorous rinsing for 48 hours. A nutritious soft diet is recommended and the use of gentle toothbrushing for oral hygiene should be prescribed.

Chlorhexidine gluconate (Peridex, PerioGard, others) rinse, 0.12%

Disp: 16-ounce bottle

Sig: 1/2-ounce rinse for 1 minute immediately before surgery, followed by 1/2-ounce gentle rinse for 1 minute, twice a day, for 1 week after surgery.

Treatment

The goal in treating AO is to reduce discomfort and promote healing. Currently, there are no products available that truly meet both these goals. Conservative therapy consists of the following:

1. Remove any sutures to allow easy access to extraction site; local anesthesia is often required for this.

2. Thoroughly irrigate the site with warm saline to loosen any debris and carefully suction the site.

3. There is no need to curette the site to incur bleeding (once AO occurs, healing will occur through secondary intention).

4. Provide and instruct the patient on the appropriate use of a curved tip plastic syringe to keep the socket site clean by irrigating with either chlorhexidine gluconate or saline.

5. Prescribe an analgesic; reassure and educate the patient on the process and the therapeutic goals.

For pain relief

> ℞ Hydrocodone 7.5-mg and ibuprofen 200-mg tablets (Vicoprofen)
> *Disp*: 20 tablets
> *Sig*: Take 1 to 2 tablets every 4 to 6 hours as needed.

STOMATITIS

Stomatitis is an encompassing term used to refer to any inflammatory condition affecting the mucosal tissues of the mouth. As such, many of the conditions addressed in this chapter qualify as forms of stomatitis. The degree of mucosal involvement in stomatitis varies greatly, depending on the predisposing and etiological factors involved. Typically, stomatitis is associated with mild-to-moderate pain and a potential for secondary bacterial and fungal infections.

DIAGNOSIS

The diagnosis of stomatitis is usually easily made based on the patient's presenting complaint and findings of the clinical examination. However, a careful and thorough discernment of the patient's history is often required to identify any and all possible etiologies.

CHEMICAL, THERMAL, AND PHYSICAL TRAUMA lesions present as white or raw bleeding, painful, desquamative (sloughing) areas. Common examples include ASA (Figure 5-21✿ on CD-ROM) and pizza burns. The heat and chemical irritants produced by excessive smoking cause erythema of the hard palate, which progresses to a grayish-white, thickened papular appearance with small red spots indicating the dilated orifices of minor salivary glands. Inadvertent gasoline exposure, which may occur with siphoning, may induce mucosal swelling and a vesiculobullous eruption. Ill-fitting removable dental prostheses may traumatize the oral mucosa, producing erythema, erosion, and ulceration. Dental prostheses that are improperly worn and/or inadequately maintained may predispose to the development of candidiasis. Finally, numerous medications including gold salts and NSAIDs have the potential to produce mucosal damage, which may range from superficial erosions to pronounced ulcerations covered with fibrin and at times surrounded by an erythematous halo.

CHEMOTHERAPY-INDUCED AND RADIATION-INDUCED STOMATITIS is perhaps the most dramatic form of stomatitis (Figures 5-22 ✿ and 5-23 ✿ on CD-ROM), because the therapeutic value of both of these modalities lies in their ability to interfere with cell replication. Chemotherapeutic agents used to eradicate malignant cells may also destroy certain normal cells, resulting in generalized mucositis. Similarly, any form of radiation has the potential to directly or indirectly interact with critical targets in the cells and initiate a chain of events that leads to tissue damage when absorbed in biological material. When the oral cavity is in the field of radiation, the rapidly dividing cells of the oral mucosa may be affected. The resultant large ulcerative lesions may make it difficult for patients to maintain an adequate nutritional intake and serve as portals for serious disseminated infection.

MANAGEMENT

Depending on the etiology and severity, the management strategies to address stomatitis will vary. For many cases, simple recognition along with patient education and reassurance is all that is necessary. For others, more aggressive therapies may be required.

Primary line of therapy

Small isolated lesions such as burns or traumatic ulcerations frequently require no specific therapy. There are numerous prescription and OTC topical gels, creams, ointments, and rinses marketed for the treatment of mouth sores (see the section on recurrent aphthous stomatitis, p. 75). However, clinicians are reminded that no validated studies exist to demonstrate the clinical superiority of any formulation over another. For cases of stomatitis thought to be caused by a medication, the patient should be advised to cease using the medication if self-prescribed. For cases possibly caused by a prescription medication, a medical consultation with the physician is warranted to consider the use of an alternative agent.

Secondary line of therapy

For more severe cases, such as may occur with radiation therapy and/or chemotherapy, strategies to provide palliation and prevent secondary infection are indicated. Patients should be instructed to carefully remove plaque either with a soft toothbrush or with a foam toothette to minimize trauma; to avoid products irritating to oral soft tissues (such as alcohol and tobacco; hot, spicy, and coarse foods; and fruits and beverages with a high acid content); to refrain from wearing removable prostheses; to eat a soft diet; and to frequently rinse with alkaline saline (sodium bicarbonate) solution. A topical anesthetic agent such as lidocaine viscous or diphenhydramine hydrochloride and, if necessary, a systemic analgesic may be prescribed. When topical anesthetics are used, the patient should be warned that these agents may increase the risk of self-induced trauma, may interfere with the pharyngeal phase of swallowing, and may lead to aspiration.

Alkaline saline mouth rinse

Disp: Mix 1/2 teaspoon each of salt and baking soda in 16 ounces of water

Sig: Gently rinse with copious amounts 4 times a day.

Diphenhydramine (Children's Benadryl) elixir, 12.5 mg/5 mL [OTC]

Disp: 8 ounces

Sig: Rinse with 1 teaspoonful every 2 hours and spit out.

Diphenhydramine (Children's Benadryl) elixir 12.5 mg/5 mL [OTC] 4 ounces mixed with Kaopectate or Maalox [OTC] 4 ounces (50% mixture by volume)

Disp: 8 ounces

Sig: Rinse with 1 teaspoonful every 2 hours and spit out.

> R̶x̶ Lidocaine (Xylocaine) viscous, 2%
> *Disp*: 100 mL
> *Sig*: Rinse with 1 teaspoonful for 1 minute, then expectorate, before meals and at bedtime.

Prevention

Misguided individuals must be advised that the topical application of medicaments such as aspirin that are compounded for systemic use is ill-advised. The adverse mucosal effects caused by tobacco use afford the practitioner a tangible opportunity to discuss and promote tobacco use cessation. Oral lesions associated with the accidental mucosal exposure to gasoline and other chemicals generally are not severe, although they may require supportive treatment, and complete healing usually occurs within 7 days. The treatment of stomatitis caused by ill-fitting or poorly maintained removable dental prostheses may require only minor denture adjustment or cleaning, or complete refabrication of the prostheses. Patients should be educated on the need to not wear the prostheses 24 hours per day. The importance of meticulous oral hygiene cannot be overemphasized as an effective preventive and therapeutic modality in the management of stomatitis.

BURNING MOUTH DISORDER

Burning mouth disorder (BMD) is a chronic, painful condition that manifests as a burning sensation affecting the oral mucosa, particularly the mucosa of the anterior tongue and lips. When limited to the tongue, BMD is often referred to as glossodynia. The etiology of BMD is unknown, but there is a predilection to afflict women (6:1).

DIAGNOSIS

An estimated 50% of cases are associated with oral dryness and dysgeusia. The clinical examination is usually unremarkable for obvious abnormalities, causing frustration for both the patient and the clinician. Numerous conditions, such as hormonal changes in women (especially in the perimenopausal or postmenopausal periods); stomatitis areata migrans; iron, folic acid, or B_{12} deficiency; diabetes mellitus–associated neuropathy; candidiasis; and neurotic glossodynia may cause burning sensations of the oral mucosa. Appropriate medical consultations may be necessary to rule out suspected comorbid factors before establishing a diagnosis of BMD.

In iron deficiency anemia, the patient's tongue may exhibit pallor and a loss of filiform papillae. Early manifestations are noted on the lateral margins and tip of the tongue. A deficiency of folic acid or vitamin B_{12} may cause a generalized atrophy of the lingual papillae. These patients may present with a painful, beefy-red tongue, often accompanied by angular cheilitis. Diabetic neuropathy may manifest as a burning sensation in the mouth. In addition, patients with poor glycemic control and others who are at high risk for candidiasis (see the section on candidiasis, p. 70) and xerostomia (see the section on xerostomia, p. 72) and those with oral lichen planus (see section on oral lichen planus, p. 78), may also experience similar symptoms.

Stomatitis areata migrans is a commonly encountered condition that usually affects the tongue. Characteristic findings are a loss of the filiform papillae, which occurs in an irregular pattern and migrates over time. This condition is usually asymptomatic, although some patients may complain of a burning sensation, especially when eating spicy foods.

Finally, neurotic glossodynia has been described in postmenopausal women and is often accompanied by cancerophobia. A presenting complaint of glossodynia, with no evidence of clinical lesions, may be the first indication of mental depression. Patients suffering from a stress disorder may complain of glossodynia, metallic taste, or pruritus (often of the scalp).

Management

The treatment of burning mucosal sensation associated with an identifiable cause is treated primarily by managing the underlying cause. BMD, being a diagnosis of exclusion, is managed with neuroleptic agents. Such medications should be prescribed in close collaboration with the patient's physician. The recommendations below are provided for completeness with the acknowledgment that many general practitioners will choose to refer such off-label therapies to the patient's physician.

Primary line of therapy

Clonazepam taken at bedtime may be effective in relieving BMD. The initial dose is low and slowly titrated up every 3 to 7 days until a therapeutic effect is observed or the maximum recommended dose is attained. For clonazepam, the maximum daily dose is 4 mg. Alternatively, a benzodiazepine such as chlordiazepoxide may be prescribed.

Clonazepam (Klonopin), 0.5-mg tablets

Disp: 100 tablets

Sig: Take 1 tablet at bedtime. Increase daily dosage by 0.5 mg after every 3 days until improvement is noted.

Chlordiazepoxide (Librium), 5-mg tablets

Disp: 50 tablets

Sig: Take 1 to 2 tablets 3 times a day.

Secondary line of therapy

For patients nonresponsive to primary therapies, the use of a tricyclic antidepressant such as desipramine may prove effective. Desipramine is preferred over amitriptyline because it induces less oral drying. The initial dose of 10 mg is increased by 10 mg weekly until therapeutic relief is attained. The maximum allowable daily dose is 50 mg.

Desipramine (Norpramin), 10-mg tablets

Disp: 50 tablets

Sig: Take 1 tablet at bedtime. Increase dose by 10 mg each week until therapeutic relief attained. Do not exceed 50 mg per day.

Tertiary line of therapy

For patients with BMD refractory to the above therapies, the use of the anticonvulsant gabapentin may be effective. Gabapentin is approved for the treatment of postherpetic neuralgia. The initial dose of 300 mg a day is steadily increased to 300 to 600 mg three times a day until relief is attained. Doses in excess of 1,800 mg per day generally show no increase in therapeutic effect.

℞ Gabapentin (Neurontin), 300-mg capsules
Disp: 50
Sig: Take 1 tablet on the first day, increase to 1 tablet twice a day on the second day and then 1 tablet 3 times a day.

NECROTIZING ULCERATIVE GINGIVITIS

Necrotizing ulcerative gingivitis (NUG) is a unique, painful bacterial infection affecting the interdental and marginal gingival tissue. Consistently implicated microorganisms include *Prevotella intermedia, Fusobacterium fusiforme, Bacteroides melaninogenicus, Treponema,* and *Selenomonas.* The positive clinical response to antibiotics tends to support the role of these organisms as etiological agents. Although bacteria underlie the etiology, NUG is not considered to be a communicable disease. There seems to be a direct relationship between the occurrence of NUG and reduced host resistance. Other established predisposing factors include malnutrition, tobacco smoking, psychological stress, preexisting gingivitis, and trauma. In some cases, particularly in those with an immunosuppressive disorder, NUG may progress to affect the deeper periodontal ligament and osseous tissues, resulting in necrotizing ulcerative periodontitis (NUP).

DIAGNOSIS

The diagnosis of NUG is usually readily made based on the characteristic clinical findings. Essential findings include the unique punched-out crater-like ulcerations affecting the interdental and marginal gingiva, spontaneous gingival hemorrhage, and pain (Figure 5-24 ✺ on CD-ROM). Other potential findings include fetor oris, the presence of a grayish-yellow pseudomembrane consisting of necrotic debris and bacteria, fever, malaise, and lymphadenopathy. Lymphadenopathy most frequently involves the submandibular nodes and to a lesser degree the cervical nodes. Clinical findings suggestive of NUP include deep interproximal crater-like defects and denudation or sequestration of alveolar bone. However, such dramatic findings may also be observed with NUG affecting a patient with attachment loss associated with preexisting periodontal disease.

MANAGEMENT

Primary line of therapy

Reinforcement of personal plaque control combined with professional débridement is undertaken to reduce the bacterial mass. Patients should be instructed on how to gently brush their teeth with a soft-bristle toothbrush. Although ultrasonic instrumentation with copious amounts of water represents an excellent choice for débridement, judicious and gentle hand scaling with copious irrigation will also suffice. The goal is to perform a simple débridement, not a thorough fine scale. In addition, the patient is instructed to rinse with a

3% hydrogen peroxide solution, diluted one-half to one-fourth strength, or with chlorhexidine gluconate. Patients should be advised to rest, avoid smoking cigarettes and drinking alcoholic beverages, eat a soft nutritious diet, and maintain adequate hydration. Prompt clinical improvement is the rule and the patient should be seen daily until the acute phase is eliminated.

Hydrogen peroxide, 3% rinse [OTC] (4 ounces of rinse mixed with 12 ounces of water)

Disp: 16 ounces

Sig: Rinse with 1 to 2 tablespoons 4 times daily and expectorate.

Chlorhexidine gluconate (Peridex, PerioGard), 0.12%

Disp: 16-ounce bottle

Sig: Rinse with 1/2 ounce twice daily for 30 seconds and expectorate. Avoid rinsing or eating for 30 minutes after use.

Secondary line of therapy

The use of a systemic antimicrobial regimen should be considered for the patient whose condition does not promptly respond to the primary line of therapy, who initially presents with constitutional signs such as lymphadenopathy and/or fever, or who initially manifests NUP. Either penicillin or metronidazole may be used and improvement should be prompt.

Penicillin V potassium (Veetids), 500-mg tablets

Disp: 40 tablets

Sig: Take 1 tablet by mouth 4 times a day until all tablets are taken.

Metronidazole (Flagyl), 500-mg tablets

Disp: 28 tablets

Sig: Take 1 tablet every 6 hours.

Tertiary line of therapy

Close follow-up is mandatory to verify adequate resolution of NUG. Nonresponsive patients should undergo further medical evaluation to rule out conditions such as leukemia, severe malnutrition, or HIV infection. A high degree of suspicion for the presence of an underlying immunosuppressive disorder is warranted for the patient who initially presents with NUP. For all patients, additional interventions may be necessary to address any residual soft tissue deformities.

CONCLUSION

The clinical manifestations of many diseases, either local or systemic, typically appear on certain areas of the face, lips, labial or buccal mucosa, palate and tonsillar areas, tongue, floor of the mouth, or gingivae. Knowledge of the more common sites of involvement of a disease assists in its diagnosis. It must be remembered, however, that no diagnostic index or outline can take into consideration the capriciousness of a disease or the different reactions of an individual host to a disease. Therefore, the evaluation and integration of the clinical appearance and characteristics of a lesion with its history of development and other appropriate diagnostic findings should always determine the final diagnosis and therapeutic approach.

BIBLIOGRAPHY

Acute Odontogenic Pain

1. Aldous JA, Engar RC. Do dentists prescribe narcotics excessively? Gen Dent 1996;44(4):332–334.

2. Cooper SA. The relative efficacy of ibuprofen in dental pain. Compend Contin Educ Dent 1986;7:578–597.

3. Gordon SM, Dionne RA. Prevention of pain. Compend Contin Educ Dent 1997;18:239–251.

4. Huynh MP, Yagiela JA. Current concepts in acute pain management. J Calif Dent Assoc 2003;31:419–427.

5. Savage MG, Henry MA. Preoperative nonsteroidal anti-inflammatory agents: review of the literature. Oral Surg Oral Med Oral Pathol Oral Radiol Endod 2004;98:146–152.

6. Wideman GL, Keffer M, Morris E, Doyle RT, Jiang JG, Beaver WT. Analgesic efficacy of a combination of hydrocodone with ibuprofen in postoperative pain. Clin Pharmacol Ther 1999;65:66–76.

Odontogenic Infections

1. Dirks SJ, Terezhalmy GT. The patient with an odontogenic infection. Quintessence Int 2004;35:482–502.

2. Kuriyama T, Karasawa T, Nakagawa K, Saiki Y, Yamamoto E, Nakamura S. Bacteriologic features and antimicrobial susceptibility in isolates from orofacial odontogenic infections. Oral Surg Oral Med Oral Pathol Oral Radiol Endod 2000; 90(5):600–608.

3. Kuriyama T, Nakagawa K, Karasawa T, Saiki Y, Yamamoto E, Nakamura S. Past administration of beta-lactam antibiotics and increase in the emergence of beta-lactamase-producing bacteria in patients with orofacial odontogenic infections. Oral Surg Oral Med Oral Pathol Oral Radiol Endod 2000;89(2):186–192.

4. Moore PA. Dental therapeutic indications for the newer long-acting macrolide antibiotics. J Am Dent Assoc 1999;130: 1341–1343.

5. Sandor GKB, Low DE, Judd PL, Davidson RJ. Antimicrobial treatment options in the management of odontogenic infections. J Can Dent Assoc 1998;64:508–514.

6. Sanford JP, Low DE, Judd PL, Davidson RJ. Antibacterial treatment options in the management of odontogenic infections. J Can Dent Assoc 1998;64:508–514.

Actinic Cheilosis

1. Abramowicz M, ed. Prevention and treatment of sunburn. Med Lett Drugs Ther 2004;46:45–46.

2. Ting WW, Vest CD, Sontheimer R. Practical and experimental consideration of sun protection in dermatology. Int J Dermatol 2003;42:505–513.

Herpetic Infections

1. Huber MA. Herpes simplex type-1 virus infection. Quintessence Int 2003;34:453–467.

2. Wynn RL, Meiller TF, Crossley HL. Drug Information Handbook for Dentistry. 10th Ed. Hudson, OH: Lexi-Comp, 2005.

Candidiasis

1. Akpan A, Morgan R. Oral candidiasis. Postgrad Med 2002;78:455–459.

2. Sherman RG, Prusinski L, Ravenel MC, Joralmon RA. Oral candidosis. Quintessence Int 2002;34:521–532.

3. Stephens M. Understanding signs, symptoms and treatment of oral candidiasis. Nurs Times 2004;100:32–34.

Xerostomia

1. Cohen-Brown G, Ship JA. Diagnosis and treatment of salivary gland disorders. Quitessence Int 2004;35:108–123.

2. Haveman CW. Xerostomia management in the head and neck radiation patient. Tex Dent J 2004;121:483–497.

Recurrent Aphthous Stomatitis

1. Carpenter WM, Silverman S Jr. Over-the-counter products for oral ulcerations. J Calif Dent Assoc 1998;26:199–201.

2. Ship JA, Chavez EM, Doerr PA, Henson BS, Sarmadi M. Recurrent aphthous stomatitis. Quintessence Int 2000;31: 95–112.

Oral Lichen Planus

1. Huber MA. Oral lichen planus. Quintessence Int 2004;35:731–752.

Erythema Multiforme

1. Ayangco L, Rogers RS III. Oral manifestations of erythema multiforme. Dermatol Clin 2003;21:195–205.

2. Léaute-Labrèze C, Lamireau, Chawki D, Maleville J, Taïeb A. Diagnosis, classification, and management of erythema multiforme and Steven-Johnson syndrome. Arch Dis Child 2000;83:347–352.

3. Wong KC, Kennedy PJ, Lee S. Clinical manifestations and outcomes in 17 cases of Stevens-Johnson syndrome and toxic epidermal necrolysis. Australasian J Dermatol 1999;40:131–134.

Cicatricial Pemphigoid

1. Scully C, Carrozzo M, Gandolfo S, Puiatti P, Monteil R. Update of mucous membrane pemphigoid. A heterogenous immune-mediated subepithelial blistering entity. Oral Surg Oral Med Oral Pathol Oral Radiol Endod 1999;88:56–68.

2. Terezhalmy GT, Bergfeld WF. Cicatricial pemphigoid (benign mucous membrane pemphigoid). Quintessence Int 1998;29: 429–437.

3. Yeh SW, Ahmed B, Sami N, Ahmed AR. Blistering disorders: diagnosis and treatment. Dermatol Ther 2003;16:214–223.

Pericoronitis

1. Ohshima A, Ariji Y, Goto M, et al. Anatomical considerations for the spread of odontogenic infection originating from the pericoronitis of impacted mandibular third molar: computed tomographic analyses. Oral Surg Oral Med Oral Pathol Oral Radiol Endod 2004;98:589–597.

2. Sixou J-L, Magaud C, Jolivet-Gougeon A, Cormier M, Bonnaure-Mallet M. Microbiology of mandibular third molar pericoronitis: incidence of β-lactamase-producing bacteria. Oral Surg Oral Med Oral Pathol Oral Radiol Endod 2003;95: 655–659.

Alveolar Osteitis

1. Alexander RE. Dental extraction wound management: a case against medicating postextraction sockets. J Oral Maxillofac Surg 2000;58:538–551.

2. Blum IR. Contemporary views on dry socket (alveolar osteitis): a clinical appraisal of standardization, aetiopathogenesis and management: a critical review. Int J Oral Maxillofac Surg 2002;31:309–317.

3. Houston JP, McCollum J, Pietz D, Schneck D. Alveolar osteitis: a review of its etiology, prevention, and treatment modalities. Gen Dent 2002;50:457–463;quiz 464–465.

Stomatitis

1. Carpenter WM, Silverman S Jr. Over-the-counter products for oral ulcerations. J Calif Dent Assoc 1998;26:199–201.

2. Huber MA, Terezhalmy GT. The head and neck radiation oncology patient. Quintessence Int 2003;34:693–717.

3. Huber MA, Terezhalmy GT. The medical oncology patient. Quintessence Int 2005;36:383–402.

Burning Mouth Disorder

1. Meiss F, Boerner D, Marsch CH, Fisher M. Gabapentin—a promising treatment of glossodynia. Clin Exp Dermatol 2002; 27:525–526.

2. Rhodus NL, Carlson CR, Miller CS. Burning mouth (syndrome) disorder. Quintessence Int 2003;34:587–593.

3. White TL, Kent PF, Kurtz DB, Emko P. Effectiveness of gabapentin for treatment of burning mouth syndrome. Arch Otolaryngol Head Neck Surg 2004;130:786–788.

Necrotizing Ulcerative Gingivitis

1. Corbet EF. Diagnosis of acute periodontal lesions. Periodontol 2000 2004;34:204–216.

2. Novak MJ. Necrotizing ulcerative periodontitis. Ann Periodontal 1999;4:74–77.

3. Research, Science and Therapy Committee of the American Academy of Periodontology. Treatment of plaque-induced gingivitis, chronic periodontitis, and other clinical conditions. J Periodontal Res 2001;72:1790–1800.

4. Rowland RW. Necrotizing ulcerative gingivitis. Ann Periodontal 1999;4:65–73.

6 Clinical Medicine

Table of Contents

INTRODUCTION

Today's clinicians treat more medically and pharmacologically compromised patients than ever before. The availability of more than a thousand active ingredients in several thousand different formulations and over 100,000 nonprescription medications, and hundreds of facts about each of them, presents a seemingly insurmountable challenge in mastering the essentials for the clinical decision-making process. Fortunately, the clinician who understands general pharmacological principles can learn to predict the behavior of each drug based on a few facts. It is better to develop a drug profile than to memorize isolated data. The best way to achieve this objective is to associate, envision, predict, and inquire. Associate each drug with information already known. Envision the course of events that would occur as a drug enters the patient's body. Predict clinical uses and adverse drug events based on the drug's mechanism of action. Inquire which fact about a drug is going to have an impact on the clinical decision-making process in dentistry.

This section is based on the top 200 drugs dispensed by U.S. community pharmacies. The list is published annually. An awareness of the various medications commonly prescribed for patients will help clinicians anticipate the most commonly encountered medical diagnoses. The information will assist clinicians in identifying high-risk patients and guiding them in the development of appropriate diagnostic, preventive, and therapeutic strategies in the oral health care setting.

THE PATIENT TAKING CARDIOVASCULAR DRUGS

The heart pumps blood through a system of blood vessels under the control of an electric conduction system to deliver oxygen to all cells of the body. When the blood volume becomes greater than the limited volume capacity of the vascular system, the patient develops hypertension. When the myocardium does not get enough oxygen because of coronary artery disease, the patient will experience angina pectoris. If oxygen deprivation to a portion of the myocardium persists, the patient may develop myocardial infarction. When the conduction system malfunctions, arrhythmias occur and the heart is unable to pump enough blood to meet the metabolic demands of the body for oxygen, and the patient is said to have developed heart failure. In addition, many of the above conditions can lead to thromboembolic complications. An awareness of the various medications commonly prescribed to patients with cardiovascular diseases will assist clinicians in anticipating the most commonly encountered diagnoses.

DIURETICS

furosemide

hydrochlorothiazide

triamterene with hydrochlorothiazide

Mechanisms of action

- Hydrochlorothiazide and furosemide inhibit sodium reabsorption and increase the excretion of water and potassium.
- Triamterene inhibits sodium reabsorption and increases the excretion of water but has a potassium-sparing effect.

Clinical indications

- Hypertension
- Edema (congestive heart failure, hepatic failure, renal failure)

ELECTROLYTE MODIFIERS

potassium chloride (Klor-Con M20, Klor-Con 10)

Mechanisms of action

Potassium is a major intracellular ion that promotes normal impulse generation in the brain and heart and maintains normal renal function, acid base balance, carbohydrate metabolism, and gastric acid secretion.

Clinical indications

- Prevention and treatment of potassium deficiency, usually secondary to diuretic therapy

BETA$_1$-ADRENERGIC RECEPTOR AGONISTS

atenolol

carvedilol (Coreg)

metoprolol (Toprol XL)

Mechanisms of action

Competitively blocks beta$_1$-adrenergic receptors and decreases heart rate and cardiac output.

Clinical indications

- Hypertension
- Angina pectoris
- Tachyarrhythmias

ANGIOTENSIN-CONVERTING ENZYME (ACE) INHIBITORS AND ANGIOTENSIN (AT) II-RECEPTOR ANTAGONISTS

ACE inhibitors	AT II-receptor antagonists
benazepril (Lotensin)	irbesartan (Avapro)
benazepril with amlodipine (Lotrel)	losartan (Cozaar)
fosinopril (Monopril)	losartan with HCTZ (Hyzaar)
lisinopril	valsartan (Diovan)
quinapril (Accupril)	valsartan with HCTZ (Diovan HCT)
ramipril (Altace)	

Mechanisms of action

- ACE inhibitors prevent the conversion of AT I to AT II and produce vasodilation, suppress aldosterone synthesis, and potentiate the vasodilation effects of bradykinin and prostaglandins.
- The AT II-receptor antagonists block AT II from interacting with its receptor site.

Clinical indications

- Hypertension
- Congestive heart failure

CALCIUM-CHANNEL BLOCKING AGENTS

amlodipine (Norvasc)

amlodipine with benazepril (Lotrel)

diltiazem (Cartia XT)

verapamil SR

Mechanisms of action

Calcium-channel blocking agents inhibit calcium ions from entering the "slow" channels (voltage-sensitive areas) of vascular smooth muscle and myocardium. Relaxation of vascular smooth muscle and myocardium increase myocardial oxygen delivery, slow conduction velocity, and cause peripheral vasodilation.

Clinical indications

- Angina pectoris
- Supraventricular tachycardia
- Hypertension

Vasodilators

clonidine

Mechanisms of action

Clonidine is an $alpha_2$-adrenergic receptor agonist. It reduces sympathetic outflow from the central nervous system.

Clinical indications

- Hypertension

Lipid-lowering agents

HMG-CoA (3-hydroxy-3-methylglutaryl coenzyme A) reductase inhibitors

atorvastatin (Lipitor)

pravastatin (Pravachol)

simvastatin (Zocor)

Others

fenofibrate (TriCor)

gemfibrozil

ezetimibe (Zetia)

Mechanisms of action

- The "statins" competitively inhibit HMG-CoA reductase, a rate-limiting enzyme in the synthesis of very low-density lipoprotein (VLDL) and low-density lipoprotein (LDL).
- Fenofibrate enhances the synthesis of lipoprotein lipase and reduces VLDL and LDL concentrations.
- Gemfibrozil inhibits lipolysis, decreases fatty acid uptake, and reduces the synthesis of VLDL and LDL.
- Ezetimibe reduces absorption of cholesterol from the small intestine, reducing LDL and triglyceride levels.

Antianginal agents

isosorbide mononitrate

Mechanisms of action

Isosorbide mononitrate dilates coronary arteries and improves collateral flow to ischemic regions. It also decreases left ventricular pressure and systemic resistance.

Clinical indications

- Angina pectoris

CARDIAC GLYCOSIDES
digoxin (Lanoxin, Digitek)
Mechanisms of action

Inhibits the sodium/potassium ATPase pump and promotes intracellular sodium-calcium exchange, which leads to increased intracellular calcium ion concentration and increased cardiac contractility.

Clinical indications
- Congestive heart failure
- To slow ventricular tachyarrhythmia associated with supraventricular tachycardia (atrial fibrillation, atrial flutter)

ANTITHROMBOTIC AGENTS
clopidogrel (Plavix)
Mechanisms of action

Clopidogrel blocks adenosine diphosphate (ADP)–dependent platelet aggregation.

Clinical indications
- To reduce thromboembolic events in susceptible patients

ORAL ANTICOAGULANTS
warfarin (Coumadin)
Mechanisms of action

Warfarin interferes with the hepatic synthesis of vitamin K–dependent coagulation factors II, VII, IX, and X.

Clinical indications
- Prevention of venous thrombosis and pulmonary embolism, embolization with atrial fibrillation, coronary occlusion, and thrombus formation and embolization with prosthetic heart valves

Principles of Dental Management

When treating a patient taking cardiovascular drugs, the goal is to develop and implement timely preventive and therapeutic strategies compatible with the patient's physical and emotional ability to undergo and respond to dental care and with the patient's social and psychological needs.

Medical history

An initial medical history must be obtained from all patients, and it should be updated at each appointment, to confirm or to rule out predictors of increased cardiovascular risk in association with noncardiac procedures. It should also be determined whether the patient has a pacemaker or an implantable cardioverter defibrillator (ICD).

Minor predictors of increased cardiovascular risk include: advanced age, atrial fibrillation, low functional capacity, history of stroke, and uncontrolled systemic hypertension.

Intermediate predictors of increased cardiovascular risk are: stable angina pectoris, previous myocardial infarction, compensated heart failure, diabetes mellitus, and renal insufficiency.

Major predictors of increased cardiovascular risk include: recent myocardial infarction, unstable angina, decompensated heart failure, severe valvular disease, and significant cardiac arrhythmias.

Functional capacity. The history should also seek to determine the patient's functional capacity (an individual's ability to perform a spectrum of common daily tasks), which is expressed in terms of metabolic equivalents (METs). Cardiac risks in association with noncardiac procedures are increased in patients unable to meet a 4-MET demand (climb a flight of stairs, walk uphill, walk on level ground at 6.4 km/hr, run a short distance).

Vital signs

Blood pressure. Blood pressure provides a useful clue that will either confirm or rule out significant cardiovascular disease. Although high blood pressure (< 180/110 mmHg) is not an independent predictor of cardiovascular risk in association with noncardiac procedures, it serves as a useful marker for coronary artery disease and myocardial ischemia and correlates with postoperative cardiac morbidity.

Pulse pressure, rate, and rhythm. The pulse pressure correlates closely with systolic blood pressure and is a reliable cofactor that will provide further evidence to either confirm or rule out significant cardiovascular disease. Pulse rate less than 50 or greater than 120 beats per minute (bpm) should be considered a medical emergency. In addition, premature ventricular contractions, characterized by a pronounced pause in an otherwise normal rhythm, in patients with cardiovascular diseases are significant findings.

Treatment strategies

Treatment strategies for patients with cardiovascular diseases take into consideration the patient's overall health as reflected by the patient's medical history and vital signs (Table 6-1). In medicine, a stepwise approach to the assessment of cardiac risk (combined incidence of nonfatal myocardial infarction, heart failure, and sudden cardiac death syndrome) for various noncardiac medical surgical procedures confirmed that different procedures are associated with different cardiac risks. Cardiac risk most often reflects such procedure-specific variables as fluid shifts, blood loss, duration of a procedure, and associated physiological and psychological stress. There are no adequately controlled or randomized clinical trials that help define cardiac risk for various dental procedures. However, there is some evidence that dental procedures, in general, are low or very low cardiac-risk procedures.

Table 6-1. Treatment Protocols for the Dental Management of Patients With Cardiovascular Disease

PREDICTORS OF CARDIOVASCULAR RISK	PHYSICAL EXAMINATION	TREATMENT OPTIONS	CONSULTATIONS/REFERRALS
	• Blood pressure < 180/110 mmHg • Normal pulse pressure, rate, and rhythm • Functional capacity > 4 METs	Comprehensive care	Routine referral to a physician for medical management and risk factor modification
Intermediate or minor	• Blood pressure < 180/110 mmHg • Normal pulse pressure, rate, and rhythm • Functional capacity < 4 METs	Limited care	Routine referral to a physician for medical management and risk factor modification
	• Blood pressure > 180/110 mmHg *and/or* • Abnormal pulse pressure, rate, or rhythm	Emergency care	If patient is asymptomatic, routine referral to a physician for medical management and risk factor modification. If patient is symptomatic, immediate referral to a physician for medical management and risk factor modification.
Major	• Establish baseline vital signs	Emergency care	Immediate referral to a physician for medical management and risk factor modification

METs, metabolic equivalents.

Local anesthesia. The physiological events associated with the "stress" of a procedure and the administration of anesthetic agents can affect cardiac function. For most procedures in dentistry, the use of local anesthesia provides the greatest margin of safety. However, in the absence of profound regional anesthesia, the patient may experience myocardial ischemia. Local anesthetic agents may contain epinephrine 1:100,000 (0.01 mg/mL), epinephrine 1:200,000 (0.005 mg/mL), epinephrine 1:50,000 (0.02 mg/mL), or levonordefrin 1:20,000 (0.05 mg/mL), which is physiologically equivalent to epinephrine 1:100,000. (Although many textbooks caution against the use of epinephrine 1:50,000, the critical issue to consider is the total dosage of epinephrine used and not the concentration.) Healthy adults can safely receive up to 0.2 mg of epinephrine per visit. As mentioned earlier, cardiac risks in association with noncardiac procedures are increased in patients unable to meet a 4-MET demand (climb a flight of stairs, walk uphill, walk on level ground at 6.4 km/hr, run a short distance). Ergometric stress testing confirmed that the hemodynamic effects of 4 METs is equivalent to that produced by 0.045 mg of epinephrine. Consequently, 4.5 mL of a local anesthetic agent with epinephrine 1:100,000, or equivalent, can be administered safely to a patient whose functional capacity is equal to or greater than 4 METs. (See Chapter 3 on CD-ROM: *Medical Management of Acute Odontogenic Pain.*) Local anesthesia may be supplemented with an oral benzodiazepine, nitrous oxide, or intravenous sedation; an opioid-based analgesic tends to contribute to postoperative cardiovascular stability.

The patient taking antithrombotic agents. Acetylsalicylic acid (ASA) is a relatively weak antithrombotic agent, inhibiting only thromboxane A_2-mediated platelet aggregation, and the intraoperative and postoperative impacts on invasive dental procedures are minimal. Similarly, clopidogrel, which inhibits platelet aggregation induced by adenosine diphosphate, has minimal effect on intraoperative or postoperative bleeding associated with dental procedures. However, the use of clopidogrel, in addition to ASA, has been associated with increased risk of bleeding, and measurement of the patient's bleeding time can be helpful in determining the degree of antithrombotic effect and its potential impact on invasive dental procedures.

The patient taking enteric anticoagulants (warfarin). A clear relationship exists between the intensity of anticoagulation and the incidence of thromboembolism on the one hand and problematic bleeding on the other. For most medical indications, a moderate-intensity anticoagulation effect with a target international normalized ratio (INR) of 2.0 to 3.0 is appropriate. At this range, most patients can undergo routine oral surgical procedures without alterations of their warfarin regimen. However, to prevent potentially serious complications, the preoperative assessment of the patient's level of anticoagulation is imperative to ensure values that may preclude problematic bleeding yet maintain therapeutic anticoagulation (INR 2.0 to 3.0). Once an acceptable therapeutic range is confirmed, one may proceed with administering local anesthesia with caution to minimize the formation of a hematoma and, using meticulous local measures such as minimal trauma, the application of local hemostatic agents and the placement of sutures to ensure hemostasis.

The patient with an implanted pacemaker or implanted cardioverter defibrillator (ICD). Current generated by medical/dental devices may affect pacing and sensing thresholds. Inhibition of both pacemakers and ICDs is documented with electrosurgical units, ultrasonic scalers, and ultrasonic cleaners. The rate and rhythm of pacing appear to be unaffected by dental handpieces, amalgamators, electric pulp testers, composite curing lights, electric toothbrushes, microwave ovens, dental units and lights, endodontic ultrasonic instruments, sonic scalers, and radiographic units.

Preventive strategies

Several studies suggest a possible link between periodontal disease and atherosclerosis. Periodontal inflammation provides an environment that supports transient bacteremia during activities of daily living such as eating, brushing, and flossing. Invasion of endothelial and smooth muscle cells of the arterial wall by bacterial pathogens could initiate and/or exacerbate the inflammatory process. Current evidence also suggests that periodontal pathogens may also play a role in the thromboembolic aspects of coronary artery disease. Although there is no evidence that treatment of periodontal disease reduces the incidence of coronary artery disease, dental management plans should include appropriate oral hygiene and the use of topical rinses and fluorides. Patients with xerostomia may also benefit from the administration of a sialagogue such as pilocarpine or cevimeline hydrochloride.

Potential medical emergencies

See the Cardiovascular Emergencies section of Chapter 7: *Management of Medical Emergencies in the Oral Health Care Setting*. Other medical emergencies may be anticipated based on the patient's medical history and vital signs.

THE PATIENT TAKING INSULIN AND ORAL HYPOGLYCEMIC AGENTS

Glucose is an optional fuel for tissues such as muscle, fat, and liver because they can also use other substances to satisfy their energy needs. However, glucose is an obligate fuel for the central nervous system (CNS). Because the brain can neither synthesize nor store more than a few minutes' supply of glucose, normal cerebral function requires a continuous infusion of glucose from the circulation. Plasma glucose concentration is closely regulated by the autonomic nervous system to maintain delivery of this crucial substance to the CNS. Insulin, a simple protein synthesized by pancreatic beta-cells, is one of two important hormones in carbohydrate metabolism. The other hormone is glucagon, synthesized by pancreatic alpha-cells. Insulin and glucagon have opposing effects on circulating glucose levels. Insulin is a hypoglycemic agent; it stimulates cellular glucose uptake. Beta-cell destruction leads to absolute insulin deficiency and the patient is labeled as having type 1 diabetes mellitus. If the patient has metabolic abnormalities characterized by resistance to the action of insulin with relative insulin deficiency, excess hepatic glucose production, or an inadequate compensatory insulin secretory response, the patient is labeled as having type 2 diabetes mellitus.

INSULIN

short-acting insulin lispro (Humalog)

intermediate-acting insulin NPH (Humulin N)

intermediate-acting insulin NPH with short-acting regular insulin (Humulin 70/30)

long-acting insulin glargine (Lantus)

Mechanisms of action

Insulin is a hypoglycemic agent; it stimulates cellular glucose uptake.

Clinical indications

• Type 1 and type 2 diabetes mellitus

ORAL HYPOGLYCEMIC AGENTS

Sulfonylureas	Biguanides	Thiazolidinediones
glimepiride (Amaryl)	metformin	pioglitazone (Actos)
glipizide (Glucotrol XL)	(Glucophage XR)	rosiglitazone (Avandia)
glyburide	metformin with	
	glyburide (Glucovance)	

Mechanisms of action

- Sulfonylureas stimulate the release of insulin from pancreatic beta-cells.
- Biguanides and thiazolidinediones decrease insulin resistance and improve insulin's effectiveness.

Clinical indications

- Type 2 diabetes mellitus

PRINCIPLES OF DENTAL MANAGEMENT

When treating a patient taking insulin and/or oral hypoglycemic agents, the goal is to develop and implement timely preventive and therapeutic strategies compatible with the patient's physical and emotional ability to undergo and respond to dental care and with the patient's social and psychological needs.

Medical history

A history of polyuria, nocturia, polydipsia, polyphagia, weakness, obesity (type 2 diabetes mellitus), weight loss without dieting (type 1 diabetes mellitus), and pruritus should suggest diabetes mellitus. However, many patients do not manifest all the classic signs and symptoms. Because microvascular disease associated with diabetes mellitus, which leads to retinopathy and renal dysfunction, begins to develop 7 years before the clinical diagnosis of type 2 diabetes mellitus, oral health care providers should recognize other evidence, such as history of repeated cutaneous infections, ulcerations of the lower extremities, gradual loss of vision, easy bruising, and oral problems suggestive of undiagnosed or uncontrolled diabetes mellitus. Patients with diabetes mellitus are also more likely to have hypertension and dyslipidemia. Diabetes mellitus causes or contributes to macrovascular disease, which significantly increases the risk of coronary artery, cerebrovascular, and peripheral vascular disease. Coronary artery disease leads to unstable coronary syndromes, heart failure, and cardiac arrhythmias. Long-term hyperglycemia also produces tissue damage, which ultimately leads to historical evidence of neuropathy. When reviewing the medical history of patients with known diabetes mellitus, oral health care providers should determine the following:

- Degree of glycemic control
  - Self-monitoring of blood glucose (SMBG) allows patients to evaluate their response to therapy and assess whether glycemic targets are met. Results of SMBG can be useful in the oral health care setting pretreatment, intratreatment, and posttreatment to prevent hypoglycemia.

○ Glycated hemoglobin (HbA1c) concentrations reflect mean glycemia over the preceding 6 to 12 weeks. It is useful in determining whether a patient's metabolic control has been reached and maintained during the preceding 3 months.

- The type of diabetes mellitus and how long the patient has had diabetes mellitus
- The frequency of visits to a physician and the purpose of those visits
- The type of insulin and oral drugs used
- Incidence of hypoglycemic reactions and other complications
- That the patient has taken his or her medication and has had an adequate intake of food
- The patient's functional capacity (see The Patient Taking Cardiovascular Drugs, p. 101)

Vital signs

Blood pressure. Hypertension and dyslipidemia (major causes of atherosclerosis) are comorbid conditions in diabetes mellitus. While high blood pressure (> 180/110 mmHg) is not an independent predictor of cardiovascular risk in association with noncardiac procedures, it serves as a useful marker for coronary artery disease, which is also a common complication of diabetes mellitus.

Pulse pressure, rate, and rhythm. The pulse pressure correlates closely with systolic blood pressure and is a reliable cofactor that will provide further evidence to either confirm or rule out significant cardiovascular disease. Pulse rate less than 50 or greater than 120 bpm should be considered a medical emergency. In addition, premature ventricular contractions, characterized by a pronounced pause in an otherwise normal rhythm, in patients with cardiovascular diseases are significant findings.

Treatment strategies

The physiological events associated with the "stress" of a dental procedure can affect both diabetic control and cardiac function. Consequently, treatment strategies for patients with diabetes mellitus should take into consideration the patient's overall health as reflected by the patient's medical history and vital signs (Table 6-2).

Timing and length of appointments. Long, stressful procedures should be avoided. Patients should preferentially be treated in the morning, after having taken their normal insulin or oral hypoglycemic agent and after having eaten a normal breakfast.

Local anesthetic agents. For most procedures in dentistry, the use of local anesthesia provides the greatest margin of safety. However, in the absence of profound regional anesthesia, the patient may experience myocardial ischemia. When indicated, the local anesthesia may be supplemented with an oral benzodiazepine, nitrous oxide, or intravenous sedation. Epinephrine has an action opposite that of insulin. However, the minute amount of epinephrine included in local anesthetic formulations as a vasoconstrictor, to ensure profound local anesthesia for an appropriate length of time, will not appreciably raise blood glucose levels. In patients with diabetes mellitus, the presence of cardiovascular risk factors in association with dental procedures and the functional capacity of the patient should be the critical determinants for the safe use of a vasoconstrictor (see The Patient Taking Cardiovascular Drugs, p. 101).

Antibacterial agents. The reciprocal relationship between infection and poor glycemic control has led some to advocate the administration of antimicro-

Table 6-2. Treatment Protocols for the Dental Management of Patients With Diabetes Mellitus

Predictors of Diabetic or Cardiovascular Risk	Physical Examination	Treatment Options	Consultations/Referrals
• FBG 70 to 200 mg/dL and/or • Intermediate or minor predictors of cardiovascular risk	• Blood pressure < 180/110 mmHg • Normal pulse pressure, rate, and rhythm • Functional capacity >4 METs	Comprehensive care	Routine referral to a physician for medical management and risk factor modification
	• Blood pressure < 180/110 mmHg • Normal pulse pressure, rate, and rhythm • Functional capacity < 4 METs	Limited care	Routine referral to a physician for medical management and risk factor modification
	• Blood pressure >180/110 mmHg and/or • Abnormal pulse pressure, rate, or rhythm	Emergency care	If patient is asymptomatic, routine referral to a physician for medical management and risk factor modification. If patient is symptomatic, immediate referral to a physician for medical management and risk factor modification.
• FBG < 70 or > 200 mg/dL and/or • Major predictors of cardiovascular risk	• Establish baseline vital signs	Emergency care	Immediate referral to a physician for medical management and risk factor modification

FBG, fasting blood glucose; METs, metabolic equivalents.

bial prophylaxis before dental therapy, particularly in the patient with poorly controlled diabetes. However, there are no studies directly supporting this recommendation. It is axiomatic that any infection in the patient with diabetes, including periodontal disease, must be managed promptly and aggressively. **Postoperative pain management.** Treatment strategies should also include effective postoperative pain management. Opioid-based analgesics effectively block not only pain, but importantly, they tend to contribute to cardiovascular stability. Possible increased hypoglycemic effect with large doses of salicylates has been reported in patients on insulin and increased hypoglycemia with large doses of salicylates has been reported in combination with chlorpropamide, a sulfonylurea. However, usual therapeutic doses of ASA have little effect. Indeed, since many patients with diabetes mellitus are taking ASA as primary or secondary therapy to prevent thromboembolic events, an opioid/ASA formulation is more appropriate than an opioid/ibuprofen formulation, which may interfere with the antiplatelet effect of ASA. Although acetaminophen (APAP) has not been implicated in these drug-drug interactions, APAP is not an anti-inflammatory agent.

Postoperative glycemic control. Procedures that may affect the patient's ability to eat must be planned in consultation with the patient's physician. It is critical that patients have a balanced intake of protein, carbohydrate, and fat in combination with an appropriate regimen of insulin and/or oral hypoglycemic agents to ensure that targeted blood glucose levels are maintained in the postoperative period.

Preventive strategies

Increased susceptibility to periodontal disease does not appear to correlate with increased levels of plaque and calculus, however, patients with diabetes mellitus are at increased risk of developing periodontal disease with age, and the severity of periodontal disease increases with increased duration of diabetes. Although hard evidence on the prevalence of caries in the diabetic patient is equivocal, investigators recently reported an association between resting salivary flow rate less than 0.01 mL/min and a slightly higher prevalence of dental caries. Consequently, dental management plans should include appropriate oral hygiene and the use of topical rinses and fluorides. Patients with xerostomia may benefit from the administration of a sialagogue such as pilocarpine or cevimeline hydrochloride.

Potential medical emergencies

See the Endocrine Emergencies section of Chapter 7: *Management of Medical Emergencies in the Oral Health Care Setting.* Other medical emergencies may be anticipated based on the patient's medical history and vital signs.

THE PATIENT TAKING GLUCOCORTICOSTEROIDS

The adrenal cortex secretes glucocorticoids and mineralocorticoids. The synthesis and secretion of glucocorticoids is under the control of corticotropin (ACTH) and the renin-angiotensin pathway controls mineralocorticoid secretion. Glucocorticosteroids regulate cell metabolism (at the level of translation and transcription), promote gluconeogenesis, and have pronounced anti-inflammatory and immunomodulatory effects. Mineralocorticoids promote sodium retention in the distal convoluted tubule of the kidney. The main glucocorticoid is cortisol, with a daily secretion of 15 mg. The main mineralocorticoid is aldosterone, with a daily secretion of 100 mcg.

DRUGS	
Systemic formulations	**Inhalants/Intranasal formulations**
prednisone	budesonide (Rhinocort AQUA)
	fluticasone (Flovent, Flonase)
	mometasone furoate (Nasonex)
	triamcinolone (Nasacort AQ)

Mechanisms of action

- Decreases inflammation by suppressing the migration of polymorphonuclear leukocytes and by reducing capillary permeability.
- Suppresses the immune system by reducing the volume and activity of lymphocytes.

Clinical indications

- Treatment of a variety of allergic, inflammatory, and autoimmune diseases
- Therapeutic immunosuppression in organ transplant patients
- Allergic rhinitis and asthma
- Neoplastic diseases
- Adrenocortical insufficiency (Addison disease)

PRINCIPLES OF DENTAL MANAGEMENT

When treating a patient taking glucocorticosteroids, the goal is to develop and implement timely preventive and therapeutic strategies compatible with the patient's physical and emotional ability to undergo and respond to dental care and with the patient's social and psychological needs.

Medical history

Hyperadrenocorticism or Cushing syndrome may result from excess endogenous ACTH and/or cortisol secretion and should be considered in patients with a history of pituitary tumors, small-cell lung carcinoma, hypothalamic abnormalities (excess corticotropin-releasing hormone [CRH]), and adrenal adenoma or carcinoma. However, most cases of Cushing syndrome are secondary to the long-term use of "therapeutic" doses of glucocorticoids prescribed or administered for the management of a variety of allergic, inflammatory, and autoimmune diseases; therapeutic immunosuppression in organ transplant patients; allergic rhinitis and asthma; certain neoplastic diseases; and adrenocortical insufficiency (Addison disease). Addison disease may also develop as a consequence of hypothalamic-pituitary-adrenal (HPA) axis suppression following the therapeutic administration of glucocorticoids and lead to an addisonian crisis characterized by hypotension and shock.

Functional capacity. The history should also seek to determine the patient's functional capacity. This is particularly important when treating patients with adrenal dysfunction, because physiological stressors (physical, metabolic, psychological) can destabilize homeostatic mechanisms (see The Patient Taking Cardiovascular Drugs, p. 101).

Vital signs

Cortisol acts in a permissive role and allows catecholamines and angiotensin II to maintain cardiac contractility, vascular tone, and blood pressure. As a result of this increased sympathomimetic activity, heart rate, blood pressure, and respirations are increased. Acute adrenal insufficiency is a medical emergency marked by hypotension, and blood pressure of 90/50 mmHg is a reliable sign of shock. Hypernatremia and hypokalemia secondary to hyperadrenocorticism lead to volume expansion and hypertension. Cortisol-induced hyperglycemia may further contribute to hypertension, dyslipidemia, and cardiovascular complications. A blood pressure in excess of 180/110 mmHg represents a hypertensive crisis. An "at rest" pulse rate below 60 or above 100 bpm in adults, if symptomatic (sweating, weakness, dyspnea, and/or chest pain), should be considered a cardiac risk in association with noncardiac procedures.

Treatment strategies

In medicine, current recommendations for glucocorticoid prophylaxis to prevent an addisonian crisis are based on the anticipated procedure-specific magnitude of physiological stress response. There appears to be universal concordance of procedure-specific cardiovascular and addisonian risk; clearly, the same procedure-specific factors (fluid shifts, blood loss, duration of a procedure, and other physiological events associated with the administration of anesthetic agents) contribute to physiological stress. In view of this, it can be concluded that the risk of an addisonian crisis in association with a dental procedure is also low or very low. Consequently, treatment strategies for a patient with adrenal dysfunction (Table 6-3) should take into consideration the patient's overall health as reflected by the patient's medical history and vital signs.

Local anesthetic agents. The physiological stress associated with the use of local anesthetic agents in patients with adrenal dysfunction is low. As mentioned earlier, cardiac risk, and by extension addisonian risk, in association with physiological stressors increases in patients unable to meet a 4-MET demand. The hemodynamic effects of 4 METs is equivalent to that produced by 0.045 mg of epinephrine. Consequently, 4.5 mL of a local anesthetic agent with epinephrine 1:100,000, or equivalent, can be administered safely to a patient whose functional capacity is equal to or greater than 4 METs. Although local anesthesia eliminates some of the undesirable effects of general anesthesia, in the absence of profound regional anesthesia, the patient may experience increased physiological stress. When indicated, the local anesthesia may be supplemented with oral benzodiazepines, nitrous oxide, or intravenous sedation. Therapeutic strategies should also include an effective postoperative analgesic regimen, importantly one that effectively blocks the stress response and contributes to cardiovascular stability, such as an opioid-based analgesic.

Corticosteroid prophylaxis in association with dental care. A consensus paper in the medical literature recommends that clinicians prescribe "stress dose" glucocorticoids in the amount equivalent to the normal physiological response to procedure-related "stress." Based on available evidence, the risk of an addisonian crisis in association with a dental procedure is low or very low. Similarly, the physiological stress associated with the use of local anesthetic agents in patients with adrenal dysfunction is also low. Consequently, the anticipated perioperative physiological stress in patients undergoing dental care (minor surgical stress) under local dental anesthesia should take only their usual daily glucocorticoid dose before dental intervention. No supplementation is justified. This recommendation also takes into consideration potential risks

Table 6-3.   Dental Management of Patients With Adrenal Dysfunction

PREDICTORS OF ADDISONIAN RISK	PHYSICAL EXAMINATION	TREATMENT OPTIONS	CONSULTATIONS/REFERRALS
	• Blood pressure < 180/110 mmHg • Normal pulse pressure, rate, and rhythm • Functional capacity >4 METs	Usual daily glucocorticoid dose during perioperative period • Comprehensive care	Routine referral to a physician for medical management and risk factor modification
Minor procedure-related stress level • Dental care AND • Local anesthesia	• Blood pressure < 180/110 mmHg • Normal pulse pressure, rate, and rhythm • Functional capacity < 4 METs	Usual daily glucocorticoid dose during perioperative period • Limited care	Routine referral to a physician for medical management and risk factor modification
	• Blood pressure >180/110 mmHg AND/OR • Abnormal pulse pressure, rate and rhythm	Usual daily glucocorticoid dose during perioperative period • Emergency care	If patient is asymptomatic, routine referral to a physician for medical management and risk factor modification. If patient is symptomatic, immediate referral to a physician for medical management and risk factor modification.

METs, metabolic equivalents.

associated with the administration of additional glucocorticosteroids such as fluid retention, hypertension, hyperglycemia, increased risk of infection, impaired wound healing, gastrointestinal bleeding, and psychiatric disturbances. If moderate or major surgical stress is anticipated under general anesthesia and the patient has documented or presumed HPA axis suppression, then appropriate "stress doses" of perioperative steroids are indicated. Topical and inhaled corticosteroids can suppress the HPA axis but rarely cause clinical adrenal insufficiency.

Preventive strategies

Hyperadrenocorticism promotes gluconeogenesis and glycogenolysis and impairs peripheral glucose use. Indeed, an estimated 2% to 3% of patients with type 2 diabetes mellitus suffer from unrecognized Cushing syndrome. Consequently, dental management plans should include appropriate oral hygiene and the use of topical rinses and fluorides. Patients with xerostomia may benefit from the administration of a sialagogue such as pilocarpine or cevimeline hydrochloride.

Potential medical emergencies

The likelihood of an addisonian crisis in the oral health care setting is extremely remote. Other medical emergencies may be anticipated based on the patient's medical history and vital signs. See Chapter 7: *Management of Medical Emergencies in the Oral Health Care Setting.*

THE PATIENT TAKING THYROID HORMONES

Thyroid-stimulating hormone (thyrotropin or TSH), produced in the anterior pituitary, stimulates the production of cyclic adenosine monophosphate (AMP) with corresponding increases in the uptake of circulating inorganic iodide by the thyroid gland. The iodine is oxidized to organic iodine, which binds to tyrosine residues of thyroglobulin to form monoiodotyrosine (MIT) and diiodotyrosine (DIT). Two DIT molecules couple to form thyroxin (T_4) or an MIT molecule couples with one DIT molecule to form triiodothyronine (T_3). Circulating concentrations of the thyroid hormones, T_3 and T_4, are maintained at physiological levels by the interaction of the secretions of the hypothalamus and pituitary and thyroid glands.

DRUGS

levothyroxine (Levothroid, Levoxyl, Synthroid)

Mechanisms of action

- Thyroid hormones are involved in the regulation of growth and development; thermoregulation and calorigenesis; the metabolism of carbohydrates, proteins, and lipids; and they increase oxygen consumption.

- Thyroid hormones act synergistically with epinephrine to enhance glycogenolysis and hyperglycemia and enhance tissue sensitivity to catecholamines possibly by up-regulation of adrenergic receptors.

Clinical indications

- Hypothyroidism

PRINCIPLES OF DENTAL MANAGEMENT

When treating a patient taking thyroid hormones, the goal is to develop and implement timely preventive and therapeutic strategies compatible with the patient's physical and emotional ability to undergo and respond to dental care and with the patient's social and psychological needs.

Medical history

Identifiable risk factors for thyroid dysfunction from the medical history include evidence of previous thyroid disease, surgery or radiotherapy of the thyroid gland, diabetes mellitus or a family history of diabetes mellitus, medications such as lithium carbonate and iodine-containing drugs, pernicious anemia, or primary adrenal insufficiency. Clinicians should also seek to determine the presence or absence of cardiovascular diseases (angina pectoris, coronary artery disease, arrhythmias, congestive heart failure). There is some evidence that patients with dyslipidemia associated with overt hypothyroidism have an increased incidence of coronary artery disease and associated angina pectoris. Furthermore, some patients with hypothyroidism cannot tolerate full replacement therapy because of angina pectoris and increased incidence of myocardial infarction and sudden death. The medical history should also seek to determine the patient's functional capacity (see section on The Patient Taking Cardiovascular Drugs, p. 101).

Vital signs

Myxedema coma is the extreme life-threatening complication of hypothyroidism. It is characterized by hypoventilation, hypotension, and bradycardia. A systolic blood pressure less than 90 mmHg is a reliable sign of shock. Thyroid storm is the extreme manifestation of hyperthyroidism. It is characterized by an elevated temperature, tachycardia, and high blood pressure. A blood pressure in excess of 180/110 mmHg represents a hypertensive crisis. An "at rest" pulse rate below 60 or above 100 bpm in adults, if symptomatic (sweating, weakness, dyspnea, and/or chest pain), should be considered a cardiac risk in association with noncardiac procedures. Respiratory rates less than 10 or greater than 20 breaths per minute may indicate respiratory distress.

Treatment strategies

Hypothyroidism and hyperthyroidism adversely affect cardiac function. Thyroid dysfunction may also be associated with diabetes mellitus (Hashimoto disease) and adrenal disease (autoimmune polyglandular syndrome type 2). Consequently, treatment strategies for a patient with thyroid dysfunction (Table 6-4) should take into consideration the patient's overall health as reflected by the patient's medical history and vital signs.

The hypothyroid patient. Well-controlled, medically supervised patients on thyroid replacement and patients with mild-to-moderate symptoms of hypothyroidism may safely undergo routine dental care under local anesthesia. However, patients with hypothyroidism are hyperreactive to central nervous system depressants (opioid analgesics, anxiolytic agents), which should be administered judiciously.

The hyperthyroid patient. Thyroid hormones appear to act synergistically with epinephrine by increasing tissue sensitivity to catecholamines and by possibly up-regulating adrenergic receptors. An additional problem associated with the use of local anesthetic agents containing epinephrine is related to the treatment of hyperthyroid symptoms with a nonselective beta-adrenergic antagonist. However, these concerns must be balanced against the value of a vasoconstrictor in inducing profound local anesthesia, which is essential in reducing

Table 6-4.	Dental Management of the Patient With Thyroid Dysfunction

- Euthyroid patient OR patient with mild-to-moderate thyroid dysfunction AND/OR minor clinical predictors (advanced age, atrial fibrillation, history of stroke) OR intermediate clinical predictors (stable angina pectoris, previous MI, compensated heart failure, renal insufficiency) of cardiovascular risk

  o Blood pressure < 180/110 mmHg; normal pulse pressure, rate, and rhythm; functional capacity > 4 METs

    ▪ Comprehensive dental care

    ▪ Routine referral for medical management and risk factor modification

  o Blood pressure < 180/110 mmHg; normal pulse pressure, rate, and rhythm; BUT functional capacity < 4 METs,

    ▪ Appropriate limited dental care

    ▪ Routine referral for medical management and risk factor modification

  o Blood pressure > 180/110 mmHg OR systolic blood pressure < 90 mmHg AND/OR abnormal pulse pressure, rate, or rhythm

    ▪ Appropriate emergency dental care

    ▪ If patient is symptomatic, immediate referral for medical management and risk factor modification

    ▪ If patient is asymptomatic, routine referral for medical management and risk factor modification

- Patient with severe hypothyroidism OR thyrotoxicosis AND/OR major clinical predictors (unstable coronary syndrome, decompensated heart failure, severe valvular disease, significant arrhythmias) of cardiovascular risk

  o Appropriate emergency dental care

  o Immediate referral for medical management and risk factor modification

METs, metabolic equivalents. MI, myocardial infaction.

the physiological stress associated with pain. For the patient with overt evidence of hyperthyroidism, the use of vasoconstrictors should be avoided. For all other situations, the cautious use of vasoconstrictors, based on the patient's functional capacity, should be considered. An amount of 4.5 mL of a local anesthetic agent with epinephrine 1:100,000, or equivalent, can be administered safely to a patient whose functional capacity is equal to or greater than 4 METs. Furthermore, combination analgesics containing acetylsalicylic acid (ASA) are contraindicated in patients with hyperthyroidism because ASA interferes with the protein binding of T_4 and T_3 (increasing their free form) and lead to thyrotoxicosis. The analgesic of choice for patients with inadequately treated or undiagnosed hyperthyroidism is an opioid-APAP combination.

Preventive strategies

Patients with hypothyroidism may have poor periodontal health. Patients with hyperthyroidism may have increased caries activity and periodontal disease. Consequently, dental management plans for patients with thyroid dysfunction should include appropriate oral hygiene. The use of a topical antibacterial agent is useful to combat gingivitis and other periodontal pathoses that result from plaque accumulation. For patients with xerostomia and a high incidence of dental caries, preventive modalities such as dietary analysis and counseling, and prophylaxis combined with over-the-counter home fluoride use should be implemented. A topical fluoride, 1.1% sodium fluoride in the form of a brush-on gel, may be preferred to a topical solution. Patients may also benefit from simple dietary measures such as eating carrots or celery, or by chewing sugarless or xylitol-containing gums. However, pilocarpine hydrochloride (Salagen) and cevimeline hydrochloride (Evoxac), both muscarinic agonists, may more predictably increase salivary activity.

Potential medical emergencies

The likelihood of myxedema coma or a thyroid crisis in the oral health care setting is extremely remote. Other medical emergencies may be anticipated based on the patient's medical history and vital signs. See Chapter 7: *Management of Medical Emergencies in the Oral Health Care Setting*.

THE PATIENT TAKING REPRODUCTIVE HORMONES

The hypothalamic luteinizing hormone-releasing hormone (LHRH) stimulates the release of both luteinizing hormone (LH) and follicle-stimulating hormone (FSH) from the anterior pituitary gland. LH induces development of ovarian follicles, causes ovulation, and brings forth corpus luteum formation and forms ovarian steroids (progesterone) in females and androgen (testosterone) in males. FSH induces development of ovarian follicles, promotes formation of ovarian steroids (estrogen), and maintains spermatogenesis. The activities of LH and FSH are in turn regulated by feedback inhibition. In addition to negative-feedback inhibition, positive-feedback regulation has been demonstrated. During the follicular phase of the menstrual cycle, the elevated level of estrogen enhances the release of LHRH and augments the responsiveness of the pituitary gland to LHRH. Moreover, the elevated level of progesterone during ovulation imposes a positive-feedback role on FSH. Indeed, the elevated level of estrogen and progesterone and the simultaneous surge of FSH and LH are the factors triggering ovulation.

PRINCIPLES OF DENTAL MANAGEMENT

When treating a patient taking reproductive hormones, the goal is to develop and implement timely preventive and therapeutic strategies compatible with the patient's physical and emotional ability to undergo and respond to dental care and with the patient's social and psychological needs.

Medical history

Confirm in the medical history that the patient is being treated for abnormalities of the female reproductive system; or that the patient may be taking oral contraceptives or hormone replacement therapy; or that the patient may be receiving treatment for breast, endometrial, uterine, prostate, or renal carcinoma; or that the patient may be receiving prophylactic hormone therapy for osteoporosis. In patients on hormone therapy the risk of venous thromboembolism, coronary heart disease, and stroke appears to increase within the first 1 to 2 years of therapy and these harmful effects are likely to exceed the long-term disease prevention benefits in women.

Oral contraceptives	**DRUGS** **Estrogens/Progestins**	**Estrogen modulators**
norgestimate/ethinyl estradiol (Ortho Tri-Cyclen)	conjugated estrogen (Premarin)	raloxifene (Evista)
levonorgestrel/ethinyl estradiol (Aviane)	conjugated estrogen with medroxyprogesterone (Prempro)	
norelgestromin/ethinyl estradiol (Ortho Evra)		
drospirenone/ethinyl estradiol (Yasmin)		

Mechanisms of action

- Estrogens and progesterones inhibit secretion of gonadotropin-releasing hormone via a negative feedback mechanism on the hypothalamus, which alters the normal pattern of FSH and LH secretion by the anterior pituitary.
- An estrogen receptor modulator can act as an estrogen receptor agonist and prevent bone loss or block some estrogen effects, such as those that lead to breast and uterine cancer.

Clinical indications

- Oral contraceptive formulations
  - Prevention of pregnancy or the treatment of hypermenorrhea, endometriosis, and female hypogonadism
- Estrogens
  - Atrophic vaginitis, hypogonadism, primary ovarian failure, menopausal symptoms, prostate carcinoma, and the prevention of osteoporosis
- Progestins
  - Secondary amenorrhea, abnormal uterine bleeding, endometrial and renal carcinoma
- Estrogen modulators
  - Prevention of osteoporosis in postmenopausal women
  - Palliative and adjunctive treatment for advanced breast and uterine cancer

Vital signs

The blood pressure reading provides a clue that will either confirm or rule out significant cardiovascular disease and serves as a useful marker for coronary artery disease and myocardial ischemia. The pulse pressure correlates closely with systolic blood pressure and is a reliable cofactor that will provide further evidence to either confirm or rule out significant cardiovascular disease (see section on The Patient Taking Cardiovascular Drugs, p. 101).

Treatment strategies

Treatment strategies for a patient with modulation/abnormality of the reproductive system should take into consideration the patient's overall health as reflected by the patient's medical history and vital signs.

Oral contraceptives and antibacterial agents. In 1991, the American Dental Association advised dental practitioners to alert all women of child-bearing age of a possible reduction in the efficacy of oral contraceptives during antibiotic therapy. A recent study reviewed the pharmacokinetic and clinical literature relative to the efficacy of oral contraceptives when taken concurrently with antibacterial agents and concluded that there are no pharmacokinetic data at this time to support the contention that oral antibacterial agents reduce the efficacy of oral contraceptives, except for rifampin, an antituberculin drug. The reviewers also concluded that there are no prospective, randomized clinical trials of oral contraceptive efficacy and the concomitant use of antibacterial agents and the case reports used to support such interactions are anecdotal, subject to recall bias, and lack adequate controls and medication documentation. In a recent decision, the United States District Court for the Northern District of California also concluded, "scientific evidence regarding the alleged interaction between antibacterial agents and oral contraceptives did not satisfy the '*Daubert* standard' of causality." However, the American Medical Association concluded that such interactions could not be completely discounted and that women should still be informed of the possibility of such interactions. Similarly, the American Dental Association Council on Scientific Affairs recommends that patients be advised of the potential risk, that patients consider alternative contraception during periods of antibacterial chemotherapy, and that patients be advised of the importance of compliance with their oral contraceptive regimen.

Preventive strategies

The actions of oral contraceptives, in a global sense, appear to mimic pregnancy. Consequently, patients may experience increased incidence of gingivitis, altered salivary flow, and potentially increased caries activity. Similarly, postmenopausal women may experience reduced salivary function, increased caries activity, gingivitis, and periodontitis, but hormone therapy appears to inhibit gingival inflammation, periodontitis, and alveolar bone loss. However, the harmful effects of hormone therapy are likely to exceed the chronic disease prevention benefits in most women. As with all patients, the importance of appropriate oral hygiene cannot be overemphasized. Such strategies should take into consideration toothbrush design and technology to increase the effectiveness of plaque removal. The use of topical antibacterial agents is useful to combat gingivitis and other periodontal pathoses that result from plaque accumulation. For patients with xerostomia and a high incidence of dental caries, preventive modalities such as dietary analysis and counseling, and prophylaxis combined with over-the-counter home fluoride use should be implemented. A topical fluoride, 1.1% sodium fluoride in the form of a brush-on gel, may be preferred to a topical solution. Patients may also benefit from simple dietary measures such as eating carrots or celery, or by chewing sugarless or xylitol-containing gums. However, pilocarpine hydrochloride (Salagen) and cevimeline hydrochloride (Evoxac), both muscarinic agonists, may more predictably increase salivary activity.

Potential medical emergencies

The likelihood of a medical emergency in the oral health care setting associated with reproductive disorders or other conditions for which a patient may be taking a reproductive hormone is extremely remote. Other medical emergencies may be anticipated based on the patient's medical history and vital signs. See Chapter 7: *Management of Medical Emergencies in the Oral Health Care Setting.*

THE PATIENT TAKING BRONCHODILATOR DRUGS

Susceptible patients (genetic predisposition) may experience intermittent, reversible chronic airway inflammation and bronchoconstriction. These events are closely linked to repeated exposure to inhaled allergens. When these antigens are recognized by the immune system, they interact with dendritic cells, the resident antigen-presenting cells of the airways. Cytokines released by T lymphocytes play a central role in orchestrating the immune response. Interleukin (IL)-4 signals B lymphocytes to produce antigen-specific immunoglobulin E (IgE), mast cell proliferation, and the expression by vascular endothelial cells of adhesion molecules for eosinophils. IL-5 prolongs the survival of eosinophils in the bronchial walls. Following subsequent exposure, the inhaled antigens are recognized by the IgE antibodies on the surface of mast cells, leading to mast cell degranulation and the release of inflammatory mediators such as histamine, prostaglandins, leukotrienes, and chemoattractants for eosinophils. These mediators cause immediate airway smooth muscle contraction (bronchospasm), stimulate microvascular leakage and mucous gland secretion (edema), and activate sensory nerve endings (reflex bronchoconstriction via vagal stimulation), and the eosinophils release proteases, which cause epithelial damage and desquamation.

DRUGS

Beta$_2$-receptor agonists	Anticholinergic agents	Leukotriene receptor antagonists (LTRAs)
albuterol	ipratropium/albuterol (Combivent)	montelukast (Singulair)
salmeterol (Advair Diskus)		

Mechanisms of action

- Albuterol is a short-acting and salmeterol is a long-acting beta$_2$-receptor agonist, which relax bronchial smooth muscle.
- Ipratropium blocks the action of acetylcholine in bronchial smooth muscle causing bronchodilation.
- Montelukast is a selective and competitive LTRA. Leukotrienes are associated with the pathophysiology of asthma, airway edema, smooth muscle contraction, and other inflammatory processes.

Clinical indications

- Asthma
- Chronic obstructive pulmonary disease (COPD)

PRINCIPLES OF DENTAL MANAGEMENT

When treating a patient taking a bronchodilator drug, the goal is to develop and implement timely preventive and therapeutic strategies compatible with the patient's physical and emotional ability to undergo and respond to dental care and with the patient's social and psychological needs.

Medical history

Asthma. Asthma most often begins in childhood, typically before 5 to 7 years of age. In most patients the symptoms are intermittent, despite the persistence of inflammation. At the other extreme are patients who suffer cough, wheezing, and/or shortness of breath virtually all the time, which interferes with daily activities and poses a risk for severe, potentially life-threatening, acute asthma attacks. In addition to the drugs noted above, depending on the severity of asthma, patients may also be on inhaled or oral glucocorticosteroids (see section on The Patient Taking Glucocorticosteroids, p. 113). About 10% of asthmatics have a triad of aspirin-induced asthma, nasal polyps, and sinusitis.

Chronic bronchitis. Chronic bronchitis is seen most commonly in smokers 35 years or older. Severe, recurrent respiratory infections as a child and air pollution may be contributing factors. Chronic bronchitis is characterized by a productive cough. Hypoxic hypoxemia, carbon dioxide retention, respiratory acidosis, and right heart failure may occur early. Chronic hypoxemia leads to polycythemia and right heart failure leads to cyanosis. The course of the disease is gradual until heart failure occurs.

Emphysema. Emphysema is usually preceded by chronic bronchitis. It has been suggested that cigarette smoke stimulates proteases and inhibits antiprotease activity. Emphysema may also be a result of a hereditary defect (lack of protease inhibitor) that allows for protease digestion of pulmonary elastic tissues. In advanced cases there is right heart failure, peripheral edema, and hepatomegaly.

Functional capacity. The history should also seek to determine the patient's functional capacity, an individual's ability to perform a spectrum of common daily tasks, which is expressed in terms of metabolic equivalents (METs). Cardiac risks in association with noncardiac procedures are increased in patients unable to meet a 4-MET demand (climb a flight of stairs, walk uphill, walk on level ground at 6.4 km/hr, run a short distance).

Vital signs

The blood pressure reading provides a clue that will either confirm or rule out significant cardiovascular disease and serves as a useful marker for coronary artery disease and myocardial ischemia. A systolic blood pressure lower than 90 mmHg is a reliable sign of shock. A blood pressure in excess of 180/110 mmHg represents a hypertensive crisis. The pulse pressure correlates closely with systolic blood pressure and is a reliable cofactor that will provide further evidence to either confirm or rule out significant cardiovascular disease. An "at rest" pulse rate below 60 or above 100 bpm in adults, if symptomatic (sweating, weakness, dyspnea, and/or chest pain), should be considered a cardiac risk in association with noncardiac procedures. The patient's respiration (rate and character) should also be monitored. Respiratory rates less than 10 or greater than 20 breaths per minute may indicate respiratory distress. Patients with asthma may experience acute respiratory distress as a result of oxygenation failure. Acute respiratory distress in patients with COPD is a complication of ventilation failure.

Treatment strategies

The clinician treating a patient with asthma or COPD must develop treatment strategies taking into consideration the patient's degree of respiratory dysfunction and the patient's overall health as reflected by the patient's medical history and vital signs. The physiological events (emotional stress) associated with a dental procedure can lead to respiratory distress. Reduce anxiety and ensure profound local anesthesia during treatment. However, high-dose local anesthetic agents, anxiolytic agents, and opioid analgesics may depress respiration, mandating their judicious use.

Preventive strategies

As with all patients, the importance of appropriate oral hygiene cannot be overemphasized. Such strategies should take into consideration effectiveness of plaque removal. The use of topical antibacterial agents is useful to combat gingivitis and other periodontal pathoses that result from plaque accumulation. For patients with xerostomia and a high incidence of dental caries, preventive modalities such as dietary analysis and counseling, and prophylaxis combined with over-the-counter home fluoride use should be implemented. A topical fluoride, 1.1% sodium fluoride in the form of a brush-on gel, may be preferred to a topical solution. Patients may also benefit from simple dietary measures such as eating carrots or celery, or by chewing sugarless or xylitol-containing gums. However, pilocarpine hydrochloride (Salagen) and cevimeline hydrochloride (Evoxac), both muscarinic agonists, may more predictably increase salivary activity.

Potential medical emergencies

See the section on Respiratory Emergencies in Chapter 7: *Management of Medical Emergencies in the Oral Health Care Setting*. Other medical emergencies may be anticipated based on the patient's medical history and vital signs.

THE PATIENT TAKING HISTAMINE$_1$-RECEPTOR ANTAGONISTS

Histamine is a biogenic amine synthesized primarily in mast cells and basophils, some cells of the gastric mucosa, and histaminergic neurons in the central nervous system (CNS). The actions of histamine are mediated by histamine binding to H_1, H_2, or H_3 receptors. H_1 receptor activation is involved chiefly in inflammation and allergic reactions. They are expressed primarily on vascular endothelial cells and smooth muscle cells. Stimulation of H_1 receptors results in edema (blood vessel dilation and increased vascular permeability), bronchospasm, and sensitization of primary efferent nerve terminals. H_2 receptors are expressed primarily on parietal cells of the gastric mucosa where they act synergistically with gastrin and acetylcholine to regulate acid secretion. H_3 receptors are expressed on presynaptic nerve terminals in the CNS and some peripheral nerves, where they are believed to cause feedback inhibition of certain effects of histamine.

DRUGS

cetirizine (Zyrtec, Zyrtec D12HR)

desloratadine (Clarinex)

fexofenadine (Allegra)

meclizine

olopatadine (Patanol)

Mechanisms of action

- Compete with histamine at H_1-receptor sites in the gastrointestinal, vascular, and respiratory systems.

Clinical indications

- Perennial and seasonal allergic rhinitis
- Urticaria and other allergic symptoms

PRINCIPLES OF DENTAL MANAGEMENT

When treating a patient who is taking an H_1-receptor antagonist, the goal is to develop and implement timely preventive and therapeutic strategies compatible with the patient's physical and emotional ability to undergo and respond to dental care and with the patient's social and psychological needs.

Medical history

Confirm in the medical history evidence of perennial and seasonal allergic rhinitis, urticaria, or other allergic symptoms. Many patients habitually take drugs for minor complaints and often do not recognize nonprescription medications as drugs and, therefore, may not mention the use of antihistamines. This is particularly important to note because most first-generation antihistamines are over-the-counter formulations. First-generation antihistamines have high lipid solubility and readily penetrate the blood-brain barrier, which accounts for the sedative effect of these drugs. Other side effects include xerostomia as a result of a weak anticholinergic effect. Second-generation H_1-receptor antagonists are ionized at physiological pH, are highly protein bound, are less likely to diffuse into the CNS, and, consequently, do not produce significant sedation.

Vital signs

Because first-generation H_1-receptor antagonists are CNS depressants, it would be prudent to establish baseline blood pressure and pulse rate and character prior to the initiation of dental care. A systolic blood pressure lower than 90 mmHg is a reliable sign of shock and a blood pressure in excess of 180/110 mmHg represents a hypertensive crisis. An "at rest" pulse rate below 60 or above 100 bpm in adults, if symptomatic (sweating, weakness, dyspnea, and/or chest pain), should be considered a cardiac risk in association with noncardiac procedures. Furthermore, because patients may be taking these medications for the treatment of allergies associated with asthma-like symptoms, the patient's respiration (rate and character) should also be recorded. Respiratory rates less than 10 or greater than 20 breaths per minute may indicate respiratory distress.

Treatment strategies

Treatment strategies for a patient taking H_1-receptor antagonists should take into consideration the patient's overall health as reflected by the patient's medical history and vital signs. Because first-generation H_1-receptor antagonists may produce sedation, the coadministration of other CNS depressants (anxiolytic agents, local anesthetic agents, opioid analgesics) may lead to further CNS depression. Monitor the dosages administered carefully.

Preventive strategies

Since a weak anticholinergic effect associated with H_1-receptor antagonists produces xerostomia, dental management plans should include appropriate oral hygiene. The use of topical antibacterial agents is useful to combat gingivitis and other periodontal pathoses that result from plaque accumulation. For patients with xerostomia and a high incidence of dental caries, preventive modalities such as dietary analysis and counseling, and prophylaxis combined with over-the-counter home fluoride use should be implemented. A topical fluoride, 1.1% sodium fluoride in the form of a brush-on gel, may be preferred to a topical solution. Patients may also benefit from simple dietary measures such as eating carrots or celery, or by chewing sugarless or xylitol-containing gums. However, pilocarpine hydrochloride (Salagen) and cevimeline hydrochloride (Evoxac), both muscarinic agonists, may more predictably increase salivary activity.

Potential medical emergencies

The likelihood of a medical emergency in the oral health care setting associated with seasonal or perennial allergic rhinitis is extremely remote. Other medical emergencies may be anticipated based on the patient's medical history and vital signs. See Chapter 7: *Management of Medical Emergencies in the Oral Health Care Setting*.

THE PATIENT TAKING HISTAMINE$_2$-RECEPTOR ANTAGONISTS AND PROTON PUMP INHIBITORS

Histamine is a biogenic amine synthesized primarily in mast cells and basophils, some cells of the gastric mucosa, and histaminergic neurons in the CNS. The actions of histamine are mediated by histamine binding to H_1, H_2, or H_3 receptors. The major function of the histamine (H_2) receptor is to mediate gastric acid secretion in the stomach. This receptor subtype is expressed on parietal cells of the gastric mucosa, where it acts synergistically with gastrin and acetylcholine. These substances bind their respective receptors on parietal cells, which increases the cytoplasmic accumulation of Ca^{2+}. Ca^{2+} activates protein kinase C, which phosphorylates and activates the H^+/K^+ ATPase (proton pump). The proton pump, by exchanging intracellular H^+ for extracellular K^+, effectively increases H^+ concentration in the gastric and duodenal lumen. Increased concentration of H^+ in the gastric and duodenal lumen and in the esophagus (secondary to reflux), in susceptible patients, may lead to epithelial cell damage.

DRUGS

Histamine$_2$-receptor antagonists	Proton pump inhibitors
ranitidine	esomeprazole (Nexium)
	lansoprazole (Prevacid)
	omeprazole (Prilosec)
	pantoprazole (Protonix)
	rabeprazole (AcipHex)

Mechanisms of action

- Histamine$_2$-receptor antagonists competitively block H_2-receptors in parietal cells, resulting in reduced gastric acid secretion.
- Proton pump inhibitors suppress gastric acid secretion by inhibiting parietal H^+/K^+ ATPase.

Clinical indications

- Gastroesophageal reflux disease (GERD)
- Peptic ulcer disease (PUD)

PRINCIPLES OF DENTAL MANAGEMENT

When treating a patient taking an H_2-receptor antagonist and/or a proton pump inhibitor, the goal is to develop and implement timely preventive and therapeutic strategies compatible with the patient's physical and emotional ability to undergo and respond to dental care and with the patient's social and psychological needs.

Medical history

Confirm in the medical history evidence of GERD and/or PUD. The drug history may reveal evidence of prior or current H_2-receptor antagonist and/or a proton pump inhibitor therapy. Note that some formulations are available over the counter and some patients may also routinely self-administer antacids. The primary determinant of GERD appears to be transient relaxation of the lower esophageal sphincter (not induced by a swallow), most commonly after meals. Episodes of transient relaxation are exacerbated in the presence of a hiatal hernia, obesity, and smoking (nicotine relaxes the lower esophageal sphincter). The typical symptom associated with GERD is substernal burning pain radiating up to the neck (relieved immediately by antacids) brought on by positions that encourage gastroesophageal reflux, mainly lying flat and stooping after a meal.

The main pathophysiological mechanisms involved in PUD are *Helicobacter pylori* infection and the use of cyclooxygenase (COX)-1 inhibitors. Stress, alcohol, caffeine, cigarette smoking, and genetic factors further exacerbate the injury. The principal symptom is abdominal pain. The patient often has a history of remissions, with complete freedom from symptoms for weeks or months. Vomiting may also occur with PUD, and the patient is predisposed to hemorrhage, perforation, and pyloric stenosis.

Vital signs

The typical symptom associated with GERD is substernal burning pain mimicking pain of cardiac origin. The blood pressure provides a clue that will either confirm or rule out significant cardiovascular disease and serves as a useful marker for coronary artery disease and myocardial ischemia. The pulse pressure correlates closely with systolic blood pressure and is a reliable cofactor that will provide further evidence to either confirm or rule out significant cardiovascular disease.

Treatment strategies

Treatment strategies for a patient taking H_2-receptor antagonists and/or proton pump inhibitors should take into consideration the patient's overall health as reflected by the patient's medical history and vital signs. COX-1 inhibitors are the drugs of choice in the medical management of odontogenic pain. However, the gastrointestinal tract is the most common target for the adverse effects of these drugs. COX-1 inhibitor–induced gastrointestinal damage is attributable to both topical as well as systemic effects. COX-1 inhibitors are weak acids that readily cross into gastric epithelial cells. In the neutral pH intracellular environment, they become ionized, accumulate (ion trapping), and cause cell damage. The systemic injury is related to decreased prostaglandin synthesis. Decreased prostaglandin synthesis leads to increased gastric acid secretion, decreased bicarbonate and mucus production, and decreased blood flow.

Preventive strategies

Dental management plans should include appropriate oral hygiene. The use of topical antibacterial agents is useful to combat gingivitis and other periodontal pathoses that result from plaque accumulation. For patients with xerostomia and a high incidence of dental caries, preventive modalities such as dietary analysis and counseling, and prophylaxis combined with over-the-counter home fluoride use should be implemented. A topical fluoride, 1.1% sodium fluoride in the form of a brush-on gel, may be preferred to a topical solution. Patients may also benefit from simple dietary measures such as eating carrots or celery, or by chewing sugarless or xylitol-containing gums. However, pilocarpine hydrochloride (Salagen) and cevimeline hydrochloride (Evoxac), both muscarinic agonists, may more predictably increase salivary activity.

Potential medical emergencies

The likelihood of a medical emergency in the oral health care setting associated with GERD or PUD is extremely remote. Other medical emergencies may be anticipated based on the patient's medical history and vital signs. See Chapter 7: *Management of Medical Emergencies in the Oral Health Care Setting*.

THE PATIENT TAKING AN ANXIOLYTIC AGENT

Excitatory and inhibitory amino acid neurotransmitters regulate a diverse array of behavioral processes. The primary inhibitory neurotransmitter in the CNS is gamma-aminobutyric acid (GABA). There are two main types of GABA receptors: $GABA_A$ and $GABA_B$. Activation of $GABA_A$ receptors results in conformational changes that open ligand-gated Cl^- ion channels. GABA binding to $GABA_B$ receptors activates G proteins, which open K^+ channels and allow for efflux K^+ ions. The inward flow of Cl^- and efflux of K^+ result in hyperpolarization and decrease the excitability of target cells. Thereby, GABAergic neurotransmission depresses the CNS.

DRUGS

alprazolam

diazepam

lorazepam

temazepam

zolpidem (Ambien)

Mechanisms of action

- The benzodiazepines potentiate GABA binding to $GABA_A$ receptors and increase the duration of Cl^- channel opening.
- Zolpidem is structurally different from the benzodiazepines, however it has a similar mechanism of action.

Clinical indications

- Anxiety
- Alcohol detoxification
- Panic attack
- Seizures
- Preoperative sedation
- Insomnia
- Muscle spasm

PRINCIPLES OF DENTAL MANAGEMENT

When treating a patient taking a $GABA_A$ receptor agonist, the goal is to develop and implement timely preventive and therapeutic strategies compatible with the patient's physical and emotional ability to undergo and respond to dental care and with the patient's social and psychological needs.

Medical history

Benzodiazepines are used as anxiolytics, hypnotics, antiepileptics, muscle relaxants, and prophylactic drugs against the symptoms of ethanol withdrawal. A significant number of patients are taking these drugs for the treatment of anxiety. Symptoms of anxiety may be associated medical (cardiovascular, metabolic, respiratory) and psychiatric illness (depressive syndrome, psychoses) or psychological anxiety (phobias). Evaluation directed toward the patient's "somatic locus" of anxiety, the system most prominently affected, provides the greatest yield to the investigating clinician.

Vital signs

When GABA$_A$ receptor agonists are prescribed for the treatment of symptoms of anxiety associated with systemic disease, determination of baseline vital signs before the initiation of dental intervention may be prudent. The blood pressure reading provides a clue that will either confirm or rule out significant cardiovascular disease and serves as a useful marker for coronary artery disease and myocardial ischemia. The pulse pressure correlates closely with systolic blood pressure and is a reliable cofactor that will provide further evidence to either confirm or rule out significant cardiovascular disease. Furthermore, since patients may be taking these medications for the treatment of anxiety associated with respiratory abnormalities, the patient's respiration (rate and character) should also be recorded. Respiratory rates less than 10 or greater than 20 breaths per minute may indicate respiratory distress.

Treatment strategies

Treatment strategies for a patient taking a GABA$_A$ receptor agonist should take into consideration the patient's overall health as reflected by the patient's medical history and vital signs. Benzodiazepines, when used alone, rarely cause significant CNS depression. However, ethanol, other CNS depressants, and opioid analgesics may enhance their CNS effect, mandating judicious concomitant use.

Preventive strategies

Dental management plans should include appropriate oral hygiene. The use of topical antibacterial agents is useful to combat gingivitis and other periodontal pathoses that result from plaque accumulation. For patients with xerostomia and a high incidence of dental caries, preventive modalities such as dietary analysis and counseling, and prophylaxis combined with over-the-counter home fluoride use should be implemented. A topical fluoride, 1.1% sodium fluoride in the form of a brush-on gel, may be preferred to a topical solution. Patients may also benefit from simple dietary measures such as eating carrots or celery, or by chewing sugarless or xylitol-containing gums. However, pilocarpine hydrochloride (Salagen) and cevimeline hydrochloride (Evoxac), both muscarinic agonists, may more predictably increase salivary activity.

Potential medical emergencies

The likelihood of a medical emergency in the oral health care setting associated with the conditions for which a patient may be taking a GABA$_A$ receptor agonist is extremely remote. Other medical emergencies may be anticipated based on the patient's medical history and vital signs. See Chapter 7: *Management of Medical Emergencies in the Oral Health Care Setting*.

THE PATIENT TAKING AN ANTICONVULSANT

Seizures are one of the most common neurological disorders affecting humans. A symptom rather than a disease, it is characterized by recurrent convulsions.

Seizures stem from acute changes in the availability of excitatory or inhibitory neurotransmitters within the brain and are accompanied by sudden disturbances in sensory and/or motor function. Seizures are classified according to their clinical manifestations as either partial (begins focally) or generalized (begins generally and involves both hemispheres). Under physiological conditions, neuronal action potentials are propagated by alternating currents of depolarizing Na^+ influx and hyperpolarizing K^+ efflux. At the same time, the firing neurons activate neighboring neurons and interneurons that transmit inhibitory (GABA) signals resulting in "surround inhibition." These events impose a limit on the frequency of firing (prevent repetitive firing). Disruption of this intricate balance (abnormal synchronous discharge) is characteristic of all forms of seizures. Finally, T-type calcium channels associated with relay neurons connecting the thalamus to the cortex, which under physiological conditions are depolarized and inactive during the awake state, may undergo paroxysmal hyperpolarization initiating absence (petit mal) seizure.

DRUGS

Na^+ channel-mediated inhibition	GABA-mediated inhibition	T-type calcium channel inhibition	Mechanism unknown
phenytoin (Dilantin)	clonazepam gabapentin (Neurontin)	valproic acid (Depakote)	topiramate (Topamax)

Mechanisms of action

Anticonvulsants, by different mechanisms of action, appear to stabilize neuronal activity.

Clinical indications

• Seizure disorders

PRINCIPLES OF DENTAL MANAGEMENT

When treating a patient taking anticonvulsants, the goal is to develop and implement timely preventive and therapeutic strategies compatible with the patient's physical and emotional ability to undergo and respond to dental care and with the patient's social and psychological needs.

Medical history

Partial seizures. Partial seizures, defined as aberrant motor or psychomotor activity, result from a local discrete spread of excitation. Simple motor seizures often follow physical injury to the head: trauma to the motor cortex is characterized by involuntary, repetitive movement; abnormal activity in the sensory cortex may produce paresthesia; and trauma to the visual cortex produces flashing lights. Consciousness is typically preserved. Psychomotor or complex partial seizures are caused by abnormal activity in the temporal or frontal lobes and are preceded by an aura, may produce altered consciousness, and are often associated with involuntary automatism such as smacking of lips or wringing of hands. Partial seizures may progress to secondary generalized seizure.

Tonic-clonic (grand mal) seizures. Tonic-clonic (grand mal) seizures are characterized by loss of consciousness usually preceded by an aura (visual, auditory, epigastric, or psychic). Initial convulsions explosively force air out of the lungs, resulting in the epileptic "cry." Generalized motor tonic-clonic seizures follow this eerie, birdlike scream. The tonic component of the seizure is characterized by opisthotonos, the arched position (convexity in the ventral body region) caused by the violent spasm of back muscles. The clonic component is characterized by rhythmic movements (contraction and relaxation of muscles) of all limbs. Postseizure depression of motor and sensory function is common.

Absence (petit mal) seizures. Absence (petit mal) seizures are a form of generalized seizure characterized by sudden, brief interruption of consciousness. They are termed absence seizures because these attacks cause the patient to simply stare off into space. Patients do not experience an aura but occasional motor symptoms such as smacking of lips or rapid blinking may be noted. Commonly seen in the prepubertal years.

Myoclonic attacks. Myoclonic attacks are generalized seizures characterized by rhythmic body jerks without loss of consciousness. Symptoms may affect individual muscles or may be generalized to all muscle groups of the body contributing to falls. Myoclonic attacks are most often seen in patients with uremia, hepatic failure, hereditary degenerative conditions, and in association with Creutzfeldt-Jacob disease.

Vital signs

Patients taking anticonvulsants may experience a seizure attack while in the oral health care setting, so determination of baseline blood pressure and pulse pressure, rate, and rhythm before the initiation of dental intervention may be prudent. Furthermore, respiratory depression is a potential serious complication of a seizure attack. Baseline respiration (rate and character) should be recorded and the respiration should be monitored closely in the postictal period. Respiratory rates less than 10 or greater than 20 breaths per minute may indicate respiratory distress.

Treatment strategies

Treatment strategies for a patient taking anticonvulsants should consider the patient's degree of seizure control and overall health as reflected by the patient's medical history and vital signs. Confirm the patient's compliance with anticonvulsant chemotherapy. Reduce anxiety and ensure profound local anesthesia during treatment. Anticonvulsants, when used alone, rarely cause significant CNS depression. However, ethanol, other CNS depressants, high-dose local anesthetic agents, and opioid analgesics may enhance their CNS effect, mandating judicious concomitant use.

Preventive strategies

Gingival hyperplasia is one of the well-known effects of phenytoin use. Consequently, dental management plans should include appropriate oral hygiene. The use of topical antibacterial agents is useful to combat gingivitis and other periodontal pathoses that result from plaque accumulation. For patients with xerostomia and a high incidence of dental caries, preventive modalities such as dietary analysis and counseling, and prophylaxis combined with over-the-counter home fluoride use should be implemented. A topical fluoride, 1.1% sodium fluoride in the form of a brush-on gel, may be preferred to a topical solution. Patients may also benefit from simple dietary measures such as eating carrots or celery, or by chewing sugarless or xylitol-containing gums. However, pilocarpine hydrochloride (Salagen) and cevimeline hydrochloride (Evoxac), both muscarinic agonists, may more predictably increase salivary activity.

Potential medical emergencies

See the section on Neurological Emergencies in Chapter 7: *The Management of Medical Emergencies in the Oral Health Care Setting.* Other medical emergencies may be anticipated based on the patient's medical history and vital signs.

THE PATIENT TAKING AN ANTIPSYCHOTIC AGENT

Peripheral adrenergic neurons and most central adrenergic neurons employ norepinephrine as their main neurotransmitter; however, some central adrenergic neurons synthesize and use dopamine. There are two main classes of dopamine receptors: D_1 and D_2. D_1 and D_2 class receptors can be found throughout the brain, but their pattern of distribution varies greatly. The cerebral cortex and limbic structures are innervated by dopaminergic cell bodies from the midbrain, which appear to play a role in motivation, goal-directed thinking, regulation of affect, and positive reinforcement (reward). In addition, serotonin ($5HT_2$) receptor activation appears to lower the threshold for neuronal firing in the CNS (particularly the cortex). The biochemical theory suggests that dysregulation of dopaminergic and/or serotonergic neurotransmission in mesolimbic and mesocortical systems appears, at least partially, to be involved in the pathogenesis of psychoses.

DRUGS

olanzapine (Zyprexa)

quetiapine (Seroquel)

risperidone

Mechanisms of action

Mixed serotonin-dopamine receptor antagonists bind to serotonin ($5HT_2$) and to dopamine (D_2) receptors. These drugs also antagonize alpha$_1$- and alpha$_2$-adrenergic, and histamine (H_1) receptors with relatively high affinity.

Clinical indications

- Psychotic disorders (schizophrenia)
- Dementia in the elderly

Principles of Dental Management

When treating a patient taking an antipsychotic agent, the goal is to develop and implement timely preventive and therapeutic strategies compatible with the patient's physical and emotional ability to undergo and respond to dental care and with the patient's social and psychological needs.

Medical history

The medical history should seek to determine evidence of major disturbances in thought content, bizarre behavior, a regression in intellectual functioning, inappropriate affective expression, and frequent hallucinations and delusions. The social history might suggest social/occupational dysfunction. Confirm the patient's compliance with antipsychotic chemotherapy.

Vital signs

Both dopamine and serotonin are in the catecholamine family of neurotransmitters. Mixed serotonin-dopamine receptor antagonist drugs also antagonize alpha$_1$- and alpha$_2$-adrenergic and histamine (H$_1$) receptors with relatively high affinity. Consequently, determination of baseline blood pressure and pulse pressure, rate, and rhythm before the initiation of dental intervention may be prudent.

Treatment strategies

Treatment strategies for a patient taking antipsychotic drugs should take into consideration the patient's degree of control and overall health as reflected by the patient's medical history and vital signs. Confirm the patient's compliance with antipsychotic chemotherapy. Patients may not understand complex treatment plans or tolerate long appointments. Reduce anxiety and ensure profound local anesthesia during treatment. Antipsychotic drugs, when used alone, rarely cause significant CNS depression. However, ethanol, other CNS depressants, high-dose local anesthetic agents, and opioid analgesics may enhance their CNS effect, mandating judicious concomitant use.

Preventive strategies

Self-care regresses markedly below the level achieved before the onset of psychosis. Consequently, dental management plans should include appropriate oral hygiene. The use of topical antibacterial agents is useful to combat gingivitis and other periodontal pathoses that result from plaque accumulation. For patients with xerostomia and a high incidence of dental caries, preventive modalities such as dietary analysis and counseling, and prophylaxis combined with over-the-counter home fluoride use should be implemented. A topical fluoride, 1.1% sodium fluoride in the form of a brush-on gel, may be preferred to a topical solution. Patients may also benefit from simple dietary measures such as eating carrots or celery, or by chewing sugarless or xylitol-containing gums. However, pilocarpine hydrochloride (Salagen) and cevimeline hydrochloride (Evoxac), both muscarinic agonists, may more predictably increase salivary activity.

Potential medical emergencies

The likelihood of a medical emergency in the oral health care setting associated with psychiatric disorders and dementia is extremely remote. Other medical emergencies may be anticipated based on the patient's medical history and vital signs. See Chapter 7: *Management of Medical Emergencies in the Oral Health Care Setting.*

THE PATIENT TAKING AN ANTIDEPRESSANT

The serotonin (5HT) and norepinephrine (NE) neurotransmitter systems are diffuse projecting systems that modulate the firing of neurons in a disuse or global manner. 5HT-containing cells within the raphe nuclei and NE-containing cells within the locus ceruleus project broadly throughout the cerebral cortex with other projections to the limbic system. The metabolic cycle of both 5HT and NE involve neurotransmitter synthesis, uptake into synaptic vesicles, exocytosis, reuptake into the cytoplasm, and reuptake into vesicles or degradation. Regulation of the levels of 5HT and NE can occur at any of these steps and 5HT and NE also autoregulate their own release. Both 5HT and NE play critical roles in regulating mood and are involved in many other complex neuropsychiatric processes.

DRUGS		
Selective serotonin reuptake inhibitors (SSRIs)	**Tricyclic antidepressants (TCAs)**	**Atypical antidepressants**
citalopram (Celexa)	amitriptyline	bupropion (Wellbutrin)
escitalopram (Lexapro)		trazodone HCl
fluoxetine		
paroxetine (Paxil, Paxil CR)		
sertraline (Zoloft)		
venlafaxine (Effexor XR)		

Mechanisms of action

- SSRIs inhibit serotonin reuptake increasing synaptic serotonin levels, causing increased 5HT receptor activation and enhanced postsynaptic responses.
- TCAs inhibit the reuptake of 5HT and NE from the synaptic cleft by blocking 5HT and NE transporters.
- Bupropion and trazodone inhibit the reuptake of 5HT and NE from the synaptic cleft by a mechanism not fully understood.

Clinical indications

- Depression
- Neuropathic pain

PRINCIPLES OF DENTAL MANAGEMENT

When treating a patient taking an antidepressant, the goal is to develop and implement timely preventive and therapeutic strategies compatible with the patient's physical and emotional ability to undergo and respond to dental care and with the patient's social and psychological needs.

Medical history

Major depressive disorder (MDD) and bipolar disorder (BPD) are both characterized by extremes in mood. MDD is characterized by recurrent major depressive events and BPD is defined by the presence of mania. The social history might suggest social/occupational dysfunction. Confirm the patient's compliance with antidepressant chemotherapy. Patients with MDD may relate a persistent depressed mood or loss of interest in nearly all activities, weight change or significant change in appetite, insomnia, psychomotor slowing, fatigue or loss of energy, impaired concentration, sense of worthlessness or guilt, and thoughts of suicide or death. An abnormally elevated mood, inflated self-esteem or grandiosity; rapid, loud, emphatic speech; and psychomotor agitation characterize a manic episode.

Vital signs

Although rare, the most serious side effects of antidepressants (serotonin syndrome) involve the cardiovascular system and are characterized by tachycardia, cardiac arrhythmia, hypertensive crisis, and stroke. Other clinical manifestations include hyperthermia, muscle rigidity, and fluctuations in mental state. Consequently, determination of baseline blood pressure and pulse pressure, rate, and rhythm before the initiation of dental intervention may be prudent.

Treatment strategies

Treatment strategies for a patient taking antidepressant drugs should take into consideration the patient's degree of control and overall health as reflected by the patient's medical history and vital signs. Confirm the patient's compliance with antidepressant chemotherapy. Patients may not understand complex treatment plans or tolerate long appointments. Reduce anxiety and ensure profound local anesthesia during treatment.

Preventive strategies

Self-care may regress with MDD. Consequently, dental management plans should include appropriate oral hygiene. The use of a topical antibacterial agent is useful to combat gingivitis and other periodontal pathoses that result from plaque accumulation. For patients with xerostomia and a high incidence of dental caries, preventive modalities such as dietary analysis and counseling, and prophylaxis combined with over-the-counter home fluoride use should be implemented. A topical fluoride, 1.1% sodium fluoride in the form of a brush-on gel, may be preferred to a topical solution. Patients may also benefit from simple dietary measures such as eating carrots or celery, or by chewing sugarless or xylitol-containing gums. However, pilocarpine hydrochloride (Salagen) and cevimeline hydrochloride (Evoxac), both muscarinic agonists, may more predictably increase salivary activity.

Potential medical emergencies

The likelihood of a medical emergency in the oral health care setting associated with MDD and BPD is extremely remote. Other medical emergencies may be anticipated based on the patient's medical history and vital signs. See Chapter 7: *Management of Medical Emergencies in the Oral Health Care Setting.*

BIBLIOGRAPHY

1. Belmaker RH. Bipolar disorder. N Engl J Med. 2004;351(5):476–486.
2. Friedlander AH, Marder SR. The psychopathology, medical management and dental implications of schizophrenia. J Am Dent Assoc. 2002;133(5):603–610.
3. Friedlander AH. The physiology, medical management and oral implications of menopause. J Am Dent Assoc. 2002; 133(1):73–81.
4. Huber MA, Terezhalmy GT. Risk stratification and dental management of the patient with adrenal dysfunction. Quintessence Int. In press.
5. Huber MA, Terezhalmy GT. Risk stratification and dental management of the patient with thyroid dysfunction. Quintessence Int. In press.
6. Levin JA, Muzyka BC, Glick M. Dental management of patients with diabetes mellitus. Compend Contin Educ Dent. 1996;17:82–103.
7. Miley DD, Terezhalmy GT. The patient with diabetes mellitus. Quintessence Int. 2005; 36(10):(in press).
8. Miller CS, Little JW, Falace DA. Supplemental corticosteroids for dental patients with adrenal insufficiency: reconsideration of the problem. J Am Dent Assoc. 2001;132(11):1570–1579.
9. Nicholson G, Burrin JM, Hall GM. Peri-operative steroid supplementation. Anesthesia. 1998;53:1091–1104.
10. Salem M, Tainsh RE, Bromberg J, Loriaux DL, Chernow B. Perioperative glucocorticoid coverag: a reassessment 42 years after emergence of a problem. Ann Surg. 1994;219(4):416–425.
11. Steinhauer T, Bsoul SA, Terezhalmy GT. Risk stratification and dental management of the patient with cardiovascular diseases. Part II: the oral disease burden and principles of dental management. Quintessence Int. 2005;36(3): 209–227.
12. Steinhauer T, Bsoul SA, Terezhalmy GT. Risk stratification and dental management of the patient with cardiovascular diseases. Part I: etiology, epidemiology, and principles of medical management. Quintessence Int. 2005;36(2): 119–137.
13. U.S. Preventive Services Task Force. Hormone therapy for the prevention of chronic conditions in postmenopausal women: recommendations from the U.S. Preventive Services Task Force. Ann Intern Med. 2005;142(10):855–860.
14. Vernillo AT. Diabetes mellitus: relevance to dental treatment. Oral Surg Oral Med Oral Pathol Oral Radiol Endod. 2001; 91(3):263–270.
15. Yaltirik M, Kocaelli H, Yargic I. Schizophrenia and dental management: review of the literature. Quintessence Int. 2004;35(4):317–320.

7 Management of Medical Emergencies in the Oral Health Care Setting

Table of Contents

INTRODUCTION

With advances in medicine, oral health care providers are called upon to provide dental care to an ever-increasing number of medically and pharmacologically compromised patients. Consequently, oral health care providers can expect to face situations that may threaten the physical well-being of their patients. Poor preparation for such an eventuality is inexcusable. Being the subject of public censure or accused of negligence is an agony best prevented. This section summarizes common medical emergencies that require immediate response in the dental office. Clinicians must recognize these common disorders and learn to act promptly. The treatment procedures included are those activities a clinician "can't afford not to do" when faced with an unexpected urgent problem.

BEING PREPARED FOR MEDICAL EMERGENCIES

Oral health care providers must be able to assess the physical and emotional ability of a patient to tolerate dental care; identify high-risk patients who may experience a medical emergency; and know how to sustain life with their hands, their breaths, a few basic therapeutic agents, and a great deal of common sense. An awareness of the medical history and the various medications commonly prescribed for patients to self-administer will assist clinicians in anticipating the most commonly encountered medical diagnoses and provide valuable information that will help in identifying high-risk patients who may experience a life-threatening medical emergency.

NEVER TREAT A STRANGER

Determine the patient's medical history prior to all therapeutic interventions.

ASSESS THE PATIENT'S VITAL SIGNS

- Blood pressure (all patients)
- Pulse pressure, rate, and character (all patients)
- Rate and character of respiration (patients with respiratory abnormalities)
- Body temperature (patients with infection)

DETERMINE THE PATIENT'S RISK STATUS

Risk status I
- No evidence of overt systemic disease
- No limitation on physical activity
- Excellent functional capacity

Risk status II
- Evidence of systemic disease
- Medically stable
- No limitation on physical activity
- Good functional capacity

Risk status III
- Evidence of systemic disease
- Medically fragile
- Limitation of physical activity
- Moderate functional capacity

Risk status IV
- Evidence of systemic disease
- Condition(s) constant threat to life
- No physical activity
- Poor functional capacity

KNOW WHAT TO LOOK FOR

Be familiar with the signs and symptoms of the various medical emergencies that may occur in the oral health care setting.

BE ALERT

Monitor the patient's physical well-being during treatment and look for evidence of adverse reactions, particularly when drugs are being administered.

CHECK EMERGENCY EQUIPMENT AND SUPPLIES REGULARLY

Ensure that the equipment is functioning properly and that the emergency drugs are not past their expiration date.

FIRST DO NO HARM

Be adequately trained in emergency medicine and practice with staff under simulated emergency conditions.

DEVELOP AN EMERGENCY TEAM

1. The dentist (emergency team supervisor)
   a. Assesses level of consciousness
   b. Performs physical examination
      i. Obtains initial vital signs
   c. Determines the course of treatment
   d. Initiates cardiopulmonary resuscitation (CPR)
2. Second member
   a. Notifies staff
   b. Gathers emergency equipment and supplies
   c. Prepares therapeutic agents for administration by the dentist
      i. Administers oxygen
   d. Assists with cardiopulmonary resuscitation (CPR)
3. Third member
   a. Monitors vital signs
   b. Records information in the patient's chart
   c. Makes phone calls
   d. Assists with CPR
   e. Performs other tasks

BASIC EMERGENCY PROCEDURES

PRIMARY SURVEY

Five fundamental steps are to be implemented in every emergency situation. Life-threatening problems identified in the primary survey must be treated immediately.

1. Assess responsiveness
   a. Alert
   b. Disoriented
   c. Unresponsive
      i. PERRLA (pupils equal, round, reactive to light, and accommodate)
         1. Constricted, as in drug overdose
         2. Dilated, as in shock
         3. Unequal, as in stroke
2. Check airway
   a. Is the airway open?
      i. Check for movement of air
         1. Look to see whether the chest rises
         2. Listen for airflow
         3. Feel the chest wall for movement
   b. Is the patient properly positioned?
   c. Are respirations effortless or labored with stridor or wheezing?
      i. Check for excessive or frothy saliva and other causes of partial obstruction
   d. Is there complete foreign body obstruction?
      i. If a complete obstruction is suspected, immediately begin procedures to remove obstruction
3. Check breathing
   a. If the patient is responsive and talking, the patient is breathing at this time
   b. Check the rate of respiration
      i. Rates less than 10 or greater that 20 breaths per minute may indicate respiratory distress
         1. In case of respiratory distress, provide positive pressure respiration
4. Check pulse rate
   a. Is there a palpable pulse?
      i. Pulse rates less than 50 beats or greater than 120 beats per minute should be considered a medical emergency
         1. Check for signs of inadequate perfusion (diaphoresis, weakness, dyspnea, chest pain)
      ii. Unresponsiveness and the absence of a palpable pulse must be assumed to be a result of cardiac arrest
         1. Call emergency medical service (EMS)
         2. Immediately begin CPR
5. Check blood pressure
   a. Blood pressure less than 90/50 mmHg
      i. Reliable sign of shock
   b. Blood pressure greater than 180/120 mmHg
      i. Hypertensive syndrome

   c. Sudden drop in blood pressure (20/10 mmHg) following abrupt positional change

      i. Postural hypotension

Nota bene

Unresponsiveness and the absence of a palpable pulse must be assumed to be a result of sudden cardiac arrest. At least 50% of the patients experiencing sudden cardiac arrest have ventricular fibrillation. Consequently, the clinician should think of defibrillation immediately after completing the primary survey.

1. Early CPR and defibrillation provide the best chance of survival for the patient

   a. Oral health care facilities should have a defibrillator and the emergency team should be trained to use it to determine whether a defibrillator shock should be administered to the patient

2. Patients with cardiac arrest who are not in ventricular fibrillation will require continued CPR until the emergency medical service team arrives

Secondary Survey

If the patient is conscious and is communicative, a focused history and physical examination will assist the clinician in identifying the cause of the acute illness. Review or determine the following:

1. Chief complaint

   a. Signs and symptoms

2. Allergies

3. Medications

4. Past medical history

5. Last oral intake of food

6. Events leading up to this incident

Nota bene

The secondary survey directs the clinician to specific problem areas so that he or she may proceed with the physical examination that focuses only on those organ systems that may be associated with the patient's complaints and/or the primary survey findings. The purpose of the secondary survey is to identify problems that are usually not immediately life threatening but require immediate stabilization.

CARDIOVASCULAR EMERGENCIES

The Patient With Vasopressor Syncope

Vasopressor syncope is defined as a sudden brief loss of consciousness. It is a result of cerebral ischemia caused by dilation of resistance vessels. Because cerebral vascular resistance cannot compensate for the dilation of resistance vessels, cerebral blood flow becomes significantly reduced and precipitates a generalized, progressive, autonomic discharge. The initial appropriate adrenergic response to precipitating factors is overwhelmed by a cholinergic response just before unconsciousness.

Predisposing factors

1. Anxiety
   a. Personal and environmental stress
2. Pain
3. Heat and humidity
4. Cardiovascular disorders
   a. Dysrhythmia
   b. Postural hypotension
5. Cerebrovascular insufficiency

Prevention

1. Identify high-risk patient
   a. Reduce stress
   b. Ensure profound local anesthesia
   c. Treat patient in a supine position
   d. Recognize presyncope

Signs and symptoms

1. Adrenergic component
   a. Feeling of anxiety
   b. Pallor
   c. Pupillary dilation
   d. Hyperventilation
   e. Tachycardia
2. Cholinergic component
   a. Perspiration
   b. Nausea
   c. Salivation
   d. Bradycardia
   e. Hypotension
   f. Loss of consciousness
   g. Convulsion (rarely)

Treatment

1. Place patient in a supine position
   a. Head and chest parallel to the floor
   b. Feet slightly elevated
2. Administer oxygen
   a. 4 to 6 L/minute by nasal cannula
3. Stimulate cutaneous reflexes
   a. Cold towel
   b. Amyl nitrate
4. Evaluate pulse rate, respiratory rate, and blood pressure every 10 minutes

5. If at any time the patient becomes unresponsive with no palpable pulse
   a. Call EMS
   b. Initiate CPR
      i. Automated external defibrillator

Nota bene
   Most cases of syncope are benign, especially in young adults who may only require reassurance. Syncope in a patient older than 50 years of age should be regarded as serious. Initiate a medical consultation to determine underlying cause.

THE PATIENT WITH POSTURAL HYPOTENSION

   Postural hypotension is defined as a decline of 20 mmHg or more in the systolic blood pressure, or a decline of 10 mmHg or more in the diastolic blood pressure, or an increase in pulse rate of 20 beats/minute or more, and the presence of accompanying symptoms of cerebral hypoperfusion following postural change from a supine to an upright position. When a patient assumes an upright posture, approximately 500 to 700 mL of blood is pooled in the lower extremities and in splanchnic and pulmonary tissues leading to a decrease in venous blood return to the heart. In susceptible patients, this reduction in blood volume and inadequate cardiovascular compensation for the decline in cardiac preload can lead to postural hypotension.

Predisposing factors

1. Impaired homeostatic mechanisms of blood pressure regulation
   a. Age-related physiological changes
   b. Disease-related physiological changes
   c. Antihypertensive medications
   d. Recent intake of food

Prevention

1. Identify high-risk patients
   a. Schedule dental appointments 30 to 60 minutes after the ingestion of meals and medications
   b. Following treatment, allow susceptible patients to assume an upright position gradually

Signs and symptoms

1. No prodromal signs and symptoms
2. Syncope when the patient assumes an upright position
3. A decline of 20 mmHg or more in the systolic blood pressure
   or
   A decline of 10 mmHg or more in the diastolic blood pressure
   or
   An increase in pulse rate of 20 beats/minute or more

Treatment

1. Return patient to supine position for 5 to 10 minutes
   a. Evaluate pulse rate, blood pressure, and respiratory rate
   b. Administer oxygen
      i. 4 to 6 L/minute by nasal cannula

2. Allow patient to assume a sitting position for at least 2 minutes
    a. Evaluate pulse rate, blood pressure, and respiratory rate
3. Allow patient to stand for 2 minutes
    a. Evaluate pulse rate, blood pressure, and respiratory rate
4. If at any time the patient becomes unresponsive with no palpable pulse
    a. Call EMS
    b. Initiate CPR
        i. Automated external defibrillator

Nota bene
Postural hypotension, often observed in older patients, may result in significant morbidity from associated falls. The lack of prodromal signs and symptoms associated with postural hypotension should prompt oral health care providers to take preemptive action.
1. A systolic blood pressure of less than 90 mmHg is a reliable sign of shock

The Patient With Hypertensive Crisis

Hypertension is defined as a systolic blood pressure greater than 140 mmHg or a diastolic blood pressure greater than 90 mmHg. Hypertensive urgency is defined as a systolic blood pressure greater than 180 mmHg or a diastolic blood pressure greater than 110 mmHg. Hypertensive emergency is defined as a systolic blood pressure greater than 200 mmHg or a diastolic blood pressure greater than 140 mmHg. The mechanisms that lead to hypertensive crises are unclear, but a rise in vascular resistance seems to be a necessary initial step. Increased vasoreactivity can be precipitated by the release of vasoconstrictive substances such as angiotensin II or norepinephrine or can occur as a result of relative hypovolemia.

Predisposing factors

1. Hypertensive emergencies in the oral health care setting are usually associated with patients with unrecognized or undertreated hypertension
    a. Primary hypertension
        i. Hereditary and environmental factors
    b. Secondary hypertension
        i. Renal disease
        ii. Adrenal disease
        iii. Coarctation of the aorta
        iv. Hyperthyroidism
        v. Pregnancy (eclampsia)
        vi. Autonomic hyperactivity
        vii. Central nervous system (CNS) disorders
        viii. Sleep apnea
        ix. Medications (drug-related and drug-induced)

Prevention

1. Identify high-risk patient
    a. Reduce anxiety

b. Determine the patient's functional capacity

    i. Use local anesthetic agents containing a vasoconstrictor with caution but ensure profound local anesthesia

Signs and symptoms

1. Restlessness
2. Flushed face
3. Headache, dizziness, tinnitus
4. Visual disturbances
5. Dyspnea
    a. Pulmonary edema/congestive heart failure
6. A "hammering" pulse
7. Blood pressure greater than 180/110 mmHg
8. Altered mental state
9. Chest pain
    a. Myocardial ischemia, infarction, or aortic dissection
10. Seizure
    a. Hypertensive encephalopathy

Treatment

1. Elevate the patient's head
2. Administer oxygen
    a. 4 to 6 L/minute by nasal cannula
3. Hypertensive urgency (blood pressure greater than 180/110 mmHg)
    a. Blood pressure should be lowered within a few hours
        i. Same day referral to a physician
4. Hypertensive emergency (blood pressure greater than 200/140 mmHg)
    a. Blood pressure should be reduced immediately
        i. Administer nitroglycerin
            1. 0.4 mg, tablet/spray, sublingual (SL)
        ii. Call EMS
        iii. Evaluate pulse rate, blood pressure, and respiratory rate every 5 minutes
        iv. If at any time the patient becomes unresponsive with no palpable pulse
            1. Initiate CPR
                a. Automated external defibrillator

Nota bene

If inadequately treated, a hypertensive syndrome (hypertensive urgency or emergency) can progress to cerebral hemorrhage, coma, and death.

THE PATIENT WITH ANGINA PECTORIS

Angina pectoris is a clinical syndrome characterized by substernal discomfort or pressure often described as heavy, squeezing, crushing, or tight, associated with transient ischemia to the myocardium. It is in response to increased cardiac oxygen demand in the presence of decreased perfusion (anoxia or hypoxia) of the myocardium.

Predisposing factors

1. Decreased perfusion of the myocardium
   a. Obstruction of the coronary arteries by fatty deposits (atherosclerosis)
2. Increased myocardial oxygen demand
   a. Physical exertion
   b. Emotional stress
   c. Cold
   d. Meals

Prevention

1. Identify high-risk patient
   a. Reduce anxiety
   b. Determine the patient's functional capacity
      i. Use local anesthetic agents containing a vasoconstrictor with caution but ensure profound local anesthesia

Signs and symptoms

1. Mild-to-moderate substernal pain of sudden onset
   a. Squeezing
   b. Tight
   c. Heavy
   d. Radiates to the left shoulder, arm, and jaw

Treatment

1. Allow patient to assume a comfortable position
2. Note the time and administer nitroglycerin
   a. 0.4 mg, tablet/spray, SL
3. Administer oxygen
   a. 2 to 4 L/minute by nasal cannula
4. Evaluate pulse rate, blood pressure, and respiratory rate
5. If pain is not relieved 5 minutes after the initial dose, repeat nitroglycerin
   a. 0.4 mg, tablet/spray, SL
6. Evaluate pulse rate, blood pressure, and respiratory rate
7. If pain is not relieved 10 minutes after the initial dose, repeat nitroglycerin
   a. 0.4 mg, tablet/spray, SL
8. Chest pain lasting more than 10 minutes must be assumed to be myocardial infarction
   a. Call EMS
9. If at any time the patient becomes unresponsive with no palpable pulse
   a. Initiate CPR
      i. Automated external defibrillator

Nota bene

Rest and nitroglycerin often relieve angina pectoris. Adverse reaction to nitroglycerin includes flushing, headache, dizziness, nausea, and vomiting. Syncope and paradoxical angina pectoris due to nitrate-induced vasodilation has been reported.

THE PATIENT WITH MYOCARDIAL INFARCTION

Myocardial infarction is caused by abrupt ischemia to a portion of the myocardium resulting in necrosis (myocardial cell death). The ischemia (hypoxia or anoxia) is primarily a result of occlusion of the large and medium-sized arteries of the heart.

Predisposing factors

1. Atherosclerotic plaques and thrombus formation
    a. When the fibrous atherosclerotic plaques are large enough, they become occlusive
    b. In later stages, atherosclerotic plaques may become disrupted and contribute to thrombus formation

Prevention

1. Identify high-risk patients
    a. Reduce anxiety
    b. Determine the patient's functional capacity
        i. Use local anesthetic agents containing a vasoconstrictor with caution, but ensure profound local anesthesia

Signs and symptoms

1. Substernal chest pain
    a. Radiates to the arms, neck, shoulders, or jaw
2. Weakness, dizziness, and palpitation
3. Nausea
4. Dyspnea, tachypnea, or apnea
5. Pallor/cyanosis
6. Diaphoresis
    a. Cool, clammy skin
7. Hypotension
    a. Systolic blood pressure less than 90 mmHg
8. Tachycardia (over 100 beats/minute)

Treatment

1. Call EMS
2. Place patient in a semireclining position
3. Administer oxygen
    a. 6 L/minute by nasal cannula
        i. In case of respiratory distress or altered mental state
            1. Provide positive pressure ventilation

4. Monitor pulse rate, blood pressure, and respiration
5. If at any time the patient becomes unresponsive with no palpable pulse
   a. Initiate CPR
      i. Automated external defibrillator

Nota bene

Signs and symptoms of myocardial infarction vary from mild, vague discomfort to cardiogenic shock, which is a life-threatening emergency with an overall mortality rate to greater than 80%. Furthermore, patient denial may minimize symptoms and elderly and diabetic patients have a higher incidence of silent myocardial infarction characterized by vague symptoms of shortness of breath, epigastric distress, hypotension, and altered mental state.

NEUROLOGICAL EMERGENCIES

THE PATIENT WITH CEREBROVASCULAR ACCIDENT

Cerebrovascular stroke (CVS) is a syndrome associated with an interruption of the blood supply to a portion of the brain resulting in transient, reversible, or irreversible ischemia. Most commonly, a CVS is secondary to an evolving blood clot associated with atherosclerosis, which progressively blocks a cerebral artery. Alternatively, it may be the result of an embolus that lodged in a cerebral artery, obstructing blood flow, or caused by hemorrhage into brain tissue from a ruptured cerebral blood vessel.

Predisposing factors

1. Cardiovascular disease
   a. Atherosclerosis
   b. Valvular disease
   c. Atrial fibrillation
   d. Recent myocardial infarction (< 6 months)
2. Dyslipidemia
3. Hypertension
4. Diabetes mellitus
5. Transient ischemic attacks
6. Drugs
   a. Amphetamines
   b. Cocaine
   c. Oral contraceptives
7. Smoking

Prevention

1. Identify high-risk patient
   a. Reduce anxiety
   b. Determine the patient's functional capacity
      i. Use local anesthetic agents containing a vasoconstrictor with caution, but ensure profound local anesthesia

Sign and symptoms

1. Headache, stiffness in the neck
2. Nausea and vomiting
3. Pupils unequal
4. Slurred speech
5. Motor dysfunction
    a. Facial drooping
    b. Hemiplegia
6. Generalized or focal seizure
7. Altered mentation
8. Blood pressure is often elevated while the heart rate is decreasing

Treatment

1. Call EMS
2. Provide a calm and quiet environment
3. Administer oxygen
    a. 2 to 4 L/minute by nasal cannula
        i. In case of respiratory distress or altered mental state
            1. Provide positive pressure ventilation
4. Monitor vital signs
    a. Blood pressure
        i. If blood pressure is high, elevate head slightly
    b. Heart rate
    c. Respiration
5. Monitor mental state

Nota bene

During the first day of a stroke, neither progression nor outcome can be predicted. Be reassuring to the patient, but do not make exaggerated claims that everything will be all right. About 20% of the patients die. Any neurological deficit noted after 6 months should be considered permanent.

THE PATIENT WITH SEIZURE

Seizure is a sudden episode of cerebral dysfunction characterized by altered motor activity, sensory phenomenon, and unconsciousness. It is the result of focal or generalized disturbance of cortical function caused by excessive discharge of cerebral neurons.

Predisposing factors

1. Epilepsy
2. Head trauma
3. Cerebrovascular accident
4. Hypoxia
5. Drug or alcohol overdose or withdrawal
6. Hypoglycemia

7. Psychogenic "hysterical" seizures
8. Exogenous factors
   a. Sensory input (sound, light, touch, smell)
   b. Anxiety
   c. Heat exhaustion (sodium depletion)

Prevention

1. Identify high-risk patient
   a. Eliminate causative or precipitating factors
   b. Confirm compliance with anticonvulsant chemotherapy
   c. Reduce anxiety
   d. Ensure profound local anesthesia

Signs and symptoms

1. Aura phase
   a. Visual and auditory disturbances
   b. Dizziness
2. Sudden loss of consciousness
3. Tonic-clonic phase
   a. Tongue biting
   b. Increased salivation
   c. Incontinence
   d. Hyperventilation
4. Postictal phase
   a. Fatigue, mental confusion, and amnesia

Treatment

1. Protect patient from injury
   a. It may be safer to leave patient in the dental chair
      i. Otherwise, lower patient to the floor
   b. Guide the extremities during seizure, but do not restrain
2. After the seizure is complete
   a. Suction if needed
   b. Position patient on his or her side (recovery position)
   c. Administer oxygen
      i. 4 to 6 L/minute by nasal cannula
         1. In case of respiratory depression or altered mental state
            a. Provide positive pressure ventilation
            b. Call EMS
   d. Monitor vital signs
      i. Blood pressure
      ii. Heart rate
      iii. Rate and character of respiration

Nota bene

In the postictal phase, monitor respiration closely. Respiratory depression can lead to death. Be prepared to initiate CPR. If the patient has a history of diabetes mellitus, rule out hypoglycemia (tachycardia, pallor, and diaphoresis).

RESPIRATORY EMERGENCIES

THE PATIENT WITH HYPERVENTILATION

Hyperventilation is a state of decreased systemic carbon dioxide concentration. Cerebral hypoxia secondary to cerebral vasoconstriction increases the rate (> 20 breaths/minute) and depth of respiration, which results in low carbon dioxide concentration and an elevated arterial pH (respiratory alkalosis).

Predisposing factors

1. Pain

2. Anxiety (personal and environmental stress)

3. Cardiopulmonary disease (cardiogenic shock, chronic obstructive pulmonary disease, pulmonary edema)

4. Stimulants (drugs, cola, coffee, tea)

Prevention

1. Identify high-risk patient

   a. Reduce anxiety

   b. Ensure profound local anesthesia

Signs and symptoms

1. Frequent, deep, and sighing respiration

2. Light-headedness and dizziness

3. Paresthesia

   a. Burning or prickling feeling of the face and extremities

4. Tonic muscle spasm

5. Tightness in the chest

6. Syncope

Treatment

1. Provide a calm and quiet environment

   a. Allow patient to assume a comfortable position

   b. Reassure the patient with soothing words

2. Instruct the patient to take in a shallow breath and hold it as long as possible

   a. Repeat this sequence 6 to 10 times

3. Alternatively, have patient rebreathe expired air from a paper bag

4. If hyperventilation is secondary to a medical condition other than anxiety

   a. Call EMS

Nota bene

The most common predisposing factor associated with hyperventilation is anxiety. Patients usually give a history of dyspnea and anxiety, often precipitated by personal or environmental stress. These patients respond well to preoperative sedation. However, hyperventilation may also be from hypoxia associated with cardiopulmonary disease. Patients who relate a history of hyperventilation secondary to a medical condition other than anxiety should not receive preoperative sedation.

The Patient With Asthma

Asthma is a clinical syndrome characterized by reversible bronchial constriction and/or excessive mucous secretions leading to too little oxygen in the blood. It is an inflammatory response to a variety of stimuli. Susceptible patients experience bronchial smooth muscle contraction, inflammatory cell infiltration into the alveoli, edema of the airway mucosa, and increased mucous secretions. The alveoli tend to increase in diameter with inhalation but collapse on exhalation, causing a pronounced extended and forced expiratory phase, and may lead to "air-trapping."

Predisposing factors

1. Extrinsic asthma

    a. Pollens and other allergens

2. Intrinsic asthma

    a. Pollutants such as smoke and dust

    b. Physical or emotional stress

    c. Infection

Prevention

1. Identify high-risk patients

    a. Reduce stress

    b. Ensure profound local anesthesia

    c. Avoid respiratory depressants

    d. Use cyclooxygenase-inhibitors with caution

Signs and symptoms

1. Coughing, wheezing, shortness of breath (dyspnea)

2. Anxiety, restlessness, agitation

3. Pallor and/or cyanosis of the lips

4. Noticeable use of the accessory muscles of respiration

5. Patient may become confused and lethargic

Treatment

1. Place patient in a sitting position

2. Provide a calm and quiet environment

    a. Allow patient to assume a comfortable position

    b. Reassure the patient with soothing words

3. Administer oxygen
    a. 2 to 4 L/minute by nasal cannula
4. Administer a short-acting beta$_2$-agonist bronchodilator
    a. Two puffs of albuterol by metered-dose inhaler
5. In case of respiratory depression or altered mental state
    a. Provide positive pressure ventilation
    b. Call EMS

Nota bene

When ventilating an asthmatic patient, squeeze the bag only until resistance is felt or the chest starts to rise and allow time for expiration. Attempting to ventilate with large volumes of air or too rapidly will increase "air-trapping" and may lead to pneumothorax. Patients with a particularly severe ongoing asthma attack (status asthmaticus) who do not respond to usual treatment may progress to acute respiratory failure and death. They must have rapid transport to an advanced life support (ALS) unit.

Acute Respiratory Distress in a Patient With Chronic Obstructive Pulmonary Disease (COPD)

Acute respiratory distress is characterized by either too little oxygen or too much carbon dioxide in the blood secondary to a functional abnormality, which interferes with gas exchange. It may result from oxygenation failure or from ventilation failure. Acute respiratory distress in patients with COPD is a complication of ventilation failure.

Predisposing factors

1. Ventilation failure
    a. COPD
        i. Progressive destruction of lung tissue
            1. Chronic bronchitis
                a. Excess mucus production in response to smoking; exposure to allergens, chemicals, and pollutants; recurrent infections
            2. Emphysema
                a. Decreased elasticity leading to distention of the alveoli, which become filled with trapped air

Prevention

1. Identify high-risk patient
    a. Reduce anxiety
    b. Ensure profound local anesthesia

Signs and symptoms

1. Shallow, labored breathing
    a. Wheezing, gasping, coughing
2. Anxiety, restlessness, agitation

3. Pallor and/or cyanosis of the lips
4. Noticeable use of the accessory muscles of respiration

Treatment

1. Place patient in a sitting position
2. Provide a calm and quiet environment
   c. Allow patient to assume a comfortable position
   d. Reassure the patient with soothing words
3. Administer oxygen
   a. 2 L/minute by nasal cannula
4. Administer a short-acting beta$_2$-agonist bronchodilator
   a. Two puffs of albuterol by metered-dose inhaler
5. In case of respiratory depression or altered mental state
   a. Provide positive pressure ventilation
   b. Call EMS

Nota bene

Patients with COPD in acute respiratory distress need oxygen, despite the possibility that raising the blood oxygen level could reduce the drive to breathe. Never withhold oxygen from a COPD patient in respiratory distress. When ventilating a patient with COPD, squeeze the bag only until resistance is felt or the chest starts to rise and allow time for expiration. Attempting to ventilate with large volumes of air or too rapidly will increase "air-trapping" and may lead to pneumothorax. Patients in severe respiratory distress who do not respond to usual treatment must have rapid transport to an ALS unit.

THE PATIENT WITH UPPER AIRWAY OBSTRUCTION

Upper airway obstruction is characterized by inspiratory retractions at supraclavicular and intercostal spaces, and diaphragmatic movements without evidence of airflow.

Predisposing factors

1. Common causes of upper airway obstruction
   a. Blood, mucus, or vomitus
   b. Foreign body
   c. Spasm or edema of the vocal cords
2. In an unconscious person, upper airway obstruction is commonly due to posterior tongue displacement into the oropharynx secondary to loss of muscle tone

Prevention

1. Identify high-risk patient
   a. Medical history
      i. Allergies (latex)
2. High-volume suctioning
3. Oropharyngeal curtain

Signs and symptoms

1. Universal sign of choking distress
2. Ineffective respiratory efforts
3. Agitated patient
4. Cyanosis
5. Loss of consciousness

Treatment

1. Position patient properly
   a. Head tilt with chin or neck lift
      i. Check for movement of air
         1. Look to see whether the chest rises
         2. Listen for airflow
         3. Feel the chest wall for movement
2. Ask the patient to speak
   a. If the patient is responsive and talking, the patient is breathing at this time
      i. If respirations are labored with stridor or wheezing
         1. Check for excessive or frothy saliva and other causes of partial obstruction
      ii. Inspiratory retractions at supraclavicular and intercostal spaces, and diaphragmatic movements without evidence of airflow suggest complete obstruction
         1. Check for evidence of foreign body or other causes of complete obstruction (angioedema)
3. Foreign body obstruction
   a. Call EMS
   b. Immediately begin procedures for the removal of foreign body
      i. Position the patient
         1. Deliver five abdominal thrusts
         2. Use finger sweep
         3. Attempt ventilation
         4. Repeat 1, 2, and 3 until airway is cleared

Nota bene

Complete airway obstruction for more than 5 minutes may lead to cardiac arrest and brain damage. However, CPR is of no value until upper airway obstruction is cleared. If complete obstruction persists for more than 5 minutes, it may be necessary to perform a cricothyroidectomy.

ALLERGIC REACTIONS

The Patient With an Anaphylactic Reaction

In susceptible patients, type I (immediate) hypersensitivity reactions follow initial exposure to an allergen, which result in antigen-specific antibody production dominated by the immunoglobulin E (IgE) isotype.

Predisposing factors

1. Following reexposure to a specific antigen, IgE antibodies bind to mast cells, basophils, and eosinophils associated with mucosal and epithelial tissues

    a. The simultaneous binding of an antigen to adjacent IgE molecules fixed to Fc receptors triggers degranulation of mast cells and basophils resulting in the production and release of histamine, leukotrienes, prostaglandins, chemokines, enzymes, and cytokines in target tissues

        i. Histamine produces peripheral vasodilatation and increased capillary permeability

        ii. Leukotrienes and prostaglandins promote smooth muscle contraction, increased vascular permeability, and increased mucous secretion

        iii. Chemokines attract leukocytes

        iv. Enzymes break down tissue matrix proteins

        v. Cytokines promote inflammatory activities

Prevention

1. Identify high-risk patient

    a. Medical history

Signs and symptoms

1. 1 to 15 minutes following exposure to a specific allergen

    a. Coughing, sneezing, wheezing

    b. Agitation, flushing, palpitation

    c. Pruritus, urticaria, angioedema

    d. Unresponsiveness, convulsion, shock

Treatment

1. Place patient in a recumbent position with legs elevated

2. Immediately treat with epinephrine 1:1000

    a. Adult: epinephrine (EpiPen), 0.3 mg, intramuscular (anterolateral thigh); may be repeated in 20 minutes if necessary

    b. Child: epinephrine (EpiPen Jr), 0.15 mg, intramuscular (anterolateral thigh); may be repeated in 20 minutes if necessary

    c. Maintain the airway and administer 100% oxygen

        i. Provide positive pressure ventilation with 100% oxygen

3. Call EMS

4. If at any time the patient becomes unresponsive with no palpable pulse

    a. Initiate CPR

        i. Automated external defibrillator

Nota bene

While patients taking beta-adrenergic blocking agents may require more epinephrine to reverse the effects of anaphylaxis, for patients with cardiovascular diseases and/or diabetes mellitus, start treatment with smaller doses of epinephrine.

THE PATIENT WITH DELAYED HYPERSENSITIVITY REACTION

Type IV (delayed) hypersensitivity reactions are closely related to cellular immunity in that specifically sensitized $CD4^+$ T lymphocytes initiate the reaction. Initial sensitization occurs slowly, over a 10- to 14-day period. Small molecular weight drugs bind covalently to host cell membrane proteins or "hapten-carrier conjugates."

Predisposing factors

1. Following reexposure to a specific antigen, the immunologically committed lymphocytes react with the allergen (antigens) and release cytokines (lymphokines)
    a. Lymphokines activate macrophages resulting in the production and release of histamine, leukotrienes, prostaglandins, chemokines, enzymes, and cytokines in target tissues

Prevention

1. Identify the high-risk patient
    a. Medical history

Signs and symptoms

1. 6 to 48 hours following exposure to a specific antigen
    a. Fever, malaise
    b. Erythema, pruritus, urticaria
    c. Perioral paresthesia, angioedema
    d. Wheezing

Treatment

1. Identify drugs and other potential allergens to which the patient may have been exposed in the clinical process
2. Verify that the onset of signs and symptoms was after the initiation of pharmacological or clinical intervention
    a. Determine the time interval between the initiation of drug therapy or clinical intervention and the onset of signs and symptoms
3. If the patient is still exposed to the suspected allergen, stop its use
4. If the patient relates wheezing, instruct patient or caretaker to call EMS
5. In the absence of respiratory distress
    a. Prescribe diphenhydramine hydrochloride, 25 to 50 mg, orally, 4 times a day
    b. Arrange supervision of the patient for at least 6 hours after the onset of signs and symptoms

Nota bene

Instruct caretaker to call EMS immediately if the patient's status deteriorates.

ENDOCRINE EMERGENCIES

THE PATIENT WITH HYPOGLYCEMIA

Hypoglycemia is defined as an abnormally low plasma glucose level. Because the brain depends on plasma glucose as its major metabolic fuel, the

CNS regulates the plasma glucose level to ensure adequate glucose transport into the brain. Plasma glucose deficiency leads to autonomic nervous system stimulation (epinephrine and glucagon release) and ultimately CNS dysfunction. Hypoglycemia is characterized by acute, rapid onset and may represent a life-threatening situation if unrecognized.

Predisposing factors

1. Most commonly treatment with insulin and an oral hypoglycemic agent
   a. Delayed, decreased, or missed meal
   b. Decreased carbohydrate content of a meal
2. Increased rates of insulin absorption as a result of increased skin temperature owing to high ambient environmental temperatures
3. Heavy exercise
4. Anxiety
5. Infection

Prevention

1. Identify high-risk patients
   a. Medical history
2. Confirm compliance
   a. Insulin
   b. Oral hypoglycemic agents
   c. Food intake
3. Reduce anxiety

Signs and symptoms

1. Weakness, hunger, dizziness, sweating
2. Tachycardia (palpitation)
3. Anxiety, tremor
4. Headaches
5. Visual and mental disturbances
6. Respiration may be normal to shallow
7. The pulse may be full and pounding
8. The blood pressure is usually normal

Treatment

1. If the patient is responsive
   a. Administer a glass of fruit juice
      or
      3 tbsp of sugar with water
2. If the patient is unresponsive
   a. Apply a spread of sucrose paste (cake icing) on oral soft tissues
      or
      Administer glucagon, 1 mg, intramuscularly or SL
   b. Call EMS
   c. Administer oxygen
      i. 4 to 6 L/minute by nasal cannula

Nota bene

Most of the signs and symptoms of hypoglycemia are caused by the hypoglycemia-induced release of epinephrine, which causes glycogenolysis and promotes gluconeogenesis and lipolysis. Visual disturbances and altered mentation are secondary to the inadequate energy supply to the brain. Distress in a patient with diabetes mellitus must always be assumed to be a result of hypoglycemia.

BIBLIOGRAPHY

1. Copass MK, Gonzales L, Eisenberg, MS, Soper RG. EMT Manual. 3rd ed. Philadelphia: WB Saunders Company, 1998.

2. Terezhalmy GT, Batizy LG, eds. Urgent Care in the Dental Office. An Essential Handbook. 1st ed. Chicago: Quintessence Publishing Co, Inc, 1998.

A to Z
to
Listing of Drugs

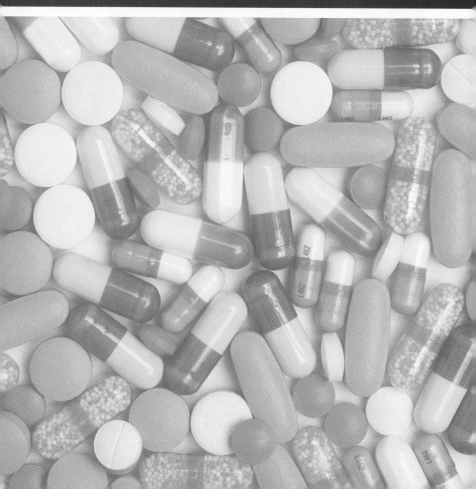

1/2 Halfprin — see aspirin

13-cis-retinoic acid — see isotretinoin

3-A Ofteno — see diclofenac

3TCZ — see lamivudine

40 Winks — see diphenhydramine HCl

5-aminosalicylic acid — see mesalamine

5-ASA — see mesalamine

642 — see propoxyphene HCl

abacavir sulfate (ab-ah-KAV-ear SULL-fate)
Ziagen

Drug Class: Antiretroviral, nucleoside reverse transcriptase inhibitor

PHARMACOLOGY
Action
Converted by cellular enzymes to carbovir triphosphate, which inhibits HIV-1 reverse transcriptase and interferes with DNA synthesis.

Uses
Treatment of HIV-1 in combination with other antiretroviral agents.

➤◆ DRUG INTERACTIONS RELATED TO DENTAL THERAPEUTICS
No documented drug-drug interactions. The absence of evidence is not evidence of safety.

ADVERSE EFFECTS
CNS: Insomnia and other sleep disorders; headache.

GI: Nausea; vomiting; diarrhea; loss of appetite; anorexia; pancreatitis.

MISC: Hypersensitivity reactions (e.g., fever, rash, fatigue, GI symptoms, malaise, lethargy, myalgia, arthralgia, edema, shortness of breath, paresthesia, hypotension, death); fever.

CLINICAL IMPLICATIONS
General
- Determine why drug is being taken. Consider implications of condition on dental treatment.
- Consider medical consult to determine disease control and influence on dental treatment.
- Anticipate oral candidiasis when HIV disease is reported.
- If GI side effects occur, consider semisupine chair position.
- Antibiotic prophylaxis should be considered when <500 PMN/mm^3 are reported; elective dental treatment should be delayed until blood values improve above this level.
- This drug is frequently prescribed in combination with one or more other antiviral agents. Side effects of all agents must be considered during the drug review process.

Oral Health Education
- Recommend frequent maintenance prophylaxis when immunosuppression is evident.
- Encourage daily plaque control procedures for effective self-care because HIV infection reduces host resistance.

Information on drug interactions adapted with permission from Handbook of Adverse Drug Interactions. New Rochelle, NY: The Medical Letter, Inc; 2005. www.medicalletter.org

abacavir sulfate/lamivudine/zidovudine (ab-ah-KAV-ear

SULL-fate/la-MIH-view-deen/zie-DOE-view-DEEN)

Trizivir

Drug Class: Antiretroviral combination

PHARMACOLOGY

Action

Inhibits replication of HIV by incorporation into HIV DNA and producing incomplete, non-functional DNA.

Uses

Use alone and in combination with other antiretroviral agents for the treatment of HIV-1 infection.

➡◀ DRUG INTERACTIONS RELATED TO DENTAL THERAPEUTICS

Fluconazole: Possible zidovudine toxicity (decreased metabolism)
- Monitor clinical status.

Clarithromycin: Possible decreased zidovudine effect (mechanism unknown)
- Avoid concurrent use.

ADVERSE EFFECTS

⚠ **ORAL:** Stomatitis; oral mucosal pigmentation; candidiasis.

CNS: Loss of appetite; anorexia; insomnia; sleep disorders; headache; malaise; fatigue; neuropathy; dizziness; depression; paresthesia; peripheral neuropathy; seizures.

GI: Nausea; vomiting; diarrhea; pancreatitis; abdominal pain; dyspepsia.

RESP: Cough; abnormal breath sounds; wheezing.

MISC: Hypersensitivity; fever; chills; musculoskeletal pain; myalgia; arthralgia; vasculitis; weakness; muscle weakness; creatine phosphokinase elevation; rhabdomyolysis.

CLINICAL IMPLICATIONS

General

- Determine why drug is being taken. Consider implications of condition on dental treatment.
- Consider medical consult to determine disease control and influence on dental treatment.
- Anticipate oral candidiasis when HIV disease is reported.
- This drug is frequently prescribed in combination with one or more other antiviral agents. Side effects of all agents must be considered during the drug review process.
- Antibiotic prophylaxis should be considered when <500 PMN/mm^3 are reported; elective dental treatment should be delayed until blood values improve above this level.

Oral Health Education

- Recommend frequent maintenance prophylaxis when immunosuppression is evident.
- Encourage daily plaque control procedures for effective self-care because HIV infection reduces host resistance.

Abenol — see acetaminophen

Abilify — see aripiprazole

Abreva — see docosanol

absorbable gelatin sponge

Gelfoam: Sponges: Size 12: 2 × 6 cm × 3 or 7 mm, Size 50: 8 × 6.25 cm, Size 100: 8 × 12.5 cm, Size 200: 8 × 25 cm; Packs: Size 2: 40 × 2 cm, Size 6: 40 × 6 cm; Dental Pack: Size 4: 2 × 2 cm

Drug Class: Hematological agents, topical

PHARMACOLOGY

Action
Provides a matrix for fibrin deposition and propagation of blood clot to control capillary or venous hemorrhage. When implanted into tissues, it is absorbed completely within 4 to 6 wk without inducing excessive scar tissue formation. When applied to bleeding areas of nasal, rectal, or vaginal mucosa, it completely liquefies within 2 to 5 days.

Uses
For use in surgical procedures as an adjunct to hemostasis when control of bleeding by ligature or conventional procedures is ineffective or impractical. Also used in oral and dental surgery as an aid in providing hemostasis. In open prostatic surgery, insertion into the prostatic cavity provides hemostasis.

Contraindications
Closure of skin incisions (may interfere with the healing of skin edges); control of postpartum bleeding or menorrhalgia.

Usual Dosage
Local bleeding associated with oral surgical procedures
SPONGES, PACKS
ADULTS AND CHILDREN: Apply pack or sponge to bleeding site with moderate pressure (may be placed into a socket).

➡◀ DRUG INTERACTIONS
No documented drug-drug interactions. The absence of evidence is not evidence of safety.

ADVERSE EFFECTS
⚠ **ORAL:** Sponge may cause infection and abscess formation.
CNS: Giant cell granuloma in the brain has occurred at implantation site, as well as brain and spinal cord compression due to sterile fluid accumulation.
MISC: Excessive fibrosis and prolonged fixation of the tendon were seen when the sponge was used at a tendon juncture.

CLINICAL IMPLICATIONS

General
- Not recommended in the presence of infection. If signs of infection or abscess develop in the area where the sponge has been placed, reoperation may be necessary to remove the infected material and allow drainage.
- Sponge may expand and impinge on nearby structures. When placing into cavities or closed tissue spaces, use minimal preliminary compression; avoid overpacking.
- Once package is opened, contents are subject to contamination.
- Do not resterilize by heat, since heating may change absorption time. Ethylene oxide is not recommended for resterilization; it may be trapped in the interstices of the foam and trace amounts may cause burns or irritation to tissue.

Pregnancy Risk Category: Category C.

Oral Health Education
- Instruct patient to inform dentist if pain, swelling, or infection develops.

Acanol — see loperamide HCl

acarbose (A-car-bose)
Precose

■✦■ **Prandase**

■◆■ **Glucobay**

Drug Class: Antidiabetic, alpha-glucosidase inhibitor

PHARMACOLOGY

Action
Inhibits intestinal enzymes that digest carbohydrates, thereby reducing carbohydrate digestion after meals. This lowers postprandial glucose elevation in diabetic patients.

Uses
Patients with type 2 diabetes mellitus who have failed dietary therapy. May be used alone or in combination with sulfonylureas, insulin, or metformin.

➜✦ DRUG INTERACTIONS RELATED TO DENTAL THERAPEUTICS
No documented drug-drug interactions. The absence of evidence is not evidence of safety.

ADVERSE EFFECTS
GI: Flatulence (74%); diarrhea (31%); abdominal pain (19%).

CLINICAL IMPLICATIONS

General
- *Hypoglycemia:* Acarbose does not produce hypoglycemia; however, hypoglycemia may develop if used together with sulfonylureas or insulin.
- Determine degree of disease control and current blood sugar levels. A_1C levels ≥8% indicate significant uncontrolled diabetes.
- The routine use of antibiotics in the dental management of diabetic patients is not indicated; however, antibiotic therapy in patients with poorly controlled diabetes has been shown to improve disease control and improve response following periodontal debridement.
- Monitor blood pressure, as hypertension and dyslipidemia (i.e., CAD) are prevalent in diabetes mellitus.
- Monitor vital signs (BP, pulse pressure, rate, and rhythm) at each appointment to assess disease control. Do not provide elective dental treatment when BP is ≥180/110 or in the presence of other high-risk CV conditions. Refer to the section entitled "The Patient Taking Cardiovascular Drugs" in Chapter 6: *Clinical Medicine.*
- *Loss of blood sugar control:* Certain medical conditions (e.g., surgery, fever, infection, trauma) and drugs (e.g., corticosteroids) affect glucose control. In these situations, it may be necessary to seek medical consultation before surgical procedures.
- Obtain patient history regarding diabetic ketoacidosis or hypoglycemia with current drug regimen.
- Observe for signs of hypoglycemia (confusion, argumentative, perspiration, altered consciousness). Be prepared to treat hypoglycemic reactions with oral glucose instead of cane sugar.
- If GI side effects occur, consider semisupine chair position.

Oral Health Education
- Explain role of diabetes in periodontal disease and the need to maintain effective plaque control and disease control.
- Advise patient to bring data on blood sugar values and A_1C levels to dental appointments.
- Encourage daily plaque control procedures for effective self-care in patients at risk for cardiovascular disease.

Accolate — see zafirlukast
Accupril — see quinapril HCl
Accurbron — see theophylline
Accutane — see isotretinoin
Accutane Roche — see isotretinoin

acebutolol HCl (ass-cee-BYOO-toe-lahl HIGH-droe-KLOR-ide)

Sectral

■✦■ **Apo-Acebutolol, Gen-Acebutolol, Gen-Acebutolol Type S, Monitan, Novo-Acebutolol, Nu-Acebutolol, Rhotral**

Drug Class: Beta$_1$-adrenergic blocker

PHARMACOLOGY

Action
Blocks beta$_1$-receptors, primarily affecting heart (slows rate), vascular musculature (decreases BP), and lungs (reduces function).

Uses
Management of hypertension and premature ventricular contractions.

➡◆ DRUG INTERACTIONS RELATED TO DENTAL THERAPEUTICS

Nonsteroidal anti-inflammatory drugs: Decreased antihypertensive effect (inhibition of prostaglandin synthesis)
- Instruct patient to monitor blood pressure.

Sympathomimetic amines: Decreased antihypertensive effect (pharmacological antagonism)
- Use local anesthetic agents with a vasoconstrictor with caution while monitoring vital signs.

ADVERSE EFFECTS

⚠ **ORAL:** Dry mouth; taste disturbance (rare).
CNS: Insomnia; fatigue; dizziness; depression; lethargy; drowsiness; forgetfulness.
CVS: Bradycardia; orthostatic hypotension (rare).
GI: Nausea; vomiting; diarrhea.
RESP: Bronchospasm; dyspnea; wheezing.
MISC: Thrombocytopenia, leukopenia (both rare).

CLINICAL IMPLICATIONS

General
- Monitor vital signs (e.g., BP, pulse pressure, rate, and rhythm) at each appointment to assess disease control. Do not provide elective dental treatment when BP is ≥180/110 or in the presence of other high-risk CV conditions. Refer to the section entitled "The Patient Taking Cardiovascular Drugs" in Chapter 6: *Clinical Medicine*.
- *Postural hypotension:* Monitor BP at the beginning and end of each appointment; anticipate syncope. Have patient sit upright for several min at the end of the dental appointment before dismissing.
- Chronic dry mouth is possible, anticipate increased caries, candidiasis, and lichenoid mucositis.
- Use local anesthetic agents with vasoconstrictor with caution based on functional capacity of the patient and use aspirating technique to prevent intravascular injection.
- Beta blockers may mask epinephrine-induced signs and symptoms of hypoglycemia in patients with diabetes.
- Determine ability to adapt to stress of dental treatment. Consider short appointments.

Oral Health Education
- If chronic dry mouth occurs, recommend home fluoride therapy and use of nonalcoholic oral health care products.
- Encourage daily plaque control procedures for effective self-care in patients at risk for cardiovascular disease.

Aceon — see perindopril erbumine

Acephen — see acetaminophen

Aceta — see acetaminophen

Aceta w/Codeine — see acetaminophen/codeine phosphate

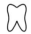 **acetaminophen** (ass-cet-ah-MEE-noe-fen)

Synonym: *n*-acetyl-p-aminophenol; APAP

Acephen, Aceta, Acetaminophen Uniserts, Apacet, Aspirin Free Anacin Maximum Strength, Aspirin Free Pain Relief, Children's Dynafed Jr., Children's Feverall, Children's Genapap, Children's Halenol, Children's Mapap, Children's Panadol, Children's Silapap, Children's Tylenol, Children's Tylenol Soft Chews, Dapacin, Extra Strength Dynafed E.X., Feverall, Feverall Junior Strength, Genapap, Genapap Infants' Drops, Genapap Extra Strength, Genebs, Genebs Extra Strength, Infants' Pain Reliever, Infants' Silapap, Liquiprin Drops for Children, Mapap Extra Strength, Mapap Infant Drops, Mapap Regular Strength, Maranox, Meda Cap, Meda Tab, Neopap, Oraphen-PD, Panadol, Panadol Infants' Drops, Redutemp, Ridenol, Tapanol Extra Strength, Tapanol Regular Strength, Tempra, Tempra 1, Tempra 2 Syrup, Tempra 3, Tylenol Arthritis, Tylenol Caplets, Tylenol Extended Relief, Tylenol Extra Strength, Tylenol Infants' Drops, Tylenol Junior Strength, Tylenol Regular Strength, Uni-Ace: Tablets: 325, 500 mg; Chewable tablets: 80, 120 mg; Gelcaps: 500 mg; Caplets: 325, 500, 650 mg; Solution: 80 mg/1.66 mL, 100 mg/mL, 160 mg/5 mL, 500 mg/15 mL; Elixir: 80 mg/2.5 mL, 80 mg/5 mL, 120 mg/5 mL, 160 mg/5 mL; Drops: 80 mg/0.8 mL; Suppositories: 80, 120, 125, 325, 650 mg

■✦■ **Abenol, Apo-Acetaminophen, Atasol, Pediatrix**

■✦■ **Algitrin, Analphen, Andox, Cilag, Datril, Febrin, Magnidol, Minofen, Neodol, Neodolito, Sedalito, Sinedol, Sinedol 500, Temperal, Tempra, Tylex, Tylex 750, Winasorb**

Drug Class: Analgesic; Antipyretic

PHARMACOLOGY
Action
Inhibits prostaglandins in CNS but lacks anti-inflammatory effects in periphery; reduces fever through direct action on hypothalamic heat-regulating center.

Uses
Relief of mild to moderate pain; treatment of fever.

Unlabeled Uses
Pain and fever prophylaxis after vaccination.

Usual Dosage
ORAL
ADULTS: *PO:* 325 to 650 mg prn q 4 to 6 hr or 1 g 3 to 4 times/day. Do not exceed 4 g/day.
CHILDREN: *PO:* 10 to 15 mg/kg dose prn q 4 to 6 hr; do not exceed 5 doses/24 hr.

Suppositories

Adults: *PR:* 650 mg q 4 to 6 hr; do not exceed 6 suppositories/24 hr.
Children 3 to 6 yr: *PR:* 120 mg q 4 to 6 hr; do not exceed 720 mg/24 hr.
Children 6 to 12 yr: *PR:* 325 mg q 4 to 6 hr; do not exceed 2.6 g/24 hr.

Pharmacokinetics

ABSORP: Rapid and complete from the GI tract. T_{max} is 0.5 to 2 hr; 4 hr after overdosage.
DIST: Distributed throughout most body fluids. Binding to plasma proteins is variable.
METAB: Primarily metabolized by hepatic conjugation (94%), and about 4% is metabolized by CYP450 oxidase to toxic metabolite.
EXCRET: $T_{1/2}$ is about 2 hr; 90% to 100% is recovered in the urine within the first day, primarily as inactive metabolites; 2% is excreted as unchanged drug.
SPECIAL POP: *Cirrhotic patients:* Half-life is slightly prolonged.

✦✦ DRUG INTERACTIONS

Cholestyramine: Decreased acetaminophen effect (unknown mechanism)
• Administer acetaminophen 1 hr before cholestyramine.
Contraceptives, combination: Possible decreased analgesic effect (increased metabolism)
• Monitor analgesia.
Isoniazid: Acetaminophen toxicity (increase in toxic metabolites)
• Avoid concurrent use.
Phenytoin: Possible increased acetaminophen toxicity (increase in toxic metabolites)
• Avoid concurrent use.
Probenecid: Possible acetaminophen toxicity (decreased metabolism and renal excretion)
• Avoid concurrent use.
Sulfinpyrazone: Possible decreased acetaminophen effect (increased metabolism)
• Monitor analgesia.

ADVERSE EFFECTS

GI: Nausea, vomiting <1%, hepatotoxicity (high doses).

CLINICAL IMPLICATIONS

General

• *Lactation:* Excreted in breast milk.
• *Hepatic failure:* Patients with chronic alcoholism should not exceed 2 g/day.
• *Persistent pain or fever:* May indicate serious illness. Consult health care provider.
• Obtain patient history, including drug history and any known allergies.
• Determine why drug is being taken. Consider implications of condition on dental treatment.
• *If used for arthritis:* Consider patient comfort and need for semisupine chair position.
• COX-1 inhibitors are the indicated analgesics for dental pain; use APAP when those cannot be used.

Pregnancy Risk Category: Category B.

Oral Health Education

• Instruct adult patients not to continue taking drug more than 10 days for pain or 3 days for fever.

---

 acetaminophen/codeine phosphate (ass-cet-ah-MEE-noe-fen with KOE-deen FOSS-fate)

Synonym: codeine phosphate/acetaminophen

Aceta w/Codeine, Capital w/Codeine, Phenaphen w/Codeine No. 3, Phenaphen w/Codeine No. 4, Tylenol w/Codeine, Tylenol w/Codeine No. 2, Tylenol w/ Codeine No. 3, Tylenol w/Codeine No. 4: Tablets: 15, 30, 60 mg codeine phosphate/300 mg APAP; Caplets: 30, 60 mg codeine phosphate/325 mg APAP; Elixir/Suspension: 12 mg codeine phosphate/120 mg APAP

■✦■ Triatec-30, Tylenol Elixir with Codeine

■✦■ Tylex CD

Drug Class: Narcotic analgesic combination

PHARMACOLOGY

Action

Inhibits synthesis of prostaglandins; binds to opiate receptors in CNS and peripherally blocks pain impulse generation; produces antipyresis by direct action on hypothalamic heat-regulating center; causes cough suppression by direct central action in medulla; may produce generalized CNS depression; does not have significant anti-inflammatory or antiplatelet effects.

Uses

Relief of mild to moderate pain; analgesic-antipyretic therapy in presence of aspirin allergy, hemostatic disturbances, bleeding diatheses, upper GI disease, and gouty arthritis.

Contraindications

Hypersensitivity to codeine phosphate or similar compounds.

Usual Dosage

Tylenol No. 2 equals 15 mg codeine, 300 mg acetaminophen. Tylenol No. 3 equals 30 mg codeine, 300 mg acetaminophen. Tylenol No. 4 equals 60 mg codeine, 300 mg acetaminophen.

Max adult dose: Codeine equals 360 mg/day; acetaminophen equals 4 g/day.

Orodental Pain

TABLETS, CAPLETS

ADULTS: *PO:* Usually 1 to 2 tablets q 4 hr (varies according to product).

CHILDREN UNDER 12 YR: *PO:* 0.5 to 1 mg codeine/kg/dose q 4 to 6 hr; 10 to 15 mg acetaminophen/kg/dose q 4 hr to max 2.6 g/24 hr.

ELIXIR/SUSPENSION

CHILDREN OLDER THAN 12 YR: *PO:* 15 mL q 4 hr.

CHILDREN 7 TO 12 YR: *PO:* 10 mL tid to qid.

CHILDREN 3 TO 6 YR: *PO:* 5 mL tid to qid.

Pharmacokinetics

Acetaminophen

ABSORP: Rapid and complete from the GI tract. T_{max} is 0.5 to 2 hr; 4 hr after overdosage.

DIST: Distributed throughout most body fluids. Binding to plasma proteins is variable.

METAB: Primarily metabolized by hepatic conjugation (94%), and about 4% is metabolized by CYP450 oxidase to toxic metabolite.

EXCRET: $T_{1/2}$ is about 2 hr. 90% to 100% is recovered in the urine within the first day, primarily as inactive metabolites. 2% is excreted as unchanged drug.

Codeine

METAB: Metabolized in the liver by undergoing *O*-demethylation, *N*-demethylation, and partial conjugation.

EXCRET: Excreted in the urine, largely as inactive metabolites, and small amounts of free and conjugated morphine. The $t_{1/2}$ is 3 hr.

ONSET: *Oral/SC:* 15 to 30 min.

PEAK: *Oral:* 60 min.

DURATION: *Oral/SC:* 4 to 6 hr.

➔◆ DRUG INTERACTIONS

See also: acetaminophen – Drug interactions

Cimetidine: Severe opioid toxicity (decreased metabolism)
  • Use with caution.

Bupivacaine: Possible respiratory depression (mechanism unknown)
  • Avoid concurrent use.

Paroxetine: Lack of analgesic activity (blocks the conversion of codeine to morphine)
- Avoid concurrent use.

Quinidine: Lack of analgesic activity (blocks the conversion of codeine to morphine)
- Avoid concurrent use.

Rifampin: Possible decreased efficacy of codeine (mechanism unknown)
- Avoid concurrent use.

ADVERSE EFFECTS
⚠ **ORAL:** Dry mouth.

CVS: Flushing; orthostatic hypotension.

CNS: Lightheadedness; dizziness; sedation; euphoria; insomnia; disorientation; incoordination.

GI: Nausea; vomiting; constipation; abdominal pain.

RESP: Dyspnea; respiratory depression; decreased cough reflex.

MISC: Histamine release.

CLINICAL IMPLICATIONS
General
When prescribed by DDS:
- *Lactation:* Excreted in breast milk.
- *Hepatic failure:* Acetaminophen intake must be limited to 2 g/day or less.
- *Sulfite sensitivity:* Caution is needed with sulfite-sensitive patients; some commercial preparations contain sodium bisulfite.
- *Overdosage:* Blood dyscrasias, respiratory depression, hepatic damage (may occur up to several days after overdose).
- Obtain patient history, including drug history and any known allergies. Note pulmonary or hepatic disease, alcoholism, head injury, Addison disease, hypothyroidism, or previous addiction to narcotic drugs.
- Assess baseline level of pain before prescribing.
- Consider related factors that may lower pain threshold (e.g., anxiety, fear, boredom, environmental stressors).
- Administer scheduled dose before pain becomes severe.

When prescribed by medical facility:
- Determine why drug is being taken. Consider implications of condition on dental treatment.
- *Postural hypotension:* Monitor BP at the beginning and end of each appointment; anticipate syncope. Have patient sit upright for several min at the end of the dental appointment before dismissing.
- If GI side effects occur, consider semisupine chair position.
- Chronic dry mouth is possible; anticipate increased caries activity and candidiasis.

Pregnancy Risk Category: Category C.

Oral Health Education
When prescribed by DDS:
- Caution patient that drug dependency or tolerance may result from long-term use.
- Caution patient to avoid intake of alcohol and other CNS depressants without consulting health care provider.
- Advise patient that drug may cause drowsiness and to use caution while driving or performing other tasks requiring mental alertness.
- Instruct patient to notify health care provider if the following signs/symptoms occur: persistence or recurrence of pain before next scheduled dose; difficulty breathing; blurred vision; increased drowsiness; severe nausea; vomiting; urinary retention; yellowing of skin, sclera, or gums.
- Warn patient that orthostatic hypotension may occur; instruct patient to change positions slowly and to sit or lie down if symptoms occur.
- Explain that diaphoresis is a common side effect and does not indicate a problem.
- Warn patient that constipation may occur. Advise patient to increase dietary fiber and fluids unless contraindicated.
- Caution patient against taking OTC medications that contain acetaminophen.

When prescribed by medical facility:
• If chronic dry mouth occurs, recommend home fluoride therapy and use of nonalcoholic oral health care products.

---

 acetaminophen/hydrocodone bitartrate (ass-eet-ah-MEE-noe-fen/HIGH-droe-KOE-dohn by-TAR-trate)

Synonym: hydrocodone bitartrate/acetaminophen

Anexsia 5/500, Duocet, Duradyne DHC, Hy-Phen, Lortab 5/500, Margesic H, Panacet 5/500, Vicodin: Tablets: 5 mg hydrocodone bitartrate/500 mg acetaminophen
Anexsia 7.5/650, Lorcet Plus: Tablets: 7.5 mg hydrocodone bitartrate/650 mg acetaminophen
Anexsia 10/660, Vicodin HP: Tablets: 10 mg hydrocodone bitartrate/660 acetaminophen
Bancap-HC, Ceta-Plus, Co-Gesic, Dolacet, Hydrocet, Hydrogesic, Lorcet-HD, Stagesic, T-Gesic: Capsules: 5 mg hydrocodone bitartrate/500 mg acetaminophen
Lorcet 10/650: Tablets: 10 mg hydrocodone bitartrate/650 mg acetaminophen
Lortab 7.5/500: Tablets: 7.5 mg hydrocodone bitartrate/500 mg acetaminophen
Lortab 10/500: Tablets: 10 mg hydrocodone bitartrate/500 mg acetaminophen
Norco: Tablets: 10 mg hydrocodone bitartrate/325 mg acetaminophen
Vicodin ES: Tablets: 7.5 mg hydrocodone bitartrate/750 mg acetaminophen
Zydone: Tablets: 7.5 mg hydrocodone bitartrate/400 mg acetaminophen, 10 mg hydrocodone bitartrate/400 mg acetaminophen

Drug Class: Narcotic analgesic
DEA Schedule: Schedule III

PHARMACOLOGY

Action
Inhibits synthesis of prostaglandins and binds to opiate receptors in CNS and peripherally blocks pain impulse generation; produces antipyresis by direct action on hypothalamic heat-regulating center; causes cough suppression by direct central action in medulla; may produce generalized CNS depression.

Uses
Management of mild to moderate pain.

Contraindications
Hypersensitivity to acetaminophen, hydrocodone, or similar compounds.

Usual Dosage
Varies according to product and strength.
ADULTS: *PO:* 1 to 2 tablets or capsules (hydrocodone 2.5 to 10 mg; acetaminophen 500 to 1000 mg) q 4 to 6 hr or 5 to 10 mL (elixir, 15 mL) q 4 to 6 hr.
CHILDREN (YOUNGER THAN 12 YR): *PO:* 10 to 15 mg acetaminophen/kg/dose q 4 hr to max of 2.6 g/24 hr.

Pharmacokinetics
Acetaminophen
ABSORP: Rapid and complete from the GI tract. T_{max} is 0.5 to 2 hr; 4 hr after overdosage.
DIST: Distributed throughout most body fluids. Binding to plasma proteins is variable.
METAB: Primarily metabolized by hepatic conjugation (94%), and about 4% is metabolized by CYP450 oxidase to toxic metabolite.
EXCRET: $T_{1/2}$ is about 2 hr. 90% to 100% is recovered in the urine within the first day, primarily as inactive metabolites. 2% is excreted as unchanged drug.

Hydrocodone
ABSORP: Hydrocodone is rapidly absorbed from the GI tract. T_{max} is achieved at 1.7 hr.

DIST: Distributed throughout the body. Not extensively protein bound.

METAB: Extensively metabolized in the liver to hydromorphone by *O*-demethylation by the CYP2D6 isoenzyme.

EXCRET: Hydrocodone and its metabolites are eliminated primarily in the kidneys.

ONSET: 30 min.

PEAK: 1.7 hr.

DURATION: 4.5 hr.

SPECIAL POP: *Severe renal insufficiency:* The effect of renal insufficiency on the pharmacokinetics of hydrocodone has not been determined.

➡️⬅ DRUG INTERACTIONS
See also: acetaminophen — Drug Interactions

No specific documented drug-drug interactions with hydrocodone. The absence of evidence is not evidence of safety.

ADVERSE EFFECTS
CVS: Hypotension; bradycardia.

CNS: Lightheadedness; dizziness; sedation; drowsiness; weakness; anxiety; fear; fatigue; dysphoria; psychological dependence; confusion.

GI: Nausea; vomiting; constipation.

RESP: Dyspnea; respiratory depression; irregular breathing.

CLINICAL IMPLICATIONS
General
When prescribed by DDS:
- *Lactation:* Excreted in breast milk.
- *Children:* Safety and effectiveness in children have not been established.
- *Hepatic failure:* Patients with chronic alcoholism should limit acetaminophen intake to less than 2 g/day.
- *Special risk:* Closely monitor elderly, debilitated patients, and those with conditions accompanied by hypoxia or hypercapnia to avoid decrease in pulmonary ventilation. Also use caution in patients sensitive to CNS depressants. Because of cough suppressant effects, exercise caution when using postoperatively or in patients with pulmonary disease.
- *Sulfite sensitivity:* Use caution in sulfite-sensitive individuals; some commercial preparations contain sodium bisulfite.
- *Overdosage:* Blood dyscrasias, respiratory depression, and hepatic necrosis (all may occur up to several days after overdose); renal tubular necrosis, hypoglycemic coma, nausea, vomiting, diaphoresis, malaise, somnolence, skeletal muscle flaccidity, bradycardia, hypotension, apnea, cardiac arrest.
- Monitor for orthostatic hypotension and supervise ambulation.
- Encourage coughing and deep breathing in patients with pulmonary problems.
- Check for reduced dosage if another CNS depressant medication is being administered concurrently.

When prescribed by medical facility:
- Determine why drug is being taken. Consider implications of condition on dental treatment.
- If GI side effects occur, consider semisupine chair position.
- Monitor vital signs.

Pregnancy Risk Category: Category C.

Oral Health Education
When prescribed by DDS:
- Instruct patient to take before pain becomes severe.
- Advise patient to take with food or milk.
- When medication is being used for acute pain, advise patient of possible addiction and explain that drug should be used for the short term only.

- Advise patient to change position slowly and to use caution when ambulating and performing other activities requiring mental alertness, such as driving or operating machinery.
- Instruct patient to eat high-fiber diet, maintain adequate fluid intake, and use stool softener or bulk laxative to prevent constipation.
- Advise patient to avoid alcohol and any other drug that causes drowsiness, such as sleeping aids and antihistamines.
- Instruct patient to discontinue drug and notify health care provider if blurred vision, rash, or yellowing of skin occurs.
- If lightheadedness, dizziness, drowsiness, nausea, or vomiting occurs, advise patient to lie down until symptoms subside and to notify health care provider if symptoms persist.

---

 acetaminophen/oxycodone HCl (ass-cet-ah-MEE-noe-fen/OX-ee-KOE-dohn HIGH-droe-KLOR-ide)

Synonym: oxycodone HCl/acetaminophen

Percocet: Tablets: 5 mg oxycodone HCl/325 mg acetaminophen, 7.5 mg oxycodone HCl/500 mg acetaminophen, 10 mg oxycodone HCl/650 mg acetaminophen
Roxicet: Tablets: 5 mg oxycodone HCl/325 mg acetaminophen; Solution, oral: 5 mg oxycodone HCl/325 mg acetaminophen
Roxicet 5/500: Caplets: 5 mg oxycodone/500 mg acetaminophen
Roxilox: Capsules: 5 mg oxycodone HCl/500 mg acetaminophen
Tylox: Capsules: 5 mg oxycodone HCl/500 mg acetaminophen
■✦■ **Percocet-Demi, ratio-Oxycocet**

Drug Class: Narcotic analgesic combination
DEA Schedule: Schedule II

PHARMACOLOGY
Action
Acetaminophen inhibits synthesis of prostaglandins centrally and peripherally blocks pain impulse generation, whereas oxycodone binds to opiate receptors in the CNS. Combination has synergistic effect in alleviating pain.

Uses
Relief of moderate to moderately severe pain.

Contraindications
Hypersensitivity to acetaminophen, oxycodone, or similar compounds.

Usual Dosage
ADULTS: *PO:* 5 mg (1 tablet, caplet, or teaspoonful) q 6 hr prn.

Pharmacokinetics
Acetaminophen
ABSORP: Rapid and complete from the GI tract. T_{max} is 0.5 to 2 hr; 4 hr after overdosage.
DIST: Distributed throughout most body fluids. Binding to plasma proteins is variable.
METAB: Primarily metabolized by hepatic conjugation (94%), and about 4% is metabolized by CYP450 oxidase to toxic metabolite.
EXCRET: $T_{1/2}$ is about 2 hr. 90% to 100% is recovered in the urine within the first day, primarily as inactive metabolites. 2% is excreted as unchanged drug.

Oxycodone
ABSORP: High oral availability due to low presystemic or first-pass metabolism. Exhibits a biphasic absorption pattern. The immediate-release oral bioavailability is 100%. The oral bioavailability is 60% to 87%. Peak plasma concentration increased by 25% with a high fat meal. Once absorbed, it is distributed to skeletal muscle, liver, intestinal tract, lungs, spleen, and brain.

DIST: The Vd is 2.6 L/kg (IV). It is found in breast milk.

METAB: Extensively metabolized in the liver to noroxycodone (a major metabolite), oxymorphone, and their glucuronides.

EXCRET: Excreted through the urine, with less than 19% as free oxycodone, less than 50% as conjugated oxycodone, and less than 14% as conjugated oxymorphone. The $t_{1/2}$ for immediate release is 0.4 hr. Clearance is 0.8 L/min. Elimination on $t_{1/2}$ is 3.2 hr (immediate release).

ONSET: 15 to 30 min.

PEAK: 1 hr.

DURATION: 4 to 6 hr.

SPECIAL POP: *Severe renal insufficiency:* For less than 60 mL/min, higher peak plasma oxycodone (50%), and noroxycodone (20%), higher AUC for oxycodone (60%), noroxycodone (50%), oxymorphone (40%). There is an increased $t_{1/2}$ of oxycodone elimination of only 1 hr.

Mild to moderate hepatic insufficiency: Peak plasma oxycodone and noroxycodone concentrations 50% and 20% higher; AUC values are 95% and 65% higher, respectively. Oxymorphone peak plasma concentration and AUC values are lower by 30% and 40%. The $t_{1/2}$ elimination for oxycodone is increased by 2.3 hr.

➡️◀ DRUG INTERACTIONS

See also: acetaminophen — Drug Interactions

Sertraline: Possible increased risk of serotonin syndrome (mechanism unknown)
- Monitor clinical status.

ADVERSE EFFECTS

⚠ **ORAL:** Dry mouth.

CVS: Hypotension; bradycardia; tachycardia.

CNS: Lightheadedness; dizziness; weakness; fatigue; sedation; euphoria; dysphoria; nervousness; headache; confusion.

GI: Nausea; vomiting; constipation; abdominal pain; anorexia; biliary spasm.

RESP: Dyspnea; respiratory depression.

MISC: Malaise; tolerance; psychological and physical dependence with long-term use.

CLINICAL IMPLICATIONS

General

When prescribed by DDS:
- Short-term use only; there is no justification for long-term use in the management of dental pain.
- *Lactation:* Undetermined.
- *Children:* Safety and efficacy not established.
- *Hepatic failure:* Chronic alcoholics should limit acetaminophen intake to less than 2 g/day.
- *Special risk:* Use with caution in elderly, debilitated patients and those with hepatic or kidney failure or conditions accompanied by hypoxia or hypercapnia; monitor carefully to avoid decrease in pulmonary ventilation. Also use cautiously in patients sensitive to CNS depressants, in all patients postoperatively, and in patients with pulmonary disease.
- *Sulfite sensitivity:* Use with caution in patients known to be sensitive, as some products contain bisulfites.
- *Dependence:* Can produce drug dependence; has abuse potential.
- *Overdosage:* Miosis, respiratory depression, CNS depression (somnolence progressing to stupor or coma), hepatic damage, circulatory collapse, cardiopulmonary arrest, death.

When prescribed by medical facility:
- Determine why drug is being taken. Consider implications of condition on dental treatment.
- Monitor vital signs.
- If GI side effects occur, consider semisupine chair position.
- Chronic dry mouth is possible; anticipate increased caries and candidiasis.

Pregnancy Risk Category: Category C.

Oral Health Education
When prescribed by DDS:
- Instruct patient to take medication before pain becomes severe for greatest effectiveness.
- Teach patient methods to prevent constipation.
- Instruct patient to make position changes slowly if lightheadedness or sedation occurs.
- Advise patient to avoid intake of alcoholic beverages or products containing alcohol while using this medication.
- Advise patient that drug may cause drowsiness, and to use caution while driving or performing other tasks requiring mental alertness.
- Caution patient that physical dependency and withdrawal symptoms may occur following discontinuation of long-term therapy.
- Instruct patient not to take any OTC medications without consulting health care provider.

When prescribed by medical facility:
- If chronic dry mouth occurs, recommend home fluoride therapy and use of nonalcoholic oral health care products.

---

acetaminophen/propoxyphene (ass-cet-ah-MEE-noe-fen/pro-POX-ee-feen)

(acetaminophen/propoxyphene HCl, acetaminophen/propoxyphene napsylate)

Synonym: propoxyphene/acetaminophen; propoxyphene HCl/acetaminophen; propoxyphene napsylate/acetaminophen

Darvocet A500, Darvocet-N 100, Darvocet-N 50, Wygesic

Drug Class: Narcotic analgesic combination

PHARMACOLOGY
Action
Propoxyphene relieves pain by stimulating opiate receptors in CNS; causes respiratory depression, peripheral vasodilation, inhibition of intestinal peristalsis, sphincter of hepato-pancreatic ampulla spasm, stimulation of receptors that cause vomiting, and increased bladder tone. Acetaminophen inhibits synthesis of prostaglandins; does not have significant anti-inflammatory effects or antiplatelet effects; produces antipyresis by direct action on the hypothalamic heat-regulating center.

Uses
Relief of mild to moderate pain; as analgesic-antipyretic in presence of aspirin allergy, hemostatic disturbances, bleeding diatheses, upper GI disease, and gouty arthritis.

➡️ DRUG INTERACTIONS RELATED TO DENTAL THERAPEUTICS
Alprazolam: Possible alprazolam toxicity with propoxyphene (decreased metabolism)
- Avoid concurrent use.

Diazepam: Possible diazepam toxicity with acetaminophen (mechanism unknown)
- Avoid concurrent use.

ADVERSE EFFECTS
CNS: Lightheadedness; weakness; fatigue; sedation; dizziness; disorientation; incoordination; paradoxical excitement; euphoria; dysphoria; insomnia; headache; hallucinations.
GI: Nausea; vomiting; constipation; anorexia; abdominal pain; biliary spasm.
RESP: Dyspnea; depression of cough reflex.
MISC: Tolerance; psychological and physical dependence with long-term use; histamine release; skin rashes.

CLINICAL IMPLICATIONS
General
- Determine why drug is being taken. Consider implications of condition on dental treatment.

- If GI side effects occur, consider semisupine chair position.
- If oral pain requires additional analgesics, consider nonopioid products.

---

acetaminophen/propoxyphene HCl — see acetaminophen/propoxyphene

acetaminophen/propoxyphene napsylate — see acetaminophen/propoxyphene

---

 # acetaminophen/tramadol HCl (ass-cet-ah-MEE-noe-fen/TRAM-uh-dole HIGH-droe-KLOR-ide)

Synonym: tramadol HCl/acetaminophen

Ultracet: Tablets: 325 mg acetaminophen/37.5 mg tramadol HCl

Drug Class: Nonnarcotic analgesic combination

PHARMACOLOGY

Action

TRAMADOL: Exact mechanism is unknown; however, it binds to certain opioid receptors and inhibits reuptake of norepinephrine and serotonin.

ACETAMINOPHEN: Inhibits prostaglandin in CNS and reduces fever through direct action on hypothalamic heat-regulating center.

Uses

Short-term (≤5 days) management of acute pain.

Contraindications

Any situation in which opioids are contraindicated, including acute intoxication with any of the following: alcohol, hypnotics, narcotics, centrally acting analgesics, opioids, or psychotropic drugs; hypersensitivity to any component of the product or opioids.

Usual Dosage

ADULTS: *PO:* 2 tablets (37.5 mg tramadol/325 mg acetaminophen/tablet) q 4 to 6 hr (max 8 tablets/day). In patients with Ccr less than 30 mL/min, it is recommended that the dosing interval be increased not to exceed 2 tablets q 12 hr.

Pharmacokinetics

ABSORP: The absolute bioavailability of tramadol after administration of a single 100-mg dose is approximately 75%. The mean peak plasma concentration of racemic tramadol occurs at approximately 2 hr. Oral absorption of acetaminophen occurs primarily in the small intestine. Peak concentrations of acetaminophen occur within 1 hr.

DIST: The Vd of tramadol is 2.6 and 2.9 L/kg in men and women, respectively, following IV administration of 100 mg. Tramadol is approximately 20% protein bound. Acetaminophen is widely distributed throughout the body tissue except fat. The Vd is approximately 0.9 L/kg. Less than 20% is bound to plasma protein.

METAB: Tramadol is extensively metabolized in the liver by a number of pathways, including CYP2D6 and 3A4, as well as by conjugation. The O-desmethyltramadol metabolite is pharmacologically active. Plasma levels of tramadol are approximately 20% higher in poor metabolizers (CYP2D6) compared with extensive metabolizers. Acetaminophen is primarily metabolized in the liver. In adults, most acetaminophen is conjugated with glucuronic acid and is not active. In premature infants, newborns, and young infants, the predominant metabolite is the sulfate conjugate.

EXCRET: Approximately 30% of the tramadol dose is excreted unchanged in the urine and 60% is excreted as metabolites. The plasma elimination $t_{1/2}$ of tramadol and the active metabolite are approximately 5 to 6 hr and 7 hr, respectively. The apparent $t_{1/2}$ of racemic tramadol increases to 7 to 9 hr with multiple dosing. The $t_{1/2}$ of acetaminophen is approximately 2 to 3 hr in adults and somewhat less in children, while being somewhat longer in neonates and patients with cirrhosis. Acetaminophen is eliminated in the urine, primarily as metabolites (less than 9% excreted unchanged).

SPECIAL POP: Use in patients with hepatic impairment is not recommended. Clearance of tramadol is 20% higher in women compared with men.

➔◆ DRUG INTERACTIONS

See also: acetaminophen — Drug Interactions

Antidepressants, tricyclic: Increased risk of seizure (additive proconvulsant effect)
• Avoid concurrent use.
Carbamazepine: Decreased tramadol effect (increased metabolism)
• Avoid concurrent use.
Citalopram: Increased risk of seizure (additive proconvulsant effect)
• Avoid concurrent use.
Fluoxetine: Increased risk of seizure (additive proconvulsant effect)
• Avoid concurrent use.
Increased risk of serotonin syndrome (additive serotonin effect)
• Avoid concurrent use.
Fluvoxamine: Increased risk of seizure (additive proconvulsant effect)
• Avoid concurrent use.
Monoamine oxidase inhibitors: Increased risk of serotonin syndrome (reduced uptake of monoamines)
• Avoid concurrent use.
Olanzapine: Possible increased risk of serotonin syndrome (mechanism nor established)
• Monitor clinical status.
Ondansetron: Possible decreased tramadol analgesia (serotonin antagonism)
• Monitor clinical status.
Paroxetine: Increased risk of seizure (additive proconvulsant effect)
• Avoid concurrent use.
Increased risk of serotonin syndrome (additive serotonin effect)
• Avoid concurrent use.
Sertraline: Increased risk of serotonin syndrome (additive serotonin effect)
• Avoid concurrent use.
Increased risk of serotonin syndrome (additive serotonin effect)
• Avoid concurrent use.
Warfarin: Bleeding into skin (mechanism unknown)
• Avoid concurrent use.

ADVERSE EFFECTS

⚠ **ORAL:** Dry mouth.
CVS: Hypertension; hypotension; arrhythmia; palpitation; tachycardia.
CNS: Somnolence; anorexia; insomnia; dizziness; headache; tremor; anxiety; confusion; euphoria; nervousness; amnesia; hallucination.
GI: Constipation; diarrhea; nausea; abdominal pain; dyspepsia; flatulence; vomiting.
RESP: Dyspnea.
MISC: Asthenia; fatigue; hot flushes; allergic reactions.

CLINICAL IMPLICATIONS

General
When prescribed by DDS:
• Short-term use only; there is no justification for long-term use in the management of dental pain.
• *Lactation:* Undetermined.
• *Children:* Safety and efficacy not established.
• *Elderly:* Use with caution, reflecting the greater frequency of decreased hepatic, renal, or cardiac function, and concomitant disease and multiple drug therapy.
• *Anaphylactoid reactions:* Serious and rarely fatal anaphylactoid reactions may occur.

- *Dependence:* Morphine-like psychic and physical dependence may occur with tramadol.
- *Hepatic disease:* Use is not recommended in patients with hepatic impairment.
- *Respiratory depression:* Use with caution in patients at risk of respiratory depression.
- *Seizures:* May occur.
- *Withdrawal:* Symptoms (e.g., anxiety, sweating, insomnia, rigors, pain, tremors) may occur if tramadol is discontinued abruptly.
- *Overdosage:* TRAMADOL: Respiratory depression, seizures, lethargy, coma, cardiac arrest, death. ACETAMINOPHEN: Anorexia, nausea, vomiting, malaise, pallor, diaphoresis, hepatic centrilobular necrosis (leading to hepatic failure and death), renal tubular necrosis, hypoglycemia, coagulation defects.

Pregnancy Risk Category: Category C.

Oral Health Education
When prescribed by DDS:
- Explain name, dose, action, and potential side effects of drug.
- Advise patient to take 2 tablets q 4 to 6 hr if needed for pain but not to take more than 8 tablets in 24 hr.
- Advise patient to take without regard to meals but to take with food if GI upset occurs.
- Caution patient to not take more tablets than prescribed or more frequently than prescribed. Serious toxicity may develop if prescribed dose is exceeded or doses are taken too close together.
- Advise patient that medication is for short-term use (≤5 days) only and if symptoms persist to contact health care provider regarding other therapies for pain control.
- Instruct patient to avoid taking acetaminophen or other acetaminophen-containing products, tramadol, or other tramadol-containing products.
- Instruct patient to avoid alcoholic beverages and other depressants while taking this medication.
- Advise patient that drug may impair judgment, thinking, or motor skills or cause dizziness and to use caution while driving or performing other tasks requiring mental alertness until tolerance is determined.
- Advise women to inform the health care provider if pregnant, planning to become pregnant, or breast feeding.
- Warn patient not to take any prescription or OTC drugs or dietary supplements without consulting the health care provider.
- Advise patient that follow-up visits may be necessary to monitor therapy and to keep appointments.

When prescribed by medical facility:
- If chronic dry mouth occurs, recommend home fluoride therapy and use of nonalcoholic oral health care products.

Acetaminophen Uniserts — see acetaminophen

acetohexamide (uh-seet-toe-HEX-uh-mide)
Dymelor
🔳✴🔳 **Dimelor**

Drug Class: Antidiabetic, sulfonylurea

PHARMACOLOGY
Action
Decreases blood glucose levels by stimulating release of insulin from pancreas.

Uses
Adjunctive therapy, used with dietary modification, in patients with type 2 diabetes mellitus for lowering blood glucose level.

➜◄ DRUG INTERACTIONS RELATED TO DENTAL THERAPEUTICS

Azole antifungal agents: Severe hypoglycemia (decreased metabolism of acetohexamide)
• Avoid concurrent use.

ADVERSE EFFECTS

CNS: Dizziness; vertigo.
GI: Nausea; epigastric fullness; heartburn; cholestatic jaundice (rare).
MISC: Disulfiram-like reaction; weakness; paresthesia; fatigue; malaise; photosensitivity; hypoglycemia.

CLINICAL IMPLICATIONS

General

• Determine degree of disease control and current blood sugar levels. A₁C levels ≥8% indicate significant uncontrolled diabetes.
• The routine use of antibiotics in the dental management of patients with diabetes is not indicated; however antibiotic therapy in patients with poorly controlled diabetes has been shown to improve disease control and improve response following periodontal debridement.
• Monitor blood pressure, as hypertension and dyslipidemia (CAD) are prevalent in diabetes mellitus. Monitor vital signs (e.g., BP, pulse pressure, rate, and rhythm) at each appointment to assess disease control. Do not provide elective dental treatment when BP is ≥180/110 or in the presence of other high-risk CV conditions. Refer to the section entitled "The Patient Taking Cardiovascular Drugs" in Chapter 6: *Clinical Medicine.*
• *Loss of blood sugar control:* Certain medical conditions (e.g., surgery, fever, infection, trauma) and drugs (e.g., corticosteroids) affect glucose control. In these situations, it may be necessary to seek medical consultation.
• Obtain patient history regarding diabetic ketoacidosis or hypoglycemia with current drug regimen.
• Observe for signs of hypoglycemia (e.g., confusion, argumentativeness, perspiration, altered consciousness). Be prepared to treat hypoglycemic reactions with oral glucose or sucrose.
• Prescribe drugs with photosensitization side effect with caution due to additive adverse effects.
• *Elderly:* Particularly susceptible to hypoglycemic effects of drug.
• *Disulfiram-like syndrome:* Alcohol may cause facial flushing and breathlessness.
• *Hypoglycemia:* May be difficult to recognize in elderly patients or in patients receiving beta-blockers.

Oral Health Education

• Explain role of diabetes in periodontal disease and the need to maintain effective plaque control and disease control.
• Advise to bring data on blood sugar values and A₁C levels to dental appointments.
• Encourage daily plaque control procedures for effective self-care in patients at risk for cardiovascular disease.

acetylsalicylic acid — see aspirin

Acifur — see acyclovir

Acimox — see amoxicillin

AcipHex — see rabeprazole sodium

acitretin (ASS-ih-TREH-tin)

Soriatane
Drug Class: Retinoid

PHARMACOLOGY

Action

Unknown.

Uses

Treatment of severe psoriasis.

➠⬅ DRUG INTERACTIONS RELATED TO DENTAL THERAPEUTICS

Tetracyclines: Increased intracranial pressure (mechanism unknown)
• Avoid concurrent use.

ADVERSE EFFECTS

⚠ **ORAL:** Dry, chapped lips (>75%); dry mouth (10% to 25%); tongue disorders, stomatitis, ulcerative stomatitis, gingival bleeding, gingivitis, increased salivation, thirst, taste disorder (1% to 10%).

CNS: Rigors (10% to 25%); headache, pain, depression, insomnia, somnolence (1% to 10%); myopathy with peripheral neuropathy, aggressive feelings and/or suicidal thoughts (postmarketing).

GI: Abdominal pain, diarrhea, nausea (1% to 10%).

MISC: Increased triglycerides (50% to 75%); increased CPK, fasting blood glucose (25% to 50%); decreased fasting blood sugar, high occult blood (10% to 25%); anorexia, edema, fatigue, hot flashes, increased appetite, photophobia, infection, decreased and increased iron, flushing (1% to 10%).

CLINICAL IMPLICATIONS

General
• Chronic dry mouth is possible; anticipate increased caries and candidiasis.
• Advise products for palliative relief of oral manifestations (e.g., stomatitis, cheilitis, xerostomia).
• If GI side effects occur, consider semisupine chair position.
• *Photophobia:* Direct dental light out of patient's eyes and offer dark glasses for comfort.

Oral Health Education
• If chronic dry mouth occurs, recommend home fluoride therapy and use of nonalcoholic oral health care products.

Aclimafel — see amoxicillin

Acromicina — see tetracycline HCl

Acroxil — see amoxicillin

ACT — see sodium fluoride

Actonel — see risedronate sodium

Actos — see pioglitazone

Acular — see ketorolac tromethamine

Acular LS — see ketorolac tromethamine

Acularen — see ketorolac tromethamine

Acupril — see quinapril HCl

---

 acyclovir (A-SIKE-low-vihr)

Acyclovir: Injection: 50 mg/mL (as sodium); Powder for injection: 500 mg/vial (as sodium); Powder for injection: 1,000 mg/vial (as sodium)
Zovirax: Tablets: 400, 800 mg; Capsules: 200 mg; Suspension: 200 mg per 5 mL; Powder for injection, lyophilized: 500 mg/vial (as sodium), 1,000 mg/vial (as sodium); Ointment: 5%; Cream: 5%

■✦■ Apo-Acyclovir, Gen-Acyclovir, Nu-Acyclovir

■✦■ Acifur, Cicloferon, Isavir, Laciken, Opthavir

Drug Class: Anti-infective; Antiviral

PHARMACOLOGY

Action
Inhibits viral DNA replication by interfering with viral DNA polymerase.

Uses
PARENTERAL: Treatment of initial or recurrent mucosal and cutaneous herpes simplex viruses (HSV) and varicella zoster infections (shingles) in immunocompromised patients; treatment of HSV-related encephalitis; treatment of severe initial clinical episodes of genital herpes; and treatment of neonatal herpes infections.

ORAL: Treatment of initial and recurrent episodes of genital herpes in certain patients; acute treatment of shingles and chickenpox.

TOPICAL: Treatment of initial episodes of herpes genitalis and non–life-threatening mucotaneous HSV infections in immunocompromised patients (ointment); recurrent herpes labialis (cold sores) (cream).

Unlabeled Uses
Treatment of cytomegalovirus and HSV infection after bone marrow or renal transplant; treatment of infectious mononucleosis, varicella pneumonia, chickenpox, and other HSV infections.

Contraindications
Hypersensitivity to acyclovir or valacyclovir.

Usual Dosage
PARENTERAL
For IV infusion only; rapid or bolus IV must be avoided.
Herpes simplex infections in immunocompromised patients
ADULTS AND ADOLESCENTS 12 YR OF AGE AND OLDER: *IV:* 5 mg/kg infused at a constant rate over 1 hr q 8 hr for 7 days.
CHILDREN YOUNGER THAN 12 YR OF AGE: *IV:* 10 mg/kg infused at a constant rate over 1 hr q 8 hr for 7 days.
ORAL
Chickenpox
ADULTS AND CHILDREN (GREATER THAN 40 KG): *PO:* 800 mg qid for 5 days.
CHILDREN 2 YR AND OLDER (40 KG OR LESS): *PO:* 20 mg/kg qid for 5 days.
Herpes zoster
ADULTS: *PO:* 800 mg q 4 hr 5 times/day for 7 to 10 days.
TOPICAL
Recurrent herpes labialis (cold sores)
ADULTS AND CHILDREN 12 YR OF AGE AND OLDER: *Cream:* Apply to lesion 5 times/day for 4 days.

Pharmacokinetics
ABSORP: *Oral:* Bioavailability is 10% to 20%. C_{max} is 0.83 to 1.61 mcg/mL (200 to 800 mg at steady state). *IV:* C_{max} is 9.8 mcg/mL (5-mg/kg dose), 22.9 mcg/mL (10 mg/kg). *Topical:* Systemic absorption is minimal.
DIST: 9% to 33% protein bound. *IV:* CSF concentrations are about 50% of plasma values.
METAB: Liver.
EXCRET: The $t_{1/2}$ is 2.5 to 3.3 hr. Cl and $t_{1/2}$ are dependent on renal function.
SPECIAL POP: *Renal failure:* Total body Cl and $t_{1/2}$ are dependent on renal function. Dosage adjustment recommended.
Elderly: Increased plasma concentrations. Dosage adjustment may be required.

➜◀ DRUG INTERACTIONS

Meperidine: Possible meperidine toxicity (decreased renal excretion)
• Monitor clinical status.

Zidovudine: Severe drowsiness and lethargy (mechanism unknown)
  • Monitor clinical status.

ADVERSE EFFECTS

⚠ **ORAL:** Burning, stinging (>10%); itching (topical cream).

CVS: Phlebitis at injection site (9%); hypotension.

CNS: Headache; agitation; coma; confusion; delirium; dizziness; hallucinations; obtundation; psychosis; seizure; somnolence.

GI: Nausea, vomiting (7%); diarrhea; GI distress; abdominal pain.

MISC: Anaphylaxis; fever; pain; peripheral edema thrombocytopenic purpura (immunocompromised patient).

CLINICAL IMPLICATIONS

General
  • *Lactation:* Excreted in breast milk.
  • *Children:* ORAL: Safety and efficacy in children younger than 2 yr of age not established. TOPICAL: Safety and efficacy not established in pediatric patients.
  • *Elderly:* Use with caution because of the greater frequency of decreased hepatic, renal, or cardiac function, and concomitant diseases or other drug therapy.
  • *Renal failure:* Dosage adjustment may be needed. With parenteral use, acyclovir may precipitate as crystals in renal tubules.
  • *Cutaneous use:* Care must be taken to avoid getting drug in eyes.
  • *Encephalopathic changes:* Patients with underlying neurological abnormalities or severe hypoxia may have increased risk of neurotoxic effects.
  • *Thrombotic thrombocytopenic purpura/hemolytic uremic syndrome:* May occur and has resulted in death in immunocompromised patients.
  • *Overdosage:* Increased BUN and serum creatinine, renal failure, convulsions, lethargy, acyclovir precipitation, renal tubules, agitation, coma.
  • Blood dyscrasias rarely reported; anticipate increased bleeding, infection, and poor healing.

Pregnancy Risk Category: Category B.

Oral Health Education
When prescribed by DDS:
  • Explain name, dose, action, and potential side effects of drug.
Topical
  • Advise patient not to cover the cold sore with a bandage or dressing.
  • Advise patient or caregiver using ointment to use finger cot or rubber glove when applying to prevent spread of infection and to wash hands with soap and water after applying ointment.
  • Advise patient or caregiver to apply enough ointment to adequately cover all lesions q 3 hr during waking hours (6 times/day) for 7 days. Advise patient or caregiver that a 1/2-inch ribbon of ointment should cover about 4 square inches.
  • Advise patient or caregiver using cream to apply to lesions 5 times/day for 4 days and to wash hands with soap and water after each application.
  • Advise patient or caregiver to notify health care provider if lesions do not appear to be improving, are getting worse, or if application site reactions (e.g., burning, stinging, redness, itching) develop.
Tablets, Capsules, or Suspension
  • Review dose and appropriate dosing schedule depending on condition being treated (e.g., shingles, chickenpox, recurrent herpes). Instruct patient to take medication exactly as prescribed and not to stop taking or change the dose unless advised by health care provider.
  • Advise patient that medication can be taken without regard to meals but to take with food if stomach upset occurs.
  • Advise patient or caregiver using suspension to shake it well before measuring dose and to measure and administer prescribed dose using a dosing syringe, dosing dropper, or medicine cup.

- Remind patient using medication for recurrent episodes of herpes to initiate therapy at the first sign or symptom or recurrence and that medication may not be effective if started more than 6 hr after onset of signs or symptoms of recurrence.
- Advise patient with herpes that this drug is not a cure for herpes and does not prevent transmission of virus.
- Advise patient to contact health care provider if medication does not seem to be controlling lesions and/or symptoms or if intolerable side effects develop.
- Advise women to notify health care provider if pregnant, planning to become pregnant, or breast feeding.
- Instruct patient not to take any prescription or OTC medications, dietary supplements, or herbal preparations unless advised by health care provider.
- Advise patient that follow-up visits may be necessary to monitor therapy and to keep appointments.

Aczone — see dapsone
Adalat — see nifedipine
Adalat CC — see nifedipine
Adalat XL — see nifedipine

---

adalimumab (ah-dah-LIM-you-mab)
Humira

Drug Class: Immunological agent

PHARMACOLOGY
Action
Blocks interaction of human tumor necrosis factor (TNF)-alpha with receptors and modulates biological responses induced or regulated by TNF.

Uses
Reduce signs and symptoms and inhibit progression of structural damage in patients with moderate to severe active rheumatoid arthritis who have had an inadequate response to one or more disease-modifying antirheumatic drugs.

➧← DRUG INTERACTIONS RELATED TO DENTAL THERAPEUTICS
No documented drug-drug interactions. The absence of evidence is not evidence of safety.

ADVERSE EFFECTS
CNS: Headache ($\geq$5%); confusion, multiple sclerosis, paresthesia, subdural hematoma, tremor (<5%).
CVS: Arrhythmia, tachycardia, atrial fibrillation, syncope, palpitation (<5%).
GI: Nausea, abdominal pain ($\geq$5%); cholecystitis, cholelithiasis, gastroenteritis, GI disorder and hemorrhage, vomiting (<5%).
RESP: URI, infection, sinusitis, flu-like syndrome ($\geq$5%); asthma, bronchospasm, dyspnea, lung disorder, decreased lung function, pleural effusion, pneumonia (<5%).
MISC: Accidental injury, back pain ($\geq$5%); fever, infection, pain in extremity, pelvic pain, sepsis, thorax pain, reactivated tuberculosis, lupus erythematosus syndrome, parathyroid disorder, adenoma, carcinoma (including breast, GI, skin, urogenital), lymphoma, malignancies, melanoma; leg thrombosis (<5%); serious infection (0.04%).

CLINICAL IMPLICATIONS
General
- *Immunosuppression:* May affect host defenses against infection and malignancies.
- Determine why drug is being taken. Consider implications of condition on dental treatment.

- If GI side effects occur, consider semisupine chair position.
- Monitor vital signs.
- *Arthritis:* Consider patient comfort and need for semisupine chair position.
- Place on frequent maintenance schedule to avoid periodontal inflammation.

Oral Health Education
- Evaluate manual dexterity; consider need for power toothbrush.

Adderall — see amphetamine and dextroamphetamine
Adderall XR — see amphetamine and dextroamphetamine
Adecur — see terazosin

---

adefovir dipivoxil (Ah-DEF-fah-vihr die-pihv-VOX-ill)
Hepsera

Drug Class: Antiviral Agent

PHARMACOLOGY
Action
Inhibits HBV DNA polymerase (reverse transcriptase) by competing with the natural substrate deoxyadenosine triphosphate and by causing DNA chain termination after its incorporation into viral DNA.

Uses
Treatment of chronic HBV infection in adults with evidence of active viral replication and evidence of persistent elevations in serum aminotransferases (ALT or AST) or histologically active disease.

➜← DRUG INTERACTIONS RELATED TO DENTAL THERAPEUTICS
No documented drug-drug interactions. The absence of evidence is not evidence of safety.

ADVERSE EFFECTS
Treatment-related adverse events reported in patients before and after transplantation include:
CNS: Headache.
GI: Nausea; vomiting; diarrhea; flatulence.
RESP: Increased cough; sinusitis.
MISC: Asthenia; abdominal pain; fever.

CLINICAL IMPLICATIONS
General
- Determine why drug is being taken. Consider implications of condition on dental treatment.
- Consider medical consult to determine disease control and influence on dental treatment.
- Anticipate oral candidiasis when HIV disease is reported.
- If GI side effects occur, consider semisupine chair position.
- Antibiotic prophylaxis should be considered when <500 PMN/mm^3 are reported; elective dental treatment should be delayed until blood values improve above this level.
- This drug is frequently prescribed in combination with one or more other antiviral agents. Side effects of all agents must be considered during the drug review process.

Oral Health Education
- Recommend frequent maintenance prophylaxis when immunosuppression is evident.
- Encourage daily plaque control procedures for effective self-care since HIV infection reduces host resistance.

Adel — see clarithromycin
Adipex-P — see phentermine HCl
Adoxa — see doxycycline hyclate
Adrenalin — see epinephrine
Adrenalin Chloride — see epinephrine
Adrucil — see fluorouracil
Adsorbocarpine — see pilocarpine HCl
Advair Diskus — see fluticasone propionate/salmeterol
Advicor — see niacin/lovastatin
Advil — see ibuprofen
Advil Liqui-Gels — see ibuprofen
Advil Migraine — see ibuprofen
Aerius — see desloratadine
Aerobec — see beclomethasone dipropionate
AeroBid — see flunisolide
AeroBid-M — see flunisolide
Aeroseb-Dex — see dexamethasone
Afeditab CR — see nifedipine
Afungil — see fluconazole
AF Valdecasas — see folic acid
Agenerase — see amprenavir
Aggrenox — see aspirin/dipyridamole
A-Hydrocort — see hydrocortisone
Airet — see albuterol
Airomir — see albuterol
Akarpine — see pilocarpine HCl
AK-Dex — see dexamethasone
Akineton — see biperiden
Akne-mycin — see erythromycin
Akorazol — see ketoconazole
AK-Pred — see prednisolone
Ala-Cort — see hydrocortisone
Ala-Scalp — see hydrocortisone
alatrofloxacin mesylate/trovafloxacin mesylate — see trovafloxacin mesylate/alatrofloxacin mesylate
Alavert — see loratadine
Alboral — see diazepam

 albuterol (al-BYOO-ter-ahl)

Airet: Solution for inhalation: 0.083% (as sulfate)

Proventil: Tablets: 2, 4 mg (as sulfate); Syrup: 2 mg (as sulfate) per 5 mL; Aerosol: Each actuation delivers 90 mcg albuterol; Solution for inhalation: 0.083%, 0.5% (as sulfate)
Proventil HFA: Aerosol: Each actuation delivers 90 mcg albuterol (as sulfate)
Ventolin: Tablets: 2, 4 mg (as sulfate); Syrup: 2 mg (as sulfate) per 5 mL; Solution for inhalation: 0.5% (as sulfate)
Ventolin Nebules: Solution for inhalation: 0.083% (as sulfate)
Ventolin Rotacaps: Capsules for inhalation: 200 mcg microfine (as sulfate)

■✦■ **Airomir, Alti-Salbutamol Sulfate, Apo-Salvent, Gen-Salbutamol Respirator Solution, Gen-Salbutamol Sterinebs P.F., Novo-Salmol, Nu-Salbutamol Solution, PMS-Salbutamol Respirator Solution, ratio-Salbutamol, Rho-Salbutamol, Rhoxal-salbutamol, Ventodisk Disk, Ventolin Diskus, Ventolin Oral Liquid**

■✦■ **Inspiryl, Salbulin, Salbutalan, Volmax**

Drug Class: Bronchodilator, sympathomimetic

PHARMACOLOGY
Action
Produces bronchodilation by relaxing bronchial smooth muscle through beta-2 receptor stimulation.

Uses
Prevention and treatment of reversible bronchospasm associated with asthma and other obstructive pulmonary diseases.

Unlabeled Uses
Adjunctive treatment of hyperkalemia in patients undergoing dialysis.

Contraindications
Cardiac tachyarrhythmias.

Usual Dosage
INHALATION AEROSOL
ADULTS AND CHILDREN AT LEAST 4 YR (AT LEAST 12 YR FOR PROVENTIL): 1 to 2 inhalations q 4 to 6 hr.
For prevention of exercise-induced bronchospasm
2 inhalations 15 min before exercise.
INHALATION SOLUTION
ADULTS AND CHILDREN AT LEAST 12 YR: 2.5 mg/dose 3 to 4 times/day by nebulization.
CHILDREN 2 TO 12 YR (ACCUNEB): 1.25 mg or 0.63 mg 3 to 4 times/day by nebulization.

Pharmacokinetics
ABSORP: *Tablets:* Rapidly absorbed; T_{max} is 2 hr; C_{max} is about 18 ng/mL. *Inhalation:* Less than 20% absorbed; T_{max} is 0.5 hr; C_{max} is 2.1 ng/mL.
EXCRET: $T_{1/2}$ is 5 to 6 hr. 76% recovered in urine over 3 days with 60% as metabolites; 4% excreted in feces.
ONSET: *Oral:* Within 30 min. *Inhalation:* Within 5 min.
DURATION: *Oral:* 4 to 8 hr. *Inhalation:* 3 to 6 hr.

➜✦ DRUG INTERACTIONS
Beta-adrenergic blockers: Decreased bronchodilator effect (antagonism)
 • Monitor clinical status.

ADVERSE EFFECTS
⚠ **ORAL:** Taste changes; dry mouth; teeth discoloration.
CVS: Palpitations; tachycardia; elevated BP; chest tightness; angina.

CNS: Tremor; dizziness; hyperactivity; nervousness; headache; insomnia; weakness; drowsiness; restlessness.

GI: Nausea; vomiting; heartburn; diarrhea.

RESP: Cough; bronchospasm; wheezing; dyspnea.

MISC: Flushing; sweating; anorexia; unusual sensory changes.

CLINICAL IMPLICATIONS

General
If prescribed by DDS:
* Monitor vital signs (e.g., BP, pulse rate, respiratory function) before and after administration. Uncontrolled disease characterized by wheezing, coughing.
* Acute bronchoconstriction can occur during dental treatment; have bronchodilator available.
* Ensure that bronchodilator inhaler is present at each dental appointment.
* Be aware that sulfites in local anesthetic with vasoconstrictor can precipitate acute asthma attack in susceptible individuals.
* Inhalants can dry oral mucosa; anticipate candidiasis, increased calculus and plaque levels, and increased caries.

Pregnancy Risk Category: Category C.

Oral Health Education
If prescribed by DDS:
* Teach patient correct method for using metered-dose inhaler. Have patient demonstrate proper technique, including timing between inhalations.
* Instruct patient in home monitoring of pulse and BP.
* Advise patient to maintain fluid intake of 2000 mL/day and to rinse mouth after each complete dose to prevent dryness.
* If chronic dry mouth occurs, recommend home fluoride therapy and use of nonalcoholic oral health care products.
* Instruct patient not to use OTC inhalers without consulting health care provider.
* Instruct patient to contact health care provider if symptoms are not relieved by normal dose.
* Tell patient to report adverse reactions or side effects.

---

albuterol sulfate/ipratropium bromide — see ipratropium bromide/albuterol sulfate

Aldactone — see spironolactone

Aldomet — see methyldopa and methyldopate HCl

---

alefacept (ah-LEE-fah-sept)
Amevive

Drug Class: Antipsoriatic; Immunosuppressant

PHARMACOLOGY

Action
Interferes with lymphocyte activation.

Uses
Treatment of adult patients with moderate to severe chronic plaque psoriasis who are candidates for systemic therapy or phototherapy.

➦◄ DRUG INTERACTIONS RELATED TO DENTAL THERAPEUTICS
No documented drug-drug interactions. The absence of evidence is not evidence of safety.

ADVERSE EFFECTS
GI: Nausea.
CNS: Dizziness.

RESP: Pharyngitis; increased cough.

MISC: Hypersensitivity reactions (e.g., urticaria, angioedema, anaphylactic reactions); malignancies; serious infections; lymphopenia; myalgia; chills; injection site reactions (e.g., pain, inflammation, bleeding, edema, nonspecific reaction, mass, skin hypersensitivity); accidental injury.

CLINICAL IMPLICATIONS

General

- *Immunosuppressive system:* Because of the risk of excessive immunosuppression, do not use with other immunosuppressive agents.
- *Serious infections:* Because alefacept is an immunosuppressive agent, it may increase the risk of infection and reactivate latent, chronic infections.
- Determine why drug is being taken. Consider implications of condition on dental treatment.
- If GI side effects occur, consider semisupine chair position.
- Consider semisupine chair position to assist respiratory function.

Oral Health Education

- Encourage daily plaque control procedures for effective self-care.
- Recommend frequent maintenance prophylaxis when immunosuppression is evident.

---

alendronate sodium (al-LEN-droe-nate SO-dee-uhm)

Fosamax

Drug Class: Bisphosphonate

PHARMACOLOGY

Action

Inhibits bone resorption and increases bone density.

Uses

Treatment of osteoporosis in postmenopausal women; prevention of osteoporosis in postmenopausal women at risk of developing osteoporosis; increase bone mass in men; treatment of glucocorticoid-induced osteoporosis in men and women; treatment of Paget disease of the bone.

➡◀ DRUG INTERACTIONS RELATED TO DENTAL THERAPEUTICS

Nonsteroidal anti-inflammatory drugs: Increased gastric ulcers (additive with alendronate)
- Avoid concurrent use.

ADVERSE EFFECTS

⚠ **ORAL:** Osteonecrosis of jaw (rare); oropharyngeal ulceration.

CNS: Headache (3%); malaise (postmarketing).

GI: Abdominal pain (7%); acid regurgitation, flatulence (4%); constipation, diarrhea, dyspepsia, nausea (3%); esophageal ulcer (2%); abdominal distention, dysphagia, gastric ulcer, gastritis (1%); duodenal ulcer, esophagitis, esophageal erosion, esophageal stricture, or perforation.

MISC: Fever, musculoskeletal pain.

CLINICAL IMPLICATIONS

General

- Determine why drug is being taken. Consider implications of condition on dental treatment.
- Patients may be high-risk candidates for pathological fractures or jaw fractures during extractions.

- This drug is used for Paget disease. Be aware of the head and neck manifestations (e.g., macrognathia, alveolar pain, bone warm to touch).
- If GI side effects occur, consider semisupine chair position.
- Osteonecrosis of the jaw is reported; consider this adverse drug effect when osteolytic disease is suspected.

Alertec — see modafinil
Aleve — see naproxen

alfuzosin HCl (al-FEW-zoe-sin HIGH-droe-KLOR-ide)
Uroxatral
Drug Class: Alpha₁-adrenergic blocker

PHARMACOLOGY
Action
Selective blockade for alpha₁-adrenergic receptors in the lower urinary tract, which cause smooth muscle relaxation in the bladder neck and prostate, resulting in improved urine flow and reduced symptoms of benign prostatic hyperplasia (BPH).

Uses
Treatment of signs and symptoms of benign prostatic hyperplasia.

➨◀ DRUG INTERACTIONS RELATED TO DENTAL THERAPEUTICS
Ketoconazole or itraconazole: Increased alfuzosin toxicity (decreased metabolism)
- Avoid concurrent use.

ADVERSE EFFECTS
CNS: Dizziness (6%); headache, fatigue (3%).
GI: Abdominal pain, dyspepsia, constipation, nausea (1% to 2%).
RESP: Upper respiratory tract infection (3%); bronchitis (1% to 2%).
MISC: Pain (1% to 2%); chest pain.

CLINICAL IMPLICATIONS
General
- If GI or respiratory side effects occur, consider semisupine chair position.

Algitrin — see acetaminophen
Alidol — see ketorolac tromethamine
Alin — see dexamethasone
Alin Depot — see dexamethasone

alitretinoin (al-ih-TRET-ih-no-in)
Panretin
Drug Class: Retinoid

PHARMACOLOGY
Action
Binds to and activates all known intracellular retinoid receptor substrates. Once activated, these receptors function as transcription factors that regulate the expression of genes that control the process of cellular differentiation and proliferation of both normal and neoplastic cells.

Uses
Topical treatment of cutaneous lesions of AIDS-related Kaposi sarcoma (KS).

➡◆ DRUG INTERACTIONS RELATED TO DENTAL THERAPEUTICS

No documented drug-drug interactions. The absence of evidence is not evidence of safety.

ADVERSE EFFECTS

MISC: Rash, pain, pruritus, edema, crusting at application site.

CLINICAL IMPLICATIONS

General

- Determine why drug is being taken. Consider implications of condition on dental treatment.
- Consider medical consult to determine disease control and influence on dental treatment.
- Anticipate oral candidiasis when HIV disease is reported.

Oral Health Education

- Recommend frequent maintenance prophylaxis when immunosuppression is evident.
- Encourage daily plaque control procedures for effective self-care.

Alka-Seltzer Flavoured — see aspirin

Allegra — see fexofenadine HCl

Allegra-D — see fexofenadine HCl/pseudoephedrine HCl

Allegra 12 Hour — see fexofenadine HCl

Allegra 24 Hour — see fexofenadine HCl

Aller-Chlor — see chlorpheniramine maleate

Allerdryl — see diphenhydramine HCl

Allergy — see chlorpheniramine maleate

AllerMax — see diphenhydramine HCl

AllerMax Maximum Strength — see diphenhydramine HCl

Allermed — see pseudoephedrine

Allernix — see diphenhydramine HCl

Allfen Jr — see guaifenesin

---

allopurinol (AL-oh-PURE-ee-nahl)

Aloprim, Zyloprim

■✦■ Apo-Allopurinol, Novo-Purol

■▨■ Atisuril, Unizuric 300, Zyloprim

Drug Class: Analgesic, Gout, Cytoprotective

PHARMACOLOGY

Action

Inhibits xanthine oxidase, the enzyme responsible for conversion of hypoxanthine to xanthine and then to uric acid.

Uses

TABLETS: Treatment of primary or secary gout, hyperuricemia resulting from chemotherapy for malignancies, recurrent calcium oxalate renal calculi.

TABLETS AND INJECTIONS: Management of patients with leukemia, lymphoma, and solid tumor malignancies when concurrently receiving cancer therapy that causes elevations of serum and urinary uric acid levels. Use injection in patients who cannot tolerate oral therapy.

Unlabeled Uses

Prevention of fluorouracil-induced stomatitis and fluorouracil-induced granulocyte suppression.

➡◀ DRUG INTERACTIONS RELATED TO DENTAL THERAPEUTICS

Penicillins: Increased incidence of rash (mechanism unknown)
• Monitor clinical status.

ADVERSE EFFECTS

⚠ **ORAL:** Taste loss; stomatitis, tongue edema, salivary gland swelling (<1%); lichenoid drug reaction (rare).

CNS: Drowsiness; headache; neuritis; paresthesias; peripheral neuropathy.

GI: Abdominal pain; diarrhea; dyspepsia; gastritis; granulomatous changes; nausea; vomiting.

MISC: Acute gouty attacks; arthralgia; fever; myopathy; necrotizing angiitis; maculopapular skin rash, thrombocytopenia (rare).

CLINICAL IMPLICATIONS

General

• If GI side effects occur, consider semisupine chair position.
• Patient may experience unilateral or bilateral TMJ pain (gouty arthritis) associated with acute exacerbation of gout.

Oral Health Education

• Gouty arthritis may affect fingers. Determine relevance to performing self-care procedures.
• Determine need for power toothbrush for self-care.

---

almotriptan malate (al-moe-TRIP-tan MAL-ate)

Axert

Drug Class: Analgesic, Migraine

PHARMACOLOGY

Action

Selective agonist for vascular serotonin (5-HT) receptor subtype, causing vasoconstriction of cranial arteries.

Uses

Acute treatment of migraine with or without aura.

➡◀ DRUG INTERACTIONS RELATED TO DENTAL THERAPEUTICS

No documented drug-drug interactions. The absence of evidence is not evidence of safety.

ADVERSE EFFECTS

⚠ **ORAL:** Dry mouth (1%).

CNS: Somnolence; headache; paresthesia; dizziness (≥1%).

CVS: Chest pain; tachycardia; hypertension (rare).

GI: Nausea (2%).

CLINICAL IMPLICATIONS

General

• This drug is used for an acute migraine attack. Patient is unlikely to come for dental treatment.

- Monitor vital signs (BP and pulse). Drugs for prevention are sympatholytic; drugs for treatment of acute attack are sympathomimetic.

Alocril — see nedocromil sodium
Aloprim — see allopurinol
Alor 5/500 — see aspirin/hydrocodone bitartrate
Alora — see estradiol

---

alosetron (al-OH-seh-trahn)
Lotronex

Drug Class: 5HT$_3$ receptor antagonist

PHARMACOLOGY

Action
Selective serotonin (5HT$_3$) receptor antagonist that inhibits serotonin receptors in the GI tract.

Uses
Treatment of irritable bowel syndrome (IBS) in women whose predominant bowel syndrome is diarrhea.

Unlabeled Uses
Treatment of IBS in men; carcinoid diarrhea.

➜⬅ DRUG INTERACTIONS RELATED TO DENTAL THERAPEUTICS
No documented drug-drug interactions. The absence of evidence is not evidence of safety.

ADVERSE EFFECTS
CNS: Sleep disorders; depressive disorders.
GI: Constipation; nausea; GI discomfort and pain; abdominal discomfort and pain; GI gaseous symptoms; viral GI infections; dyspeptic symptoms; abdominal distention; hemorrhoids.
RESP: Allergic rhinitis; throat and tonsil discomfort and pain; bacterial ear, nose, and throat infections.

CLINICAL IMPLICATIONS

General
- This drug was removed from the market in 2000; only physicians who have completed training in monitoring adverse drug effects associated with the product may prescribe it.
- If GI side effects occur, consider semisupine chair position.

---

alprazolam (al-PRAY-zoe-lam)

Alprazolam Intensol: Oral solution: 1 mg/mL
Niravam: Orally disintegrating tablets: 0.25, 0.5, 1, 2 mg
Xanax: Tablets: 0.25, 0.5, 1, 2 mg
Xanax XR: Tablets, extended-release: 0.5, 1, 2, 3 mg

■✦■ **Apo-Alpraz, Apo-Alpraz TS, Gen-Alprazolam, Novo-Alprazol, Nu-Alpraz, ratio-Alprazolam, Xanax TS**

■✦■ **Tafil**

Drug Class: Antianxiety, benzodiazepine
DEA Schedule: Schedule IV

PHARMACOLOGY

Action
Potentiates action of GABA, an inhibitory neurotransmitter, resulting in increased neuronal inhibition and CNS depression, especially in limbic system and reticular formation.

Uses
Treatment of panic disorders with or without agoraphobia (Niravam, Xanax, Xanax XR); management of anxiety disorders or for short-term relief of symptoms of anxiety, including anxiety associated with depression (Niravam, immediate-release tablets and oral solution).

Unlabeled Uses
Treatment of irritable bowel syndrome, depression, premenstrual syndrome.

Contraindications
Hypersensitivity to other benzodiazepines; acute narrow-angle glaucoma; patients receiving itraconazole or ketoconazole.

Usual Dosage
Anxiety disorder
IMMEDIATE-RELEASE TABLETS AND ORAL SOLUTION
ADULTS: *PO:* Immediate-release tablets and oral solution: 0.25 to 0.5 mg tid (max, 4 mg/day in divided doses). Extended-release tablets: Start with 0.5 mg daily and gradually increase if needed (suggested total daily dose range 3 to 6 mg/day).

Pharmacokinetics
ABSORP: Readily absorbed; T_{max} is 1 to 2 hr; C_{max} is 8 to 37 ng/mL (0.5 to 3 mg doses).
DIST: 80% protein bound. Crosses the placenta and is excreted in breast milk.
METAB: Metabolized in the liver to alpha-hydroxy-alprazolam (activity is approximately 50% that of alprazolam) and a benzophenone derivative (inactive).
EXCRET: The $t_{1/2}$ is approximately 16.3 hr. Excreted in the urine.
SPECIAL POP: *Hepatic failure:* The $t_{1/2}$ is approximately 19.7 hr in those with alcoholic liver disease.
Elderly: The $t_{1/2}$ is approximately 16.3 hr.
Obese: The $t_{1/2}$ is approximately 21.8 hr.

➜← DRUG INTERACTIONS
Alcohol: Increased CNS depression (additive and decreased metabolism of alprazolam)
• Avoid concurrent use.
Ketoconazole and itraconazole: Possible alprazolam toxicity (decreased metabolism)
• Monitor clinical status.
Fluoxetine: Possible increased impairment of skills related to driving (decreased metabolism)
• Warn patients of the risk.
Propoxyphene: Possible alprazolam toxicity (decreased metabolism)
• Avoid concurrent use.

ADVERSE EFFECTS
⚠ **ORAL:** Dry mouth (15%); increased salivation (6%).
CVS: Tachycardia (15%); hypotension (5%); palpitation (≥1%).
CNS: Drowsiness (77%); fatigue/tiredness (49%); sedation (45%); irritability, memory impairment (33%); cognitive disorder (29%); somnolence (23%); light-headedness (21%); decreased libido (14%); depression (12%); dysarthria (11%); confusional state (10%); abnormal coordination (9%); ataxia, mental impairment (7%); disturbed attention, impaired balance, disinhibition (3%); disorientation, paresthesia, dyskinesia, talkativeness, derealization, abnormal dreams, lethargy (2%); anxiety, hypesthesia, hypersomnia, fear, warm feeling (1%); malaise, weakness, headache, dizziness, tremor, irritability, insomnia, nervousness, increased libido, restlessness, agitation, depersonalization, nightmare (≥1%).
GI: Constipation (26%); nausea/vomiting (22%); diarrhea (21%); abdominal distress (18%); dry mouth (15%); increased salivation (6%); dyspepsia, abdominal pain (≥1%).

RESP: URI (4%); dyspnea (2%); hyperventilation (≥1%).
MISC: Chest pain (≥1%); hyperprolactinemia.

CLINICAL IMPLICATIONS
General
When prescribed by DDS:
- *Lactation:* Excreted in breast milk.
- *Children:* Safety and efficacy in children younger than 18 yr of age not established.
- *Elderly:* Use smallest effective dose to preclude development of ataxia or overdosage.
- *Renal failure:* Caution is needed to avoid accumulation of drug.
- *Hepatic failure:* Caution is needed to avoid accumulation of drug.
- *Dependence:* Prolonged use can lead to physical and psychological dependence. Withdrawal syndrome has occurred within 4 to 6 wk of treatment, especially if abruptly discontinued. Cautious use and tapering of dosage are necessary.
- *Fetal harm:* There is a risk of fetal harm (e.g., congenital abnormalities) when used during pregnancy.
- *Impaired pulmonary function:* Death has been reported in patients with pulmonary disease shortly after starting alprazolam treatment.
- *Interdose symptoms:* Early morning anxiety and emergence of anxiety symptoms have been reported between doses in patients with panic disorder.
- *Mania:* Hypomania and mania have been reported.
- *Psychiatric disorders:* Not intended for patients with primary depressive disorder, psychoses, or disorders in which anxiety is not prominent.
- *Seizures:* May occur during abrupt drug discontinuation or dose reduction.
- *Suicide:* Use with caution in patients with suicidal tendencies; do not allow access to large quantities of drug.
- *Overdosage:* Somnolence, confusion, impaired coordination, diminished reflexes, coma, death.

When prescribed by medical provider:
- Monitor vital signs.
- If GI side effects occur, consider semisupine chair position.
- Blood dyscrasias rarely reported; anticipate increased bleeding, infection, and poor healing.
- Chronic dry mouth is possible; anticipate increased caries and candidiasis.
- Determine ability to adapt to stress of dental treatment. Consider short appointments.
- Depressed or anxious patients may neglect self-care. Monitor for plaque control effectiveness.

Pregnancy Risk Category: Category D.
Oral Health Education
When prescribed by DDS:
- Explain name, dose, action, and potential side effects of drug.
- Advise patient or caregiver to read the *Patient Information* leaflet before starting therapy and with each refill.
- Advise patient that medication is usually started at a low dose and then gradually increased until maximum benefit is obtained.
- Caution patient that medication may be habit forming and to take as prescribed and not to increase the dose or frequency of use unless advised by health care provider.
- Advise patient to take each dose without regard to meals but to take with food if stomach upset occurs.
- Advise patient using extended-release tablets to take prescribed dose once daily, preferably in the morning. Caution patient to swallow tablets whole and not to crush, chew, divide, or break the tablet.
- Advise patient or caregiver using oral solution to measure prescribed dose using calibrated dropper and then add solution to a liquid (e.g., juice, water, soda) or semisolid food (e.g., applesauce, pudding), stir for a few sec then immediately take (give) the entire mixture. Caution patient or caregiver not to prepare mixtures ahead of time and store.
- Advise patient using orally disintegrating tablet to remove tablet from bottle immediately before administration using dry hands and to place the tablet on top of tongue where it

will disintegrate and be swallowed with saliva. Advise patient that administration with liquid is not required. Instruct patient to discard any cotton that was included in the bottle and to reseal the bottle tightly after removing tablet(s) to prevent introducing moisture into bottle (which can cause the tablets to disintegrate).

- Caution patient using half of a scored orally disintegrating tablet to discard the unused portion of the tablet and not to save for future use, because the remaining tablet portion may not be stable.
- Advise patient that if a dose is missed to skip that dose and take the next one at the regularly scheduled time. Caution patient to never take two doses at the same time.
- Advise patient that if medication needs to be discontinued it will be slowly withdrawn for a period of 2 wk or more unless safety concerns (e.g., rash) require a more rapid withdrawal. Caution patient not to stop taking the medication abruptly or decrease the dose unless advised by health care provider because of the risk of withdrawal symptoms occurring.
- Instruct patient to avoid alcoholic beverages and other depressants while taking this medication.
- Advise patient with anxiety to take as needed and to seek alternative methods for controlling or preventing anxiety (e.g., stress reduction, counseling).
- Instruct patient to contact health care provider if symptoms do not appear to be getting better, worsen, or if bothersome side effects (e.g., drowsiness, memory impairment) occur.
- Advise patient that drug may cause drowsiness or impair judgment, thinking, or reflexes and to use caution while driving or performing other tasks requiring mental alertness until tolerance is determined.
- Advise women to notify health care provider if pregnant, planning to become pregnant, or breastfeeding.
- Warn patient not to take any prescription or OTC drugs, herbal preparations, or dietary supplements without consulting health care provider.
- Advise patient that follow-up visits may be necessary to monitor therapy and to keep appointments.

When prescribed by medical provider:
- If chronic dry mouth occurs, recommend home fluoride therapy and use of nonalcohol oral products.
- Encourage daily plaque control procedures for effective self-care.

Alprazolam Intensol — see alprazolam

Altace — see ramipril

Alti-Pindolol — see pindolol

Alti-Piroxicam — see piroxicam

Alti-Prazosi — see prazosin HCl

Alti-Prednisone — see prednisone

Alti-Ranitidine HCl — see ranitidine HCl

Alti-Salbutamol Sulfate — see albuterol

Alti-Trazodone — see trazodone HCl

Alti-Trazodone Dividose — see trazodone HCl

Alti-Triazolam — see triazolam

Alti-Valproic — see valproic acid and derivatives

Alti-Verapamil — see verapamil HCl

Altoprev — see lovastatin

Altruline — see sertraline HCl
Alupent — see metaproterenol sulfate

amantadine HCl (uh-MAN-tuh-deen HIGH-droe-KLOR-ide)

Amantadine HCl, Symmetrel

■✦■ **Endantadine, Gen-Amantadine, Symmetrel**

Drug Class: Antiparkinson; Antiviral

PHARMACOLOGY

Action
Exact mechanism is unknown; thought to facilitate dopamine release from intact dopaminergic terminals, increasing dopamine concentration at dopaminergic terminals. Exhibits antiviral activity against influenza A virus by inhibiting entry of virus into host cell.

Uses
Symptomatic treatment of several forms of Parkinson disease or syndrome and drug-induced extrapyramidal reactions; prevention and treatment of influenza A viral respiratory illness, especially in high-risk patients.

➜◄ DRUG INTERACTIONS RELATED TO DENTAL THERAPEUTICS
No documented drug-drug interactions. The absence of evidence is not evidence of safety.

ADVERSE EFFECTS
⚠ **ORAL:** Dry mouth (10%).
CNS: Dizziness, lightheadedness, insomnia (5% to 10%); depression, anxiety, irritability, hallucinations, confusion, headache, somnolence, nervousness, abnormal dreams, agitation (1% to 5%); coma; stupor; delusions; aggressive behavior; paranoid reaction; manic reaction; involuntary muscle contractions; abnormal gait; paresthesia; EEG changes; tremor.
CVS: Orthostatic hypotension (infrequent); tachycardia; mild bradycardia.
GI: Nausea (5% to 10%); constipation, diarrhea (1% to 5%); dysphagia.
RESP: Acute respiratory failure; pulmonary edema; tachypnea.
MISC: Ataxia, livedo reticularis, peripheral edema, fatigue (1% to 5%); allergic reactions (including anaphylactic reactions, edema, and fever); neuroleptic malignant syndrome.

CLINICAL IMPLICATIONS

General
- Determine why drug is being taken. Consider implications of condition on dental treatment.
- Prolonged use can lead to significant xerostomia. Anticipate increased caries, candidiasis, and oral discomfort.
- Monitor vital signs due to potential CV side effects.
- *Postural hypotension:* Monitor BP at the beginning and end of each appointment; anticipate syncope. Have patient sit upright for several min at the end of the dental appointment before dismissing.

Oral Health Education
- If chronic dry mouth occurs, recommend home fluoride therapy and use of nonalcoholic oral products.
- Parkinson disease can cause tremors and neuromuscular problems. Determine need for power toothbrush for self-care.

Amaryl — see glimepiride

ambenonium Cl (am-be-NOE-nee-um)
Mytelase

Drug Class: cholinesterase inhibitor

PHARMACOLOGY

Action
Inhibits destruction of acetylcholinesterase, which facilitates transmission of impulses across the myoneural junction.

Uses
Cholinergic for treatment of myasthenia gravis.

➡← DRUG INTERACTIONS RELATED TO DENTAL THERAPEUTICS
No documented drug-drug interactions. The absence of evidence is not evidence of safety.

ADVERSE EFFECTS
⚠ **ORAL:** Increased salivation; dysphagia.
CNS: Dizziness; loss of consciousness; convulsions; drowsiness; speech disturbances.
CVS: Arrhythmia; bradycardia; hypotension; tachycardia (uncommon); cardiac arrest; syncope.
GI: Nausea; vomiting; diarrhea; abdominal cramps.
RESP: Increased bronchial secretions; laryngospasm; dyspnea; respiratory arrest.
MISC: Muscle weakness; muscle cramps; diaphoresis; flushing.

CLINICAL IMPLICATIONS

General
- Excessive salivation may complicate crown and bridge impression procedures; anticipate need for suction control. Avoid drugs that reduce salivary flow, as they may antagonize this drug.
- Disease may cause patient to be unable to keep mouth open for long periods; anticipate need for short appointments.
- Monitor vital signs. Follow protocol to avoid postural hypotension at end of appointment.
- If GI side effects occur, consider semisupine chair position.

Oral Health Education
- Determine need for power toothbrush for self-care.

Ambien — see zolpidem tartrate

Ambotetra — see tetracycline HCl

Amcort — see triamcinolone

Ameblin — see metronidazole

Amen — see medroxyprogesterone acetate

Amerge — see naratriptan

Americaine Anesthetic Lubricant — see benzocaine

A-Methapred — see methylprednisolone

amethopterin — see methotrexate

Ametop — see tetracaine HCl

Amevive — see alefacept

Amicar — see aminocaproic acid

amiloride HCl (uh-MILL-oh-ride HIGH-droe-KLOR-ide)

Midamor

Drug Class: Potassium-sparing diuretic

PHARMACOLOGY

Action

Interferes with sodium reabsorption at distal tubule, resulting in increased excretion of water and sodium and decreased excretion of potassium.

Uses

Treatment of CHF or hypertension (in combination with thiazide or loop diuretics) and diuretic-induced hypokalemia.

Unlabeled Uses

Reduction of lithium-induced polyuria; slowed reduction of pulmonary function in patients with cystic fibrosis (aerosol form).

➡◀ DRUG INTERACTIONS RELATED TO DENTAL THERAPEUTICS

No documented drug-drug interactions. The absence of evidence is not evidence of safety.

ADVERSE EFFECTS

⚠ **ORAL:** Dry mouth; thirst.

CNS: Headache; dizziness; encephalopathy; paresthesia; tremors; vertigo; nervousness; mental confusion; insomnia; decreased libido; depression.

CVS: Irregular heartbeat (hyperkalemia); orthostatic hypotension, angina pectoris, palpitation ($<$1%).

GI: Nausea; anorexia; diarrhea; vomiting; abdominal pain; gas pain; appetite changes; constipation; GI bleeding; abdominal fullness; heartburn; flatulence.

RESP: Cough; dyspnea.

MISC: Musculoskeletal (e.g., weakness; fatigue; muscle cramps; joint/back/chest pain; neck or shoulder ache).

CLINICAL IMPLICATIONS

General

- Determine why drug is being taken. Consider implications of condition on dental treatment.
- Monitor vital signs (e.g., BP, pulse pressure, rate, and rhythm) at each appointment to assess disease control. Do not provide elective dental treatment when BP is ≥180/110 or in the presence of other high-risk CV conditions.
- Monitor pulse rhythm to assess for electrolyte imbalance.
- Use local anesthetic agents with vasoconstrictor with caution based on functional capacity of the patient and use aspirating technique to prevent intravascular injection.
- *Postural hypotension:* Monitor BP at the beginning and end of each appointment; anticipate syncope. Have patient sit upright for several min at the end of the dental appointment before dismissing.
- If GI side effects occur, consider semisupine chair position.
- Chronic dry mouth is possible. Anticipate increased caries, candidiasis, and lichenoid mucositis.
- Determine ability to adapt to stress of dental treatment. Consider short appointments.

Oral Health Education

- If chronic dry mouth occurs, recommend home fluoride therapy and use of nonalcoholic oral products.

aminocaproic acid (uh-mee-no-kuh-PRO-ik AS-id)

Amicar: Injection: 250 mg/mL; Tablets: 500 mg, Dose form: Syrup, 250 mg/mL
Drug Class: Hemostatic

PHARMACOLOGY

Action
Inhibits fibrinolysis to stop bleeding.

Uses
Treatment of excessive bleeding from systemic hyperfibrinolysis and urinary fibrinolysis.

Unlabeled Uses
Prevention of recurrence of subarachnoid hemorrhage; management of amegakaryocytic thrombocytopenia; abortion; or prevention of attacks of hereditary angioneurotic edema.

Contraindications
Active intravascular clotting; disseminated intravascular coagulation; administration to newborns.

Usual Dosage
ADULTS: *IV/PO:* 4 to 5 g in first hr; then 1 to 1.25 g/hr for 8 hr or until bleeding is controlled. Dosage over 30 g/24 hr is not recommended.

Pharmacokinetics
ABSORP: *Oral:* Zero order process; absorption rate of 5.2 g/hr. C_{max} is about 164 mcg/mL; T_{max} is about 1.2 hr.
DIST: *Oral:* Vd is about 23.1 L. *IV:* Vd is about 30 L.
METAB: Metabolite is adipic acid.
EXCRET: Renally eliminated; 65% is recovered in the urine as unchanged drug and 11% as the metabolite adipic acid. Renal clearance is 116 mL/min and total body clearance is 169 mL/min. $T_{1/2}$ is about 2 hr.
DURATION: 3 hr for single IV dose.

➡◀ DRUG INTERACTIONS
No documented drug-drug interactions. The absence of evidence is not evidence of safety.

ADVERSE EFFECTS
CVS: Bradycardia; hypotension; peripheral ischemia; thrombosis intracranial hypertension; stroke; syncope.
CNS: Dizziness; headache; delirium; hallucinations; confusion.
GI: Nausea; diarrhea; abdominal pain; vomiting.
RESP: Dyspnea; nasal congestion; pulmonary embolism.
MISC: Injection site reaction; pain and necrosis; myalgia; myositis; myopathy (characterized by muscle weakness, fatigue, elevated creatinine phosphokinase, rhabdomyolysis associated with myoglobinuria and renal failure); edema; allergic and anaphylactic reactions; anaphylaxis; malaise.

CLINICAL IMPLICATIONS

General
When used by DDS:
- *Lactation:* Undetermined.
- *Children:* Safety and efficacy not established.
- *Overdosage:* Hypotension, severe acute renal failure.
- Obtain patient history, including drug history and any known allergies.
- Determine baseline BP and pulse before starting IV infusion.
- Assess patient's respiratory and neurological status.

- Note presence of menstrual bleeding.
- Monitor serum potassium levels, clotting factors, and platelet counts.
- Monitor vital signs, especially BP and pulse, and respiratory and neurological status throughout therapy.
- Monitor input and output. Note any increase or decrease in urinary output.
- Observe for signs of internal bleeding (e.g., petechiae, gingival oozing, hematuria, epistaxis, ecchymosis).
- Have vitamin K or protamine sulfate available for emergency use.

Pregnancy Risk Category: Category C.

Oral Health Education
When used by DDS:
- Caution patient to avoid sudden position changes to prevent orthostatic hypotension.
- Advise patient to use soft toothbrush or sponge for dental care.
- Instruct patient to report the following symptoms to health care provider: gingival bleeding, epistaxis, hematuria, skin changes (e.g., ecchymosis, petechiae), difficulty in urination, reddish-brown urine, chest or leg pain, or difficulty breathing.

aminophylline (am-in-AHF-ih-lin)
Synonym: theophylline ethylenediamine

Phyllocontin, Truphylline

◼◆◼ **Phyllocontin, Phyllocontin-350**

◼◆◼ **Drafilyn**

Drug Class: Bronchodilator; Xanthine derivative

PHARMACOLOGY
Action
Relaxes bronchial smooth muscle and pulmonary blood vessels; stimulates central respiratory drive; increases diaphragmatic contractility.

Uses
Prevention or treatment of reversible bronchospasm associated with asthma or COPD.

Unlabeled Uses
Treatment of apnea and bradycardia of prematurity.

➡◆ DRUG INTERACTIONS RELATED TO DENTAL THERAPEUTICS
Diazepam, alprazolam, or midazolam: Decreased effect with aminophylline (mechanism unknown)
- Avoid concurrent use.

Erythromycin, clarithromycin, or azithromycin: Possible aminophylline toxicity (decreased metabolism)
- Avoid concurrent use.

ADVERSE EFFECTS
CNS: Irritability; headache; insomnia; muscle twitching; seizures.
CVS: Hypotension; tachycardia; ventricular arrhythmia (i.e., toxicity).
GI: Nausea; vomiting; anorexia; diarrhea; gastroesophageal reflux; epigastric pain.
RESP: Tachypnea; respiratory arrest.
MISC: Fever; flushing; hyperglycemia; inappropriate antidiuretic hormone secretion; sensitivity reactions (e.g., exfoliative dermatitis, urticaria).

CLINICAL IMPLICATIONS
General
- *Toxicity:* Patients with liver impairment or cardiac failure and those older than 55 yr are at greatest risk.

- Monitor vital signs (e.g., BP, pulse rate) and respiratory function. Uncontrolled disease characterized by wheezing, coughing.
- Acute bronchoconstriction can occur during dental treatment; have bronchodilator inhaler available.
- Ensure that bronchodilator inhaler is present at each dental appointment.
- Be aware that sulfites in local anesthetic with vasoconstrictor can precipitate acute asthma attack in susceptible individuals.
- Therapeutic doses may induce GERD while in supine position, increasing risk of aspiration and bronchospasm. Use semisupine chair position.

Oral Health Education
- Advise patient not to smoke. If patient changes smoking habits or stops smoking, dosage adjustment may be necessary.

---

aminosalicylate sodium (uh-MEE-no-suh-LIS-ih-late SO-dee-uhm)

Synonym: para-aminosalicylate sodium; PAS

Paser

Drug Class: Anti-infective; Antitubercular

PHARMACOLOGY

Action
Competitively antagonizes metabolism of para-aminobenzoic acid, resulting in bacteriostatic activity against *Mycobacterium tuberculosis*.

Uses
Treatment of tuberculosis (in combination with other antituberculous drugs) caused by susceptible strains of tubercle bacilli.

➡◀ DRUG INTERACTIONS RELATED TO DENTAL THERAPEUTICS
No documented drug-drug interactions. The absence of evidence is not evidence of safety.

ADVERSE EFFECTS
GI: Nausea; vomiting; diarrhea; abdominal pain.
MISC: Hypersensitivity (e.g., fever, skin eruptions, infectious mononucleosis–like syndrome, leukopenia, agranulocytosis, thrombocytopenia, hemolytic anemia, jaundice, hepatitis, encephalopathy, Löffler syndrome, vasculitis).

CLINICAL IMPLICATIONS

General
- Determine why drug is being taken (prevention or treatment). Consider implications of condition on dental treatment.
- Complete medical consultation to ensure noninfectious state exists before providing dental treatment. For dental emergencies: follow special precautions to minimize disease transmission (particulate respirators) or refer patient to a hospital-based dental facility.
- If GI side effects occur, consider semisupine chair position.
- Blood dyscrasias rarely reported; anticipate increased bleeding, infection, and poor healing.
- Monitor patient for signs of active disease (e.g., cough, blood in sputum, night sweats, fever). If positive for signs, refer for medical evaluation.
- *CDC advises to ensure noninfectiousness by these criteria:* Anti-TB drugs have been taken for >3 wk and culture confirmed susceptibility to TB organism; patient is not coughing; two consecutive sputum smears were negative for TB organism.

amiodarone (uh-MEE-oh-duh-rone)

Cordarone, Pacerone

■✦■ Gen-Amiodarone, Novo-Amiodarone, ratio-Amiodarone, Rhoxal-amiodarone

■✦■ Braxan, Cardiorona, Cordarone

Drug Class: Antiarrhythmic

PHARMACOLOGY

Action

Prolongs action potential duration and refractory period in myocardial cells; acts as non-competitive inhibitor of alpha- and beta-adrenergic receptors.

Uses

ORAL: Treatment of life-threatening recurrent ventricular arrhythmias (i.e., ventricular fibrillation and hemodynamically unstable ventricular tachycardia) that do not respond to other antiarrhythmic agents. Use only in patients with the indicated life-threatening arrhythmias because its use is accompanied by substantial toxicity.

PARENTERAL: Initiation of treatment and prophylaxis of frequently recurring ventricular fibrillation and hemodynamically unstable ventricular tachycardia in patients refractory to other therapy; treatment of ventricular tachycardia and fibrillation when oral amiodarone is indicated but patient is unable to take oral medication.

Unlabeled Uses

Conversion of atrial fibrillation and maintenance of sinus rhythm; treatment of supraventricular tachycardia; IV amiodarone has been used to treat AV nodal reentry tachycardia.

➦← DRUG INTERACTIONS RELATED TO DENTAL THERAPEUTICS

Fentanyl: Increased cardiotoxicity with amiodarone (mechanism unknown)
 • Monitor vital signs.

ADVERSE EFFECTS

⚠ ORAL: Abnormal salivation (1% to 3%); bitter or metallic taste.

CNS: Fatigue; malaise; tremor/abnormal involuntary movements; lack of coordination; abnormal gait/ataxia; dizziness; paresthesias; decreased libido; insomnia; headache; sleep disturbances; abnormal sense of smell.

CVS: Bradycardia; arrhythmia; hypotension (<1%).

GI: Nausea, vomiting, constipation, anorexia, abdominal pain, abnormal salivation (oral); diarrhea (parenteral).

RESP: Pulmonary inflammation or fibrosis, progressive dyspnea, pulmonary toxicosis, and death (oral); lung edema, respiratory disorder (parenteral).

MISC: Edema, photosensitivity (10%); photophobia, hyperthyroidism, or hypothyroidism (oral); fever (parenteral).

CLINICAL IMPLICATIONS

General

 • Monitor vital signs (e.g., BP, pulse pressure, rate, and rhythm) at each appointment to assess disease control. Do not provide elective dental treatment when BP is ≥180/110 or in the presence of other high-risk CV conditions.
 • Patients taking this drug have significant CV disease. Medical consult to determine patient's ability to withstand stress of dental treatment is recommended.
 • If GI or respiratory side effects occur, consider semisupine chair position.
 • As needed for photophobia, direct dental light out of patient's eyes and offer dark glasses for comfort.

Oral Health Education

- Encourage daily plaque control procedures for effective self-care in patients at risk for cardiovascular disease.

Amitriptyline — see amitriptyline HCl

---

amitriptyline HCl (am-ee-TRIP-tih-leen HIGH-droe-KLOR-ide)

Amitriptyline, Elavil

APO-Amitriptyline

Anapsique, Tryptanol

Drug Class: Tricyclic antidepressant

PHARMACOLOGY

Action

Inhibits presynaptic reuptake of norepinephrine and serotonin in CNS.

Uses

Relief of depression. Endogenous depression is more likely to be alleviated than are other depressive states.

Unlabeled Uses

Management of chronic pain associated with migraine, tension headache, phantom limb syndrome pain, tic douloureux, diabetic neuropathy, peripheral neuropathy, cancer, or arthritis; treatment of panic and eating disorders.

DRUG INTERACTIONS RELATED TO DENTAL THERAPEUTICS

Fluconazole: Possible amitriptyline toxicity (decreased metabolism)
- Monitor clinical status.

Diazepam: Increased impairment of skills related to driving (additive)
- Warn patients of the risk of driving.

Propoxyphene: Possible amitriptyline toxicity (decreased metabolism)
- Avoid concurrent use.

Pentazocine: Possible respiratory depression (additive)
- Monitor clinical status.

Tramadol: Increased risk of seizure (additive)
- Avoid concurrent use.

Sympathomimetic amines: Hypertension or hypertensive crisis (inhibition of epinephrine/norepinephrine uptake)
- Use local anesthetic agents with a vasoconstrictor with caution while monitoring vital signs.

ADVERSE EFFECTS

⚠ **ORAL:** Dry mouth (>10%); taste disturbance.

CNS: Confusion; hallucinations; disturbed concentration; decreased memory; delusions; nervousness; restlessness; agitation; panic; insomnia; nightmares; mania; exacerbation of psychosis; drowsiness; dizziness; weakness; emotional lability; numbness; tremors; extrapyramidal symptoms (e.g., pseudoparkinsonism, movement disorders, akathisia); seizures.

CVS: Orthostatic hypotension.

GI: Nausea; vomiting; anorexia; GI distress; diarrhea; flatulence; constipation.

RESP: Pharyngitis; rhinitis; sinusitis; cough.

MISC: Breast enlargement agranulocytosis, blood dyscrasias (rare).

CLINICAL IMPLICATIONS

General

- Depressed or anxious patients may neglect self-care. Monitor for plaque control effectiveness.

- Chronic dry mouth is possible; anticipate increased caries and candidiasis.
- *Postural hypotension:* Monitor BP at the beginning and end of each appointment; anticipate syncope. Have patient sit upright for several min at the end of the dental appointment before dismissing.
- Blood dyscrasias rarely reported; anticipate increased bleeding, infection, and poor healing.
- Determine ability to adapt to stress of dental treatment. Consider short appointments.
- If GI side effects occur, consider semisupine chair position.
- Avoid using epinephrine-impregnated gingival reaction cord concurrently.
- Extrapyramidal behaviors can complicate performance of oral procedures. If present, consult with MD to consider medication changes.

Oral Health Education
- If chronic dry mouth occurs, recommend home fluoride therapy and use of nonalcoholic oral products.
- Evaluate manual dexterity; consider need for power toothbrush.

amlodipine (am-LOW-dih-PEEN)
Norvasc

▐▪▐ Norvas

Drug Class: Calcium channel blocker

PHARMACOLOGY
Action
Inhibits movement of calcium ions across cell membrane in systemic and coronary vascular smooth muscle.

Uses
Hypertension; chronic stable angina; vasospastic (Prinzmetal or variant) angina.

➡◀ DRUG INTERACTIONS RELATED TO DENTAL THERAPEUTICS
No documented drug-drug interactions. The absence of evidence is not evidence of safety.

ADVERSE EFFECTS
⚠ **ORAL:** Dry mouth, thirst, gingival hyperplasia (<1%).
CNS: Headache; dizziness; lightheadedness; fatigue; lethargy; somnolence.
CVS: Edema (14.5%); palpitations (4.5%); postural hypotension (<1%); flushing (4.5%).
GI: Nausea; abdominal discomfort; cramps; dyspepsia.
RESP: Shortness of breath; dyspnea; wheezing.
MISC: Flushing; sexual difficulties; muscle cramps, pain, or inflammation.

CLINICAL IMPLICATIONS
General
- Monitor vital signs (e.g., BP, pulse pressure, rate, and rhythm) at each appointment to assess disease control. Do not provide elective dental treatment when BP is ≥180/110 or in the presence of other high-risk CV conditions.
- *Postural hypotension:* Monitor BP at the beginning and end of each appointment; anticipate syncope. Have patient sit upright for several min at the end of the dental appointment before dismissing.
- If GI side effects occur, consider semisupine chair position.
- Use local anesthetic agents with vasoconstrictor with caution based on functional capacity of the patient and use aspirating technique to prevent intravascular injection.
- Chronic dry mouth is possible; anticipate increased caries, candidiasis, and lichenoid mucositis.

Oral Health Education
- If chronic dry mouth occurs, recommend home fluoride therapy and use of nonalcoholic oral health care products.

- Encourage daily plaque control procedures for effective self-care in patients at risk for cardiovascular disease.

---

amlodipine/benazepril HCl (am-LOW-dih-PEEN/ben-AZE-uh-pril HIGH-droe-CLOR-ide)

Synonym: benazepril HCl/amlodipine

Lotrel

Drug Class: Calcium channel blocker; Antihypertensive; ACE inhibitor

PHARMACOLOGY

Action

AMLODIPINE: Inhibits movement of calcium ions across cell membrane in systemic and coronary vascular smooth muscle.

BENAZEPRIL: Competitively inhibits angiotensin I–converting enzyme, resulting in the prevention of angiotensin I conversion to angiotensin II, a potent vasoconstrictor that stimulates aldosterone secretion. This action results in a decrease in sodium and fluid retention, an increase in diuresis, and a decrease in blood pressure.

Uses

Treatment of hypertension.

DRUG INTERACTIONS RELATED TO DENTAL THERAPEUTICS

See *amlodipine:* Drug Interactions Related to Dental Therapeutics

See *benazepril:* Drug Interactions Related to Dental Therapeutics

ADVERSE EFFECTS

⚠ **ORAL:** Dry mouth.

CNS: Headache; dizziness; somnolence; fatigue; insomnia; nervousness; anxiety; tremor; decreased libido.

CVS: Palpitations; flushing; dizziness; hypotension.

GI: Nausea; abdominal pain; constipation; diarrhea; dyspepsia.

RESP: Cough; pharyngitis.

MISC: Edema; flushing; hot flashes; angioedema; asthenia; back pain; other musculoskeletal pain; cramps; muscle cramps; neutropenia, agranulocytosis (rare).

CLINICAL IMPLICATIONS

General

- Monitor vital signs (e.g., BP, pulse pressure, rate and rhythm) at each appointment to assess disease control. Do not provide elective dental treatment when BP is ≥180/110 or in the presence of other high-risk CV conditions. Refer to the section entitled "The Patient Taking Cardiovascular Drugs" in Chapter 6: *Clinical Medicine*.
- Use local anesthetic agents with vasoconstrictor with caution based on functional capacity of the patient, and use aspirating technique to prevent intravascular injection.
- If coughing is problematic, consider semisupine chair position for treatment.
- Susceptible patient with DM may experience severe recurrent hypoglycemia.
- *Postural hypotension:* Monitor BP at the beginning and end of each appointment; anticipate syncope. Have patient sit upright for several min at the end of the dental appointment before dismissing.
- Determine ability to adapt to stress of dental treatment. Consider short appointments.
- Blood dyscrasias rarely reported; anticipate increased bleeding, infection, and poor healing.

Oral Health Education

- Encourage daily plaque control procedures for effective self-care in patients at risk for cardiovascular disease.

amoxicillin (uh-MOX-ih-sil-in)

Amoxil: Tablets, chewable: 200, 400 mg (as trihydrate); Tablets: 500, 875 mg (as trihydrate); Capsules: 250, 500 mg (as trihydrate); Powder for oral suspension: 125 mg/5 mL, 200 mg/5 mL, 250 mg/5 mL, 400 mg/5 mL (as trihydrate) when reconstituted
Amoxil Pediatric Drops: Powder for oral suspension: 50 mg/mL (as trihydrate) when reconstituted
Trimox: Tablets, chewable: 125, 250 mg (as trihydrate); Capsules: 250, 500 mg (as trihydrate); Powder for oral suspension: 125 mg/5 mL, 250 mg/5 mL (as trihydrate) when reconstituted

■✦■ **APO-Amoxi, Gen-Amoxicillin, Lin-Amox, Novamoxin, Nu-Amoxi**

■✦■ **Acimox, Aclimafel, Acroxil, Amoxifur, Amoxinovag, Amoxisol, Amoxivet, Ampliron, Ardine, Eumetinex, Flemoxon, Gimalxina, Grunicina, Hidramox, Moxlin, Penamox, Polymox, Servamox, Solciclina, Xalyn-Or**

Drug Class: Antibiotic, penicillin

PHARMACOLOGY

Action
Inhibits bacterial cell wall mucopeptide synthesis.

Uses
Treatment of ear, nose, throat, GU, skin and skin structure, lower respiratory tract, and acute uncomplicated gonorrhea infections caused by susceptible strains of specific organisms.

Contraindications
Hypersensitivity to penicillins, cephalosporins, or imipenem. Not used to treat severe pneumonia, empyema, bacteremia, pericarditis, meningitis, and purulent or septic arthritis during acute stage.

Usual Dosage
Orodental infections
ADULTS AND CHILDREN WEIGHING AT LEAST 40 KG:
   Mild to Moderate Infections: *PO:* 500 mg q 12 hr or 250 mg q 8 hr.
   Severe Infections: *PO:* 875 mg q 12 hr or 500 mg q 8 hr.
CHILDREN (OLDER THAN 3 MO AND WEIGHING LESS THAN 40 KG):
   Mild to Moderate Infections: *PO:* 25 mg/kg/day in divided doses q 12 hr or 20 mg/kg/day in divided doses q 8 hr.
   Severe Infections: *PO:* 45 mg/kg/day in divided doses q 12 hr or 40 mg/kg/day in divided doses q 8 hr.

Pharmacokinetics
ABSORP: Rapidly absorbed. T_{max} is 1 to 2 hr; C_{max} is 3.5 mcg/mL (250-mg dose), 5 mcg/mL (500-mg dose), and approximately 13.8 mcg/mL (875-mg dose).
DIST: Diffuses into most body tissues and fluids; penetration in CNS is poor unless meninges are inflamed. Approximately 20% protein bound.
METAB: Liver.
EXCRET: $T_{1/2}$ is 61.3 min; approximately 60% excreted in the urine within 6 to 8 hr as unchanged drug.
PEAK: 1 to 2 hr.
DURATION: 6 to 8 hr.

➤◆ DRUG INTERACTIONS

Warfarin or acenocoumarol: Increased anticoagulant effect (decreased metabolism)
- Avoid concurrent use.

Methotrexate: Possible methotrexate toxicity (decreased excretion)
- Avoid concurrent use.

ADVERSE EFFECTS

⚠ **ORAL:** Glossitis; stomatitis; discolored tongue; taste disturbance; dry mouth.

CNS: Dizziness; fatigue; insomnia; reversible hyperactivity.

CVS: Tachycardia; hypotension; syncope; palpitations; vasodilation.

GI: Gastritis; anorexia; nausea; vomiting; abdominal pain or cramps; epigastric distress; diarrhea or bloody diarrhea; rectal bleeding; flatulence; enterocolitis; pseudomembranous colitis.

MISC: Hyperthermia.

CLINICAL IMPLICATIONS

General

When prescribed by DDS:
- *Lactation:* Excreted in breast milk.
- *Hypersensitivity:* Reactions range from mild to life threatening. Use cautiously in cephalosporin-sensitive patients because of possible cross-allergenicity.
- *Superinfection:* May result in overgrowth of nonsusceptible bacterial or fungal organisms.
- *Overdosage:* Hyperexcitability, convulsions.
- Ensure patient knows how to take the drug, how long it should be taken, and to immediately report adverse effects (e.g., rash, difficult breathing, diarrhea, GI upset).
- Antibiotic-associated diarrhea can occur. Have patient contact DDS immediately if signs develop.
- Prolonged use of antibiotics may result in bacterial or fungal overgrowth of nonsusceptible microorganisms; anticipate candidiasis.

When prescribed by medical facility:
- Determine why drug is being taken. If oral infection occurs that requires antibiotic therapy, select an appropriate product from a different class of anti-infectives.
- If GI side effects occur, consider semisupine chair position.
- Monitor vital signs.

Pregnancy Risk Category: Category B.

Oral Health Education

When prescribed by DDS:
- Instruct patient to time doses evenly over a 24-hr period.
- Inform patient that the medication works best on empty stomach but may be taken with food if there is GI upset.
- Instruct patient to increase fluid intake to 2,000 to 3,000 mL/day unless contraindicated.
- Advise patient to discard oral liquid preparations that are more than 14 days old.
- If therapy is changed because of allergic reaction, explain significance of penicillin allergy and inform patient of potential sensitivity to cephalosporins.
- Instruct patient to report the following symptoms to health care provider: rash, difficulty breathing.

---

 amoxicillin/clavulanate potassium (uh-MOX-ih-sil-in/CLAV-you-lah-nate poe-TASS-ee-uhm)

Synonym: clavulanate potassium/amoxicillin

Augmentin: Tablets: 250, 500, 875 mg amoxicillin and 125 mg clavulanic acid; Chewable tablets: 125 mg amoxicillin and 31.25 mg clavulanic acid, 200 mg amoxicillin and 28.5 mg clavulanic acid, 250 mg amoxicillin and 62.5 mg clavulanic acid, 400 mg amoxicillin and 57 mg clavulanic acid; Powder for oral suspension: 125 mg amoxicillin and 31.25 mg clavulanic acid per 5 mL, 200 mg amoxicillin and 28.5 mg clavulanic acid per 5 mL, 250 mg amoxicillin and 62.5 mg clavulanic acid per 5 mL, 400 mg amoxicillin and 57 mg clavulanic acid per 5 mL

Augmentin ES-600: Powder for oral suspension: 600 mg amoxicillin (as trihydrate) and 42.9 mg clavulanic acid per 5 mL (as the potassium salt)

Augmentin XR: Tablets: 1,000 mg amoxicillin and 62.5 mg clavulanic acid

■✦■ **Apo-Amoxi-Clav, Clavulin, ratio-Amoxi Clav**

■✦■ **Amoxiclav, Clavulin, Servamox Clv**

Drug Class: Antibiotic, aminopenicillin

PHARMACOLOGY

Action

Amoxicillin inhibits bacterial cell wall mucopeptide synthesis. Clavulanic acid inactivates a wide range of beta-lactam enzymes found in bacteria resistant to penicillins and cephalosporins.

Uses

Treatment of infections of lower respiratory tract, otitis media, sinusitis, skin and skin structure infections, UTIs, and community-acquired pneumonia caused by susceptible microorganisms.

Contraindications

History of penicillin allergy; history of amoxicillin and clavulanate-associated cholestatic jaundice or liver disease. AUGMENTIN XR: Severe renal impairment (Ccr less than 30 mL/min);
hemodialysis patients.

Usual Dosage

Strengths listed below are based on amoxicillin content.

AUGMENTIN TABLETS

Warning: Because 250- and 500-mg tablets contain the same amount of clavulanate, two 250-mg tablets are not equivalent to one 500-mg tablet.

ADULTS AND CHILDREN WEIGHING 40 KG OR MORE: *PO:* One 500-mg tablet q 12 hr or one 250-mg tablet q 8 hr. For more severe infections and infections of the respiratory tract, give one 875-mg tablet q 12 hr or one 500-mg tablet q 8 hr.

Adult patients with severely impaired renal function (glomerular filtration rate [GFR] 10 to 30 mL/min) should receive 500 mg or 250 mg q 12 hr, depending on severity of infection. Patients with GFR less than 10 mL/min should receive 500 mg or 250 mg q 24 hr, depending on severity of infection. Hemodialysis patients should receive 500 mg or 250 mg q 24 hr, depending on severity of infection. They should receive an additional dose during and at the end of dialysis.

AUGMENTIN EXTENDED-RELEASE TABLETS (XR)

Warning: Because Augmentin XR contains 62.5 mg of clavulanate, Augmentin tablets cannot be used to provide the same dosages as Augmentin XR.

ADULTS AND CHILDREN 16 YR OF AGE AND OLDER: *PO:* Recommended daily dose is 4,000 mg amoxicillin and 250 mg clavulanate potassium daily.

AUGMENTIN ORAL SUSPENSION AND CHEWABLE TABLETS

Warning: Augmentin ES-600 (5 mL) does not contain the same amount of clavulanic acid as any of the other Augmentin suspensions (5 mL). Therefore, Augmentin ES-600 and Augmentin are not interchangeable. Because Augmentin 250-mg chewable tablets and Augmentin 250-mg tablets do not contain the same amount of clavulanic acid, they are not interchangeable and should not be substituted for each other.

ADULTS: *PO:* See dose for Augmentin tablets.

Adults who have trouble swallowing may be given 125 mg per 5 mL or 250 mg per 5 mL suspension in place of the 500-mg tablet. The 200 mg per 5 mL suspension or the 400 mg per 5 mL suspension may be used in place of the 875-mg tablet.

CHILDREN WEIGHING 40 KG OR MORE: *PO:* Should be dosed according to the adult recommendations.

Pharmacokinetics

ABSORP: Rapidly absorbed. T_{max} is 1 to 2 hr; C_{max} is 3.5 mcg/mL (250 mg dose), 5 mcg/mL (500 mg dose), and approximately 13.8 mcg/mL (875 mg dose).
DIST: Diffuses into most body tissues and fluids; penetration in CNS is poor unless meninges are inflamed. Approximately 20% protein bound.
METAB: Liver.
EXCRET: $T_{1/2}$ is 61.3 min; approximately 60% excreted in the urine within 6 to 8 hr as unchanged drug.
PEAK: 1–2 hr.
DURATION: 6–8 hr.

➡◆ DRUG INTERACTIONS

Anticoagulants, oral: Increased anticoagulant effect (decreased metabolism)
• Avoid concurrent use or monitor INR.

ADVERSE EFFECTS

⚠ **ORAL:** Oral candidiasis.
CNS: Agitation; anxiety; behavioral changes; confusion; convulsions; dizziness; fatigue; headache; insomnia; reversible hyperactivity.
GI: Diarrhea/loose stools (9%); nausea (3%); vomiting (1%); abdominal pain or cramps; anorexia; bloody diarrhea; enterocolitis; epigastric distress; flatulence; gastritis; pseudomembranous colitis; rectal bleeding.
MISC: Hyperthermia; superinfection.

CLINICAL IMPLICATIONS

General
• Determine why drug is being taken. If oral infection occurs that requires antibiotic therapy, select an appropriate product from a different class of anti-infectives.
• Prolonged use of antibiotics may result in bacterial or fungal overgrowth of nonsusceptible microorganisms; anticipate candidiasis.

When prescribed by DDS:
• Ensure patient knows how to take the drug, how long it should be taken, and to immediately report adverse effects (e.g., rash, difficult breathing, diarrhea, GI upset). See Chapter 4: *Medical Management of Odontogenic Infections.*
• Antibiotic-associated diarrhea can occur. Have patient contact DDS immediately if signs develop.
• *Lactation:* Secreted into breast milk.
• *Children:* AUGMENTIN TABLETS: Safety and efficacy of 250-mg tablet not established in children weighing less than 40 kg. AUGMENTIN XR TABLETS: Safety and efficacy not established in children younger than 16 yr of age. AUGMENTIN ES-600: Safety and efficacy not established in children younger than 3 mo of age. Safety and efficacy has not been established for treatment of otitis media in infants and children 3 mo to 12 yr of age. AUGMENTIN ORAL SUSPENSION AND CHEWABLE TABLETS: Modify dosage for children younger than 12 wk of age.
• *Hypersensitivity:* Serious and sometimes fatal reactions have been reported in patients on penicillin therapy. Also, there are reports of severe reactions in patients treated with a cephalosporin who have a history of penicillin hypersensitivity.
• *Renal failure:* Dose reduction or q 12 hr recommended with severe impairment.
• *Hepatic failure:* Use with caution.
• *Superinfection:* May result in overgrowth of nonsusceptible bacterial or fungal organisms.
• *Adults:* Safety and efficacy of Augmentin ES-600 not established.
• *Mononucleosis patients:* Increased risk of skin rash. Use not recommended.
• *Phenylalanine:* Contains phenylalanine in 200- and 400-mg chewable tablets, 200 mg per 5 mL, 400 mg per 5 mL, and 600 mg per 5 mL oral suspensions.
• *Pseudomembranous colitis:* Consider the possibility in patients who develop diarrhea.
• *Overdosage:* Stomach and abdominal pain; vomiting; diarrhea; rash; hyperactivity; drowsiness; interstitial nephritis, resulting in oliguric renal failure; crystalluria, which may lead to renal failure.

Pregnancy Risk Category: Category B.

Oral Health Education

When prescribed by DDS:

- Inform patient that antibacterial drug regimens must be followed to completion.
- Explain name, dose, action, and potential side effects of drug.
- Review dosing schedule (q 8 or 12 hr) and prescribed length of therapy with patient or caregiver. Advise patient or caregiver that dose, dosing frequency, and duration of therapy are dependent on the site and cause of infection and strength of antibiotic being used.
- Reinforce to patient or caregiver the need to take exactly as prescribed and to complete the entire course of therapy, even if symptoms of infection have disappeared. Caution patient or caregiver that skipping doses or not completing the full course of therapy may allow the infection to worsen and increase the possibility that the bacteria will become resistant to the antibiotic and may cause infections that will not be treatable in the future.
- Instruct patient to take each dose at the start of a meal or snack to minimize intestinal side effects.
- Advise patient using the nonscored extended-release tablet to swallow tablet whole. Caution patient not to break, crush, or chew the tablet.
- Advise patient using the scored extended-release tablet that the tablet may be split and taken as 2 halves. Advise patient that half tablets should be swallowed whole. Caution patient not to crush, chew, or break half tablets.
- Instruct patient or caregiver administering suspension to do the following: keep suspension refrigerated; shake well before each use; use dosing syringe, dosing spoon, or dosing cup when measuring and administering dose; and discard any unused suspension at end of treatment period.
- Advise patient or caregiver using chewable tablets to swallow whole or crush or chew before swallowing. Advise patient or caregiver to follow each dose with water.
- Instruct patient to notify health care provider if infection does not appear to be improving or is worsening.
- Advise patient or caregiver to notify health care provider if severe diarrhea or diarrhea lasting 2 or 3 days occurs.
- Warn patient that diarrhea containing blood or pus may be a sign of a serious disorder and to seek medical care if noted and not try to treat at home.
- Advise patient or caregiver to report signs of superinfection to health care provider: black "furry" tongue, white patches in mouth, foul-smelling stools, or vaginal itching or discharge.
- Advise patient, family, or caregiver to discontinue therapy and contact health care provider immediately if skin rash, hives, itching, or shortness of breath occurs.
- Advise women to notify health care provider if pregnant, planning to become pregnant, or breast feeding.
- Instruct patient not to take any prescription or OTC medications, herbal preparations, or dietary supplements unless advised by health care provider.
- Advise patient or caregiver that follow-up examinations and laboratory tests may be required to monitor therapy and to keep appointments.

Amoxiclav — see amoxicillin/clavulanate potassium

Amoxifur — see amoxicillin

Amoxil — see amoxicillin

Amoxil Pediatric Drops — see amoxicillin

Amoxinovag — see amoxicillin

Amoxisol — see amoxicillin

Amoxivet — see amoxicillin

amphetamine and dextroamphetamine (am-FET-uh-meen DEX-troe-am-FET-uh-meen)

Synonym: amphetamine sulfate, aspartate; dextroamphetamine and amphetamine

Adderall, Adderall XR

Drug Class: CNS stimulant; Amphetamine
DEA Schedule: Schedule II

PHARMACOLOGY

Action

Activates noradrenergic neurons, causing CNS and respiratory stimulation; stimulates satiety center in brain, causing appetite suppression.

Uses

Narcolepsy; attention deficit hyperactivity disorder; short-term (i.e., no longer than a few weeks) exogenous obesity adjunct used only when alternative therapy has been ineffective.

➤◀ DRUG INTERACTIONS RELATED TO DENTAL THERAPEUTICS

No documented drug-drug interactions. The absence of evidence is not evidence of safety.

ADVERSE EFFECTS

⚠ **ORAL:** Dry mouth; unpleasant taste.
CNS: Hyperactivity; dizziness; restlessness; tremors; insomnia; euphoria; headache.
CVS: Palpitations, hypertension, tachycardia, arrhythmia (high doses).
GI: Diarrhea; constipation; anorexia.

CLINICAL IMPLICATIONS

General

- Determine why drug is being taken. Consider implications of condition on dental treatment.
- Monitor vital signs.
- Chronic dry mouth is possible; anticipate increased caries and candidiasis.
- Use local anesthetic agents with vasoconstrictors with caution based on functional capacity of the patient and use aspirating technique to prevent intravascular injection.
- Patients with ADHD may have short attention spans; consider short appointment.

Oral Health Education

- If chronic dry mouth occurs, recommend home fluoride therapy and use of nonalcoholic oral health care products.

---

amphetamine sulfate — see amphetamine and dextroamphetamine

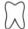 **ampicillin** (am-pih-SILL-in)

Ampicillin Sodium: Powder for injection: 250 mg, 500 mg, 1 g, 2 g
Principen: Capsules: 250, 500 mg (as trihydrate); Powder for oral suspension: 125 mg/5 mL, 259 mg/5mL (as trihydrate) when reconstituted

■✦■ **APO-Ampi, Novo Ampicillin, Nu-Ampi**

■◗■ **Anglopen, Binotal, Dibacilina, Flamicina, Lampicin, Marovilina, Omnipen, Pentrexyl, Sinaplin**

Drug Class: Antibiotic, penicillin

PHARMACOLOGY

Action
Inhibits bacterial cell wall mucopeptide synthesis.

Uses
Treatment of respiratory, GI, and GU tract and soft tissue infections, bacterial meningitis and enterococcal endocarditis, septicemia and gonococcal infections caused by susceptible microorganisms.

Unlabeled Uses
Prophylaxis during cesarean section in certain high-risk patients.

Contraindications
Hypersensitivity to penicillins, cephalosporins, or imipenem. Oral form not used to treat severe pneumonia, empyema, bacteremia, pericarditis, meningitis, and purulent or septic arthritis during acute stage.

Pharmacokinetics
ABSORP: Well absorbed from GI tract. C_{max} is approximately 3 mcg/mL (500-mg capsules) and 3.4 mcg/mL (500-mg oral suspension). Food affects absorption; take on empty stomach.

DIST: Diffuses readily into most body tissues and fluids; penetrates into the cerebrospinal fluid and brain only when meninges are inflamed. Approximately 20% protein bound; excreted in breast milk.

EXCRET: Excreted largely unchanged in the urine.

SPECIAL POP: *Renal failure:* $T_{1/2}$ may be prolonged. Dosing interval adjustments may be necessary.

➡◀ DRUG INTERACTIONS
No documented drug-drug interactions. The absence of evidence is not evidence of safety.

ADVERSE EFFECTS
⚠ **ORAL:** Discolored tongue; glossitis; stomatitis; dry mouth; taste disturbance.
CVS: Thrombophlebitis at injection site; tachycardia; hypotension; syncope.
CNS: Dizziness; fatigue; insomnia; reversible hyperactivity; neurotoxicity (e.g., lethargy, neuromuscular irritability, hallucinations, convulsions, seizures).
GI: Diarrhea; pseudomembranous colitis.
MISC: Pain at injection site; hyperthermia.

CLINICAL IMPLICATIONS

General
- Determine why drug is being taken. Take precautions to avoid cross-contamination of microorganisms.
- If oral infection occurs that requires antibiotic therapy, select an appropriate product from a different class of anti-infectives.
- If GI side effects occur, consider semisupine chair position.
- Monitor vital signs.
- Anticipate oral candidiasis when long-term use is reported.

Pregnancy Risk Category: Category B.

Ampicillin Sodium — see ampicillin

Ampliron — see amoxicillin

---

amprenavir (am-PREN-ah-veer)
Agenerase
Drug Class: Antiretroviral, protease inhibitor

PHARMACOLOGY

Action
Inhibits HIV protease, the enzyme required to form functional proteins in HIV-infected patients.

Uses
Treatment of HIV-1 infection in combination with other antiretroviral agents.

➜✦ DRUG INTERACTIONS RELATED TO DENTAL THERAPEUTICS
Midazolam or triazolam: Possible serious life-threatening toxicity (decreased metabolism)
  • Avoid concurrent use.
Lidocaine: Possible serious life-threatening toxicity with lidocaine (decreased metabolism)
  • Avoid concurrent use.

ADVERSE EFFECTS
⚠ **ORAL:** Taste disturbance, perioral paresthesia.
CNS: Depression; paresthesia.
GI: Nausea; vomiting; diarrhea; abdominal pain.

CLINICAL IMPLICATIONS

General
• Determine why drug is being taken. Consider implications of condition on dental treatment.
• Consider medical consult to determine disease control and influence on dental treatment.
• Anticipate oral candidiasis when HIV disease is reported.
• If GI side effects occur, consider semisupine chair position.
• Antibiotic prophylaxis should be considered when <500 PMN/mm³ are reported; elective dental treatment should be delayed until blood values improve above this level.
• This drug is frequently prescribed in combination with one or more other antiviral agents. Side effects of all agents must be considered during the drug review process.

Oral Health Education
• Recommend frequent maintenance prophylaxis when immunosuppression is evident.
• Encourage daily plaque control procedures for effective self-care since HIV infection reduces host resistance.
• Recommend frequent maintenance prophylaxis when immunosuppression is evident.

---

 amyl nitrite (A-mill NYE-trite)

Amyl Nitrite Aspirols, Amyl Nitrite Vaporole: Inhalant: 0.3 mL
Drug Class: Antianginal

PHARMACOLOGY

Action
Relaxes smooth muscle of venous and arterial vasculature.

Uses
Relief of angina pectoris.

Contraindications
Hypersensitivity to nitrates; pregnancy; severe anemia; closed-angle glaucoma; orthostatic hypotension; head trauma; cerebral hemorrhage.

Usual Dosage
ADULT: Inhalation 0.3 mL prn; 1 to 6 inhalations from 1 capsule are usually sufficient. May be repeated in 3 to 5 min.

Pharmacokinetics
EXCRET: Approximately 33% excreted in the urine.
ONSET: 0.5 min
DURATION: 3 to 5 min.

➡◀ DRUG INTERACTIONS
Diazoxide: Severe hypotension (additive)
 • Monitor clinical status.
Diltiazem: Hypotension (additive)
 • Monitor clinical status.

ADVERSE EFFECTS
⚠ **ORAL:** Stinging of nasal mucosa.
CVS: Tachycardia; palpitations; hypotension; orthostatic hypotension; syncope; arrhythmias; edema.
CNS: Headache; apprehension; weakness; vertigo; dizziness; agitation; insomnia.
GI: Nausea; vomiting; diarrhea; dyspepsia.
RESP: Bronchitis; pneumonia.
MISC: Arthralgia; perspiration; pallor; cold sweat.

CLINICAL IMPLICATIONS
General
 • This drug is used for emergency procedures related to unconsciousness in the dental office.
 • *Children:* Safety and efficacy not established.
 • *Angina:* May aggravate angina caused by hypertrophic cardiomyopathy.
 • *Drug abuse:* May be abused for sexual stimulation or for effects of lightheadedness, dizziness, and euphoria.
 • *Glaucoma:* May increase intraocular pressure.
 • *Orthostatic hypotension:* May occur even with small doses; alcohol accentuates this reaction.
 • *Withdrawal:* Dose is gradually reduced to prevent withdrawal reaction.
 • *Overdosage:* Severe headache, severe hypotension, flushing, tachycardia, vertigo, confusion, syncope, nausea, slow breathing or dyspnea, cyanosis, metabolic acidosis, convulsions, coma, death.

Pregnancy Risk Category: Category X.
Oral Health Education
 • Caution patient to avoid sudden position changes to prevent orthostatic hypotension.
 • Instruct patient to avoid intake of alcoholic beverages or other CNS depressants and aspirin.

Amyl Nitrite Aspirols — see amyl nitrite
Amyl Nitrite Vaporole — see amyl nitrite
Anafranil — see clomipramine HCl
Analfin — see morphine sulfate
Analphen — see acetaminophen
Anapenil — see penicillin V
Anaprox — see naproxen
Anaprox DS — see naproxen
Anapsique — see amitriptyline HCl
Anaspaz — see hyoscyamine sulfate
Ancef — see cefazolin sodium

Andox — see acetaminophen
Androxicam — see piroxicam
Anestacon — see lidocaine HCl
Anexate — see flumazenil
Anexsia 5/500 — see acetaminophen/hydrocodone bitartrate
Anexsia 7.5/650 — see acetaminophen/hydrocodone bitartrate
Anexsia 10/660 — see acetaminophen/hydrocodone bitartrate
Angiotrofin — see diltiazem HCl
Angiotrofin AP — see diltiazem HCl
Angiotrofin Retard — see diltiazem HCl
Anglix — see nitroglycerin
Anglopen — see ampicillin
Ansaid — see flurbiprofen
Antabuse — see disulfiram
Antalgin — see indomethacin
Antepsin — see sucralfate
Antiphlogistine Rub A-535 Capsaicin — see capsaicin
Antispas — see dicyclomine HCl
Anti-Tuss — see guaifenesin
Antivert — see meclizine
Antrizine — see meclizine
Anucort-HC — see hydrocortisone
Anumed HC — see hydrocortisone
Anusol-HC — see hydrocortisone
Anusol HC-1 Hydrocortisone Anti-Itch — see hydrocortisone
Apacet — see acetaminophen
APAP — see acetaminophen
Apo-Acebutolol — see acebutolol HCl
Apo-Acetaminophen — see acetaminophen
Apo-Acyclovir — see acyclovir
Apo-Allopurinol — see allopurinol
Apo-Alpraz — see alprazolam
Apo-Alpraz TS — see alprazolam
APO-Amitriptyline — see amitriptyline HCl
APO-Amoxi — see amoxicillin
Apo-Amoxi-Clav — see amoxicillin/clavulanate potassium
APO-Ampi — see ampicillin
Apo-Atenol — see atenolol
Apo-Azathioprine — see azathioprine
Apo-Beclomethasone — see beclomethasone dipropionate

Apo-Bromocriptine — see bromocriptine mesylate
Apo-Buspirone — see buspirone HCl
APO-Capto — see captopril
APO-Carbamazepine — see carbamazepine
Apo-Cefaclor — see cefaclor
Apo-Cefadroxil — see cefadroxil
Apo-Cefuroxime — see cefuroxime
APO-Cephalex — see cephalexin
Apo-Cetirizine — see cetirizine
Apo-Chlordiazepoxide — see chlordiazepoxide
Apo-Chlorhexidine — see chlorhexidine gluconate
APO-Chlorpropamide — see chlorpropamide
Apo-Chlorthalidone — see chlorthalidone
Apo-Cimetidine — see cimetidine
Apo-Clomipramine — see clomipramine HCl
Apo-Clonazepam — see clonazepam
APO-Clonidine — see clonidine HCl
Apo-Clorazepate — see clorazepate dipotassium
Apo-Cromolyn Nasal Spray — see cromolyn sodium
Apo-Cromolyn Sterules — see cromolyn sodium
Apo-Cyclobenzaprine — see cyclobenzaprine HCl
Apo-Desipramine — see desipramine HCl
Apo-Diazepam — see diazepam
Apo-Diclo — see diclofenac
Apo-Diclo Rapide — see diclofenac
Apo-Diclo SR — see diclofenac
Apo-Diflunisal — see diflunisal
Apo-Diltiaz — see diltiazem HCl
Apo-Diltiaz CD — see diltiazem HCl
Apo-Diltiaz Injectable — see diltiazem HCl
Apo-Diltiaz SR — see diltiazem HCl
Apo-Dimenhydrinate — see dimenhydrinate
Apo-Divalproex — see valproic acid and derivatives
Apo-Doxazosin — see doxazosin mesylate
Apo-Doxepin — see doxepin HCl
Apo-Doxy — see doxycycline hyclate
Apo-Doxy-Tabs — see doxycycline hyclate
Apo-Erythro Base — see erythromycin
Apo-Erythro E-C — see erythromycin
Apo-Erythro-ES — see erythromycin

Apo-Erythro-S — see erythromycin
Apo-Etodolac — see etodolac
Apo-Famotidine — see famotidine
Apo-Fenofibrate — see fenofibrate
Apo-Feno-Micro — see fenofibrate
Apo-Ferrous Sulfate — see ferrous salts
Apo-Fluconazole — see fluconazole
Apo-Fluconazole-150 — see fluconazole
Apo-Flunisolide — see flunisolide
Apo-Fluoxetine — see fluoxetine HCl
Apo-Fluphenazine — see fluphenazine
Apo-Fluphenazine Decanoate Injection — see fluphenazine
Apo-Flurazepam — see flurazepam HCl
Apo-Flurbiprofen — see flurbiprofen
Apo-Fluvoxamine — see fluvoxamine maleate
Apo-Folic — see folic acid
Apo-Furosemide — see furosemide
Apo-Gabapentin — see gabapentin
APO-Gain Topical Solution — see minoxidil
Apo-Gemfibrozil — see gemfibrozil
Apo-Glyburide — see glyburide
Apo-Haloperidol — see haloperidol
Apo-Haloperidol Decanoate Injection — see haloperidol
Apo-Hydralazine — see hydralazine HCl
Apo-Hydro — see hydrochlorothiazide
Apo-Hydroxyzine — see hydroxyzine
Apo-Ibuprofen — see ibuprofen
Apo-Imipramine — see imipramine HCl
Apo-Indapamide — see indapamide
Apo-Indomethacin — see indomethacin
Apo-Ipravent — see ipratropium bromide
APO-ISDN — see isosorbide dinitrate
APO-K — see potassium products
APO-Keto — see ketoprofen
APO-Keto SR — see ketoprofen
Apo-Ketoconazole — see ketoconazole
APO-Keto-E — see ketoprofen
Apo-Ketorolac — see ketorolac tromethamine
Apo-Ketorolac Injection — see ketorolac tromethamine
Apo-Labetalol — see labetalol HCl

Apo-Levocarb — see levodopa/carbidopa
Apo-Lisinopril — see lisinopril
Apo-Loperamide — see loperamide HCl
Apo-Loratadine — see loratadine
Apo-Lorazepam — see lorazepam
Apo-Lovastatin — see lovastatin
Apo-Mefenamic — see mefenamic acid
Apo-Metformin — see metformin HCl
Apo-Methyldopa — see methyldopa and methyldopate HCl
APO-Metoclop — see metoclopramide
Apo-Metoprolol — see metoprolol
Apo-Metoprolol (Type L) — see metoprolol
Apo-Metronidazole — see metronidazole
Apo-Midazolam — see midazolam HCl
Apo-Minocycline — see minocycline HCl
Apo-Misoprostol — see misoprostol
Apo-Nabumetone — see nabumetone
Apo-Nadol — see nadolol
Apo-Napro-Na — see naproxen
Apo-Napro-Na DS — see naproxen
Apo-Naproxen — see naproxen
Apo-Naproxen SR — see naproxen
Apo-Nefazodone — see nefazodone HCl
Apo-Nifed — see nifedipine
Apo-Nifed PA — see nifedipine
Apo-Nitrofurantoin — see nitrofurantoin
Apo-Nizatidine — see nizatidine
Apo-Norflox — see norfloxacin
Apo-Nortriptyline — see nortriptyline HCl
Apo-Oflox — see ofloxacin
Apo-Oxaprozin — see oxaprozin
Apo-Oxazepam — see oxazepam
Apo-Oxybutynin — see oxybutynin Cl
APO-Pen VK — see penicillin V
Apo-Perphenazine — see perphenazine
APO-Pindol — see pindolol
Apo-Piroxicam — see piroxicam
Apo-Pravastatin — see pravastatin sodium
APO-Prazo — see prazosin HCl
Apo-Prednisone — see prednisone

Apo-Primidone — see primidone
Apo-Procainamide — see procainamide HCl
APO-Propranolol — see propranolol HCl
Apo-Quinidine — see quinidine
Apo-Ranitidine — see ranitidine HCl
Apo-Salvent — see albuterol
Apo-Selegiline — see selegiline HCl
Apo-Sertraline — see sertraline HCl
Apo-Sotalol — see sotalol HCl
Apo-Sulfatrim — see trimethoprim/sulfamethoxazole
APO-Sulin — see sulindac
Apo-Tamox — see tamoxifen citrate
Apo-Temazepam — see temazepam
Apo-Terazosin — see terazosin
Apo-Terbinafine — see terbinafine
Apo-Tetra — see tetracycline HCl
Apo-Theo LA — see theophylline
Apo-Thioridazine — see thioridazine HCl
Apo-Ticlopidine — see ticlopidine HCl
Apo-Timol — see timolol maleate
Apo-Timop — see timolol maleate
Apo-Tolbutamide — see tolbutamide
Apo-Trazodone — see trazodone HCl
Apo-Trazodone D — see trazodone HCl
APO-Triazo — see triazolam
Apo-Trifluoperazine — see trifluoperazine HCl
Apo-Valproic — see valproic acid and derivatives
APO-Verap — see verapamil HCl
Apo-Warfarin — see warfarin
APO-Zidovudine — see zidovudine
Apresolina — see hydralazine HCl
Apresoline — see hydralazine HCl
Aprovel — see irbesartan
Aquachloral Supprettes — see chloral hydrate
Aquacort — see hydrocortisone
Aquavit E — see vitamin E
Aralen — see chloroquine
Aralen HCl — see chloroquine
Aralen Phosphate — see chloroquine

Arava — see leflunomide
Ardine — see amoxicillin
Arestin — see minocycline HCl
Aricept — see donepezil

aripiprazole (A-rih-PIP-ray-zole)
Abilify
Drug Class: Atypical antipsychotic

PHARMACOLOGY
Action
Partial agonist at dopamine D_2 and serotonin 5-HT_{1A} receptors, and antagonist at serotonin 5-HT_{2A} receptors.

Uses
Treatment of schizophrenia; treatment of acute manic and mixed episodes associated with bipolar disorder.

➡◀ DRUG INTERACTIONS RELATED TO DENTAL THERAPEUTICS
No documented drug-drug interactions. The absence of evidence is not evidence of safety.

ADVERSE EFFECTS
⚠ **ORAL:** Increased salivation (>1%).
CNS: Headache (32%); anxiety, agitation (25%); insomnia (24%); akathisia, somnolence (12%); lightheadedness (11%); extrapyramidal syndrome (6%); tremor (4%); depression, nervousness, hostility, suicidal thought, manic reaction, abnormal gait, confusion, cogwheel rigidity (≥1%).
GI: Nausea (16%); dyspepsia (15%); vomiting (12%); constipation (11%); anorexia (≥1%).
RESP: Coughing (3%); dyspnea, pneumonia (≥1%).
MISC: Asthenia (8%); accidental injury (5%); myalgia (4%); fever (2%); flu-like symptoms, peripheral edema, chest pain, neck pain, neck rigidity, muscle cramp (≥1%).

CLINICAL IMPLICATIONS
General
- Determine why drug is being taken. Consider implications of condition on dental treatment.
- Determine ability to adapt to stress of dental treatment. Consider short appointments.
- Depressed or anxious patients may neglect self-care. Monitor for plaque control effectiveness.
- Extrapyramidal behaviors can complicate performance of oral procedures. If present, consult with MD to consider medication changes.
- If GI side effects occur, consider semisupine chair position.

Oral Health Education
- Encourage patient to follow daily plaque control procedures for effective self-care.
- Evaluate manual dexterity; consider need for power toothbrush.

Aristocort — see triamcinolone
Aristocort A — see triamcinolone
Aristocort Intralesional — see triamcinolone
Aristocort Parenteral — see triamcinolone
Aristocort Syrup — see triamcinolone

Aristospan — see triamcinolone
Aristospan Intra-articular — see triamcinolone
Aristospan Intralesional — see triamcinolone
Armour Thyroid — see thyroid, desiccated
Aropax — see paroxetine
Arthritis Foundation Pain Reliever — see aspirin

 articaine HCl (AR-ti-kane HIGH-droe-KLOR-ide)

Septocaine, Zorcaine 4%: Injection: 4% with 1:100,000 epinephrine
▌✦▌**Astracaine, Astracaine Forte, Ultracaine-DS**

PHARMACOLOGY

Action
Inhibits sodium ion fluxes across membrane to block nerve action potential.

Uses
For local, infiltrative, or conductive anesthesia in simple and complex dental and periodontal procedures.

Contraindications
Hypersensitivity to local anesthetics or any components of the products, para-aminobenzoic acid (esters only) or parabens; congenital or idiopathic methemoglobinemia.

Usual Dosage
To prevent pain during dental procedures
INJECTION
ADULTS: The dose of local anesthetic administered varies with the procedure, vascularity of the tissues, depth of anesthesia, degree of required muscle relaxation, duration of anesthesia desired, and the physical condition of the patient. Not to exceed 7 mg/kg of body weight.
CHILDREN: Articaine is not indicated in children younger than 4 yr of age. For children older than 4 yr, not to exceed 7 mg/kg of body weight.

Pharmacokinetics
METAB: Plasma carboxylesterase and liver (P450 enzymes 5% to 10%).
EXCRET: Urinary.
ONSET: 1 to 6 min.
DURATION: 1 hr.
SPECIAL POP: Repeated doses may cause accumulation of the drug or its metabolites or slow metabolic degradation. Give reduced doses. Use anesthetics with caution in patients with severe disturbances of cardiac rhythm, hypotension, shock, or heart block. Also, use local anesthetics with caution in patients with impaired cardiovascular function because they may be less able to compensate for functional changes associated with the prolongation of AV conduction produced by these drugs.
Elderly: Repeated doses may cause accumulation of the drug or its metabolites or slow metabolic degradation; give reduced doses.
Hepatic failure: Because amide-type local anesthetics are metabolized primarily in the liver and ester-type local anesthetics are hydrolyzed by plasma cholinesterase produced by the liver, patients with hepatic disease, especially severe hepatic disease, may be more susceptible to potential toxicity. Use cautiously in such patients.

➜← DRUG INTERACTIONS

Intercurrent use: Mixtures of local anesthetics are sometimes employed to compensate for the slower onset of one drug and the shorter duration of action of the second drug. Toxicity is probably additive with mixtures of local anesthetics, but some experiments suggest synergy. Exercise caution regarding toxic equivalence when mixtures of local anesthetics are employed. Some preparations contain vasoconstrictors. Keep this in mind when using concurrently with other drugs that may interact with vasoconstrictors.

Sedatives: If employed to reduce patient apprehension during dental procedures, use reduced doses, since local anesthetics used in combination with CNS depressants may have additive effects. Give young children minimal doses of each agent.

ADVERSE EFFECTS

⚠ **ORAL:** Injection site reactions; dry mouth; increased salivation; glossitis; gingival hemorrhage; mouth ulceration; stomatitis; tongue edema; tooth disorder.

CNS: Dizziness; facial paralysis; hyperesthesia; nervousness; neuropathy; paresthesia; somnolence.

CVS: Hemorrhage; migraine; syncope; tachycardia.

GI: Abdominal pain; constipation; diarrhea; dyspepsia; nausea; vomiting.

RESP: Pharyngitis; rhinitis.

MISC: Accidental injury; asthenia; back pain; dysmenorrhea; injection site pain; malaise; neck pain.

CLINICAL IMPLICATIONS

General

- *Dosage:* Use the lowest dosage that results in effective anesthesia to avoid high plasma levels and serious adverse effects. Inject slowly, with frequent aspirations before and during the injection, to avoid intravascular injection. Perform syringe aspirations before and during each supplemental injection in continuous (intermittent) catheter techniques. During the administration of epidural anesthesia, it is recommended that a test dose be administered initially and that the patient be monitored for CNS toxicity and cardiovascular toxicity, as well as for signs of unintended intrathecal administration, before proceeding.
- *Inflammation or sepsis:* Use local anesthetic procedures with caution when there is inflammation or sepsis in the region of proposed injection.
- *CNS toxicity:* Monitor cardiovascular and respiratory vital signs and state of consciousness after each injection. Restlessness, anxiety, incoherent speech, lightheadedness, numbness, and tingling of the mouth and lips, metallic taste, tinnitus, dizziness, blurred vision, tremors, twitching, or drowsiness may be early signs of CNS toxicity.
- *Malignant hyperthermia:* Many drugs used during anesthesia are considered potential triggering agents for familial malignant hyperthermia. It is not known whether local anesthetics may trigger this reaction and the need for supplemental general anesthesia cannot be predicted in advance; therefore, have a standard protocol for management available.
- *Vasoconstrictors:* Use solutions containing a vasoconstrictor with caution and in carefully circumscribed quantities in areas of the body supplied by end arteries or having otherwise compromised blood supply (e.g., digits, nose, external ear, penis). Use with extreme caution in patients whose medical history and physical evaluation suggest the existence of hypertension, peripheral vascular disease, arteriosclerotic heart disease, cerebral vascular insufficiency, or heart block; these individuals may exhibit exaggerated vasoconstrictor response. Serious dose-related cardiac arrhythmias may occur if preparations containing a vasoconstrictor such as epinephrine are employed in patients during or following the administration of potent inhalation agents.
- *Lactation:* Safety for use in the nursing mother has not been established.
- Monitor vital signs (e.g., BP, pulse pressure, rate, and rhythm) prior to using vasoconstrictor to assess CV status. Do not provide elective dental treatment when BP is

≥180/110 or in presence of other high-risk CV conditions. Refer to the section entitled "The Patient Taking Cardiovascular Drugs" in Chapter 6: *Clinical Medicine*.

Pregnancy Risk Category: Category C. Safety for use in pregnant women, other than those in labor, has not been established. Local anesthetics rapidly cross the placenta.

Oral Health Education

- Advise the patient to exert caution to avoid inadvertent trauma to the lips, tongue, cheek, mucosae, or soft palate when these structures are anesthetized. The ingestion of food should therefore be postponed until normal function returns.
- Advise the patient to consult the dentist if anesthesia persists or a rash develops.

Artinor — see piroxicam

Artosin — see tolbutamide

Artrenac — see diclofenac

Artron — see naproxen

Artyflam — see piroxicam

ASA — see aspirin

ASA 500 — see aspirin

ASA/codeine phosphate — see aspirin/codeine phosphate

Asacol — see mesalamine

Asaphen — see aspirin

Asaphen E.C. — see aspirin

Asmalix — see theophylline

Asmanex Twisthaler — see mometasone furoate

aspartate — see amphetamine and dextroamphetamine

A-Spas S/L — see hyoscyamine sulfate

Aspergum — see aspirin

---

 aspirin (ASS-pihr-in)

Synonym: acetylsalicylic acid; ASA

Arthritis Foundation Pain Reliever, Aspergum, Bayer Children's Aspirin, Bayer Low Adult Strength, Easprin, Ecotrin, Ecotrin Adult Low Strength, Ecotrin Maximum Strength, Empirin, Extended Release Bayer 8-Hour, Extra Strength Bayer Enteric 500 Aspirin, Genprin, Genuine Bayer, 1/2 Halfprin, Halfprin 81, Heartline, Maximum Bayer, Norwich Extra-Strength, St. Joseph Adult Chewable Aspirin, ZORprin: Tablets: 325, 500 mg; Chewable tablets: 81 mg; Enteric-coated tablets: 81, 165, 325, 500 mg; Delayed-release tablets: 81 mg; Controlled-release tablets: 800 mg; Gum: 227.5 mg

■✦■ **Alka-Seltzer Flavoured, Asaphen, Asaphen E.C., Entrophen, MSD Enteric Coated ASA, Novasen**

■✦■ **ASA 500, Aspirina Protect**

Drug Class: Analgesic; Salicylate

PHARMACOLOGY

Action

Inhibits prostaglandin synthesis, resulting in analgesia, anti-inflammatory activity, and platelet aggregation inhibition; reduces fever by acting on the brain's heat-regulating center to promote vasodilation and sweating.

Uses

Treatment of mild to moderate pain; fever; various inflammatory conditions; reduction of risk of death or MI in patients with previous infarction or unstable angina pectoris or recurrent transient ischemia attacks or stroke in men who have had transient brain ischemia caused by platelet emboli.

Unlabeled Uses

Prevention of cataract formation; prevention of toxemia of pregnancy; improvement of inadequate uteroplacental blood flow in pregnancy.

Contraindications

Hypersensitivity to salicylates or NSAIDs; hemophilia, bleeding ulcers, or hemorrhagic states.

Usual Dosage

Analgesic/antipyretic

ADULTS: *PO:* 325 to 650 mg q 4 hr; 500 mg q 3 hr; 1000 mg q 6 hr.
CHILDREN (2 TO 12 YR): *PO:* 10 to 15 mg/kg/dose q 4 hr (up to 80 mg/kg/day).

Pharmacokinetics

ABSORP: Rapidly and completely absorbed. T_{max} is 1 to 2 hr (salicylic acid).
DIST: Widely distributed to all tissues and fluids including CNS, breast milk, and fetal tissues. Approximately 90% of salicylate is protein bound at concentrations of less than 100 mcg/mL and approximately 75% is bound at concentrations of more than 400 mcg/mL.
METAB: Rapidly hydrolyzed to salicylic acid (active). Salicylic acid is conjugated in the liver to the metabolites.
EXCRET: Salicylic acid plasma $t_{1/2}$ is approximately 6 hr but may exceed 20 hr in higher doses. $T_{1/2}$ is approximately 15 to 20 min for aspirin. Elimination follows zero-order kinetics. Renal elimination of unchanged drug depends on urine pH. A pH of more than 6.5 increases renal clearance of free salicylate from less than 5% to more than 80%.

➨◀ DRUG INTERACTIONS

Angiotensin-converting enzyme inhibitors: Decreased antihypertensive effect (inhibition of prostaglandin synthesis)
• Monitor blood pressure.
Anticoagulants, oral: Increased bleeding (platelet inhibition)
• Avoid concurrent use.
Cimetidine or nizatidine: Possible salicylate toxicity (decreased metabolism)
• Avoid concurrent use.
Clopidogrel: Increased gastrointestinal bleeding (additive effect on platelet function)
• Avoid concurrent use.
Heparin: Increased bleeding (platelet inhibition)
• Avoid concurrent use.
Ibuprofen: Inhibition of antiplatelet effect of aspirin (blocks access to active site on platelets)
• Avoid concurrent use.
Lithium: Lithium toxicity (decreased renal excretion)
• Avoid concurrent use.
Methotrexate: Possible methotrexate toxicity (decreased renal clearance)
• Avoid concurrent use.

Quinidine: Increased bleeding (additive antiplatelet effect)
- Avoid concurrent use.

Spironolactone: Decreased antihypertensive effect (inhibition of prostaglandin synthesis)
- Monitor blood pressure.

Valproate: Possible valproate toxicity (displacement from binding site)
- Avoid concurrent use.

Zafirlukast: Possible zafirlukast toxicity (decreased metabolism)
- Avoid concurrent use.

ADVERSE EFFECTS
⚠ **ORAL:** Increased bleeding.
GI: Nausea; dyspepsia; heartburn; bleeding.
MISC: Hypersensitivity reactions may include urticaria, hives, rashes, angioedema, and anaphylactic shock.

CLINICAL IMPLICATIONS
General
When recommended by DDS:
- *Lactation:* Excreted in breast milk.
- *Children:* Reye syndrome has been associated with aspirin administration to children (including teenagers) with acute febrile (viral) illness.
- *Hypersensitivity:* Reaction may include bronchospasm and generalized urticaria or angioedema; patients with asthma or nasal polyps have greatest risk.
- *Renal failure:* May decrease renal function or aggravate kidney diseases.
- *Hepatic failure:* May cause hepatotoxicity in patients with impaired liver function.
- *GI disorders:* Can cause gastric irritation and bleeding.
- *Surgical patients:* Aspirin may increase risk of postoperative bleeding. If possible, avoid use 1 wk before surgery. No significantly increased risk of hemorrhage after oral surgery.
- *Overdosage:* Nausea, vomiting, tinnitus, dizziness, respiratory alkalosis, metabolic acidosis, hemorrhage, convulsions.

Pregnancy Risk Category: Category D.

Oral Health Education
When recommended by DDS:
- Instruct patient to take drug with food or after meals and with full glass of water. Explain that antacids should be avoided within 1 to 2 hr after ingestion of enteric-coated tablets.
- Instruct patient to report ringing in ears or unusual bleeding, bruising, or persistent GI pain.
- Tell patient on sodium-restricted diet to limit use of effervescent or buffered aspirin preparations.
- Caution parents to avoid giving aspirin to children or teenagers with flu-like symptoms or chickenpox without first consulting health care provider.
- Instruct patient to avoid intake of alcoholic beverages or other CNS depressants.

Aspirina Protect — see aspirin

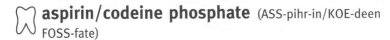 **aspirin/codeine phosphate** (ASS-pihr-in/KOE-deen FOSS-fate)

Synonym: ASA/codeine phosphate; codeine phosphate/ASA; codeine phosphate/aspirin

Empirin with Codeine #2: Tablet: Aspirin 325 mg and codeine 15 mg
Empirin with Codeine #3: Tablet: Aspirin 325 mg and codeine 30 mg
Empirin with Codeine #4: Tablet: Aspirin 325 mg and codeine 60 mg

Drug Class: Narcotic analgesic combined with nonsteroidal anti-inflammatory analgesic

PHARMACOLOGY

Uses

Relief of mild to moderate pain.

Contraindications

Hypersensitivity to local anesthetics or any components of the products, para-aminobenzoic acid (esters only), or parabens; congenital or idiopathic methemoglobinemia; spinal and caudal anesthesia in septicemia; existing neurologic disease; spinal deformities; severe hypertension; hemorrhage; shock; or heart block.

Usual Dosage

Mild to moderate pain
ADULTS: One to 2 tablets every 4 to 6 hr; not to exceed 12 tablets in a 24-hr period.
CHILDREN: Not recommended for pediatric use.

Pharmacokinetics

Aspirin
ABSORP: Rapidly and completely absorbed. T_{max} is 1 to 2 hr (salicylic acid).
DIST: Widely distributed to all tissues and fluids including CNS, breast milk, and fetal tissues. Approximately 90% of salicylate is protein bound at concentrations of less than 100 mcg/mL and approximately 75% is bound at concentrations of more than 400 mcg/mL.
METAB: Rapidly hydrolyzed to salicylic acid (active). Salicylic acid is conjugated in the liver to the metabolites.
EXCRET: Salicylic acid plasma $t_{1/2}$ is approximately 6 hr but may exceed 20 hr in higher doses. $T_{1/2}$ is approximately 15 to 20 min for aspirin. Elimination follows zero order kinetics. Renal elimination of unchanged drug depends on urine pH. A pH of more than 6.5 increases renal clearance of free salicylate from less than 5% to more than 80%.

Codeine
METAB: Metabolized in the liver by undergoing *O*-demethylation, *N*-demethylation, and partial conjugation.
EXCRET: Excreted in the urine, largely as inactive metabolites, and small amounts of free and conjugated morphine. The $t_{1/2}$ is 3 hr.
ONSET: *Oral/SC*: 15 to 30 min.
PEAK: *Oral*: 60 min.
DURATION: *Oral/SC*: 4 to 6 hr.

➥← DRUG INTERACTIONS

See also: aspirin — Drug Interactions
Codeine is additive with other CNS depressants
Bupivacaine: Possible respiratory depression (mechanism unknown)
• Use bupivacaine with caution.

ADVERSE EFFECTS

⚠ **ORAL:** Taste alteration, dry mouth, dysphagia (codeine); gingival bleeding (ASA).
CNS: Lightheadedness; dizziness; sedation; disorientation; incoordination; euphoria; delirium.
CVS: Bradycardia; postural hypotension; arrhythmia.
GI: Nausea, vomiting, abdominal pain, constipation, anorexia, biliary tract spasm (codeine); nausea, dyspepsia, abdominal pain, bleeding (ASA).
MISC: Tolerance; psychological and physical dependence with chronic use (codeine); hypersensitivity skin reactions such as rash, edema, urticaria, anaphylaxis, angioedema (ASA).

CLINICAL IMPLICATIONS

General

• *Lactation:* Undetermined.
• Assess patient for GI and general side effects. Inform health care provider if noted and significant.

- Determine why drug is being taken. Consider implications of condition on dental treatment.
- If oral pain requires additional analgesics, consider nonopioid products.
- Chronic dry mouth is possible; anticipate increased caries and candidiasis.
- If GI side effects occur, consider semisupine chair position.
- *Postural hypotension:* Monitor BP at the beginning and end of each appointment; anticipate syncope. Have patient sit upright for several min at the end of the dental appointment before dismissing.
- *When prescribed by DDS:* Short-term use only; there is no justification for long-term use in the management of dental pain.
- *Geriatric patients:* Use lower dose of opioid.

Pregnancy Risk Category: Category C (codeine); category D (ASA).

Oral Health Education
- If chronic dry mouth occurs, recommend home fluoride therapy and use of nonalcoholic oral health care products.
- *If prescribed by DDS:* Warn patient not to drive, sign important papers, or operate mechanical equipment.

---

aspirin/dipyridamole (ASS-pihr-in/dye-peer-ID-a-mole)

Synonym: dipyridamole/aspirin

Aggrenox

Drug Class: Antiplatelet

PHARMACOLOGY

Action
Antithrombotic action resulting from additive antiplatelet effects.

Uses
Reduces the risk of stroke in patients who have had transient ischemia of the brain or complete ischemic stroke caused by thrombosis.

➡◀ DRUG INTERACTIONS RELATED TO DENTAL THERAPEUTICS

Ibuprofen: Inhibits the antiplatelet effect of aspirin (blocks receptor site)
- Avoid concurrent use.

ADVERSE EFFECTS

⚠ **ORAL:** Taste loss.

CNS: Headache; amnesia; convulsions; anorexia; somnolence; confusion; coma; cerebral, subarachnoid, and intracranial hemorrhage; fatigue (5.8%).

CVS: Hypotension, tachycardia, palpitation, arrhythmia (<1%); syncope.

GI: Abdominal pain; dyspepsia; nausea; vomiting; diarrhea; melena; rectal hemorrhage; GI hemorrhage; hemorrhoids; perforation; Reye syndrome.

RESP: Coughing; URI.

MISC: Arthralgia; arthritis; myalgia; arthrosis; pain; back pain; asthenia; neoplasm; malaise; anaphylaxis; laryngeal edema; rhabdomyolysis; hemorrhage (3.2%), epistaxis (2.4%), thrombocytopenia, purpura, prolonged PT.

CLINICAL IMPLICATIONS

General
- Determine why drug is being taken. Consider implications of condition on dental treatment.
- Determine bleeding time before completing procedures that may result in significant bleeding. Safe levels are <20 min.
- Monitor vital signs (e.g., BP, pulse pressure, rate, and rhythm) at each appointment to assess disease control. Do not provide elective dental treatment when BP ≥180/110 or in presence of other high-risk CV conditions. Refer to the section entitled "The Patient Taking Cardiovascular Drugs" in Chapter 6: *Clinical Medicine.*

- Monitor vital signs.
- If GI side effects or back pain occur, consider semisupine chair position.
- If uncontrolled bleeding develops, use hemostatic agents and positive pressure to induce hemostasis. Do not dismiss patient until bleeding is controlled.

Oral Health Education
- Encourage daily plaque control procedures for effective self-care in patients at risk for cardiovascular disease.

Aspirin Free Anacin Maximum Strength — see acetaminophen
Aspirin Free Pain Relief — see acetaminophen

 # aspirin/hydrocodone bitartrate (ASS-pihr-in/HIGH-droe-KOE-dohn by-TAR-TRATE)

Synonym: hydrocodone bitartrate/aspirin

Alor 5/500, Lortab ASA, Panasol 5/500: Tablets: 5 mg hydrocodone bitartrate, 500 mg ASA

Drug Class: Opioid Analgesic Combination

Usual Dosage
Odontogenic pain
TABLETS
ADULTS: Two tablets every four to six hr (maximum 8 tablets in 24 hr).

Pharmacokinetics
Aspirin
ABSORP: Rapidly and completely absorbed. T_{max} is 1 to 2 hr (salicylic acid).
DIST: Widely distributed to all tissues and fluids including CNS, breast milk, and fetal tissues. Approximately 90% of salicylate is protein bound at concentrations of less than 100 mcg/mL and approximately 75% is bound at concentrations of more than 400 mcg/mL.
METAB: Rapidly hydrolyzed to salicylic acid (active). Salicylic acid is conjugated in the liver to the metabolites.
EXCRET: Salicylic acid plasma $t_{1/2}$ is approximately 6 hr but may exceed 20 hr in higher doses. $T_{1/2}$ is approximately 15 to 20 min for aspirin. Elimination follows zero-order kinetics. Renal elimination of unchanged drug depends on urine pH. A pH of more than 6.5 increases renal clearance of free salicylate from less than 5% to more than 80%.

Hydrocodone
ABSORP: Hydrocodone is rapidly absorbed from the GI tract. T_{max} is achieved at 1.7 hrs.
DIST: Distributed throughout the body. Not extensively protein bound.
METAB: Extensively metabolized in the liver to hydromorphone by *O*-demethylation by the CYP2D6 isoenzyme.
EXCRET: Hydrocodone and its metabolites are eliminated primarily in the kidneys.
ONSET: 30 min.
PEAK: 1.7 hr.
DURATION: 4.5 hr.
SPECIAL POP: *Severe renal insufficiency:* The effect of renal insufficiency on the pharmacokinetics of hydrocodone has not been determined.

➡◀ DRUG INTERACTIONS
See also: acetaminophen – Drug Interactions
No specific documented drug-drug interactions with hydrocodone. The absence of evidence is not evidence of safety.

ADVERSE EFFECTS
⚠ **ORAL:** Dry mouth; bleeding.
CNS: Dizziness; lightheadedness; euphoria; dysphoria; convulsions (overdose).
CVS: Circulatory depression; palpitations; changes in blood pressure.

GI: Nausea; vomiting.
RESP: Respiratory depression.
MISC: Tinnitus; blurred vision; miosis.

CLINICAL IMPLICATIONS

General
- Monitor vital signs.
- *Elderly:* Use lower dose of opioid.
- *When prescribed by DDS:* Short-term use only; there is no justification for long-term use in the management of dental pain.

Pregnancy Risk Category: Category C.

Oral Health Education
- *When prescribed by DDS:* Warn patient not to drive, sign important papers, or operate mechanical equipment.

---

 aspirin/oxycodone HCl (ASS-pihr-in/OX-ee-KOE-dohn HIGH-droe-KLOR-ide)

Synonym: oxycodone HCl/aspirin

Percodan: Tablets: 4.5 mg oxycodone HCl/ 0.38 mg oxycodone terephthalate/ 325 mg aspirin

▮✦▮ ratio-Oxycodan

Drug Class: Narcotic analgesic

DEA Schedule: Schedule II

PHARMACOLOGY

Action
OXYCODONE: Relieves pain by stimulating opiate receptors in CNS.
ASPIRIN: Inhibits prostaglandin synthesis, resulting in analgesia, anti-inflammatory activity, and inhibition of platelet aggregation.

Uses
For the relief of moderate to moderately severe pain.

Contraindications
Hypersensitivity to any component of the product.

Usual Dosage
ADULTS: *PO:* Usual dose is 1 tablet q 6 hr prn for pain (max, 12 tablets [4 g aspirin] q 24 hr).

Pharmacokinetics
Aspirin
ABSORP: Rapidly and completely absorbed. T_{max} is 1 to 2 hr (salicylic acid).
DIST: Widely distributed to all tissues and fluids including CNS, breast milk, and fetal tissues. Approximately 90% of salicylate is protein bound at concentrations of less than 100 mcg/mL and approximately 75% is bound at concentrations of more than 400 mcg/mL.
METAB: Rapidly hydrolyzed to salicylic acid (active). Salicylic acid is conjugated in the liver to the metabolites.
EXCRET: Salicylic acid plasma $t_{1/2}$ is approximately 6 hr but may exceed 20 hr in higher doses. $T_{1/2}$ is approximately 15 to 20 min for aspirin. Elimination follows zero order kinetics. Renal elimination of unchanged drug depends on urine pH. A pH of more than 6.5 increases renal clearance of free salicylate from less than 5% to more than 80%.
Oxycodone
ABSORP: High oral availability due to low presystemic or first-pass metabolism. Exhibits a biphasic absorption pattern. The immediate-release oral bioavailability is 100%. The oral

bioavailability is 60% to 87%. Peak plasma concentration increased by 25% with a high fat meal. Once absorbed, it is distributed to skeletal muscle, liver, intestinal tract, lungs, spleen, and brain.

DIST: The Vd is 2.6 L/kg (IV). It is found in breast milk.

METAB: Extensively metabolized in the liver to noroxycodone (a major metabolite), oxymorphone, and their glucuronides.

EXCRET: Excreted through the urine, with less than 19% as free oxycodone, less than 50% as conjugated oxycodone, and less than 14% as conjugated oxymorphone. The $t_{1/2}$ for immediate release is 0.4 hr. Clearance is 0.8 L/min. Elimination on $t_{1/2}$ is 3.2 hr (immediate release).

ONSET: 15 to 30 min.

PEAK: 1 hr.

DURATION: 4 to 6 hr.

SPECIAL POP: *Severe renal insufficiency:* For less than 60 mL/min, higher peak plasma oxycodone (50%), and noroxycodone (20%), higher AUC for oxycodone (60%), noroxycodone (50%), oxymorphone (40%). There is an increased $t_{1/2}$ of oxycodone elimination of only 1 hr.

Mild to moderate hepatic insufficiency: Peak plasma oxycodone and noroxycodone concentrations 50% and 20% higher; AUC values are 95% and 65% higher, respectively. Oxymorphone peak plasma concentration and AUC values are lower by 30% and 40%. The $t_{1/2}$ elimination for oxycodone is increased by 2.3 hr.

➡️⬅ DRUG INTERACTIONS

See also: aspirin — Drug Interactions

Sertraline: Possible increased risk of serotonin syndrome (mechanism unknown)
  • Monitor clinical status.

ADVERSE EFFECTS

⚠️ **ORAL:** Dry mouth, increased bleeding.

CNS: Lightheadedness; dizziness; sedation; euphoria; dysphoria.

CVS: Hypotension; bradycardia; tachycardia.

GI: Nausea; vomiting; constipation.

RESP: Dyspnea; respiratory depression.

MISC: Malaise; tolerance; psychological and physical dependence with chronic use.

CLINICAL IMPLICATIONS

General

When prescribed by DDS:

• Short-term use only; there is no justification for long-term use in the management of dental pain.

• If oral pain requires additional analgesics, consider nonopioid products.

• *Children:* Safety and efficacy not established. Reye syndrome has been associated with aspirin administration to children (including teenagers) with acute febrile illness.

• *Special risk:* Use with caution in the elderly or debilitated and in patients with severe impairment of hepatic or renal function, peptic ulcers, hypothyroidism, Addison disease, and prostatic hypertrophy or urethral stricture.

• *Acute abdominal conditions:* Diagnosis or clinical course may be obscured.

• *Ambulatory patients:* Mental and physical abilities may be impaired.

• *Dependency:* Oxycodone has abuse potential.

• *Peptic ulcers:* Use with caution in the presence of peptic ulcer.

• *Overdosage:* Respiratory depression, extreme somnolence progressing to stupor or coma, skeletal muscle flaccidity, cold and clammy skin, bradycardia, hypotension, apnea, circulatory collapse, cardiac arrest, death.

When prescribed by medical facility:

• Determine why drug is being taken. Consider implications of condition on dental treatment.

• Monitor vital signs.

• If GI side effects occur, consider semisupine chair position.

• Chronic dry mouth is possible; anticipate increased caries activity and candidiasis.

Pregnancy Risk Category: Category B. Category D if used for prolonged periods.

Oral Health Education

When prescribed by DDS:

- Explain name, dose, action, and potential side effects of drug.
- Advise patient to take 1 tablet q 6 hr or as prescribed if needed for pain but to not take more than 12 tablets in 24 hr.
- Advise patient to take without regard to meals but to take with food if GI upset occurs.
- Instruct patient to avoid alcoholic beverages and other depressants while taking this medication.
- Advise patient that drug may impair judgment, thinking, or motor skills or cause drowsiness, and to use caution while driving or performing other tasks requiring mental alertness until tolerance is determined.
- Advise patient to stop taking the drug and notify health care provider if any of the following occurs: allergic reaction; unusual bleeding or bruising; shortness of breath; black or tarry stools; vomiting of blood or coffee grounds–like material; excessive sedation.
- Advise women to notify health care provider if pregnant, planning to become pregnant, or breast feeding.
- Warn patient not to take any prescription or OTC drugs or dietary supplements without consulting health care provider.
- Advise patient that follow-up visits may be necessary to monitor therapy and to keep appointments.

When prescribed by medical facility:

- If chronic dry mouth occurs, recommend home fluoride therapy and use of nonalcoholic oral health care products.

Astelin — see azelastine HCl

Astracaine — see articaine HCl

Astracaine Forte — see articaine HCl

Astramorph PF — see morphine sulfate

Atacand — see candesartan cilexetil

Atasol — see acetaminophen

---

atazanavir sulfate (At-ah-zah-NAH-veer SULL-fate)

Reyataz

Drug Class: Antiviral

PHARMACOLOGY

Action

Inhibits human immunodeficiency virus (HIV) protease, the enzyme required to form functional proteins in HIV-infected cells.

Uses

In combination with other antiretroviral agents for the treatment of HIV-1 infection.

DRUG INTERACTIONS RELATED TO DENTAL THERAPEUTICS

No documented drug-drug interactions. The absence of evidence is not evidence of safety.

ADVERSE EFFECTS

⚠ **ORAL:** Aphthous stomatitis; dental pain (unspecified); esophageal ulcer; esophagitis.

CNS: Headache (14%); depression (4%); dizziness, insomnia (3%); peripheral neurological symptoms (1%); abnormal dreams; abnormal gait; agitation; amnesia; anxiety; confusion; convulsion; decreased libido; emotional lability; hallucination; hostility; hyperkinesia; hypesthesia; increased reflexes; nervousness; psychosis; sleep disorder; somnolence; suicide attempt; twitch.

GI: Nausea (16%); vomiting, abdominal pain, diarrhea (6%); acholia; anorexia; colitis; constipation; dyspepsia; enlarged abdomen; flatulence; gastritis; gastroenteritis; GI disorder; hepatitis; hepatomegaly; hepatosplenomegaly, increased appetite; liver damage; liver fatty deposit; pancreatitis; peptic ulcer.

RESP: Increased cough; dyspnea; hiccup; hypoxia.

MISC: Rash (9%); fever (4%); increased cough, pain (3%); back pain, fatigue (2%); lipodystrophy (1%); bone pain; extremity pain; muscle atrophy; myalgia; myasthenia; myopathy; allergic reactions; angioedema; asthenia; burning sensation; chest pain; dysplasia; ecchymosis; edema; facial atrophy; generalized edema; heat sensitivity; infection; malaise; pallor; peripheral edema; photosensitivity; purpura; substernal chest pain; sweating.

CLINICAL IMPLICATIONS

General
- Determine why drug is being taken. Consider implications of condition on dental treatment.
- Consider medical consult to determine disease control and influence on dental treatment.
- Anticipate oral candidiasis when HIV disease is reported.
- If GI side effects occur, consider semisupine chair position.
- This drug is frequently prescribed in combination with one or more other antiviral agents. Side effects of all agents must be considered during the drug review process.
- Antibiotic prophylaxis should be considered when <500 PMN/mm^3 are reported; elective dental treatment should be delayed until blood values improve above this level.

Oral Health Education
- Recommend frequent maintenance prophylaxis when immunosuppression is evident.
- Encourage daily plaque control procedures for effective self-care since HIV infection reduces host resistance.

Atemperator-S — see valproic acid and derivatives

---

atenolol (ah-TEN-oh-lahl)

Tenormin

■✦■ **Apo-Atenol, Gen-Atenolol, Med-Atenolol, Novo-Atenol, Nu-Atenol, PMS-Atenolol, ratio-Atenolol, Rhoxal-atenolol**

■✦■ **Blokium, Tenormin**

Drug Class: Beta$_1$-adrenergic blocker

PHARMACOLOGY

Action
Blocks beta$_1$ receptors, primarily affecting heart (slows rate), vascular system (decreases BP), and, to a lesser extent, lungs (reduces function).

Uses
Treatment of hypertension (used alone or in combination with other drugs), angina pectoris resulting from coronary atherosclerosis, acute MI.

Unlabeled Uses
Migraine prophylaxis; alcohol withdrawal syndrome; ventricular arrhythmias; supraventricular arrhythmias or tachycardias; esophageal varices rebleeding; anxiety.

➡◆ DRUG INTERACTIONS RELATED TO DENTAL THERAPEUTICS

Nonsteroidal anti-inflammatory drugs: Decreased antihypertensive effect (inhibition of prostaglandin synthesis)
- Monitor blood pressure.

Sympathomimetic amines: Decreased antihypertensive effect (pharmacological antagonism)
- Use local anesthetic agents with a vasoconstrictor with caution while monitoring vital signs.

ADVERSE EFFECTS
⚠ **ORAL:** Dry mouth; taste disturbance; taste loss.
CNS: Insomnia; fatigue; dizziness; depression; lethargy; drowsiness; forgetfulness; slurred speech.
CVS: Hypotension; bradycardia; arrhythmia; postural hypotension.
GI: Nausea; vomiting; diarrhea.
RESP: Bronchospasm; dyspnea; wheezing.
MISC: Weight changes; facial swelling; muscle weakness; hyperglycemia; hypoglycemia; antinuclear antibodies; hyperlipidemia.

CLINICAL IMPLICATIONS
General
- Monitor vital signs (e.g., BP, pulse pressure, rate, and rhythm) at each appointment to assess disease control. Do not provide elective dental treatment when BP is ≥180/110 or in the presence of other high-risk CV conditions.
- Chronic dry mouth is possible. Anticipate increased caries, candidiasis, and lichenoid mucositis.
- If GI side effects occur, consider semisupine chair position.
- Use local anesthetic agents with vasoconstrictor with caution based on functional capacity of the patient and use aspirating technique to prevent intravascular injection.
- Beta blockers may mask epinephrine-induced signs and symptoms of hypoglycemia in patient with diabetes.
- Determine ability to adapt to stress of dental treatment. Consider short appointments.

Oral Health Education
- If chronic dry mouth occurs, recommend home fluoride therapy and use of nonalcoholic oral health care products.
- Encourage daily plaque control procedures for effective self-care in patients at risk for cardiovascular disease.

Athos — see dextromethorphan HBr
Atiflan — see naproxen
Atiquim — see naproxen
Atisuril — see allopurinol
Ativan — see lorazepam

---

atomoxetine (AT-oh-MOX-ah-teen)
Strattera
Drug Class: Psychotherapeutic

PHARMACOLOGY
Action
Selective inhibition of the presynaptic norepinephrine transporter is suspected.

Uses
Treatment of attention deficit hyperactivity disorder (ADHD).

➡◀ DRUG INTERACTIONS RELATED TO DENTAL THERAPEUTICS
No documented drug-drug interactions. The absence of evidence is not evidence of safety.

ADVERSE EFFECTS
⚠ **ORAL:** Dry mouth.

CNS: Aggression; irritability; somnolence; fatigue; dizziness; mood swings; headache; crying; fatigue; insomnia; sedation; depression; decreased libido; abnormal dreams; paresthesia; sleep disorder; sinus headache; lethargy.

GI: Vomiting; dyspepsia; nausea; abdominal pain; decreased appetite; constipation; diarrhea; anorexia; viral gastroenteritis; flatulence.

RESP: Cough; rhinorrhea; sinus congestion; upper respiratory tract infection.

MISC: Allergic hypersensitivity (e.g., angioneurotic edema, urticaria, rash); influenza; early morning awakening; tearfulness; arthralgia; tremor; myalgia; pyrexia; rigors; peripheral coldness.

CLINICAL IMPLICATIONS

General
- Determine why drug is being taken. Consider implications of condition on dental treatment.
- Chronic dry mouth is possible; anticipate increased caries and candidiasis.
- Patients with ADHD may have a short attention span; consider short appointment.

Oral Health Education
- If chronic dry mouth occurs, recommend home fluoride therapy and use of nonalcoholic oral health care products.

---

atorvastatin calcium (ah-TORE-vah-STAT-in KAL-see-uhm)

Lipitor

Drug Class: Antihyperlipidemic, HMG-CoA reductase inhibitor

PHARMACOLOGY

Action
Increases rate at which body removes cholesterol from blood and reduces production of cholesterol by inhibiting enzyme that catalyzes early rate-limiting step in cholesterol synthesis; increases HDL; reduces LDL, VLDL, and triglycerides.

Uses
Elevated serum triglyceride, heterozygous familial hypercholesterolemia in pediatric patients, homozygous familial hypercholesterolemia, hypercholesterolemia, type III familial hyperlipoproteinemia.

➜⬅ DRUG INTERACTIONS RELATED TO DENTAL THERAPEUTICS

Itraconazole: Possible atorvastatin toxicity (decreased metabolism)
- Avoid concurrent use.

ADVERSE EFFECTS

CNS: Headache (17%); insomnia, dizziness (≥2%).

GI: Diarrhea (4%); abdominal pain (4%); constipation (3%); nausea (≥2%).

RESP: Bronchitis (≥2%).

MISC: Back pain, asthenia, myalgia (4%); flu-like symptoms (3%); chest pain (≥2%); anaphylaxis, angioneurotic edema, bullous rashes (including erythema multiforme, Stevens-Johnson syndrome, toxic epidermal necrolysis), rhabdomyolysis.

CLINICAL IMPLICATIONS

General
- High LDL cholesterol concentration is the major cause of atherosclerosis that leads to CAD (angina, MI); determine degree of CV health and ability to withstand stress of dental treatment.
- Monitor vital signs (e.g., BP, pulse pressure, rate, and rhythm) at each appointment to assess disease control. Do not provide elective dental treatment when BP is ≥180/110 or in the presence of other high-risk CV conditions.
- If GI side effects occur, consider semisupine chair position.

Oral Health Education
- Encourage daily plaque control procedures for effective self-care in patients at risk for cardiovascular disease.

---

atovaquone (uh-TOE-vuh-KWONE)
Mepron

Drug Class: Anti-infective; Antiprotozoal

PHARMACOLOGY

Action
Inhibits mitochondrial electron transport in metabolic enzymes of microorganisms. This may cause inhibition of nucleic acid and adenosine triphosphate synthesis.

Uses
Treatment of mild to moderate *Pneumocystis carinii* pneumonia (PCP) in patients who are intolerant of trimethoprim-sulfamethoxazole and acute oral treatment of mild to moderate PCP in patients who are intolerant to trimethoprim-sulfamethoxazole (TMP-SMZ).

➜◀ DRUG INTERACTIONS RELATED TO DENTAL THERAPEUTICS
No documented drug-drug interactions. The absence of evidence is not evidence of safety.

ADVERSE EFFECTS
⚠ **ORAL:** Candidiasis.
CNS: Headache; insomnia; dizziness; anxiety.
GI: Nausea; diarrhea; vomiting; abdominal pain; constipation; anorexia; dyspepsia.
RESP: Cough increased.
MISC: Fever; sweating; weakness; decreased sodium concentration; elevated amylase; allergic reaction; rhinitis; asthenia; infection; dyspnea.

CLINICAL IMPLICATIONS

General
- Determine why drug is being taken. Consider implications of condition on dental treatment.
- If GI side effects occur, consider semisupine chair position.
- Anticipate oral candidiasis when HIV disease is reported.
- This drug is frequently prescribed in combination with one or more other antiviral agents. Side effects of all agents must be considered during the drug review process.
- Antibiotic prophylaxis should be considered when <500 PMN/mm³ are reported; elective dental treatment should be delayed until blood values improve above this level.

Oral Health Education
- Encourage daily plaque control procedures for effective self-care since HIV infection reduces host resistance.

Atridox — see doxycycline hyclate
AtroPen — see atropine

---

 atropine (AT-troe-peen)

Sal-Tropine: Dental Tablets: 0.4 mg
AtroPen, Atropine-1, Atropine Sulfate, Atropine Sulfate Ophthalmic, Isopto Atropine

■✲■ **Atropine, Atropine Injection, Atropine Ointment, Minims Atropine**

Drug Class: Anticholinergic; Antispasmodic

PHARMACOLOGY

Action

Inhibits action of acetylcholine or other cholinergic stimuli at postganglionic cholinergic receptors, including smooth muscles, secretory glands, and CNS sites.

Uses

Antisialagogue.

Contraindications

Hypersensitivity to anticholinergics; narrow-angle glaucoma; primary glaucoma or tendency toward glaucoma (ophthalmic); adhesions between iris and lens; prostatic hypertrophy; obstructive uropathy; myocardial ischemia; unstable cardiac status caused by hemorrhage; tachycardia; myasthenia gravis; pyloric or intestinal obstruction; asthma; hyperthyroidism; renal disease; hepatic disease; toxic megacolon; intestinal atony; or paralytic ileus.

Usual Dosage

Reduced oral secretions

ADULTS: 0.4 to 0.6 mg (usually single-dose use by DDS).
CHILDREN: *PO:* Use lowest effective dose.
   7 to 16 lb: 0.1 mg
   17 to 24 lb: 0.15 mg
   24 to 40 lb: 0.2 mg
   40 to 65 lb: 0.3 mg
   65 to 90 lb: 0.4 mg
   Over 90 lb: 0.4 mg

Pharmacokinetics

ABSORP: Rapidly absorbed after oral administration.
DIST: Readily crosses blood-brain barrier.
EXCRET: The $t_{1/2}$ is 3 hr (IV); 94% of dose is eliminated through urine in 24 hr.

➔← DRUG INTERACTIONS

Sympathomimetic amines: Tachyarrhythmia (autonomic imbalance)
   • Avoid concurrent use.

ADVERSE EFFECTS

⚠ **ORAL:** Dry mouth, excessive thirst; tongue chewing.
CVS: Altered ST-T waves; systole; atrial arrhythmia; atrial ectopic beats; atrial fibrillation; bigeminal beats; bradycardia; cardiac dilation; cardiac syncope; decreased BP; flattening of T wave; increased BP; intermittent nodal rhythm (no P wave); labile BP; left ventricular failure; MI; nodal extrasystole; palpitations; prolongation of sinus node recovery time; prolonged P wave; prolonged QT interval; retrograde conduction; R on T phenomenon; shortened PR segment; shortened RT duration; supraventricular extrasystole; tachycardia (sinus, supraventricular, junctional); transient AV dissociation; trigeminal beats; ventricular arrhythmia; ventricular extrasystole; ventricular fibrillation; ventricular flutter; ventricular premature contractions; weak or impalpable pulses; widening and flattening of QRS complex.
CNS: Abnormal movements; agitation; amnesia; anxiety; ataxia; Babinski reflex/Chaddock reflex; behavioral changes; coma; confusion; delirium; depression; difficulty concentrating; diminished tendon reflex; dizziness; dysarthria; dysmetria; fatigue; hallucinations; headache; hyperreflexia; hypertonia; insomnia; lethargy; locomotor difficulties; loss of libido; mania; mental disorder; muscle clonus; muscle twitching; opisthotonos; paranoia; restlessness; seizures; sensation of intoxication; somnolence; stupor; tremor; vertigo; weakness; withdrawal behavior.
GI: Abdominal distention; abdominal pain; constipation; decreased bowel sounds; decreased food absorption; delayed gastric emptying; distended abdomen; dysphagia; nausea; paralytic ileus; vomiting.
RESP: Breathing difficulty; inspiratory stridor; labored respirations; laryngospasm; pulmonary edema; respiratory failure; shallow respiration; slow respiration; subcostal recession; syncope; tachypnea.
MISC: Chest pain; feeling hot; heat intolerance; hyperpyrexia.

CLINICAL IMPLICATIONS

General

When prescribed by DDS:

- *Lactation:* Excreted in breast milk.
- *Special risk:* Use with caution in the elderly, in patients with Down syndrome, brain damage, spastic paralysis, disorders of heart rhythm (e.g., atrial flutter), severe narrow angle glaucoma, pyloric stenosis, prostatic hypertrophy, significant renal failure, or who have suffered a recent MI.
- *Anticholinergic psychosis:* Has occurred in sensitive patients.
- *Overdosage:* Dry mouth, thirst, vomiting, nausea, abdominal distention, CNS stimulation, delirium, drowsiness, restlessness, stupor, fever, seizures, hallucinations, convulsions, coma, circulatory failure, tachycardia, weak pulse, hypertension, hypotension, respiratory depression, palpitations, urinary urgency, blurred vision, dilated pupils, photophobia, rash, dry and hot skin.
- Dim room lights or provide sunglasses if patient experiences photophobia.

Pregnancy Risk Category: Category C.

Oral Health Education

- *When prescribed by DDS:* Explain name, dose, action, and potential side effects of drug.

Atropine-1 — see atropine

Atropine Injection — see atropine

Atropine Ointment — see atropine

Atropine Sulfate — see atropine

Atropine Sulfate Ophthalmic — see atropine

Atrovent — see ipratropium bromide

A/T/S — see erythromycin

augmented betamethasone dipropionate — see betamethasone

Augmentin — see amoxicillin/clavulanate potassium

Augmentin ES-600 — see amoxicillin/clavulanate potassium

Augmentin XR — see amoxicillin/clavulanate potassium

---

auranofin (or-RAIN-oh-fin)

Ridaura

Drug Class: Analgesic; Antirheumatic, Gold compound

PHARMACOLOGY

Action

Gold compounds relieve symptoms of arthritis but do not cure this disease; decreases rheumatoid factor concentrations and immunoglobulins.

Uses

Relief of symptoms of active adult rheumatoid arthritis poorly controlled with other therapies.

Unlabeled Uses

Treatment of pemphigus and psoriatic arthritis.

➔← DRUG INTERACTIONS RELATED TO DENTAL THERAPEUTICS

No documented drug-drug interactions. The absence of evidence is not evidence of safety.

ADVERSE EFFECTS

Reactions can occur months after therapy is discontinued.

⚠ **ORAL:** Stomatitis (13%).

CNS: Confusion; hallucinations; seizures.

GI: Diarrhea; abdominal pain; anorexia; dyspepsia; flatulence; GI bleeding; enterocolitis; gastritis; colitis; tracheitis.

RESP: Interstitial pneumonitis; pulmonary fibrosis.

MISC: Vaginitis; glossitis; leukopenia, thrombocytopenia (1%).

CLINICAL IMPLICATIONS

General

- *Arthritis:* Consider patient comfort and need for semisupine chair position.
- If GI side effects occur, consider semisupine chair position.
- Blood dyscrasias rarely reported; anticipate increased bleeding, infection, and poor healing.
- Be aware that patient may be taking COX inhibitors and other analgesics.

Oral Health Education

- Review oral hygiene, including use of soft toothbrush; daily flossing; and avoidance of strong, commercial mouthwashes. If mild stomatitis develops, an isotonic NaCl and sodium bicarbonate solution may be used.

Aurolate — see gold sodium thiomalate

Avandamet — see rosiglitazone maleate/metformin HCl

Avandia — see rosiglitazone maleate

Avapro — see irbesartan

Avelox — see moxifloxacin HCl

Avelox IV — see moxifloxacin HCl

Aventyl HCl — see nortriptyline HCl

Aventyl HCl Pulvules — see nortriptyline HCl

Avita — see tretinoin

Avitene — see microfibrillar collagen hemostat

Axert — see almotriptan malate

Axid AR — see nizatidine

Axid Pulvules — see nizatidine

Aygestin — see norethindrone acetate

Azasan — see azathioprine

---

azathioprine (AZE-uh-THIGH-oh-preen)

Azasan, Imuran

▮✦▮ **Apo-Azathioprine, Gen-Azathioprine, ratio-Azathioprine**

▮✦▮ **Azatrilem, Imuran**

Drug Class: Immunosuppressive

PHARMACOLOGY

Action

Suppresses cell-mediated hypersensitivities; alters antibody production and may reduce inflammation.

Uses

Adjunct for prevention of rejection in renal homotransplantation; treatment in adults for severe, active, erosive rheumatoid arthritis not responsive to conventional management.

Unlabeled Uses

Treatment of chronic ulcerative colitis, Crohn disease, myasthenia gravis, and Behçet syndrome.

➡️⬅️ DRUG INTERACTIONS RELATED TO DENTAL THERAPEUTICS

No documented drug-drug interactions. The absence of evidence is not evidence of safety.

ADVERSE EFFECTS

GI: Nausea; vomiting (>10%).
CNS: Fever, chills (>10%).
MISC: Serious infections; neoplasias; thrombocytopenia, leukopenia, anemia (>10%).

CLINICAL IMPLICATIONS

General

- Determine why drug is being taken. Consider implications of condition on dental treatment.
- Serious infections are a potential complication of chronic immunosuppression; oral infection should be treated aggressively with antibiotic therapy.
- Medical consultation for CBC, including platelet count, should be completed.
- Blood dyscrasias are reported; anticipate increased bleeding, infection, and poor healing.
- This drug may be used with corticosteroids for additive effect.
- If GI side effects occur, consider semisupine chair position.

Oral Health Education

- Encourage daily plaque control procedures for effective self-care.

Azatrilem — see azathioprine

---

azelastine HCl (ah-ZELL-ass-teen HIGH-droe-KLOR-ide)

Astelin, Optivar

Drug Class: Antihistamine, H1

PHARMACOLOGY

Action

Competitively antagonizes histamine at H_1 receptor sites.

Uses

Treatment of symptoms of seasonal allergic rhinitis, such as rhinorrhea, sneezing, and nasal pruritus; treatment of symptoms of vasomotor rhinitis, such as rhinorrhea, nasal congestion, and postnasal drip (nasal inhalation); treatment of ocular itching associated with allergic conjunctivitis (ophthalmic).

➡️⬅️ DRUG INTERACTIONS RELATED TO DENTAL THERAPEUTICS

No documented drug-drug interactions. The absence of evidence is not evidence of safety.

ADVERSE EFFECTS

⚠️ **ORAL:** Bitter taste, dry mouth (3%); aphthous stomatitis, taste loss (<2%).
CNS: Headache (15%); somnolence (12%); fatigue, dizziness (2%); hyperkinesias, hypoesthesia, vertigo, anxiety, depersonalization, depression, nervousness, sleep disturbances, abnormal thinking (<2%); confusion.
OPHTHALMIC: Headache (15%); fatigue (1% to 10%).
CVS: Flushing, hypertension, tachycardia (<2%).
GI: Nausea (3%); constipation, gastroenteritis, ulcerative stomatitis, vomiting, abdominal pain (<2%); diarrhea.
RESP: Cough (11%); asthma (5%); bronchospasm (<2%); dyspnea (postmarketing).

OPHTHALMIC: Asthma, dyspnea (1% to 10%).

MISC: Dysesthesia (8%); myalgia, cold symptoms, temporomandibular dislocation, allergic reaction, back pain, herpes simplex, viral infection, pain in extremities, malaise (<2%); anaphylactoid reaction, chest pain, facial edema, involuntary muscle contractions, paresthesia, tolerance.
OPHTHALMIC: Influenza-like symptoms (1% to 10%).

CLINICAL IMPLICATIONS

General
- Consider semisupine chair position to control effects of postnasal drainage.
- Be aware that patients with multiple allergies are at increased risk for allergy to dental drugs.
- Chronic dry mouth is possible; anticipate increased caries activity and candidiasis.
- Monitor vital signs (e.g., BP, pulse rate) and respiratory function. Uncontrolled disease characterized by wheezing, coughing.

Oral Health Education
- If chronic dry mouth occurs, recommend home fluoride therapy and use of nonalcoholic oral health care products.

---

azidothymidine — see zidovudine

---

 azithromycin (UHZ-ith-row-MY-sin)

Zithromax: Tablets: 250, 500, 600 mg (as dihydrate); Powder for injection, lyophilized: 500 mg; Powder for oral suspension: 100 mg per 5 mL, 200 mg per 5 mL, 1 g/packet (as dihydrate)
Zmax: Tablets, extended release: 2 g

■✦■ Z-Pak

■◆■ Azitrocin

Drug Class: Antibiotic, macrolide

PHARMACOLOGY

Action
Interferes with microbial protein synthesis.

Uses
ADULTS: Treatment of infections of the respiratory tract, acute bacterial sinusitis, acute bacterial exacerbations of COPD, community-acquired pneumonia, *Mycobacterium avium* complex, pelvic inflammatory disease, pharyngitis/tonsillitis, skin and skin structure infections, and sexually transmitted diseases caused by susceptible organisms; extended release form single dose treatment for mild to moderate acute bacterial sinusitis or community-acquired pneumonia.
CHILDREN: Treatment of acute bacterial sinusitis, acute otitis media caused by susceptible organisms, community-acquired pneumonia, pharyngitis/tonsillitis caused by *Streptococcus pyogenes* in patients who cannot use first-line therapy.

Contraindications
Hypersensitivity to azithromycin, erythromycin, or to any macrolide antibiotic.

Usual Dosage
Bacterial infections
ADULTS: *PO:* 500 mg as single dose on first day, then 250 mg/day on days 2 through 5.

Pharmacokinetics

ABSORP: *Oral:* Rapidly absorbed. *IV:* C_{max} is approximately 3.63 mcg/mL; C_{min} is approximately 0.2 mcg/mL (at 24 hr), AUC_{24} is approximately 9.6 mcg hr/mL.

DIST: Widely distributed into body (skin, lung, sputum, cervix, tonsils) but distributes poorly in the cerebrospinal fluid. Higher concentrations in tissues than in plasma or serum. V_d is 31.1 L/kg (oral) and 33.3 L/kg (IV). Protein binding is 7% to 50% (concentration dependent).

EXCRET: The $t_{1/2}$ is approximately 68 hr. Plasma Cl is 630 mL/min (oral) and 10.18 mL/min/kg (IV). Excreted primarily in bile, predominantly as unchanged drug. Approximately 6% is excreted in urine as unchanged drug (oral); approximately 11% is excreted in the urine after first dose and 14% after fifth dose (IV).

➔← DRUG INTERACTIONS

Digitoxin: Possible digitoxin toxicity (mechanism unknown)
- Avoid concurrent use.

Nelfinavir: Possible increased azithromycin toxicity (inhibition of P-glycoprotein)
- Avoid concurrent use.

Theophylline: Possible theophylline toxicity (decreased metabolism)
- Avoid concurrent use.

ADVERSE EFFECTS

⚠ **ORAL:** Oral candidiasis; tongue discoloration.

CVS: Palpitations; chest pain; arrhythmias; hypotension; QT prolongation; torsades de pointes.

CNS: Dizziness; headache; vertigo; somnolence; fatigue; agitation; aggressive behavior; anxiety; asthenia; convulsions; hyperactivity; malaise; nervousness; paresthesia; syncope.

GI: Diarrhea; nausea; vomiting; abdominal pain; dyspepsia; flatulence; melena; anorexia; constipation; pseudomembranous colitis; pancreatitis.

MISC: Angioedema; anaphylaxis; edema.

CLINICAL IMPLICATIONS

General

When prescribed by DDS:
- *Lactation:* Undetermined.
- *Hypersensitivity:* Serious reactions, including anaphylaxis, have occurred.
- *Renal failure:* Use cautiously.
- *Hepatic failure:* Use cautiously.
- *Cardiac effects:* Serious CV events have occurred with other macrolide antibiotics, including prolonged cardiac repolarization and QT interval.
- *Pneumonia:* Only effective for mild community-acquired pneumonia.
- *Pseudomembranous colitis:* May be factor in patients who develop diarrhea.
- *Superinfection:* Prolonged use of antibiotics may result in bacterial or fungal overgrowth of nonsusceptible microorganisms.
- Ensure patient knows how to take the drug, how long it should be taken, and to report adverse effects (e.g., rash, difficult breathing, diarrhea, GI upset) immediately.
- Antibiotic-associated diarrhea can occur. Have patient contact DDS immediately if signs develop.

When prescribed by medical facility:
- Determine why drug is being taken. If oral infection occurs that requires antibiotic therapy, select an appropriate product from a different class of anti-infectives.
- If GI side effects occur, consider semisupine chair position.

Pregnancy Risk Category: Category B.

Oral Health Education

When prescribed by DDS:
- Explain name, dose, action, and potential side effects of drug.
- Review dosing schedule and prescribed length of therapy with patient. Advise patient that dose, dosing frequency, and duration of therapy are dependent on site and cause of infection.

- Instruct patient using tablet form to take prescribed dose with a full glass of water.
- Instruct patient or caregiver using oral suspension to shake suspension well and then measure and administer prescribed dose using dosing spoon, dosing syringe, or medicine cup.
- Advise patient to take prescribed dose without regard to meals but to take with food if stomach upset occurs.
- Advise patient to take 2 hr before or after antacids containing aluminum or magnesium.
- Instruct patient to complete entire course of therapy, even if symptoms of infection have disappeared.
- Advise patient to discontinue therapy and contact health care provider immediately if skin rash, hives, itching, or shortness of breath occurs.
- Advise women to notify health care provider if pregnant, planning to become pregnant, or breast feeding.
- Advise patient to report signs of superinfection to health care provider: black "furry" tongue, white patches in mouth, foul-smelling stools, or vaginal itching or discharge.
- Warn patient that diarrhea containing blood or pus may be a sign of a serious disorder and to seek medical care if noted and not treat at home.
- Caution patient not to take any prescription or OTC medications, herbal preparations, or dietary supplements unless advised by health care provider.
- Advise patient that follow-up examinations and lab tests may be required to monitor therapy and to keep appointments.

Azitrocin — see azithromycin

Azmacort — see triamcinolone

AZT — see zidovudine

Azulfidine — see sulfasalazine

Azulfidine EN-tabs — see sulfasalazine

B3 — see niacin

Bactrim — see trimethoprim/sulfamethoxazole

Bactrim D.S. — see trimethoprim/sulfamethoxazole

Bactrim IV — see trimethoprim/sulfamethoxazole

Bactrim Pediatric — see trimethoprim/sulfamethoxazole

Bactrim Roche — see trimethoprim/sulfamethoxazole

Bactroban — see mupirocin

Bactroban Nasal — see mupirocin

Balcoran — see vancomycin

Balminil Decongestant Syrup — see pseudoephedrine

Balminil DM — see dextromethorphan HBr

Balminil DM Children — see dextromethorphan HBr

Balminil Expectorant — see guaifenesin

Bancap-HC — see acetaminophen/hydrocodone bitartrate

Banophen — see diphenhydramine HCl

Banophen Allergy — see diphenhydramine HCl

Bayer Children's Aspirin — see aspirin

Bayer Low Adult Strength — see aspirin

beclomethasone dipropionate (BEK-low-METH-uh-zone die-PRO-pee-oh-NATE)

QVAR, Vanceril, Beconase, Vancenase Pockethaler

■✚■ **Apo-Beclomethasone, Gen-Beclo Aq., Nu-Beclomethasone, Rivanase AQ**

■⦿■ **Aerobec, Beconase Aqua, Becotide**

Drug Class: Corticosteroid

PHARMACOLOGY

Action

Has potent anti-inflammatory effect on respiratory tract and in nasal passages.

Uses

ORAL/NASAL INHALATION: Maintenance prophylactic treatment of asthma in patients 5 yr and older; asthma patients requiring systemic corticosteroid administration in which adding an inhaled corticosteroid may reduce or eliminate need for systemic corticosteroids.

➡✚ DRUG INTERACTIONS RELATED TO DENTAL THERAPEUTICS

Aspirin: Decreased aspirin effect (mechanism unknown)
 • Avoid concurrent use.
Metronidazole: Decreased metronidazole effect (increased metabolism)
 • Avoid concurrent use.
COX-1 inhibitors: Increased risk of peptic ulcer disease (additive)
 • Avoid concurrent use.

ADVERSE EFFECTS

⚠ **ORAL:** Dry mouth; facial and tongue edema.

CNS: Headache; lightheadedness; agitation; depression; mental disturbances. QVAR: Headache (≥3%).

GI: Dyspepsia; nausea; vomiting. QVAR: Nausea (≥3%).

RESP: Coughing; wheezing; pulmonary infiltrates. QVAR: Upper respiratory tract infections (≥3%); coughing (1% to 3%).

MISC: Hypersensitivity reaction with rash, urticaria, angioedema, and bronchospasm; pruritus; wheezing; dyspnea; acneiform lesions; atrophy; bruising; localized *Candida* or *Aspergillus* infections; cushingoid features; growth velocity reduction in children; weight gain. QVAR: Increased asthma symptoms, oral symptoms (inhalation route), pain, back pain, dysphonia (≥3%).

CLINICAL IMPLICATIONS

General

 • Determine why drug is being taken. Consider implications of condition on dental treatment.
 • Acute bronchoconstriction can occur during dental treatment, have bronchodilator inhaler available.
 • Ensure that bronchodilator inhaler is present at each dental appointment.
 • Be aware that sulfites in local anesthetic with vasoconstrictor can precipitate acute asthma attack in susceptible individuals.
 • Inhalants can dry oral mucosa; anticipate candidiasis, increased calculus and plaque levels, and increased caries.
 • Because of the anticipated perioperative physiological stress in patients undergoing dental care (minor surgical stress) under local anesthesia, such patients should take only

their usual daily glucocorticoid dose before dental intervention. No supplementation is justified.

Oral Health Education
• Rinse mouth with water after bronchodilator use to prevent dryness.

Beconase — see beclomethasone dipropionate
Beconase Aqua — see beclomethasone dipropionate
Becotide — see beclomethasone dipropionate
Beepen-VK — see penicillin V
Bekidiba Dex — see dextromethorphan HBr
Bellatal — see phenobarbital
Bemote — see dicyclomine HCl
Benadryl Allergy — see diphenhydramine HCl
Benadryl Children's Allergy — see diphenhydramine HCl
Benadryl Children's Dye Free — see diphenhydramine HCl
Benadryl Dye Free Allergy Liqui Gels — see diphenhydramine HCl

---

benazepril HCl (BEN-AZE-uh-prill HIGH-droe-KLOR-ide)
Lotensin

Drug Class: ACE inhibitor; Antihypertensive

PHARMACOLOGY
Action
Competitively inhibits angiotensin I–converting enzyme, resulting in the prevention of angiotensin I conversion to angiotensin II, a potent vasoconstrictor that stimulates aldosterone secretion. Results in decrease in sodium and fluid retention, decrease in BP, and increase in diuresis.

Uses
Treatment of hypertension.

➜← DRUG INTERACTIONS RELATED TO DENTAL THERAPEUTICS
COX-1 inhibitors: Decreased antihypertensive effect (decreased prostaglandin synthesis)
• Monitor blood pressure.

ADVERSE EFFECTS
CNS: Headache (6%); dizziness (4%); fatigue (3%), somnolence.
CVS: Postural dizziness (2%); hypotension.
GI: Nausea (1%).
RESP: Chronic dry cough (1%).
MISC: Anaphylactoid reactions; angioedema.

CLINICAL IMPLICATIONS
General
• Monitor vital signs (e.g., BP, pulse pressure, rate, and rhythm) at each appointment to assess disease control. Do not provide elective dental treatment when BP is ≥180/110 or in the presence of other high-risk CV conditions. Refer to the section entitled "The Patient Taking Cardiovascular Drugs" in Chapter 6: *Clinical Medicine*.

- Use local anesthetic agents with vasoconstrictors with caution based on functional capacity of the patient and use aspirating technique to prevent intravascular injection.
- If coughing is problematic, consider semisupine chair position for treatment.
- Susceptible patient with DM may experience severe recurrent hypoglycemia.
- *Postural hypotension:* Monitor BP at the beginning and end of each appointment; anticipate syncope. Have patient sit upright for several min at the end of the dental appointment before dismissing.
- Determine ability to adapt to stress of dental treatment. Consider short appointments.

Oral Health Education
- Encourage daily plaque control procedures for effective self-care in patients at risk for cardiovascular disease.

---

benazepril HCl/amlodipine — see amlodipine/benazepril HCl

Benecid — see probenecid

Benicar — see olmesartan medoxomil

Bentyl — see dicyclomine HCl

Bentylol — see dicyclomine HCl

Benuryl — see probenecid

Benylin Adult — see dextromethorphan HBr

Benylin Decongestant — see pseudoephedrine

Benylin DM — see dextromethorphan HBr

Benylin DM 12 Hour — see dextromethorphan HBr

Benylin DM for Children — see dextromethorphan HBr

Benylin DM for Children 12 Hour — see dextromethorphan HBr

Benylin E Extra Strength — see guaifenesin

Benylin Pediatric — see dextromethorphan HBr

---

 benzocaine (BEN-zoe-kane)

Americaine Anesthetic Lubricant: Gel: Benzocaine 20%
Benzocaine: Cream: Benzocaine 5%
Hurricaine: Gel: Benzocaine 20%; Spray: Benzocaine 20%
Orajel Mouth-Aid: Liquid: Benzocaine 20%; Gel: Benzocaine 20%
Solarcaine Medicated First-Aid Spray: Spray: Benzocaine 20% with 0.13% triclosan, alcohol

Drug Class: Local anesthetic, topical

PHARMACOLOGY

Action
Blocks the influx of sodium ions into axons preventing depolarization.

Uses
For local anesthesia of accessible mucous membranes, including oral, nasal, and laryngeal mucous membranes, and respiratory or urinary tracts. Also for the treatment of pruritus ani, pruritus vulvae, and hemorrhoids.

For topical anesthesia in local skin disorders, including pruritus and pain due to minor burns, skin manifestations of systemic disease (e.g., chickenpox), prickly heat, abrasions, sunburn, plant poisoning, insect bites, eczema.

Contraindications
Hypersensitivity to any component of these products; ophthalmic use.

Usual Dosage
Topical anesthesia in the oral health care setting
GEL, 20%
ADULTS AND CHILDREN OLDER THAN 2 YR: Dosage varies depending on the area to be anesthetized and the vascularity of the area; do not use in children for more than 2 days.
CHILDREN YOUNGER THAN 2 YR: Do not administer to children younger than 2 yr of age.

Pharmacokinetics
PEAK: Less than 5 min.
DURATION: 15 to 45 min.

➧◀ DRUG INTERACTIONS
No documented drug-drug interactions. The absence of evidence is not evidence of safety.

ADVERSE EFFECTS
⚠ **ORAL:** Numbness, tingling.
MISC: Urethritis with and without bleeding. In a few case reports, methemoglobinemia characterized by cyanosis has followed topical application of benzocaine.

CLINICAL IMPLICATIONS
General
- Use the lowest dose effective for anesthesia to avoid high plasma levels and serious adverse effects.
- Benzocaine should not be used in those rare patients with congenital or idiopathic methemoglobinemia and in infants younger than 12 mo of age who are receiving treatment with methemoglobin-inducing agents. Very young patients or patients with glucose-6–phosphate deficiencies are more susceptible to methemoglobinemia.
- Do not use benzocaine in infants younger than 2 yr of age.
- *Lactation:* Exercise caution when administering during lactation.
- Use cautiously in patients with known drug sensitivities or in patients with severely traumatized mucosa and sepsis in the region of the application. If irritation or rash occurs, discontinue treatment and institute appropriate therapy.
- Topical anesthetics may impair swallowing and enhance danger of aspiration. Do not ingest food for 1 hr after anesthetic use in mouth or throat. This is particularly important in children because of their frequency of eating.
- Do not use for topical anesthesia if medical history reveals allergy to procaine, p-aminobenzoic acid (PABA), parabens, or other ester-type local anesthetics.
- Avoid applying to large areas of mucosa to prevent excessive systemic absorption and potential toxicity.

Pregnancy Risk Category: Category C.

Oral Health Education
- Do not ingest food for 1 hr following use of oral topical anesthetic preparations in the mouth or throat. Topical anesthesia may impair swallowing, thus enhancing the danger of aspiration.
- Numbness of the tongue or buccal mucosa may increase the danger of biting trauma. Do not eat or chew gum while the mouth or throat area is anesthetized.

Betacort — see betamethasone
Betadine — see povidone iodine
Betagen — see povidone iodine

Betaloc — see metoprolol
Betaloc Durules — see metoprolol

 betamethasone (BAY-tuh-METH-uh-zone)
(augmented betamethasone dipropionate, betamethasone dipropionate, betamethasone valerate, betamethasone sodium phosphate, betamethasone acetate)

Valisone: Ointment: 0.1%; Lotion: 0.1%; Cream: 0.1%
Beta-Val, Celestone, Celestone Phosphate, Celestone Soluspan, Diprolene, Diprolene AF, Diprosone, Luxiq, Maxivate, Teladar

■✦■ **Betnesol, Valisone Scalp Lotion, Betacort, Celestoderm-V, Celestoderm-V/2, Prevex B, Betaprolene, Diprolene Glycol, Taro-Sone, Topilene, ratio-Topilene, ratio-Topisone**

Drug Class: Adrenal corticosteroid; Glucocorticoid

PHARMACOLOGY

Action
Synthetic, long-acting glucocorticoid that depresses formation, release, and activity of endogenous mediators of inflammation, including prostaglandins, kinins, histamine, liposomal enzymes, and complement system. Also modifies body's immune response.

Uses
TOPICAL: Relief of inflammatory and pruritic manifestations of corticosteroid-responsive mucocutaneous conditions and dermatoses.

Contraindications
TOPICAL: Do not use as monotherapy in primary bacterial infections.

Usual Dosage
TOPICAL (BETAMETHASONE DIPROPIONATE, BETAMETHASONE VALERATE)
Apply sparingly to affected areas 2 to 4 times/day.

➡️⬅️ DRUG INTERACTIONS

ADVERSE EFFECTS
⚠️ ORAL: TOPICAL: Ulcerative esophagitis; thinning of mucosa.

CLINICAL IMPLICATIONS

General
When prescribed by DDS:
- *Topical:* Apply sparingly with cotton tip applicator.
- *Infections:* May mask signs of infection. May decrease host-defense mechanisms.
- *Ocular effects:* Use cautiously in ocular herpes simplex because of possible corneal perforation.
- *Sulfites:* Some products contain sulfites, which may cause allergic-type reactions in susceptible individuals.

Pregnancy Risk Category: Safety not established (systemic). Category C (topical).

Oral Health Education
When prescribed by DDS:
- Ensure patient understands how to use product, amount to apply, method of application, and signs of adverse effects.
Topical
- Demonstrate proper technique for cleaning affected area before applying medication and for applying sparingly as a thin film.
- Tell patient to avoid contact with eyes and to avoid tight-fitting clothing on treated area.

- Explain that preparations that contain alcohol should not be applied to affected area because of drying/irritation.
- Caution patient to discontinue medication and notify health care provider if affected area worsens or develops irritation, redness, burning, swelling, or stinging.

---

betamethasone acetate — see betamethasone
betamethasone dipropionate — see betamethasone
betamethasone sodium phosphate — see betamethasone
betamethasone valerate — see betamethasone
Betapace — see sotalol HCl
Betapace AF — see sotalol HCl
Betaprolene — see betamethasone
Beta-Val — see betamethasone

---

betaxolol HCl (BAY-TAX-oh-lahl HIGH-droe-KLOR-ide)

Betoptic, Betoptic S, Kerlone

Drug Class: Beta$_1$-adrenergic blocker

PHARMACOLOGY

Action
Blocks beta$_1$ receptors, primarily affecting cardiovascular system (decreases heart rate, cardiac contractility, and BP) and lungs (promotes bronchospasm). Ophthalmic use reduces intraocular pressure, probably by reducing aqueous production.

Uses
Hypertension.
OPHTHALMIC PREPARATION: Lowering intraocular pressure; ocular hypertension; chronic open-angle glaucoma.

➔← DRUG INTERACTIONS RELATED TO DENTAL THERAPEUTICS

COX-1 inhibitors: Decreased antihypertensive effect (prostaglandin synthesis inhibition)
- Monitor blood pressure.

Sympathomimetic amines: Decreased antihypertensive effect (pharmacological antagonism)
- Use local anesthetic agents containing a vasoconstrictor with caution.

ADVERSE EFFECTS

CNS: Insomnia; fatigue; dizziness; depression; lethargy; drowsiness; forgetfulness; headache.
CVS: Bradycardia; postural hypotension (rare).
GI: Nausea; vomiting; diarrhea; constipation.
RESP: Bronchospasm; dyspnea; wheezing.
MISC: Weight changes; fever; facial swelling; muscle weakness; leukopenia, thrombocytopenia (rare). Ophthalmic betaxolol may produce the same adverse drug reactions seen with systemic use; antinuclear antibodies may develop.

CLINICAL IMPLICATIONS

General
- Monitor vital signs (e.g., BP, pulse pressure, rate, and rhythm) at each appointment to assess disease control. Do not provide elective dental treatment when BP is ≥180/110 or in the presence of other high-risk CV conditions.

- Use local anesthetic agents with vasoconstrictor with caution based on functional capacity of the patient and use aspirating technique to prevent intravascular injection.
- Beta blockers may mask epinephrine-induced signs and symptoms of hypoglycemia in patients with diabetes.
- Determine ability to adapt to stress of dental treatment. Consider short appointments.

Oral Health Education

- Encourage daily plaque control procedures for effective self-care in patients at risk for cardiovascular disease.

---

bethanechol chloride (beth-AN-ih-kole KLOR-ide)

Duvoid, Myotonachol, Urecholine

▮✦▮ PMS-Bethanechol

Drug Class: Cholinergic stimulant; Urinary tract product

PHARMACOLOGY

Action

Stimulates parasympathetic nervous system, increasing tone to muscles of urinary bladder; stimulates gastric motility and tone and may restore rhythmic peristalsis.

Uses

Treatment of acute postoperative and postpartum nonobstructive urinary retention and neurogenic atony of the urinary bladder with retention.

Unlabeled Uses

Diagnosis and treatment of reflux esophagitis.

➡◀ DRUG INTERACTIONS RELATED TO DENTAL THERAPEUTICS

No documented drug-drug interactions. The absence of evidence is not evidence of safety.

ADVERSE EFFECTS

⚠ **ORAL:** Increased salivation.
CNS: Headache; malaise.
CVS: Orthostatic hypotension (high doses).
GI: Abdominal cramps or discomfort; colicky pain; nausea; belching; diarrhea; rumbling and gurgling of stomach.
RESP: Bronchial constriction; asthmatic attacks.

CLINICAL IMPLICATIONS

General

- If GI side effects occur, consider semisupine chair position.
- *Postural hypotension:* Monitor BP at the beginning and end of each appointment; anticipate syncope. Have patient sit upright for several min at the end of the dental appointment before dismissing.

Betimol — see timolol maleate

Betnesol — see betamethasone

Betoptic — see betaxolol HCl

Betoptic S — see betaxolol HCl

Biaxin — see clarithromycin

Biaxin BID — see clarithromycin

Biaxin XL — see clarithromycin

Bidhist — see brompheniramine

Bilem — see tamoxifen citrate

Binotal — see ampicillin
Biocef — see cephalexin
Biodine Topical — see povidone iodine

---

biperiden (by-PURR-ih-den)
Akineton
Drug Class: Antiparkinson; Anticholinergic

PHARMACOLOGY

Action
Biperiden is a weak peripheral anticholinergic agent and possesses nicotinolytic activity.

Uses
Treatment of all forms of parkinsonism; control of extrapyramidal disorders secary to neuroleptic drug therapy.

➡◀ DRUG INTERACTIONS RELATED TO DENTAL THERAPEUTICS
No documented drug-drug interactions. The absence of evidence is not evidence of safety.

ADVERSE EFFECTS
⚠ ORAL: Dry mouth.
CNS: Drowsiness; euphoria; disorientation; agitation; memory loss; disturbed behavior.
CVS: Orthostatic hypotension.
GI: Constipation; GI irritation.
MISC: Hyperthermia; heat stroke; photophobia.

CLINICAL IMPLICATIONS

General
- Extrapyramidal behaviors can complicate performance of oral procedures. If present, consult with MD to consider medication changes.
- Anticholinergics have strong xerostomic effects. Anticipate increased caries and candidiasis.
- *Postural hypotension:* Monitor BP at the beginning and end of each appointment; anticipate syncope. Have patient sit upright for several min at the end of the dental appointment before dismissing.
- *Photophobia:* Direct dental light out of patient's eyes and offer dark glasses for comfort.

Oral Health Education
- If chronic dry mouth occurs, recommend home fluoride therapy and use of nonalcoholic oral health care products.

Biquin Durules — see quinidine
Bismatrol — see bismuth subsalicylate
Bismatrol Extra Strength — see bismuth subsalicylate

---

bismuth subsalicylate (BISS-muth sub-suh-LIS-ih-late)
Bismatrol, Bismatrol Extra Strength, Pepto-Bismol, Pepto-Bismol Maximum Strength, Pink Bismuth
■✦■ Pink Bismuth
Drug Class: Antidiarrheal

PHARMACOLOGY

Action

Produces antisecretory and antimicrobial effects; may have anti-inflammatory effect.

Uses

Treatment of indigestion without causing constipation, nausea, abdominal cramps; control of diarrhea, including traveler's diarrhea.

Unlabeled Uses

Treatment of recurrent ulcers, chronic infantile diarrhea, gastroenteritis associated with Norwalk virus; prevention of traveler's diarrhea.

➤◀ DRUG INTERACTIONS RELATED TO DENTAL THERAPEUTICS

Tetracyclines: Decreased tetracycline effect (decreased absorption)
• Avoid concurrent use.

ADVERSE EFFECTS

⚠ **ORAL:** Chalky taste; gray discoloration of tongue.
GI: Discoloration of stools; impaction.

CLINICAL IMPLICATIONS

General

• Determine why drug is being taken. Consider implications of condition on dental treatment.

---

bisoprolol fumarate (bis-OH-proe-lol)

Zebeta, Ziac (with hydrochlorothiazide)

Drug Class: Selective beta₁-adrenergic blocking agent

PHARMACOLOGY

Action

Blocks beta$_1$-adrenergic receptors to lower BP without reflex tachycardia or significant reduction in heart rate, and with high doses, blocks beta$_1$-adrenergic receptors in bronchial and vascular smooth muscle.

Uses

Antihypertensive, beta blocker.

Unlabeled Uses

Stable angina pectoris, stable CHF.

➤◀ DRUG INTERACTIONS RELATED TO DENTAL THERAPEUTICS

COX-1 inhibitors: Decreased antihypertensive effect (decreased prostaglandin synthesis)
• Monitor blood pressure.
Sympathomimetic amines: Decreased antihypertensive effect (pharmacological antagonism)
• Monitor blood pressure.

ADVERSE EFFECTS

⚠ **ORAL:** Dry mouth; taste distortion; stomatitis.
CNS: Dizziness; vertigo; fatigue; change in behavior; altered consciousness; disorientation; ataxia.
CVS: Bradycardia; ventricular arrhythmias; postural hypotension; angina; presyncope; syncope; tachycardia; palpitation.
GI: GI pain; nausea; flatulence; indigestion.
RESP: Bronchospasm; dyspnea; cough.
MISC: Dry eyes; visual disturbance; arthralgia; myalgia.

CLINICAL IMPLICATIONS
General
- Monitor vital signs (e.g., BP, pulse pressure, rate and rhythm) at each appointment to assess disease control. Do not provide elective dental treatment when BP ≥180/110 or in presence of other high-risk CV conditions.
- Chronic dry mouth is possible; anticipate increased caries, candidiasis, and lichenoid mucositis.
- If GI side effects occur, consider semisupine chair position.
- Use local anesthetic agents with vasoconstrictor with caution based on functional capacity of the patient and use aspirating technique to prevent intravascular injection.
- Beta blockers may mask epinephrine-induced signs and symptoms of hypoglycemia in patient with diabetes.
- Determine ability to adapt to stress of dental treatment. Consider short appointments.
- Direct dental light out of patient's eyes and offer dark glasses for comfort.

Oral Health Education
- If chronic dry mouth occurs, recommend home fluoride therapy and use of nonalcoholic oral health care products.
- Encourage daily plaque control procedures for effective self-care in patient at risk for cardiovascular disease.

Bladuril — see flavoxate

Blocadren — see timolol maleate

Blocan — see cimetidine

Blokium — see atenolol

Bonamine — see meclizine

B & O Supprettes No. 15A Suppositories — see narcotic analgesic combinations

B & O Supprettes No. 16A Suppositories — see narcotic analgesic combinations

Braccoprial — see pyrazinamide

Braxan — see amiodarone

Breonesin — see guaifenesin

Brethaire — see terbutaline sulfate

Brethine — see terbutaline sulfate

Brexicam — see piroxicam

Bricanyl — see terbutaline sulfate

Bricanyl Turbuhaler — see terbutaline sulfate

Brispen — see dicloxacillin sodium

bromocriptine mesylate (BROE-moe-KRIP-teen MEH-sih-LATE)
Parlodel

■✦■ Apo-Bromocriptine, Parlodel, PMS-Bromocriptine

■✦■ Cryocriptina, Parlodel, Serocryptin

Drug Class: Antiparkinson

PHARMACOLOGY
Action
Stimulates dopamine receptors in the corpus striatum, relieving parkinsonian symptoms. Inhibits prolactin, which is responsible for lactation; lowers elevated blood levels of growth hormone in acromegaly.

Uses

Treatment of hyperprolactinemia-associated disorders (e.g., amenorrhea with or without galactorrhea, infertility, hypogonadism) in patients with prolactin-secreting adenomas; therapy for female infertility associated with hyperprolactinemia; treatment of acromegaly; therapy for Parkinson disease (idiopathic or postencephalitic).

Unlabeled Uses

Treatment of hyperprolactinemia associated with pituitary adenomas; therapy for neuroleptic malignant syndrome; treatment of cocaine addiction.

➡◆ DRUG INTERACTIONS RELATED TO DENTAL THERAPEUTICS

Sympathomimetic amines: Cardiac arrhythmias (mechanism unknown)
- Use local anesthetic agents containing a vasoconstrictor with caution.

ADVERSE EFFECTS

⚠ **ORAL:** Dry mouth (high doses).

CNS: Headache; dizziness; fatigue; lightheadedness; fainting; drowsiness; psychosis; seizures; abnormal involuntary movements; hallucinations; confusion; dyskinesia, ataxia; insomnia; depression; vertigo; "on-off" phenomenon.

CVS: Orthostatic hypotension.

GI: Nausea; vomiting; abdominal cramps; constipation; diarrhea; anorexia; indigestion/dyspepsia; GI bleeding.

RESP: Shortness of breath; pulmonary infiltrates; pleural effusion; pleural thickening.

MISC: Exacerbation of Raynaud syndrome; asthenia.

CLINICAL IMPLICATIONS

General

- Determine why drug is being taken. Consider implications of condition on dental treatment.
- *Postural hypotension:* Monitor BP at the beginning and end of each appointment; anticipate syncope. Have patient sit upright for several min at the end of the dental appointment before dismissing.
- If GI side effects occur, consider semisupine chair position.
- Extrapyramidal behaviors can complicate performance of oral procedures. If present, consult with MD to consider medication changes.
- Chronic dry mouth is possible; anticipate increased caries and candidiasis.

Oral Health Education

- If chronic dry mouth occurs, recommend home fluoride therapy and use of nonalcoholic oral health care products.

---

brompheniramine (brome-fen-AIR-uh-meen)

Bidhist, BroveX, BroveX CT, Lodrane 24, Lodrane XR, LoHist 12, VaZol

Drug Class: Antihistamine

PHARMACOLOGY

Action

Competitively antagonizes histamine at H_1 receptor sites.

Uses

Relief of sneezing, itchy, watery eyes, itchy nose or throat, and runny nose because of hay fever (allergic rhinitis) or other respiratory allergies. VaZol is also indicated for temporary relief of runny nose and sneezing caused by the common cold; treatment of allergic and nonallergic pruritic symptoms; temporary relief of mild, uncomplicated urticaria and angioedema; amelioration of allergic reactions to blood or plasma loss; adjunctive therapy of anaphylactic reactions.

➡⬅ DRUG INTERACTIONS RELATED TO DENTAL THERAPEUTICS

No documented drug-drug interactions. The absence of evidence is not evidence of safety.

ADVERSE EFFECTS

⚠ **ORAL:** Dry mouth, nose and throat.

CVS: Hypotension; palpitations; tachycardia; extrasystoles.

CNS: Drowsiness; headache; sedation; sleepiness; dizziness; disturbed coordination; fatigue; confusion; restlessness; excitation; nervousness; tremor; irritability; insomnia; euphoria; paresthesia; vertigo; hysteria; neuritis; convulsions.

GI: Epigastric distress; anorexia; nausea; vomiting; diarrhea; constipation.

RESP: Thickening of bronchial secretions; tightness of chest and wheezing.

MISC: Anaphylactic shock; photosensitivity; excessive perspiration; chills.

CLINICAL IMPLICATIONS

General

- Determine why drug is being taken. Consider implications of condition on dental treatment.
- Additional photosensitization is possible if tetracyclines are prescribed by DDS.
- Chronic dry mouth is possible; anticipate increased caries and candidiasis.
- Consider semisupine chair position to control effects of postnasal drainage.
- Be aware that patients with multiple allergies are at increased risk for allergy to dental drugs.
- Monitor vital signs.
- If GI side effects occur, consider semisupine chair position.

Oral Health Education

- If chronic dry mouth occurs, recommend home fluoride therapy and use of nonalcoholic oral health care products.

Bronkodyl — see theophylline

BroveX — see brompheniramine

BroveX CT — see brompheniramine

---

budesonide (byoo-DESS-oh-nide)

Entocort EC, Pulmicort Respules, Pulmicort Turbuhaler, Rhinocort Aqua

▮✚▮ **Entocort Capsules, Entocort Enema, Gen-Budesonide AQ, Pulmicort Nebuamp, Rhinocort Turbuhaler**

Drug Class: Corticosteroid

PHARMACOLOGY

Action

Exhibits wide range of inhibitory activities against multiple cell types and mediators involved in allergic-mediated inflammation.

Uses

INTRANASAL: Management of seasonal and perennial allergic rhinitis symptoms in adults and children (Rhinocort Aqua).

ORAL INHALATION: For the maintenance treatment of asthma as prophylactic therapy in adults and children and for patients requiring oral corticosteroid therapy for asthma (inhaler).

INHALATION SUSPENSION: Maintenance treatment of asthma and prophylactic therapy in children 12 mo to 8 yr of age.

ORAL CAPSULE: Crohn disease.

➤← DRUG INTERACTIONS RELATED TO DENTAL THERAPEUTICS

Ketoconazole or itraconazole: Possible budesonide toxicity (decreased metabolism)
- Avoid concurrent use.

Metronidazole: Decreased metronidazole effect (increased metabolism)
- Avoid concurrent use.

COX-1 inhibitors: Increased risk of peptic ulcer disease (additive)
- Avoid concurrent use.

ADVERSE EFFECTS

⚠ **ORAL:** ORAL INHALATION: Dry mouth; tongue edema; tooth disorder (unspecified). ORAL CAPSULE: Impaired wound healing; oral candidiasis.

CNS: ORAL CAPSULE: Headache; dizziness; fatigue; hyperkinesis; paresthesia; tremor; agitation; increased appetite; confusion; insomnia; nervousness; sleep disorder; somnolence.

GI: ORAL CAPSULE: Indigestion; nausea; dyspepsia; abdominal pain; flatulence; vomiting; enteritis; epigastric pain; intestinal obstruction.

RESP: ORAL INHALATION: Increased cough; respiratory tract infection; bronchitis; dyspnea.

MISC: ORAL CAPSULE: Symptoms of hypercorticism; back pain; pain; asthenia; chest pain; dependent edema; face edema; flu-like symptoms; malaise; aggravated arthritis; cramps; myalgia; moniliasis; flushing.

CLINICAL IMPLICATIONS

General
- Determine why drug is being taken. Consider implications of condition on dental treatment.
- Acute bronchoconstriction can occur during dental treatment; have bronchodilator inhaler available.
- Ensure that bronchodilator inhaler is present at each dental appointment.
- Be aware that sulfites in a local anesthetic with vasoconstrictor can precipitate acute asthma attack in susceptible individuals.
- Inhalants can dry oral mucosa; anticipate candidiasis, increased calculus and plaque levels, and increased caries.
- Because of the anticipated perioperative physiological stress, patients undergoing dental care (i.e., minor surgical stress) under local anesthesia should take only their usual daily glucocorticoid dose before dental intervention. No supplementation is justified.

Oral Health Education
- Rinse mouth with water after bronchodilator use to prevent dryness.

Bumedyl — see bumetanide

---

bumetanide (BYOO-MET-uh-nide)

Bumex

■✦■ **Burinex**

■▨■ **Bumedyl, Drenural, Miccil**

Drug Class: Loop diuretic

PHARMACOLOGY

Action
Inhibits reabsorption of sodium and chloride in proximal tubules and loop of Henle.

Uses
Treatment of edema associated with CHF, cirrhosis, and renal disease.

Unlabeled Uses
Relief of adult nocturia.

➟◆ DRUG INTERACTIONS RELATED TO DENTAL THERAPEUTICS

COX-1 inhibitors: Decreased antihypertensive effect (inhibition of prostaglandin synthesis)
* Monitor blood pressure.

ADVERSE EFFECTS
⚠ **ORAL:** Dry mouth; increased thirst.
CNS: Asterixis; encephalopathy with preexisting liver disease; vertigo; headache; dizziness.
CVS: Postural hypotension; irregular heartbeat (hypokalemia).
GI: Upset stomach; nausea; vomiting; diarrhea; pain.
RESP: Hyperventilation.
MISC: Musculoskeletal weakness; arthritic pain; pain; muscle cramps; fatigue; dehydration; sweating.

CLINICAL IMPLICATIONS
General
* Determine why drug is being taken. Consider implications of condition on dental treatment.
* Monitor vital signs (e.g., BP, pulse pressure, rate, and rhythm) at each appointment to assess disease control. Do not provide elective dental treatment when BP is ≥180/110 or in the presence of other high-risk CV conditions. Refer to the section entitled "The Patient Taking Cardiovascular Drugs" in Chapter 6: *Clinical Medicine*.
* Use local anesthetic agents with vasoconstrictor with caution based on functional capacity of the patient and use aspirating technique to prevent intravascular injection.
* Monitor pulse rhythm to assess for electrolyte imbalance.
* Chronic dry mouth is possible; anticipate increased caries, candidiasis, and lichenoid mucositis.
* Determine ability to adapt to stress of dental treatment. Consider short appointments.
* *Postural hypotension:* Monitor BP at the beginning and end of each appointment; anticipate syncope. Have patient sit upright for several min at the end of the dental appointment before dismissing.

Oral Health Education
* If chronic dry mouth occurs, recommend home fluoride therapy and use of nonalcoholic oral health care products.
* Encourage daily plaque control procedures for effective self-care in patients at risk for cardiovascular disease.

Bumex — see bumetanide

---

 bupivacaine (byoo-PIH-vah-cane)

Bupivacaine HCl: Injection: bupivacaine 0.25%, 0.5%, 0.75%
Bupivacaine HCl with Epinephrine 1:200,000: Injection: bupivacaine 0.25%, 0.5%, 0.75% with 1:200,000 epinephrine
Bupivacaine Spinal: Injection: bupivacaine 0.75% in 8/25% dextrose
Marcaine: Injection: bupivacaine 0.25%, 0.5%, 0.75%, bupivacaine 0.25%, 0.5%, 0.75% with 1:200,000 epinephrine
Sensorcaine: Injection: bupivacaine 0.25%, 0.5%, 0.75%, bupivacaine 0.25%, 0.5% with 1:200,000 epinephrine
Sensorcaine MPF: Injection: bupivacaine 0.25%, 0.5%, 0.75%, bupivacaine 0.25%, 0.5% with 1:200,000 epinephrine
Sensorcaine-MPF Spinal: Injection: bupivacaine 0.75% in 8/25% dextrose

▮▮ Buvacaina

Drug Class: Injectable local anesthetic, amide

PHARMACOLOGY

Action

Inhibits ion fluxes across membranes to block nerve action potential.

Uses

LOCAL INFILTRATION AND SYMPATHETIC BLOCK: 0.25% solution.
LUMBAR EPIDURAL: 0.25%, 0.5%, and 0.75% solutions (0.75% nonobstetrical).
SUBARACHNOID BLOCK: 0.75% solution in 8.25% dextrose.
CAUDAL BLOCK: 0.25% and 0.5% solutions.
PERIPHERAL NERVE BLOCK: 0.25% and 0.5% solutions.
RETROBULBAR BLOCK: 0.75% solution.
DENTAL BLOCK AND EPIDURAL TEST DOSE: 0.5% solution with epinephrine.

Contraindications

Hypersensitivity to local anesthetics or any components of the products, para-aminobenzoic acid (esters only) or parabens; spinal and caudal anesthesia in septicemia; existing neurological disease; spinal deformities; and severe hypertension, hemorrhage, shock, or heart block. Obstetrical paracervical block anesthesia (such use has resulted in fetal bradycardia and death); IV regional anesthesia (Bier block; cardiac arrest and death have occurred).

Usual Dosage

Intraoperative local anesthesia for dental procedures
INJECTION, 0.5% WITH EPINEPHRINE 1:200,000
ADULTS: For infiltration and block injection in the maxillary and mandibular areas when a longer duration of local anesthetic action is desired, such as for oral surgical procedures generally associated with significant postoperative pain, an average dose of 1.8 mL (9 mg) per injection site usually will suffice; an occasional sec dose of 1.8 mL (9 mg) may be used if necessary to produce adequate anesthesia after making allowance for a 2- to 10-min onset time. The total dose for all injection sites spread out over a single dental sitting usually should not exceed 90 mg for a healthy adult patient (ten 1.8-mL injections). Inject slowly and with frequent aspirations.
CHILDREN: Because of lack of clinical experience, the administration of bupivacaine to children younger than 12 yr of age and bupivacaine 0.75% in dextrose to children younger than 18 yr of age is not recommended.

Pharmacokinetics

METAB: Liver.
EXCRET: Kidney (metabolites).
ONSET: 5 min.
DURATION: 2 to 4 hr.
SPECIAL POP: *Elderly:* Repeated doses may cause accumulation of the drug or its metabolites or slow metabolic degradation; give reduced doses.
Hepatic failure: Because amide-type local anesthetics are metabolized primarily in the liver and ester-type local anesthetics are hydrolyzed by plasma cholinesterase produced by the liver, patients with hepatic disease, especially severe hepatic disease, may be more susceptible to potential toxicity. Use cautiously in such patients.

➕ DRUG INTERACTIONS

Intercurrent use: Mixtures of local anesthetics are sometimes employed to compensate for the slower onset of one drug and the shorter duration of action of the sec drug. Toxicity is probably additive with mixtures of local anesthetics, but some experiments suggest synergisms. Exercise caution regarding toxic equivalence when mixtures of local anesthetics are employed. Some preparations contain vasoconstrictors. Keep this in mind when using concurrently with other drugs that may interact with vasoconstrictors

Sedatives: If employed to reduce patient apprehension during dental procedures, use reduced doses, since local anesthetics used in combination with CNS depressants may have additive effects. Give young children minimal doses of each agent.

Captopril: Possible increased risk of hypotension and bradycardia (mechanism unknown)
- Monitor clinical status.

Itraconazole: Possible bupivacaine toxicity (decreased metabolism)
- Monitor clinical status.

Cimetidine and ranitidine: Possible bupivacaine toxicity (decreased metabolism)
- Monitor clinical status.

Lidocaine: Possible lidocaine toxicity (displacement from binding site)
- Avoid concurrent use.

Mepivacaine: Possible mepivacaine toxicity (displacement from binding site)
- Avoid concurrent use.

Narcotics, morphine-like: Possible respiratory depression (mechanism unknown)
- Monitor clinical status.

ADVERSE EFFECTS

⚠ **ORAL:** Trismus; tingling.
CNS: Convulsions, loss of consciousness (overdose).
CVS: Myocardial depression; cardiac arrest; dysrhythmias; bradycardia.
RESP: Status asthmaticus, respiratory arrest, anaphylaxis (allergy).
MISC: Discoloration at injection site; tissue necrosis.

CLINICAL IMPLICATIONS

General

- *Lactation:* Safety for use during lactation has not been established. Bupivacaine has been reported to be excreted in breast milk. However, it is not known whether local anesthetic drugs are excreted in breast milk.
- Use the lowest dosage that results in effective anesthesia to avoid high plasma levels and serious adverse effects. Inject slowly, with frequent aspirations before and during the injection, to avoid intravascular injection. Perform syringe aspirations before and during each supplemental injection in continuous (intermittent) catheter techniques. During the administration of epidural anesthesia, it is recommended that a test dose be administered initially and that the patient be monitored for CNS toxicity and cardiovascular toxicity, as well as for signs of unintended intrathecal administration, before proceeding.
- *Inflammation or sepsis:* Use local anesthetic procedures with caution when there is inflammation or sepsis in the region of proposed injection.
- *CNS toxicity:* Monitor cardiovascular and respiratory vital signs and state of consciousness after each injection. Restlessness, anxiety, incoherent speech, lightheadedness, numbness, and tingling of the mouth and lips, metallic taste, tinnitus, dizziness, blurred vision, tremors, twitching, depression, or drowsiness may be early signs of CNS toxicity.
- *Malignant hyperthermia:* Many drugs used during anesthesia are considered potential triggering agents for familial malignant hyperthermia. It is not known whether local anesthetics may trigger this reaction and the need for supplemental general anesthesia cannot be predicted in advance; therefore, have a standard protocol for management available.
- *Vasoconstrictors:* Use solutions containing a vasoconstrictor with caution and in carefully circumscribed quantities in areas of the body supplied by end arteries or having otherwise compromised blood supply (e.g., digits, nose, external ear, penis). Use with extreme caution in patients whose medical history and physical evaluation suggest the existence of hypertension, peripheral vascular disease, arteriosclerotic heart disease, cerebral vascular insufficiency, or heart block; these individuals may exhibit exaggerated vasoconstrictor response. Serious dose-related cardiac arrhythmias may occur if preparations containing a vasoconstrictor such as epinephrine are employed in patients during or following the administration of potent inhalation agents.

Pregnancy Risk Category: Category C.

Oral Health Education

- Advise the patient to exert caution to avoid inadvertent trauma to the lips, tongue, cheek, mucosae, or soft palate when these structures are anesthetized. The ingestion of food should therefore be postponed until normal function returns.
- Advise the patient to consult the dentist if anesthesia persists or a rash develops.

Bupivacaine HCl — see bupivacaine
Bupivacaine HCl with Epinephrine 1:200,000 — see bupivacaine
Bupivacaine Spinal — see bupivacaine
Buprenex — see buprenorphine HCl

---

buprenorphine HCl (BYOO-preh-NAHR-feen HIGH-droe-KLOR-ide)
Buprenex, Subutex

■✛■ **Temgesic**

Drug Class: Narcotic agonist-antagonist analgesic
DEA Schedule: Schedule III

PHARMACOLOGY

Action
Analgesic effect caused by binding to opiate receptors in the CNS. Antagonist effects decrease abuse potential.

Uses
TABLET: Treatment of opioid dependence.
INJECTION: Relief of moderate to severe pain.

➥✛ DRUG INTERACTIONS RELATED TO DENTAL THERAPEUTICS

Benzodiazepines: Increased CNS depression (additive)
- Avoid concurrent use.

ADVERSE EFFECTS

⚠ **ORAL:** Dry mouth.
CNS: Sedation; dizziness/vertigo; headache; confusion; dreaming; psychosis; euphoria; weakness/fatigue; malaise; hallucinations; depersonalization; coma; tremor; dysphoria; agitation; convulsions; lack of muscle coordination; insomnia.
GI: Nausea; vomiting; constipation; dyspepsia; flatulence; loss of appetite; diarrhea; abdominal pain.
RESP: Hypoventilation.
MISC: Chronic and acute hypersensitivity; infection.

CLINICAL IMPLICATIONS

General
- Determine why drug is being taken. Consider implications of condition on dental treatment.
- If oral pain requires additional analgesics, consider nonopioid products.
- Chronic dry mouth is possible; anticipate candidiasis.

Oral Health Education
- If chronic dry mouth occurs, recommend home fluoride therapy and use of nonalcoholic oral health care products.

buprenorphine HCl/naloxone HCl (BYOO-preh-NAHR-feen HIGH-droe-KLOR-ide/NAL-ox-ohn HIGH-droe-KLOR-ide)

Synonym: naloxone HCl/buprenorphine HCl

Suboxone

Drug Class: Narcotic agonist-antagonist analgesic

PHARMACOLOGY

Action

BUPRENORPHINE: Analgesic effect caused by binding to opiate receptors in the CNS, while antagonist effects decrease abuse potential.

NALOXONE: Possibly antagonizes opioid effects by competing for the same receptor sites.

Uses

Treatment of opioid dependence.

➡◀ DRUG INTERACTIONS RELATED TO DENTAL THERAPEUTICS

Benzodiazepines: Increased CNS depression (additive)
- Avoid concurrent use.

ADVERSE EFFECTS

⚠ **ORAL:** Dry mouth (<1%).

CNS: Headache; insomnia; anxiety; depression; dizziness; nervousness; somnolence.

CVS: Hypotension (1% to 5%).

GI: Abdominal pain; constipation; diarrhea; nausea; vomiting; dyspepsia.

RESP: Increased cough.

MISC: Pain; back pain; withdrawal symptoms; abscess; asthenia; chills; fever; flu-like syndrome; infection; accidental injury.

CLINICAL IMPLICATIONS

General

- Determine why drug is being taken. Consider implications of condition on dental treatment.
- Avoid prescribing opioids for dental pain. Acetaminophen is appropriate if GI bleeding is present.
- Monitor vital signs.
- Chronic dry mouth is possible; anticipate increased caries and candidiasis.
- Be aware that substance abusers are at increased risk for blood-borne diseases.

Oral Health Education

- If chronic dry mouth occurs, recommend home fluoride therapy and use of nonalcoholic oral health care products.

---

bupropion HCl (byoo-PRO-pee-ahn HIGH-droe-KLOR-ide)

Wellbutrin, Wellbutrin SR, Wellbutrin XL, Zyban

Drug Class: Antidepressant; Smoking deterrent

PHARMACOLOGY

Action

Exact mechanism of antidepressant activity or as a smoking deterrent unknown; does not inhibit MAOs.

Uses

Treatment of depression; aid to smoking cessation treatment.

➜← DRUG INTERACTIONS RELATED TO DENTAL THERAPEUTICS

Corticosteroids: Increased risk of seizures with systemic corticosteroids (additive)
 • Monitor clinical status.

ADVERSE EFFECTS

⚠ **ORAL:** Dry mouth (24%); taste perversion (4%).

CNS: Headache (26%); insomnia (16%); dizziness (11%); agitation (9%); confusion (8%); anxiety, tremor, hostility (6%); nervousness (5%); impaired sleep quality, sensory disturbances (4%); somnolence, irritability, decreased memory, decreased libido (3%); paresthesia, CNS stimulation (2%).

GI: Nausea (18%); constipation (10%); diarrhea (7%); anorexia (5%); increased appetite, dyspepsia, gustatory disturbance (3%); dysphagia (2%); vomiting.

RESP: Sinusitis (3%); increased cough (2%).

MISC: Infection, abdominal pain (9%); asthenia, chest pain (4%); fever (2%).

CLINICAL IMPLICATIONS

General

 • Determine why drug is being taken. Consider implications of condition on dental treatment.
 • Depressed or anxious patients may neglect self-care. Monitor for plaque control effectiveness.
 • Determine ability to adapt to stress of dental treatment. Consider short appointments.
 • Chronic dry mouth is possible; anticipate increased caries and candidiasis.
 • If GI side effects occur, consider semisupine chair position.

Oral Health Education

 • If chronic dry mouth occurs, recommend home fluoride therapy and use of nonalcoholic oral health care products.

Burinex — see bumetanide

Burn-o-Jel — see lidocaine HCl

BuSpar — see buspirone HCl

---

buspirone HCl (byoo-SPY-rone HIGH-droe-KLOR-ide)

BuSpar

■✦■ **Apo-Buspirone, Gen-Buspirone, Lin-Buspirone, Novo-Buspirone, Nu-Buspirone, PMS-Buspirone, ratio-Buspirone**

■✦■ **Neurosine**

Drug Class: Antianxiety

PHARMACOLOGY

Action

Mechanism unknown; does not exert anticonvulsant or muscle relaxant effects.

Uses

Treatment of anxiety disorders; short-term relief of anxiety symptoms.

Unlabeled Uses

Reduction of symptoms of premenstrual syndrome.

➜← DRUG INTERACTIONS RELATED TO DENTAL THERAPEUTICS

Itraconazole: Possible buspirone toxicity (decreased metabolism)
 • Avoid concurrent use.

ADVERSE EFFECTS

⚠ **ORAL:** Dry mouth.

CNS: Dizziness (12%); drowsiness (10%); headache (6%); nervousness (5%); lightheadedness (3%); excitement, numbness, anger/hostility, confusion, weakness (2%); paresthesia, incoordination, tremor (1%); dream disturbances (≥1%); cogwheel rigidity; dizziness; dystonic reactions; ataxia; extrapyramidal effects; dyskinesias (acute and tardive); emotional lability; serotonin syndrome; difficulty in recall.

GI: Nausea (8%); diarrhea (2%).

MISC: Allergic reactions (including urticaria); angioedema.

CLINICAL IMPLICATIONS

General

- Determine why drug is being taken. Consider implications of condition on dental treatment.
- Extrapyramidal behaviors can complicate performance of oral procedures. If present, consult with MD to consider medication changes.
- Chronic dry mouth is possible; anticipate increased caries and candidiasis.
- If GI side effects occur, consider semisupine chair position.

Oral Health Education

- If chronic dry mouth occurs, recommend home fluoride therapy and use of nonalcoholic oral health care products.

Buvacaina — see bupivacaine

Byclomine — see dicyclomine HCl

Calan — see verapamil HCl

Calan SR — see verapamil HCl

Calcijex — see calcitriol

Calcimar — see calcitonin-salmon

---

calcitonin-salmon (kal-sih-TOE-nin-SAM-un)

Calcimar, Fortical, Miacalcin, Osteocalcin, Salmonine

■✦■ **Caltine, Miacalcin NS**

■✦■ **Miacalcic, Oseum, Tonocalcin**

Drug Class: Hormone

PHARMACOLOGY

Action

Decreases rate of bone turnover, presumably by regulating bone metabolism (blocking bone resorption). In conjunction with parathyroid hormone, endogenous calcitonin regulates serum calcium.

Uses

Treatment of moderate to severe Paget disease, postmenopausal osteoporosis, hypercalcemia. Nasal spray for treatment of symptomatic Paget disease.

➡◀ DRUG INTERACTIONS RELATED TO DENTAL THERAPEUTICS

No documented drug-drug interactions. The absence of evidence is not evidence of safety.

ADVERSE EFFECTS

⚠ **ORAL:** Salty taste, dry mouth.

GI: Nausea with or without vomiting (decreases with continued administration); anorexia; diarrhea; epigastric discomfort; abdominal pain.

RESP: Rhinitis (12%); nasal bleeding (intranasal spray).

CVS: Hypertension; tachycardia.

MISC: Feverish sensation; back and joint pain.

CLINICAL IMPLICATIONS

General

- Determine why drug is being taken. Consider implications of condition on dental treatment.
- Patient may be high-risk candidate for pathological fractures or jaw fractures during extractions.
- If GI side effects occur, consider semisupine chair position.
- Monitor vital signs.

---

calcitriol (kal-si-TRYE-ole)

Calcijex, Calcitriol Injection, Rocaltrol

■◆■ Tirocal

Drug Class: Fat-soluble vitamin D

PHARMACOLOGY

Action

Supply of vitamin D depends mainly on exposure to ultraviolet rays of the sun for conversion of 7-dehydrocholesterol in the skin to vitamin D_3 (cholecalciferol). Vitamin D_3 is activated in the liver and kidney before becoming fully active as a regulator of calcium and phosphorus metabolism at target tissues.

Uses

ORAL: Dialysis, predialysis, hypoparathyroidism.

IV: Dialysis.

Unlabeled Uses

Decreased severity of psoriatic lesions with an initial oral dose of 0.25 mcg bid and topically 0.1 to 0.5 mcg/g petrolatum.

➡◀ DRUG INTERACTIONS RELATED TO DENTAL THERAPEUTICS

No documented drug-drug interactions. The absence of evidence is not evidence of safety.

ADVERSE EFFECTS

⚠ **ORAL:** Dry mouth; metallic taste.

GI: Nausea; vomiting; constipation.

CNS: Weakness; headache; somnolence.

CVS: Arrhythmia; hypertension.

MISC: Muscle pain; bone pain; photophobia.

CLINICAL IMPLICATIONS

General

- Determine why drug is being taken. Consider implications of condition on dental treatment.

- Chronic dry mouth is possible; anticipate increased caries and candidiasis.
- If GI side effects occur, consider semisupine chair position.
- Monitor vital signs.
- *Photophobia:* Direct dental light out of patient's eyes and offer dark glasses for comfort.

Oral Health Education

- If chronic dry mouth occurs, recommend home fluoride therapy and use of nonalcoholic oral health care products.

Calcitriol Injection — see calcitriol
Caldecort Hydrocortisone Anti-Itch — see hydrocortisone
Calm-X — see dimenhydrinate
Caltine — see calcitonin-salmon

---

candesartan cilexetil (kan-deh-SAHR-tan sigh-LEX-eh-till)

Atacand

Drug Class: Angiotensin II antagonist; Antihypertensive

PHARMACOLOGY

Action

Antagonizes the angiotensin II effect (vasoconstriction and aldosterone secretion) by blocking the angiotensin II receptor (AT$_1$ receptor) in vascular smooth muscle and the adrenal gland, producing decreased BP.

Uses

Treatment of hypertension.

➡◀ DRUG INTERACTIONS RELATED TO DENTAL THERAPEUTICS

No documented drug-drug interactions. The absence of evidence is not evidence of safety.

ADVERSE EFFECTS

CNS: Headache; dizziness; fatigue.
CVS: Tachycardia; palpitations.
GI: Nausea; abdominal pain; diarrhea; vomiting.
RESP: URI; bronchitis; cough.
MISC: Back pain; chest pain; edema; arthralgia; albuminuria.

CLINICAL IMPLICATIONS

General

- Monitor vital signs (e.g., BP, pulse pressure, rate, and rhythm) at each appointment to assess disease control. Do not provide elective dental treatment when BP is ≥180/110 or in the presence of other high-risk CV conditions. Refer to the section entitled "The Patient Taking Cardiovascular Drugs" in Chapter 6: *Clinical Medicine.*
- Use local anesthetic agents with vasoconstrictor with caution based on functional capacity of the patient and use aspirating technique to prevent intravascular injection.
- If coughing is problematic, consider semisupine chair position for treatment.
- Determine ability to adapt to stress of dental treatment. Consider short appointments.

Oral Health Education

- Encourage daily plaque control procedures for effective self-care in patients at risk for cardiovascular disease.

Candimon — see clotrimazole
Candistatin — see nystatin
Canef — see fluvastatin

Canesten — see clotrimazole

capecitabine (cap-eh-SITE-ah-bean)
Xeloda
Drug Class: Antimetabolite; Pyrimidine

PHARMACOLOGY
Action
Capecitabine is an oral systemic prodrug that is enzymatically converted to 5-fluorouracil (5-FU). Healthy and tumor cells metabolize 5-FU to 5-fluoro-2-deoxyuridine monophosphate (FdUMP) and 5-fluorouridine triphosphate (FUTP). These metabolites cause cell injury by two different mechanisms. First, they inhibit the formation of thymidine triphosphate, which is essential for the synthesis of DNA. Second, nuclear transcriptional enzymes can mistakenly incorporate FUTP during the synthesis of RNA. This metabolic error can interfere with RNA processing and protein synthesis.

Uses
Treatment of resistant metastatic breast cancer used alone or in combination with docetaxel; treatment of colorectal cancer.

➡◆ DRUG INTERACTIONS RELATED TO DENTAL THERAPEUTICS
Metronidazole: Metronidazole toxicity (decreased metabolism)
- Avoid concurrent use.

ADVERSE EFFECTS
⚠ **ORAL:** Taste disturbances (6%); oral discomfort (unspecified) (10%); stomatitis (25%); candidiasis.

CNS: Paresthesia (21%); peripheral sensory neuropathy, headache (10%); dizziness (8%); insomnia (7%); mood alteration, depression (5%).

CVS: Edema.

GI: Diarrhea (55%); nausea (43%); abdominal pain (35%); vomiting (27%); decreased appetite (26%); constipation (14%); GI motility disorder, upper GI inflammatory disorders, dyspepsia (8%); GI hemorrhage, ileus (6%).

RESP: Dyspnea (14%); cough (7%); epistaxis (3%).

MISC: Fatigue/weakness (42%); pyrexia (18%); edema (15%); pain (12%); back pain (10%); myalgia (9%); arthralgia (8%); chest pain, pain in limb (6%); viral infections (5%); anemia (72%); neutropenia (26%); lymphopenia (94%).

CLINICAL IMPLICATIONS
General
- Determine why drug is being taken. Consider implications of condition on dental treatment.
- Advise products for palliative relief of oral manifestations (e.g., stomatitis, mucositis, xerostomia).
- Consider medical consult to determine disease control and influence on dental treatment.
- Blood dyscrasias reported; anticipate increased bleeding, infection, and poor healing.
- Anticipate oral candidiasis and need for antifungal therapy.
- If GI side effects occur, consider semisupine chair position.

Oral Health Education
- Encourage daily plaque control procedures for effective self-care, recommending soft-bristle toothbrushes.

Capital w/Codeine — see acetaminophen/codeine phosphate
Capitral — see captopril

Capoten — see captopril
Capotena — see captopril

capsaicin (kap-SAY-uh-sin)

Capsin, Capzasin P, Dolorac, No Pain-HP, Pain Doctor, Pain-X, R-Gel, Zostrix, Zostrix-HP

■✤■ **Antiphlogistine Rub A-535 Capsaicin, Capsaicin HP**

Drug Class: Analgesic, topical

PHARMACOLOGY

Action
May deplete and prevent reaccumulation of substance P, principal transmitter of pain impulses, from periphery to CNS.

Uses
Temporary relief of pain from rheumatoid arthritis and osteoarthritis; relief of neuralgias (e.g., pain after shingles, diabetic neuropathy).

Unlabeled Uses
Temporary relief of pain of psoriasis, vitiligo, intractable pruritus, postmastectomy and postamputation neuroma (phantom limb syndrome), vulvar vestibulitis, apocrine chromidrosis, reflex sympathetic dystrophy.

➜← DRUG INTERACTIONS RELATED TO DENTAL THERAPEUTICS
No documented drug-drug interactions. The absence of evidence is not evidence of safety.

ADVERSE EFFECTS
RESP: Cough; respiratory irritation.
MISC: Local burning at application site.

CLINICAL IMPLICATIONS

General
- Determine why drug is being taken. Consider implications of condition on dental treatment.

Capsaicin HP — see capsaicin
Capsin — see capsaicin

captopril (KAP-toe-prill)

Capoten

■✤■ **APO-Capto, Gen-Captopril, Novo-Captoril, Nu-Capto, PMS-Captopril, ratio-Captopril**

■✤■ **Capitral, Capotena, Captral, Cardipril, Cryopril, Ecapresan, Ecaten, Kenolan, Lenpryl, Precaptil, Romir**

Drug Class: Antihypertensive; ACE inhibitor

PHARMACOLOGY

Action
Competitively inhibits angiotensin I–converting enzyme, preventing conversion of angiotensin I to angiotensin II, a potent vasoconstrictor that also stimulates aldosterone secretion. Results in decreased BP, potassium retention, and reduced sodium reabsorption.

Uses

Treatment of hypertension, CHF, left ventricular dysfunction after MI, diabetic nephropathy.

Unlabeled Uses

Treatment of hypertensive crisis, neonatal and childhood hypertension, rheumatoid arthritis, diagnosis of anatomic renal artery stenosis and primary aldosteronism, treatment of hypertension related to scleroderma renal crisis and Takayasu disease, idiopathic edema, Bartter and Raynaud syndromes, asymptomatic left ventricular dysfunction after MI.

✦◆ DRUG INTERACTIONS RELATED TO DENTAL THERAPEUTICS

Bupivacaine: Possible increased risk of hypotension and bradycardia (mechanism unknown)
- Avoid concurrent use.

COX-1 inhibitors: Decreased antihypertensive effect (decreased prostaglandin synthesis)
- Monitor blood pressure.

ADVERSE EFFECTS

⚠ **ORAL:** Taste disturbance; aphthous ulcers; dry mouth; angioedema, oral infection associated with agranulocytosis (rare).

CNS: Headache; sleep disturbances; paresthesias; dizziness; fatigue; malaise; ataxia; confusion; depression; nervousness.

CVS: Hypotension; tachycardia; palpitation; orthostatic hypotension.

GI: Nausea; abdominal pain; vomiting; gastric irritation; peptic ulcer; jaundice; cholestasis; diarrhea; anorexia; constipation.

RESP: Chronic dry cough; dyspnea; eosinophilic pneumonitis.

MISC: Gynecomastia; myasthenia; photosensitivity; neutropenia, agranulocytosis (rare).

CLINICAL IMPLICATIONS

General

- Monitor vital signs (e.g., BP, pulse pressure, rate, and rhythm) at each appointment to assess disease control. Do not provide elective dental treatment when BP is ≥180/110 or in the presence of other high-risk CV conditions. Refer to the section entitled "The Patient Taking Cardiovascular Drugs" in Chapter 6: *Clinical Medicine.*
- Use local anesthetic agents with vasoconstrictor with caution based on functional capacity of the patient and use aspirating technique to prevent intravascular injection.
- If coughing is problematic, consider semisupine chair position for treatment.
- Susceptible patients with DM may experience severe recurrent hypoglycemia.
- *Postural hypotension:* Monitor BP at the beginning and end of each appointment; anticipate syncope. Have patient sit upright for several min at the end of the dental appointment before dismissing.
- Determine ability to adapt to stress of dental treatment. Consider short appointments.
- Chronic dry mouth is possible; anticipate increased caries, candidiasis, and lichenoid mucositis.
- If GI side effects occur, consider semisupine chair position.

Oral Health Education

- If chronic dry mouth occurs, recommend home fluoride therapy and use of nonalcoholic oral health care products.
- Encourage daily plaque control procedures for effective self-care in patients at risk for cardiovascular disease.

Captral — see captopril

Capzasin P — see capsaicin

Carac — see fluorouracil

Carafate — see sucralfate
Carbac — see loracarbef

carbamazepine (KAR-bam-AZE-uh-peen)

Carbatrol, Epitol, Tegretol, Tegretol XR

▮✦▮ APO-Carbamazepine, Gen-Carbamazepine CR, Novo-Carbamaz, Nu-Carbamazepine, PMS-Carbamazepine CR, Taro-Carbamazepine

▮✦▮ Carbazep, Carbazina, Clostedal, Neugeron

Drug Class: Anticonvulsant

PHARMACOLOGY

Action

Mechanism appears to act by reducing polysynaptic responses and blocks posttetanic potentiation.

Uses

Treatment of epilepsy (e.g., partial seizures with complex symptoms, generalized tonic-clonic seizures [grand mal], mixed seizure patterns, other partial or generalized seizures) in patients refractory to or intolerant of other agents. Treatment of pain associated with trigeminal neuralgia.

Unlabeled Uses

Treatment of certain psychiatric disorders; management of alcohol withdrawal; relief of restless legs syndrome; treatment of postherpetic neuralgia.

➡◀ DRUG INTERACTIONS RELATED TO DENTAL THERAPEUTICS

Fluconazole, ketoconazole, or itraconazole: Possible carbamazepine toxicity (decreased metabolism)
• Monitor clinical status.
Alprazolam or clonazepam: Decreased alprazolam or clonazepam effect (increased metabolism)
• Monitor clinical status.
Metronidazole: Possible carbamazepine toxicity (decreased metabolism)
• Monitor clinical status.
Tramadol: Decreased tramadol effect (increased metabolism)
• Monitor clinical status.
Doxycycline: Decreased doxycycline effect (increased metabolism)
• Avoid concurrent use.
  May decrease valproic acid levels; may alter carbamazepine levels.

ADVERSE EFFECTS

⚠ **ORAL:** Dry mouth; glossitis; stomatitis.

CNS: Dizziness; drowsiness; unsteadiness; confusion; headache; hyperacusis; fatigue; speech disturbances; abnormal involuntary movements; peripheral neuritis and paresthesias; depression with agitation; talkativeness; behavior changes (children); paralysis.

CVS: Hypertension or hypotension; arrhythmia; syncope; CHF.

GI: Nausea; vomiting; gastric distress; abdominal pain; diarrhea; constipation; anorexia.

RESP: Pulmonary hypersensitivity (e.g., fever, dyspnea, pneumonitis, pneumonia).

MISC: Aching joints and muscles; leg cramps; adenopathy; lymphadenopathy; fever; chills; syndrome of inappropriate antidiuretic hormone secretion.

CLINICAL IMPLICATIONS

General

• Determine why drug is being taken. Consider implications of condition on dental treatment.

- Determine level of disease control, type and frequency of seizure, and compliance with medication regimen.
- Chronic dry mouth is possible; anticipate increased caries and candidiasis.
- Monitor vital signs.
- If GI side effects occur, consider semisupine chair position.
- Determine ability to adapt to stress of dental treatment. Consider short appointments.

Oral Health Education

- Evaluate manual dexterity; consider need for power toothbrush.
- If chronic dry mouth occurs, recommend home fluoride therapy and use of nonalcoholic oral health care products.

Carbatrol — see carbamazepine

Carbazep — see carbamazepine

Carbazina — see carbamazepine

Carbex — see selegiline HCl

carbidopa/levodopa — see levodopa/carbidopa

Carbocaine — see mepivacaine HCl

Carbocaine with Neo-Cobefrin — see mepivacaine HCl

Carbolit — see lithium

Carbolith — see lithium

Cardene — see nicardipine HCl

Cardene I.V. — see nicardipine HCl

Cardene SR — see nicardipine HCl

Cardinit — see nitroglycerin

Cardioquin — see quinidine

Cardiorona — see amiodarone

Cardipril — see captopril

Cardizem — see diltiazem HCl

Cardizem CD — see diltiazem HCl

Cardizem LA — see diltiazem HCl

Cardura — see doxazosin mesylate

Cardura-1 — see doxazosin mesylate

Cardura-2 — see doxazosin mesylate

Cardura-4 — see doxazosin mesylate

---

cargteolol HCl (CAR-tee-oh-lahl HIGH-droe-KLOR-ide)

Cartrol, Cartrol, Ocupress

Drug Class: Beta-adrenergic blocker

PHARMACOLOGY

Action
Blocks beta-receptors, primarily affecting cardiovascular system (e.g., decreases heart rate, cardiac contractility, BP) and lungs (promotes bronchospasm). Ophthalmic use reduces intraocular pressure, probably by decreasing aqueous production.

Uses
Management of hypertension. Ophthalmic preparation for control of intraocular hypertension and lowering of intraocular pressure in chronic open-angle glaucoma.

Unlabeled Uses
Treatment of angina.

➡◆ DRUG INTERACTIONS RELATED TO DENTAL THERAPEUTICS

COX-1 inhibitors: Decreased antihypertensive effect (decreased prostaglandin synthesis)
* Monitor blood pressure.

Sympathomimetic amines: Decreased antihypertensive effect (pharmacological antagonism)
* Use local anesthetic agents containing a vasoconstrictor with caution.
* Monitor blood pressure.

ADVERSE EFFECTS

⚠ **ORAL:** Dry mouth; taste disturbance; oral ulceration (unspecified).

CNS: Insomnia; fatigue; dizziness; depression; lethargy; drowsiness; forgetfulness; headache.

CVS: Bradycardia; arrhythmia; palpitations; hypertension or hypotension orthostatic hypotension.

GI: Nausea; vomiting; diarrhea; constipation.

RESP: Bronchospasm; shortness of breath; wheezing.

MISC: Weight changes; fever; facial swelling; cramps; muscle weakness. Antinuclear antibodies may develop; blood dyscrasias (rare).

CLINICAL IMPLICATIONS

General
* Monitor vital signs (e.g., BP, pulse pressure, rate, and rhythm) at each appointment to assess disease control. Do not provide elective dental treatment when BP is ≥180/110 or in the presence of other high-risk CV conditions. Refer to the section entitled "The Patient Taking Cardiovascular Drugs" in Chapter 6: *Clinical Medicine.*
* Use local anesthetic agents with vasoconstrictor with caution based on functional capacity of the patient and use aspirating technique to prevent intravascular injection.
* Beta blockers may mask epinephrine-induced signs and symptoms of hypoglycemia in patient with diabetes.
* *Postural hypotension:* Monitor BP at the beginning and end of each appointment; anticipate syncope. Have patient sit upright for several min at the end of the dental appointment before dismissing.
* Determine ability to adapt to stress of dental treatment. Consider short appointments.
* Chronic dry mouth is possible; anticipate increased caries, candidiasis, and lichenoid mucositis.
* If GI or respiratory side effects occur, consider semisupine chair position.
* Blood dyscrasias rarely reported; anticipate increased bleeding, infection, and poor healing.

Oral Health Education
* If chronic dry mouth occurs, recommend home fluoride therapy and use of nonalcoholic oral health care products.
* Encourage daily plaque control procedures for effective self-care in patients at risk for cardiovascular disease.

---

carisoprodol (car-eye-so-PRO-dole)

Soma

Drug Class: Skeletal muscle relaxant, centrally acting

PHARMACOLOGY

Action
Produces skeletal muscle relaxation, probably as result of its sedative properties.

Uses
Adjunctive treatment of acute, painful musculoskeletal conditions (e.g., muscle strain).

➔← DRUG INTERACTIONS RELATED TO DENTAL THERAPEUTICS

No documented drug-drug interactions. The absence of evidence is not evidence of safety.

ADVERSE EFFECTS

CNS: Dizziness; drowsiness; vertigo; ataxia; tremor; agitation; irritability; headache; depressive reactions; syncope; insomnia.

CVS: Postural hypotension; tachycardia.

GI: Nausea; vomiting; hiccups; epigastric distress.

RESP: Asthma.

MISC: Allergic or idiosyncratic reactions within first to fourth doses, including skin rash, erythema multiforme, pruritus, eosinophilia, and fixed drug eruption; more severe reactions include fever, weakness, dizziness, angioneurotic edema, and anaphylactoid shock.

CLINICAL IMPLICATIONS

General

- Determine why drug is being taken. Consider implications of condition on dental treatment.
- *For back pain:* Consider semisupine chair position for patient comfort.
- *Postural hypotension:* Monitor BP at the beginning and end of each appointment; anticipate syncope. Have patient sit upright for several min at the end of the dental appointment before dismissing.
- If GI side effects occur, consider semisupine chair position.

Carnotprim — see metoclopramide

Cartia XT — see diltiazem HCl

Cartrol — see cargteolol HCl

---

carvedilol (CAR-veh-DILL-ole)

Coreg

◼▦◼ Dilatrend

Drug Class: Alpha-adrenergic blocker; Beta-adrenergic blocker

PHARMACOLOGY

Action

Blocks alpha$_1$-receptors and nonselective beta-receptors to decrease BP.

Uses

Management of essential hypertension; treatment of mild to severe heart failure of ischemic or cardiomyopathic origin. Reduce cardiovascular mortality in clinically stable patients who have survived the acute phase of MI and have a left ventricular ejection fraction of 40% or less.

Unlabeled Uses

Angina pectoris.

➔← DRUG INTERACTIONS RELATED TO DENTAL THERAPEUTICS

COX-1 inhibitors: Decreased antihypertensive effect (decreased prostaglandin synthesis)
- Monitor blood pressure.

Sympathomimetic amines: Decreased antihypertensive effect (pharmacological antagonism)
- Use local anesthetic agents containing a vasoconstrictor with caution.
- Monitor blood pressure.

ADVERSE EFFECTS

⚠ **ORAL:** Periodontitis (1% to 3%); dry mouth.

CNS: Dizziness (32%); fatigue (24%); headache (8%); lung edema (for treatment of left ventricular dysfunction following MI [>3%]); somnolence, vertigo, hypesthesia, paresthesia, depression, insomnia (1% to 3%).

CVS: Bradycardia, postural hypotension, edema (2%).

GI: Diarrhea (12%); nausea (9%); vomiting (6%); melena, GI pain (1% to 3%).

RESP: Upper respiratory tract infection (18%); increased cough (8%); sinusitis, bronchitis (5%); rales (4%); dyspnea (for treatment of LVD following MI [>3%]).

MISC: Asthenia (11%); pain (9%); edema generalized, arthralgia (6%); edema dependent (4%); allergy, malaise, hypovolemia, fever, leg edema, infection, viral infection, back pain muscle cramps, arthritis, hypotonia, flu-like syndrome, peripheral vascular disorder (1% to 3%).

CLINICAL IMPLICATIONS

General

- Determine why drug is being taken. Consider implications of condition on dental treatment.
- Monitor vital signs (e.g., BP, pulse pressure, rate, and rhythm) at each appointment to assess disease control. Do not provide elective dental treatment when BP is ≥180/110 or in the presence of other high-risk CV conditions. Refer to the section entitled "The Patient Taking Cardiovascular Drugs" in Chapter 6: *Clinical Medicine.*
- Evaluate respiratory function.
- Use local anesthetic agents with vasoconstrictor with caution based on functional capacity of the patient and use aspirating technique to prevent intravascular injection.
- Beta blockers may mask epinephrine-induced signs and symptoms of hypoglycemia in patients with diabetes.
- Determine ability to adapt to stress of dental treatment. Consider short appointments.
- *Postural hypotension:* Monitor BP at the beginning and end of each appointment; anticipate syncope. Have patient sit upright for several min at the end of the dental appointment before dismissing.
- If GI or respiratory side effects occur, consider semisupine chair position.
- Chronic dry mouth is possible; anticipate increased caries, candidiasis, and lichenoid mucositis.

Oral Health Education

- If chronic dry mouth occurs, recommend home fluoride therapy and use of nonalcoholic oral health care products.
- Encourage daily plaque control procedures for effective self-care in patients at risk for cardiovascular disease.

Cataflam — see diclofenac

Catapres — see clonidine HCl

Catapresan-100 — see clonidine HCl

Catapres-TTS-1 — see clonidine HCl

Catapres-TTS-2 — see clonidine HCl

Catapres-TTS-3 — see clonidine HCl

Ceclor — see cefaclor

Ceclor Pulvules — see cefaclor

Cedax — see ceftibuten

---

cefaclor (SEFF-uh-klor)

Ceclor, Ceclor Pulvules

■✦■ Apo-Cefaclor, Novo-Cefaclor, Nu-Cefaclor, PMS-Cefaclor

Drug Class: Antibiotic, cephalosporin

PHARMACOLOGY

Action
Inhibits mucopeptide synthesis in bacterial cell wall.

Uses
Treatment of infections of respiratory tract, urinary tract, skin and skin structures; treatment of otitis media caused by susceptible strains of specific microorganisms.

➡◀ DRUG INTERACTIONS RELATED TO DENTAL THERAPEUTICS
No documented drug-drug interactions. The absence of evidence is not evidence of safety.

ADVERSE EFFECTS
⚠ **ORAL:** Tongue discoloration; candidiasis; thirst; glossitis; swollen tongue; taste disturbance.

GI: Nausea; vomiting; diarrhea; anorexia; abdominal pain or cramps; flatulence; colitis, including pseudomembranous colitis.

RESP: Asthma; bronchitis.

CNS: Dizziness; lethargy; confusion; nervousness.

CVS: Hypotension; palpitations; syncope.

MISC: Hypersensitivity, including Stevens-Johnson syndrome, erythema multiforme and toxic epidermal necrolysis; serum sickness–like reactions (e.g., skin rash, polyarthritis, arthralgia, fever); candidal overgrowth; various blood dyscrasias (rare).

CLINICAL IMPLICATIONS

General
- Determine why drug is being taken. Take precautions to avoid cross-contamination of microorganisms.
- If oral infection occurs that requires antibiotic therapy, select an appropriate product from a different class of anti-infectives.
- If prescribed by the DDS, ensure patient knows how to take the drug, how long it should be taken, and to immediately report adverse effects (e.g., rash, difficult breathing, diarrhea, GI upset). See Chapter 4: *Medical Management of Odontogenic Infections.*
- Antibiotic-associated diarrhea can occur. Have patient contact DDS immediately if signs develop.
- Oral candidiasis is possible; determine need for antifungal therapy.
- Blood dyscrasias rarely reported; anticipate increased bleeding, infection, and poor healing.

Oral Health Education
- Encourage daily plaque control procedures for effective nontraumatic self-care.

---

 cefadroxil (SEFF-uh-DROX-ill)

Duricef: Capsules: 500 mg (as monohydrate); Tablets: 1 g (as monohydrate); Powder for Oral Suspension: 125, 250, 500 mg/5 mL

■✚■ **Apo-Cefadroxil, Novo-Cefadroxil**

■▨■ **Cefamox, Duracef**

Drug Class: Antibiotic, cephalosporin

PHARMACOLOGY

Action
Inhibits mucopeptide synthesis in bacterial cell wall.

Uses

Treatment of infections of urinary tract, skin, and skin structures; treatment of pharyngitis and tonsillitis caused by susceptible strains of specific microorganisms.

Contraindications

Hypersensitivity to cephalosporins.

Usual Dosage

ADULTS: *PO:* 1 to 2 g/day in single dose or 2 divided doses.
CHILDREN: *PO:* 30 mg/kg/day in single dose or 2 divided doses.

Pharmacokinetics

ABSORP: Rapidly absorbed. C_{max} is about 16 mcg/mL (500-mg dose) and 28 mcg/mL (1000-mg dose).
DIST: 20% protein bound.
EXCRET: More than 90% is excreted in the urine as unchanged drug within 24 hr; $t_{1/2}$ is 78 to 96 min.
SPECIAL POP: *Renal failure:* The $t_{1/2}$ is increased. Adjust dosage.

➜← DRUG INTERACTIONS

No documented drug-drug interactions significant to dentistry. The absence of evidence is not evidence of safety.

ADVERSE EFFECTS

⚠ **ORAL:** Tongue discoloration; candidiasis; thirst; glossitis; swollen tongue; taste disturbance.
GI: Nausea; vomiting; diarrhea; anorexia; abdominal pain or cramps; flatulence; colitis, including pseudomembranous colitis.
RESP: Asthma; bronchitis.
CNS: Dizziness; lethargy; confusion; nervousness.
CVS: Hypotension; palpitation; syncope.
MISC: Hypersensitivity, including Stevens-Johnson syndrome, erythema multiforme and toxic epidermal necrolysis; serum sickness–like reactions (e.g., skin rash, polyarthritis, arthralgia, fever); candidal overgrowth; blood dyscrasias (rare).

CLINICAL IMPLICATIONS

General

- Determine why drug is being taken. If oral infection occurs that requires antibiotic therapy, select an appropriate product from a different class of anti-infectives.
- Prolonged use of antibiotics may result in bacterial or fungal overgrowth of nonsusceptible microorganisms; anticipate candidiasis.
- *If prescribed by the DDS:* Ensure patient knows how to take the drug, how long it should be taken, and to report adverse effects (e.g., rash, difficult breathing, diarrhea, GI upset) immediately. See Chapter 4: *Medical Management of Odontogenic Infections.*
- Antibiotic-associated diarrhea can occur. Have patient contact DDS immediately if signs develop.
- Blood dyscrasias rarely reported; anticipate increased bleeding, infection, and poor healing.
- *Lactation:* Excreted in breast milk.
- *Children:* In infants, consider benefits relative to risks. Drug may accumulate in newborns.
- *Hypersensitivity:* Reactions range from mild to life-threatening. Administer drug with caution to penicillin-sensitive patients because of possible cross-reactivity.
- *Renal failure:* Use drug with caution in patients with renal impairment. Dosage adjustment based on renal function may be required.
- *Superinfection:* May result in bacterial or fungal overgrowth of nonsusceptible microorganisms.
- *Pseudomembranous colitis:* Consider in patients in whom diarrhea develops.
- *Overdosage:* Seizures.

Pregnancy Risk Category: Category B.

Oral Health Education

When prescribed by DDS:

- Instruct patient to complete full course of therapy.
- Instruct patient to check body temperature daily. If fever persists more than a few days or if high fever (~102°F) or shaking chills are noted, notify health care provider immediately.
- Advise patient to maintain normal fluid intake while using this medication.
- Advise diabetic patient to use enzyme-based tests (e.g., Clinistix, Testape) for monitoring urine glucose because drug may give false results with other test methods.
- Instruct patient to report the following symptoms to health care provider: nausea, vomiting, diarrhea, skin rash, hives, or muscle or joint pain.
- Instruct patient to report signs of superinfection: black "furry" tongue, white patches in mouth, foul-smelling stools, or vaginal itching or discharge.
- Warn patient that diarrhea that contains blood or pus may be a sign of serious disorders. Tell patient to seek medical care and not to treat at home. Instruct patient to seek emergency care immediately if wheezing or difficulty in breathing occurs.

Cefamezin — see cefazolin sodium

Cefamox — see cefadroxil

---

 cefazolin sodium (seff-UH-zoe-lin SO-dee-uhm)

Ancef: Injection: 500 mg, 1 g (2.1 mEq sodium/g); Powder for Injection: 500 mg, 1, 5, 10 g (2.1 mEq sodium/g)
Zolicef: Powder for Injection: 500 mg (2.1 mEq sodium/g), 1 g (2.1 mEq sodium/g)

■▪■ Cefamezin

Drug Class: Antibiotic, cephalosporin

PHARMACOLOGY

Action

Inhibits mucopeptide synthesis in bacterial cell wall.

Uses

Treatment of infections of respiratory tract, genitourinary tract, skin and skin structures, biliary tract, bones and joints; perioperative prophylaxis; treatment of septicemia and endocarditis caused by susceptible strains of specific microorganisms.

Contraindications

Hypersensitivity to cephalosporins.

Usual Dosage

Perioperative prophylaxis

ADULTS: *IV/IM:* 1 g 30 min to 1 hr prior to surgery; 0.5 to 1 g at appropriate intervals (at least 2-hr) during surgery; 0.5 to 1 g q 6 to 8 hr for 24 hr (up to 5 days) after surgery.
CHILDREN OVER 1 MO: *IV/IM:* 25 to 50 mg/kg/day divided into 3 to 4 equal doses; (max, 100 mg/kg/day).

Pharmacokinetics

ABSORP: *IV:* C_{max} is about 185 mcg/mL.
DIST: 80% to 86% protein bound. Crosses the placenta. Very low concentrations are found in breast milk.
EXCRET: The $t_{1/2}$ is approximately 1.8 hr (IV) and approximately 2 hr (IM); 70% to 80% is excreted unchanged in the urine.
SPECIAL POP: *Renal failure:* The $t_{1/2}$ is increased. Dosage adjustment is needed.

➜◄ DRUG INTERACTIONS
Methyldopa: Pustular eruption (mechanism unknown)
- Avoid concurrent use.

ADVERSE EFFECTS
GI: Nausea; vomiting; diarrhea; anorexia; abdominal pain or cramps; colitis, including pseudomembranous colitis.
MISC: Hypersensitivity, including Stevens-Johnson syndrome, erythema multiforme, toxic epidermal necrolysis; candidal overgrowth; serum sickness–like reactions (e.g., skin rash, polyarthritis, arthralgia, fever); phlebitis, thrombophlebitis, and pain at injection site.

CLINICAL IMPLICATIONS
General
- This drug is used in patients at risk for bacterial endocarditis who cannot swallow oral antibiotics. It would be administered by physician prior to a dental appointment during which significant bleeding is expected.

Pregnancy Risk Category: Category B.

cefdinir (SEFF-dih-ner)
Omnicef
Drug Class: Antibiotic, cephalosporin

PHARMACOLOGY
Action
Inhibits mucopeptide synthesis in bacterial cell wall.

Uses
Treatment of community-acquired pneumonia, acute exacerbations of chronic bronchitis, acute maxillary sinusitis, pharyngitis, and tonsillitis, uncomplicated skin and skin structure infections, and otitis media (pediatric patients only) caused by susceptible strains of specific microorganisms.

➜◄ DRUG INTERACTIONS RELATED TO DENTAL THERAPEUTICS
No documented drug-drug interactions. The absence of evidence is not evidence of safety.

ADVERSE EFFECTS
⚠ **ORAL:** Tongue discoloration; candidiasis; thirst; glossitis; swollen tongue; taste disturbance.
CNS: Headache; dizziness; lethargy; confusion; nervousness.
CVS: Hypotension; palpitations; syncope.
GI: Diarrhea; nausea; vomiting; abdominal pain.
RESP: Asthma; bronchitis.
MISC: Elevated liver enzymes; proteinuria; RBCs in urine; eosinophilia; elevated urine pH.

CLINICAL IMPLICATIONS
General
- Determine why drug is being taken. Take precautions to avoid cross-contamination of microorganisms.
- If oral infection occurs that requires antibiotic therapy, select an appropriate product from a different class of anti-infectives.
- If prescribed by the DDS, ensure patient knows how to take the drug, how long it should be taken, and to report adverse effects (e.g., rash, difficult breathing, diarrhea, GI upset) immediately. See Chapter 4: *Medical Management of Odontogenic Infections.*
- Antibiotic-associated diarrhea can occur. Have patient contact DDS immediately if signs develop.

- Oral candidiasis is possible; determine need for antifungal therapy.
- Blood dyscrasias rarely reported; anticipate increased bleeding, infection, and poor healing.

---

cefditoren pivoxil (SEFF-dih-TORE-ehn pih-VOX-ill)
Spectracef

Drug Class: Antibiotic, cephalosporin

PHARMACOLOGY

Action
Inhibits mucopeptide synthesis in bacterial cell wall.

Uses
Treatment of mild to moderate infections of acute bacterial exacerbation of chronic bronchitis, pharyngitis, tonsillitis, and uncomplicated skin and skin-structure infections caused by susceptible strains of specific microorganisms.

➡◀ DRUG INTERACTIONS RELATED TO DENTAL THERAPEUTICS
No documented drug-drug interactions. The absence of evidence is not evidence of safety.

ADVERSE EFFECTS
⚠ **ORAL:** Thirst; glossitis; candidiasis.

CNS: Headache; reversible hyperactivity; seizures.

CVS: Hypotension; syncope; palpitation.

GI: Diarrhea; nausea; abdominal pain; dyspepsia; vomiting; pseudomembranous colitis; colitis.

RESP: Asthma; bronchitis; dyspnea.

MISC: Allergic reactions; anaphylaxis; drug fever; hypertonia; superinfection; serum sickness-like reaction; blood dyscrasias (leukopenia, thrombocytopenia, others), interference with vitamin K–dependent clotting factors.

CLINICAL IMPLICATIONS

General
- Determine why drug is being taken. Take precautions to avoid cross-contamination of microorganisms.
- If oral infection occurs that requires antibiotic therapy, select an appropriate product from a different class of anti-infectives.
- If prescribed by the DDS, ensure patient knows how to take the drug, how long it should be taken, and to report adverse effects (e.g., rash, difficult breathing, diarrhea, GI upset) immediately. See Chapter 4: *Medical Management of Odontogenic Infections.*
- Antibiotic-associated diarrhea can occur. Have patient contact DDS immediately if signs develop.
- Oral candidiasis is possible; determine need for antifungal therapy.
- Blood dyscrasias rarely reported; anticipate increased bleeding, infection, and poor healing.
- Monitor vital signs.

Oral Health Education
- Encourage daily plaque control procedures for effective, nontraumatic self-care.

---

cefixime (SEFF-IKS-eem)
Suprax

■◆■ **Denvar, Novacef**

Drug Class: Antibiotic, cephalosporin

PHARMACOLOGY

Action
Inhibits mucopeptide synthesis in bacterial cell wall.

Uses
Treatment of uncomplicated UTIs, otitis media, pharyngitis, tonsillitis, acute bronchitis, acute exacerbations of chronic bronchitis, and uncomplicated gonorrhea caused by susceptible strains of specific organisms.

➜← DRUG INTERACTIONS RELATED TO DENTAL THERAPEUTICS

ADVERSE EFFECTS
⚠ **ORAL:** Tongue discoloration; candidiasis; thirst; glossitis; swollen tongue; taste disturbance.
CNS: Headaches, dizziness, seizures (<2%).
CVS: Hypotension; palpitations; syncope.
GI: Diarrhea (16%); nausea (7%); loose or frequent stools (6%); flatulence (4%); abdominal pain, dyspepsia (3%); vomiting (<2%).
RESP: Asthma; bronchitis.
MISC: Hypersensitivity, including Stevens-Johnson syndrome, erythema multiforme, and toxic epidermal necrolysis; serum sickness–like reactions (e.g., skin rash, polyarthritis, arthralgia, fever); candidal overgrowth; various blood dyscrasias (rare).

CLINICAL IMPLICATIONS

General
- Determine why drug is being taken. Take precautions to avoid cross-contamination of microorganisms.
- If oral infection occurs that requires antibiotic therapy, select an appropriate product from a different class of anti-infectives.
- If prescribed by the DDS, ensure patient knows how to take the drug, how long it should be taken, and to report adverse effects (e.g., rash, difficult breathing, diarrhea, GI upset) immediately. See Chapter 4: *Medical Management of Odontogenic Infections.*
- Antibiotic-associated diarrhea can occur. Have patient contact DDS immediately if signs develop.
- Oral candidiasis is possible; determine need for antifungal therapy.
- Blood dyscrasias rarely reported; anticipate increased bleeding, infection, and poor healing.

Oral Health Education
- Encourage daily plaque control procedures for effective, nontraumatic self-care.

---

cefpodoxime proxetil (SEF-pode-OX-eem PROX-uh-til)
Vantin

◼◼ Orelox

Drug Class: Antibiotic, cephalosporin

PHARMACOLOGY

Action
Inhibits mucopeptide synthesis in bacterial cell wall.

Uses
Treatment of infections of respiratory tract, urinary tract, skin, and skin structures; treatment of sexually transmitted diseases caused by susceptible strains of specific microorganisms.

➡️⬅️ DRUG INTERACTIONS RELATED TO DENTAL THERAPEUTICS

No documented drug-drug interactions. The absence of evidence is not evidence of safety.

ADVERSE EFFECTS

⚠️ **ORAL:** Tongue discoloration; candidiasis; thirst; glossitis; swollen tongue; taste disturbance.

GI: Nausea; vomiting; diarrhea; anorexia; abdominal pain or cramps; flatulence; colitis, including pseudomembranous colitis.

RESP: Asthma; bronchitis.

CNS: Dizziness; lethargy; confusion; nervousness.

CVS: Hypotension; palpitations; syncope.

MISC: Hypersensitivity, including Stevens-Johnson syndrome, erythema multiforme, toxic epidermal necrolysis; serum sickness–like reactions (e.g., skin rashes, polyarthritis, arthralgia, fever); candidal overgrowth; various blood dyscrasias (rare).

CLINICAL IMPLICATIONS

General

- Determine why drug is being taken. Take precautions to avoid cross-contamination of microorganisms.
- If oral infection occurs that requires antibiotic therapy, select an appropriate product from a different class of anti-infectives.
- If prescribed by the DDS, ensure patient knows how to take the drug, how long it should be taken, and to report adverse effects (e.g., rash, difficult breathing, diarrhea, GI upset) immediately. See Chapter 4: *Medical Management of Odontogenic Infections*.
- Antibiotic-associated diarrhea can occur. Have patient contact DDS immediately if signs develop.
- Oral candidiasis is possible; determine need for antifungal therapy.
- Blood dyscrasias rarely reported; anticipate increased bleeding, infection, and poor healing.

Oral Health Education

- Encourage daily plaque control procedures for effective, nontraumatic self-care.

---

cefprozil (SEFF-pro-zill)

Cefzil

◼️◼️ **Procef**

Drug Class: Antibiotic, cephalosporin

PHARMACOLOGY

Action

Inhibits mucopeptide synthesis in bacterial cell wall.

Uses

Treatment of infections of skin and skin structures, bronchitis, pharyngitis, tonsillitis, and otitis media caused by susceptible strains of specific microorganisms.

➡️⬅️ DRUG INTERACTIONS RELATED TO DENTAL THERAPEUTICS

No documented drug-drug interactions. The absence of evidence is not evidence of safety.

ADVERSE EFFECTS

⚠️ **ORAL:** Tongue discoloration; candidiasis; thirst; glossitis; swollen tongue; taste disturbance.

CNS: Headache; dizziness; fatigue; paresthesia; confusion; nervousness; sleeplessness; insomnia.

CVS: Hypotension; palpitation; syncope.

GI: Nausea; vomiting; diarrhea; abdominal pain or cramps; flatulence; colitis, including pseudomembranous colitis.

RESP: Asthma; bronchitis.

MISC: Hypersensitivity, including Stevens-Johnson syndrome, erythema multiforme, toxic epidermal necrolysis; candidal overgrowth; serum sickness–like reactions (e.g., skin rashes, polyarthritis, arthralgia, fever); various blood dyscrasias (rare).

CLINICAL IMPLICATIONS
General
- Determine why drug is being taken. Take precautions to avoid cross-contamination of microorganisms.
- If oral infection occurs that requires antibiotic therapy, select an appropriate product from a different class of anti-infectives.
- If prescribed by the DDS, ensure patient knows how to take the drug, how long it should be taken, and to report adverse effects (e.g., rash, difficult breathing, diarrhea, GI upset) immediately. See Chapter 4: *Medical Management of Odontogenic Infections.*
- Antibiotic-associated diarrhea can occur. Have patient contact DDS immediately if signs develop.
- Prolonged use of antibiotics may result in bacterial or fungal overgrowth of nonsusceptible microorganisms; anticipate candidiasis.
- Blood dyscrasias rarely reported; anticipate increased bleeding, infection, and poor healing.

Oral Health Education
- Encourage daily plaque control procedures for effective, nontraumatic self-care.

ceftibuten (seff-TIE-byoo-ten)
Cedax
Drug Class: Antibiotic, cephalosporin

PHARMACOLOGY
Action
Inhibits mucopeptide synthesis in bacterial cell wall.

Uses
Treatment of pharyngitis/tonsillitis caused by *Streptococcus pyogenes*; otitis media caused by *Moraxella catarrhalis*, *Haemophilus influenzae* (including beta-lactamase-producing strains) or *S. pyogenes;* and acute bacterial exacerbation of chronic bronchitis caused by *S. pneumoniae* (penicillin-susceptible strains), *H. influenzae* (including betalactamase-producing strains), or *M. catarrhalis* (including beta-lactamase-producing strains).

➪← DRUG INTERACTIONS RELATED TO DENTAL THERAPEUTICS
No documented drug-drug interactions. The absence of evidence is not evidence of safety.

ADVERSE EFFECTS
⚠ **ORAL:** Thirst; glossitis; candidiasis.

GI: Nausea; vomiting; diarrhea; anorexia; abdominal pain or cramps; flatulence; colitis.

RESP: Asthma; bronchitis; dyspnea.

CNS: Headache; reversible hyperactivity; seizures.

CVS: Hypotension; syncope; palpitation.

MISC: Hypersensitivity, including Stevens-Johnson syndrome, erythema multiforme, and toxic epidermal necrolysis; serum sickness–like reactions (e.g., skin rash, polyarthritis, arthralgia, fever); candidal overgrowth; blood dyscrasias (leukopenia, thrombocytopenia, others), interference with vitamin K–dependent clotting factors.

CLINICAL IMPLICATIONS
General
- Determine why drug is being taken. Take precautions to avoid cross-contamination of microorganisms.

- If oral infection occurs that requires antibiotic therapy, select an appropriate product from a different class of anti-infectives.
- If prescribed by the DDS, ensure patient knows how to take the drug, how long it should be taken, and to report adverse effects (e.g., rash, difficult breathing, diarrhea, GI upset) immediately. See Chapter 4: *Medical Management of Odontogenic Infections.*
- Antibiotic-associated diarrhea can occur. Have patient contact DDS immediately if signs develop.
- Oral candidiasis is possible; determine need for antifungal therapy.
- Blood dyscrasias rarely reported; anticipate increased bleeding, infection, and poor healing.
- Monitor vital signs.

Oral Health Education

- Encourage daily plaque control procedures for effective, nontraumatic self-care.

Ceftin — see cefuroxime
Cefuracet — see cefuroxime

---

cefuroxime (SEFF-yur-OX-eem)

Ceftin, Zinacef

■✚■ Apo-Cefuroxime

■▄■ Cefuracet, Cetoxil, Froxal, Zinnat

Drug Class: Antibiotic, cephalosporin

PHARMACOLOGY

Action

Inhibits mucopeptide synthesis in bacterial cell wall.

Uses

ORAL FORM: Treatment of infections of lower respiratory tract, urinary tract, skin, and skin structures; treatment of uncomplicated gonorrhea, otitis media, pharyngitis, and tonsillitis caused by susceptible strains of specific microorganisms. Treatment of early Lyme disease, pharyngitis/tonsillitis, and impetigo.

PARENTERAL FORM: Treatment of infections of lower respiratory tract, urinary tract, skin, and skin structures, bone and joint; preoperative prophylaxis; treatment of septicemia, gonorrhea, and meningitis caused by susceptible strains of specific microorganisms.

➔✚ DRUG INTERACTIONS RELATED TO DENTAL THERAPEUTICS

No documented drug-drug interactions. The absence of evidence is not evidence of safety.

ADVERSE EFFECTS

⚠ **ORAL:** Tongue discoloration; candidiasis; thirst; glossitis; swollen tongue; taste disturbance.

GI: Nausea; vomiting; diarrhea; anorexia; abdominal pain or cramps; flatulence; colitis, including pseudomembranous colitis.

RESP: Asthma; bronchitis.

CNS: Dizziness, lethargy; confusion; nervousness.

CVS: Hypotension; palpitation; syncope.

MISC: Hypersensitivity, including Stevens-Johnson syndrome, erythema multiforme, toxic epidermal necrolysis; candidal overgrowth; serum sickness–like reactions (e.g., skin rashes, polyarthritis, arthralgia, fever); phlebitis, thrombophlebitis, and pain at injection site; various blood dyscrasias (rare).

CLINICAL IMPLICATIONS

General
- Determine why drug is being taken. Take precautions to avoid cross-contamination of microorganisms.
- If oral infection occurs that requires antibiotic therapy, select an appropriate product from a different class of anti-infectives.
- If prescribed by the DDS, ensure patient knows how to take the drug, how long it should be taken, and to report adverse effects (e.g., rash, difficult breathing, diarrhea, GI upset) immediately. See Chapter 4: *Medical Management of Odontogenic Infections.*
- Antibiotic-associated diarrhea can occur. Have patient contact DDS immediately if signs develop.
- Prolonged use of antibiotics may result in bacterial or fungal overgrowth of nonsusceptible microorganisms; anticipate candidiasis.
- Blood dyscrasias rarely reported; anticipate increased bleeding, infection, and poor healing.

Oral Health Education
- Encourage daily plaque control procedures for effective, nontraumatic self-care.

Cefzil — see cefprozil

Celebrex — see celecoxib

---

celecoxib (sel-eh-cox-ib)
Celebrex
Drug Class: COX-2 inhibitor

PHARMACOLOGY

Action
Reduces inflammation (e.g., pain, redness, swelling, heat), fever, and pain by inhibiting chemicals in the body that cause inflammation, fever, and pain. This is probably caused by the inhibition of prostaglandin synthesis, primarily via inhibition of COX-2 isoenzyme.

Uses
Relief of symptoms of osteoarthritis; relief of symptoms of rheumatoid arthritis in adults; management of acute pain in adults; treatment of primary dysmenorrhea; reduction of the number of adenomatous colorectal polyps in familial adenomatous polyposis (FAP), as an adjunct to usual care (e.g., endoscopic surveillance, surgery).

➡◀ DRUG INTERACTIONS RELATED TO DENTAL THERAPEUTICS

Fluconazole: Possible celecoxib toxicity (decreased metabolism)
- Avoid concurrent use.

COX-1 inhibitors: Increased incidence of peptic ulcer disease (additive)
- Avoid concurrent use.

ADVERSE EFFECTS
⚠ **ORAL:** Taste disturbance, herpes simplex, nonspecified tooth disorder, dry mouth, stomatitis (<2%).

CNS: Dizziness; insomnia; fatigue; migraine; anxiety; anorexia; increased appetite; depression; nervousness; somnolence.

CVS: Palpitation, tachycardia (<2%).

GI: Abdominal pain; diarrhea; dyspepsia; flatulence; constipation; diverticulitis; dysphagia; eructation; gastritis; gastroenteritis; gastroesophageal reflux; hemorrhoids; hiatal hernia; melena; tenesmus; vomiting.

RESP: Pharyngitis; URI; bronchitis; bronchospasm; aggravated bronchospasm; coughing; dyspnea; pneumonia.

MISC: Peripheral edema; accidental injury; allergic reaction; asthenia; chest pain; generalized edema; facial edema; fever; hot flushes; flu-like symptoms; pain; peripheral pain; leg cramps; hypertonia; hypesthesia; neuralgia; neuropathy; paresthesia; vertigo; arthralgia; arthrosis; bone disorder; accidental fracture; myalgia; neck stiffness; synovitis; tendinitis; anemia, ecchymosis, thrombocytopenia (<2%).

CLINICAL IMPLICATIONS

General
- Determine why drug is being taken. Consider implications of condition on dental treatment.
- Chronic dry mouth is possible; anticipate increased caries, candidiasis, and lichenoid mucositis.
- Use COX inhibitors with caution; they may exacerbate PUD and GERD.
- *Arthritis:* Consider patient comfort and need for semisupine chair position.
- If GI or respiratory side effects occur, consider semisupine chair position.
- Blood dyscrasias reported; anticipate increased bleeding and poor healing.

Oral Health Education
- If chronic dry mouth occurs, recommend home fluoride therapy and use of nonalcoholic oral health care products.
- Encourage daily plaque control procedures for effective, nontraumatic self-care.
- Evaluate manual dexterity; consider need for power toothbrush.

Celestoderm-V — see betamethasone

Celestoderm-V/2 — see betamethasone

Celestone — see betamethasone

Celestone Phosphate — see betamethasone

Celestone Soluspan — see betamethasone

Celexa — see citalopram

CellCept — see mycophenolate mofetil/mycophenolic acid

CellCept I.V. — see mycophenolate mofetil/mycophenolic acid

Cenafed — see pseudoephedrine

Cena-K — see potassium products

Cenestin — see estrogens, synthetic conjugated, a or b

Cepacol Viractin — see tetracaine HCl

---

 cephalexin (seh-fuh-LEX-in)

Biocef: Capsules: 500 mg; Powder for Oral Suspension: 125, 250 mg/5 mL
Keflex: Capsules: 250, 500 mg; Powder for Oral Suspension: 125, 250 mg/5 mL
Keftab: Tablets: 500 mg (as HCl monohydrate)

█✦█ APO-Cephalex, Novo-Lexin, Nu-Cephalex

█▸█ Ceporex, Naxifelar

Drug Class: Antibiotic, cephalosporin

PHARMACOLOGY

Action
Inhibits mucopeptide synthesis in bacterial cell wall.

Uses
Treatment of infections of respiratory tract, urinary tract, skin and skin structures, and bone; treatment of otitis media caused by susceptible strains of specific microorganisms.

Contraindications
Hypersensitivity to cephalosporins.

Usual Dosage
ADULTS: *PO*: 1 to 4 g/day in divided doses (max, 4 g/day).
CHILDREN: *PO*: (cephalexin monohydrate only) 25 to 100 mg/kg/day in divided doses.

Pharmacokinetics
ABSORP: Cephalexin is rapidly absorbed. C_{max} is about 9 to 32 mcg/mL (250-mg to 1-g doses). T_{max} is 1 hr.
DIST: Cephalexin is 10% protein bound.
EXCRET: More than 90% is excreted unchanged in the urine within 8 hr. The $t_{1/2}$ is 50 to 80 min.

➔← DRUG INTERACTIONS
No documented drug-drug interactions significant to dentistry. The absence of evidence is not evidence of safety.

ADVERSE EFFECTS
⚠ **ORAL:** Tongue discoloration; candidiasis; thirst; glossitis; swollen tongue; taste disturbance.
GI: Nausea; vomiting; diarrhea; anorexia; abdominal pain or cramps; flatulence; colitis, including pseudomembranous colitis.
RESP: Asthma; bronchitis.
CNS: Dizziness; lethargy; confusion; nervousness.
CVS: Hypotension; palpitations; syncope.
MISC: Hypersensitivity, including Stevens-Johnson syndrome, erythema multiforme, toxic epidermal necrolysis; candidal overgrowth; serum sickness–like reactions (e.g., skin rash, polyarthritis, arthralgia, fever); blood dyscrasias (rare).

CLINICAL IMPLICATIONS
General
- Determine why drug is being taken.
- If oral infection occurs that requires antibiotic therapy, select an appropriate product from a different class of anti-infectives.
- *If prescribed by DDS:* Ensure patient knows how to take the drug, how long it should be taken, and to report adverse effects (e.g., rash, difficult breathing, diarrhea, GI upset) immediately. See Chapter 4: *Medical Management of Odontogenic Infections.*
- This drug is used for antibiotic prophylaxis in patients at risk for joint infection who have had TJR, as an alternative to amoxicillin.
- *Lactation:* Excreted in breast milk.
- *Children:* Safety and efficacy of cephalexin HCl monohydrate (Keftab) in children not established.
- *Hypersensitivity:* Reactions range from mild to life threatening. Administer drug with caution to penicillin-sensitive patients because of possible cross-reactivity.
- Assess for signs and symptoms of anaphylaxis (e.g., shortness of breath, wheezing, laryngeal spasm). Have resuscitation equipment available.

Pregnancy Risk Category: Category B.

Oral Health Education
When prescribed by DDS:
- Instruct patient to complete full course of therapy.
- Instruct patient to seek emergency care immediately if wheezing or difficulty breathing occurs.

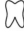 **cephradine** (SEFF-ruh-deen)

Velosef: Capsules: 250, 500 mg; Powder for Oral Suspension: 125, 500 mg/5 mL
Drug Class: Antibiotic, cephalosporin

PHARMACOLOGY

Action
Inhibits mucopeptide synthesis in bacterial cell wall.

Uses
Treatment of infections of respiratory tract, urinary tract, skin, and skin structure; treatment of otitis media caused by susceptible strains of microorganisms.

Contraindications
Hypersensitivity to cephalosporins.

Usual Dosage
ADULTS: *PO:* 250 mg to 1 g q 6 to 12 hr.
CHILDREN: *PO:* 25 to 100 mg/kg/day in equally divided doses q 6 to 12 hr (max, 4 g/day).

Pharmacokinetics
ABSORP: Cephradine is rapidly absorbed. C_{max} is about 9 mcg/mL (250 mg) to 24.2 mcg/mL (1 g). T_{max} is 1 hr. Food delays absorption.
DIST: 8% to 17% protein bound.
EXCRET: More than 90% is excreted unchanged in the urine. The $t_{1/2}$ is 48 to 80 min.
SPECIAL POP: *Renal failure:* The $t_{1/2}$ is prolonged. Dosage adjustment is recommended.

➜← DRUG INTERACTIONS
No documented drug-drug interactions significant to dentistry. The absence of evidence is not evidence of safety.

ADVERSE EFFECTS
⚠ **ORAL:** Tongue discoloration; candidiasis; thirst; glossitis; swollen tongue; taste disturbance.
GI: Nausea; vomiting; diarrhea; anorexia; abdominal pain or cramps; flatulence; colitis, including pseudomembranous colitis.
RESP: Asthma; bronchitis.
CNS: Dizziness; lethargy; confusion; nervousness.
CVS: Hypotension; palpitation; syncope.
MISC: Hypersensitivity, including Stevens-Johnson syndrome, erythema multiforme, toxic epidermal necrolysis; candidal overgrowth; serum sickness–like reactions (e.g., skin rash, polyarthritis, arthralgia, fever); various blood dyscrasias (rare).

CLINICAL IMPLICATIONS

General
- Determine why drug is being taken.
- If oral infection occurs that requires antibiotic therapy, select an appropriate product from a different class of anti-infectives.
- Prolonged use of antibiotics may result in bacterial or fungal overgrowth of nonsusceptible microorganisms; anticipate candidiasis.
- Blood dyscrasias rarely reported; anticipate increased bleeding, infection, and poor healing.
- This drug may be prescribed by DDS for antibiotic prophylaxis when the patient is at risk for joint infection following TJR.
- *If prescribed by DDS:* Ensure patient knows how to take the drug, how long it should be taken, and to immediately report adverse effects (e.g., rash, difficult breathing, diarrhea, GI upset). See Chapter 4: *Medical Management of Odontogenic Infections.*
- *Lactation:* Excreted in breast milk.
- *Hypersensitivity:* Reactions range from mild to life-threatening. Administer drug with caution to penicillin-sensitive patients because of possible cross-reactivity.
- Assess for signs and symptoms of anaphylaxis (e.g., shortness of breath, wheezing, laryngeal spasm). Have resuscitation equipment available.

Pregnancy Risk Category: Category B.

Oral Health Education
When prescribed by DDS:
- Instruct patient to complete full course of therapy.
- Advise patient to take with food or milk if GI distress occurs.
- Advise patient to maintain normal fluid intake while using this medication.
- Remind patient with diabetes to use enzyme-based tests (e.g., Clinistix or Testape) for monitoring urine glucose because drug may give false results with other test types.
- Instruct patient to seek emergency care immediately if wheezing or difficulty in breathing occurs.

Ceporex — see cephalexin
C.E.S. — see estrogens, conjugated or esterified
Cetacort — see hydrocortisone
Ceta-Plus — see acetaminophen/hydrocodone bitartrate

cetirizine (seh-TEER-ih-zeen)
Zyrtec

■✸■ Apo-Cetirizine, Reactine

■◆■ Virlix

Drug Class: Antihistamine

PHARMACOLOGY
Action
Competitively antagonizes histamine at the H_1-receptor site.

Uses
Symptomatic relief of symptoms (e.g., nasal, nonnasal) associated with seasonal and perennial allergic rhinitis; treatment of uncomplicated skin manifestations of chronic idiopathic urticaria.

➔✦ DRUG INTERACTIONS RELATED TO DENTAL THERAPEUTICS
No documented drug-drug interactions. The absence of evidence is not evidence of safety.

ADVERSE EFFECTS
⚠ **ORAL:** Dry mouth (5%); salivation, ulcerative stomatitis, caries, tongue discoloration, tongue edema, taste perversion, taste loss (<2%).
CNS: Somnolence, headache (14%); fatigue (6%); dizziness (2%); paresthesia, confusion, hyperkinesia, hypertonia, migraine, tremor, vertigo, ataxia, dystonia, abnormal coordination, hyperesthesia, hypoesthesia, myelitis, paralysis, twitching, insomnia, sleep disorder, nervousness, depression, emotional lability, impaired concentration, anxiety, depersonalization, paroniria, abnormal thinking, agitation, amnesia, decreased libido, euphoria, dysphonia, ptosis (<2%); convulsions; hallucinations; orofacial dyskinesia; suicidal ideation.
CVS: Postural hypotension; palpitation.
GI: Abdominal pain (6%); nausea, diarrhea, vomiting (3%); anorexia, increased appetite, dyspepsia, flatulence, constipation, gastritis, rectal hemorrhage, hemorrhoids, melena, eructation, enlarged abdomen, (<2%).
RESP: Coughing, epistaxis (4%); bronchospasm (3%); bronchitis, rhinitis, dyspnea, URI, hyperventilation, increased sputum, pneumonia, respiratory disorder (<2%).
MISC: Flushing, edema (e.g., facial, leg, peripheral, and generalized), lymphadenopathy, back pain, malaise, fever, asthenia, rigors, pain, chest pain, leg cramps, increased weight, pallor, hot flashes (<2%); anaphylaxis.

CLINICAL IMPLICATIONS
General
- Determine why drug is being taken. Consider implications of condition on dental treatment.

- Consider semisupine chair position to control effects of postnasal drainage.
- Be aware that patients with multiple allergies are at increased risk for allergy to dental drugs.
- Chronic dry mouth is possible; anticipate increased caries and candidiasis.
- *Postural hypotension:* Monitor BP at the beginning and end of each appointment; anticipate syncope. Have patient sit upright for several min at the end of the dental appointment before dismissing.

Oral Health Education

- If chronic dry mouth occurs, recommend home fluoride therapy and use of nonalcoholic oral health care products.

---

cetirizine HCl/pseudoephedrine HCl (seh-TIH-rih-zeen HIGH-droe-klor-ide SUE-doe-eh-FED-rin)

Synonym: pseudoephedrine HCl/cetirizine HCl

Zyrtec-D 12 Hour

Drug Class: Antihistamine; Adrenergic

PHARMACOLOGY

Action

Competitive antagonist for H1 receptors (cetirizine HCl); activates alpha-receptors to cause vasoconstriction and reduced secretions (pseudoephedrine).

Uses

Upper respiratory combination, decongestant, antihistamine.

➡️◀ DRUG INTERACTIONS RELATED TO DENTAL THERAPEUTICS

No documented drug-drug interactions. The absence of evidence is not evidence of safety.

ADVERSE EFFECTS

⚠ **ORAL:** CETIRIZINE: Dry mouth; nose, throat.
PSEUDOEPHEDRINE: Dry mouth.
CNS: CETIRIZINE: Dizziness; drowsiness; fatigue.
PSEUDOEPHEDRINE: Dizziness; tremor.
CVS: PSEUDOEPHEDRINE: Arrhythmia, tachycardia, palpitations, transient hypertension.
GI: CETIRIZINE: Nausea.
MISC: CETIRIZINE: Photophobia.
PSEUDOEPHEDRINE: Leukopenia; agranulocytosis; thrombocytopenia (rare hypersensitivity reaction).

CLINICAL IMPLICATIONS

General

- Consider semisupine chair position for patient comfort when respiratory symptoms occur.
- Chronic dry mouth is possible; anticipate increased caries activity and candidiasis.
- Monitor vital signs.
- *Photophobia:* direct dental light out of patient's eyes and offer dark glasses for comfort.
- Blood dyscrasias rarely reported; anticipate increased bleeding, infection, and poor healing.

Oral Health Education

- If chronic dry mouth occurs, recommend home fluoride therapy and use of nonalcoholic oral health care products.

Cetoxil — see cefuroxime

cevimeline HCl (seh-vih-MEH-leen HIGH-droe-KLOR-ide)

Evoxac: Gelatin capsules: 30 mg
Drug Class: Cholinergic agonist

PHARMACOLOGY

Action
Cevimeline is a cholinergic agonist that binds to muscarinic receptors. Muscarinic agonists in sufficient dosage can increase secretion of exocrine glands, such as salivary and sweat glands, and increase tone of the smooth muscle in the GI and urinary tracts.

Uses
Relieves dry mouth in patients with Sjögren syndrome.

Contraindications
Patients with uncontrolled asthma, hypersensitivity to cevimeline, or any condition in which miosis could be harmful (e.g., acute iritis, narrow-angle glaucoma).

Usual Dosage
Dry mouth with Sjögren syndrome
ADULTS: *PO:* 30 mg tid.

Dosage adjustments
ADULTS: *PO:* Because cevimeline is eliminated extensively in the urine, dosage adjustments may be required for patients with severe renal failure. However, specific recommendations are not established.

Pharmacokinetics
ABSORP: Cevimeline is rapidly absorbed. T_{max} is 1.5 to 2 hr. Food decreases the rate of absorption and C_{max} (by 17.3%).
DIST: V_d is about 6 L/kg. Cevimeline is less than 20% protein bound. It is extensively bound to tissues.
METAB: Cevimeline is metabolized by CYP2D6 and CYP3A3/4.
EXCRET: After 24 hr, 84% is excreted in the urine (16% as unchanged drug). The $t_{1/2}$ is about 5 hr.

➦◀ DRUG INTERACTIONS
No documented drug-drug interactions. The absence of evidence is not evidence of safety.

ADVERSE EFFECTS
⚠ **ORAL:** Salivation.
CNS: Dizziness; fatigue.
CVS: Hot flushes.
GI: Nausea; vomiting; diarrhea; dyspepsia.
RESP: Sinusitis; URI; rhinitis; cough.
MISC: Drugs that inhibit CYP2D6 and CYP3A3/4 also inhibit the metabolism of cevimeline. Use with caution in patients known or suspected to be deficient of CYP2D6 activity.

CLINICAL IMPLICATIONS

General
When prescribed by DDS:
• *Lactation:* Undetermined.

- *Children:* Safety and efficacy not established.
- *Elderly:* Exercise special care when cevimeline treatment is initiated in an elderly patient, considering the greater frequency of decreased hepatic, renal, or cardiac function, and of concomitant disease or other drug therapy in the elderly.
- *Biliary tract:* Administer with caution to patients with a history of nephrolithiasis.
- *CV:* Cevimeline can potentially alter cardiac conduction or heart rate. Use with caution in patients with a history of CV disease evidenced by angina pectoris or MI.
- *Ocular:* Ophthalmic formulations of muscarinic agonists have been reported to cause visual blurring that may result in decreased visual acuity (especially at night and in patients with central lens changes) and impairment of depth perception. Advise caution while driving at night or performing hazardous activities in reduced lighting.
- *Pulmonary:* Cevimeline can potentially increase airway resistance, bronchial smooth muscle tone, and bronchial secretions. Administer with caution to patients with asthma, chronic bronchitis, or COPD.
- *Renal colic:* Administer with caution to patients with a history of nephrolithiasis.
- *Overdosage:* Headache, visual disturbance, lacrimation, sweating, respiratory distress, GI spasm, nausea, vomiting, diarrhea, AV block, tachycardia, bradycardia, hypotension, hypertension, shock, mental confusion, cardiac arrhythmia, and tremors.

When prescribed by medical facility:
- Determine why drug is being taken. Consider implications of condition on dental treatment.
- If GI or respiratory side effects occur, consider semisupine chair position.

Pregnancy Risk Category: Category C.

Oral Health Education
When prescribed by DDS:
- Inform patient that cevimeline may cause visual disturbances, especially at night, which could impair their ability to drive safely.
- If a patient sweats excessively while taking cevimeline, consult health care provider and advise the patient to drink extra water as dehydration may develop.

Chibroxin — see norfloxacin
Children's Advil — see ibuprofen
Children's Congestion Relief — see pseudoephedrine
Children's Dramamine — see dimenhydrinate
Children's Dynafed Jr. — see acetaminophen
Children's Feverall — see acetaminophen
Children's Genapap — see acetaminophen
Children's Halenol — see acetaminophen
Children's Mapap — see acetaminophen
Children's Motrin — see ibuprofen
Children's Panadol — see acetaminophen
Children's Silapap — see acetaminophen
Children's Silfedrine — see pseudoephedrine
Children's Tylenol — see acetaminophen
Children's Tylenol Soft Chews — see acetaminophen
Chlo-Amine — see chlorpheniramine maleate

---

 chloral hydrate (KLOR-uhl HIGH-drate)

Aquachloral Supprettes: Suppositories: 324, 648 mg
■✚■ **PMS-Chloral Hydrate**

Drug Class: Sedative and hypnotic, nonbarbiturate
DEA Schedule: Schedule IV

PHARMACOLOGY

Action
Exact mechanism is unknown; can produce mild CNS depression.

Uses
Management of short-term insomnia; sedation; adjunctive to anesthesia, analgesia; prevention or suppression of alcohol withdrawal symptoms (rectal).

Unlabeled Uses
Conscious sedation in pediatric dentistry.

Contraindications
Hypersensitivity to chloral derivatives; severe renal or hepatic impairment; gastritis (oral forms); severe cardiac disease.

Usual Dosage
Premedication
ADULTS: *PO:* 500 mg to 1 g 30 min before procedure.
Dental sedation
CHILDREN: 75 mg/kg; supplementation with nitrous oxide may provide better sedation than manufacturer's recommended dosage.

Pharmacokinetics
ABSORP: Readily absorbed.
DIST: 35% to 41% protein bound (trichloroethanol). Excreted in breast milk.
METAB: Metabolized to trichloroethanol (active), which is then converted in liver and kidney to trichloroacetic acid (inactive).
EXCRET: The $t_{1/2}$ is 7 to 10 hr (trichloroethanol). Metabolites are excreted in urine and bile.

➡️ DRUG INTERACTIONS
Anticoagulants, oral: Increased anticoagulant effect (displacement from binding site)
• Avoid concurrent use.

ADVERSE EFFECTS
⚠ **ORAL:** Unpleasant taste.
CNS: Somnambulism; ataxia; dizziness; headache; "hangover" effect.
GI: Stomach pain; nausea; vomiting; diarrhea; flatulence.
RESP: Respiratory depression.
MISC: Hypersensitivity (e.g., rash, itching, erythema multiforme, fever).

CLINICAL IMPLICATIONS

General
When used by DDS:
• *Lactation:* Excreted in breast milk.
• *Tartrazine sensitivity:* Some products contain tartrazine, which can cause allergic-type reactions in some individuals.
• *Overdosage:* Stupor, coma, pinpoint pupils, hypotension, slow or rapid and shallow respirations, hypothermia, muscle flaccidity; also nausea, vomiting, gastritis, hemorrhagic gastritis, and gastric necrosis caused by drug's corrosive action.

Pregnancy Risk Category: Category C.

Oral Health Education
When used by DDS:
• Instruct patient to take medication exactly as prescribed. Warn that taking doses too close together could result in overdose. Omit missed doses.

- Advise patient that drug may cause drowsiness or dizziness and to use caution when driving or performing other tasks requiring mental alertness.
- Caution patient to avoid intake of alcoholic beverages and other CNS depressants such as barbiturates and narcotics.
- Instruct patient not to take OTC medications without consulting health care provider.

---

chlordiazepoxide (klor-DIE-aze-ee-POX-ide)

Librium: Capsules: 5, 10, 25 mg; Powder for Injection: 100 mg

■✦■ **Apo-Chlordiazepoxide**

Drug Class: Antianxiety, benzodiazepine

DEA Schedule: Schedule IV

PHARMACOLOGY

Action
Potentiates action of GABA to produce CNS depression.

Uses
Management of anxiety disorders; relief of acute alcohol withdrawal symptoms; relief of preoperative apprehension and anxiety.

Unlabeled Uses
Treatment of irritable bowel syndrome.

Contraindications
Hypersensitivity to benzodiazepines; psychoses; acute narrow-angle glaucoma; shock; coma.

Usual Dosage
Individualize dosage. Acute symptoms may be rapidly controlled IM or IV, with subsequent oral treatment (max, 300 mg/day).
CHILDREN OVER 6 YR: *PO:* 5 mg bid to qid; may be increased to 10 mg bid to tid.
CHILDREN OVER 12 YR: *IM:* 25 to 50 mg
Mild to Moderate Anxiety
ADULTS: *PO:* 5 to 10 mg tid or qid.
Severe Anxiety
ADULTS: *PO:* 20 to 25 mg tid or qid.
INITIAL DOSE: *IM/IV:* 50 to 100 mg, then 25 to 50 mg tid or qid.
ELDERLY OR DEBILITATED PATIENTS: *PO:* 5 mg bid to qid. *IM/IV:* 25 to 50 mg.
Preoperative Apprehension/Anxiety
ADULTS: *PO:* 5 to 10 mg tid or qid on days preceding surgery. *IM:* 50 to 100 mg 1 hr prior to surgery.

Pharmacokinetics
ABSORP: T_{max} is 0.5 to 4 hr.
DIST: 96% protein bound.
METAB: Metabolized in the liver to the major metabolite desmethylchlordiazepoxide and to several inactive intermediate metabolites.
EXCRET: The $t_{1/2}$ is 5 to 30 hr. Excreted in the urine, with 1% to 2% as unchanged drug and 3% to 6% as a conjugate.

➡✦ DRUG INTERACTIONS
Ketoconazole: Possible chlordiazepoxide toxicity (decreased metabolism)
- Avoid concurrent use.

Cimetidine: Possible chlordiazepoxide toxicity (decreased metabolism)
- Avoid concurrent use.

Contraceptives, combination: Possible chlordiazepoxide toxicity (mechanism unknown)
• Avoid concurrent use.

Disulfiram: Possible chlordiazepoxide toxicity (decreased metabolism)
• Avoid concurrent use.

Levodopa: Decreased levodopa effect (mechanism unknown)
• Avoid concurrent use.

ADVERSE EFFECTS

⚠ **ORAL:** Dry mouth; coated tongue.

CVS: CV collapse; hypotension, orthostatic hypotension; hypertension; tachycardia; brady-cardia; edema; phlebitis or thrombosis at IV sites.

CNS: Drowsiness; confusion; ataxia; dizziness; fatigue; apathy; memory impairment; disorientation; anterograde amnesia; restlessness; headache; slurred speech; loss of voice; stupor; coma; euphoria; irritability; vivid dreams; psychomotor retardation; paradoxical reactions (e.g., anger, hostility, mania, insomnia, muscle spasms); syncope; extrapyramidal symptoms.

GI: Constipation; diarrhea; nausea; anorexia; vomiting.

MISC: Dependency/withdrawal syndrome.

CLINICAL IMPLICATIONS

General

When used or prescribed by DDS:

• Geriatric, debilitated, and pediatric patients are more sensitive to the CNS effects of benzodiazepines.
• Depressed or anxious patients may neglect self-care. Monitor for plaque control effectiveness.
• Place on frequent maintenance schedule to avoid periodontal inflammation.
• Determine ability to adapt to stress of dental treatment. Consider short appointments.
• *Lactation:* Excreted in breast milk.
• *Children:* Initial dose should be small and gradually increased. Oral form not recommended in children younger than 6 yr; parenteral form not recommended in children younger than 12 yr.
• *Elderly:* Initial dose should be small and gradually increased. Use with caution in patients with limited pulmonary reserve.
• *Renal failure:* Observe caution to avoid accumulation of drug.
• *Hepatic failure:* Observe caution to avoid accumulation of drug.
• *Debilitated patients:* Initial dose should be small and gradually increased. Use with caution in patients with limited pulmonary reserve.
• *Drug dependency:* Prolonged use can lead to dependency. Withdrawal syndrome has occurred within 4 to 6 wk of treatment, especially if drug is abruptly discontinued. For discontinuation after long-term treatment, use caution and taper dosage.
• *Psychiatric disorders:* Not intended for patients with primary depressive disorder, psychosis, or disorders in which anxiety is not prominent.
• *Parenteral administration:* Reserved primarily for acute states.
• *Suicide:* Use with caution in patients with suicidal tendencies; do not allow access to large quantities of drug.
• *Overdosage:* Drowsiness, confusion, somnolence, impaired coordination, diminished reflexes, lethargy, ataxia, hypotonia, hypotension, hypnosis, coma, death.
• *Injection:* Ensure that a benzodiazepine-receptor antagonist (e.g., flumazenil), oxygen, and resuscitation and intubation equipment are available when medication is administered by IV injection.

Pregnancy Risk Category: Category D.

Oral Health Education

When used or prescribed by DDS:

• May produce sedation, interfere with eye-hand coordination, and the ability to operate mechanical equipment. Inform patient not to drive, sign important papers, or operate mechanical equipment.
• Warn patient not to drink alcoholic beverages while taking the drug.

- Explain name, dose, action, and potential side effects of drug.
- Advise patient or caregiver to read the *Patient Information* leaflet before starting therapy and with each refill.
- Advise patient that medication is usually started at a low dose and then gradually increased until maximum benefit is obtained.
- Caution patient that medication may be habit forming and to take as prescribed and not to stop taking nor change the dosage unless advised to do so by health care provider.
- Advise patient to take each dose without regard to meals but to take with food if stomach upset occurs.
- Advise patient that if a dose is missed to skip that dose and take the next dose at the regularly scheduled time. Caution patient to never take two doses at the same time.
- Advise patient that if medication needs to be discontinued, it will be slowly withdrawn unless safety concerns (e.g., rash) require a more rapid withdrawal.
- Instruct patient to avoid alcoholic beverages and other depressants while taking this medication.
- Advise patient with anxiety to take medication as needed and to seek alternative methods for controlling or preventing anxiety (e.g., stress reduction, counseling).
- Instruct patient to contact health care provider if symptoms do not appear to be getting better, are getting worse, or if bothersome side effects (e.g., drowsiness, memory impairment) occur.
- Advise patient that drug may cause drowsiness or impair judgment, thinking, or reflexes and to use caution while driving or performing other tasks requiring mental alertness until tolerance is determined.
- Advise women to notify health care provider if pregnant, planning to become pregnant, or breast feeding.
- Warn patient not to take any prescription or OTC drugs or dietary supplements without consulting health care provider.
- Advise patient that follow-up visits and lab tests may be necessary to monitor therapy and to keep appointments.

Injection:
- Advise patient or caregiver that medication will be prepared by a health care provider and administered in a health care setting under close observation when oral therapy is not feasible.

---

 chlorhexidine gluconate (klor-HEX-ih-deen GLUE-koe-nate)

Peridex: Oral Rinse: 0.12%
PerioGard: Oral Rinse: 0.12%
PerioChip: Chip: 2.5 mg

■✦■ Apo-Chlorhexidine
Drug Class: Antiseptic, germicide

PHARMACOLOGY

Action
Provides antimicrobial effect against a wide range of microorganisms.

Uses
Oral rinse for gingivitis; an adjunct to scaling and root planning procedures for reduction of pocket depth in adults with periodontitis.

Unlabeled Uses
Treatment of acne vulgaris. Amelioration of oral mucositis associated with cytoreductive therapy for bone marrow transplant candidates.

Contraindications
Standard considerations.

Usual Dosage
Periodontitis
2.5 mg (1 chip) inserted into periodontal pocket with probing depth at least 5 mm.

Oral rinse for gingivitis
15 mL (1 capful) bid for 30 sec, morning and evening after brushing teeth. Expectorate after rinsing; do not swallow.

➡◄ DRUG INTERACTIONS
No documented drug-drug interactions. The absence of evidence is not evidence of safety.

ADVERSE EFFECTS
⚠ **ORAL:** Staining of teeth and oral surfaces; increased calculus formation; minor irritation and superficial desquamation of oral mucosa; taste disturbance.

CLINICAL IMPLICATIONS
General
When prescribed by DDS:
* *Lactation:* Undetermined.
* *Overdosage:* Gastric distress, alcohol intoxication.
* Obtain patient history, including drug history and any known allergies.
* Monitor for allergic reactions (e.g., urticaria, bronchospasm, cough, shortness of breath).
* Monitor skin and mouth for irritation.

Pregnancy Risk Category: Category B (oral rinse).

Oral Health Education
When prescribed or used by DDS:
* Inform patient that staining of teeth, dental work, tongue, and oral tissue may occur. Staining does not adversely affect health and can usually be removed by professional techniques.
* Caution patient that taste perception may be altered during treatment; permanent taste alteration has not been noted.
* Inform patient that oral rinse contains alcohol.
* Instruct patient to avoid having medication come into contact with ears and eyes, which could cause permanent damage.
* Instruct patient not to swallow product but to expectorate after oral rinsing.
* Advise patient to avoid eating 2 to 3 hr after treatment.

Chip
* Advise patients to avoid dental floss at the site of chip insertion for 10 days after placement because flossing might dislodge the chip.
* Instruct patient to notify dentist promptly if chip dislodges.
* Advise patient that although mild to moderate sensitivity is normal during the first wk after placement of the chip, notify dentist if pain, swelling, or other problems occur.

---

chloroquine (KLOR-oh-kwin)
(chloroquine HCl, chloroquine phosphate)
Aralen HCl, Aralen Phosphate
∎✸∎ Aralen

Drug Class: Anti-infective; Antimalarial

PHARMACOLOGY
Action
Inhibits parasite growth, possibly by concentrating within parasite acid vesicles, raising pH.

Uses
Prophylaxis and treatment of acute attacks of malaria caused by *Plasmodium vivax, P. malariae, P. ovale,* and susceptible strains of *P. falciparum*; extraintestinal amebiasis.

Unlabeled Uses
Treatment of rheumatoid arthritis, systemic and discoid lupus erythematosus, porphyria cutanea tarda, scleroderma, pemphigus, lichen planus, polymyositis, and sarcoidosis.

➔← DRUG INTERACTIONS RELATED TO DENTAL THERAPEUTICS

Acetaminophen: Possible chloroquine toxicity (mechanism unknown)
• Monitor clinical status.

ADVERSE EFFECTS

⚠ **ORAL:** Lichen planus–like eruptions.
CNS: Headache; neuropathy; seizures; psychotic episodes.
CVS: Hypotension.
GI: Anorexia; nausea; vomiting; diarrhea; abdominal cramps.
MISC: Muscle weakness; photophobia; agranulocytosis; blood dyscrasia.

CLINICAL IMPLICATIONS

General
• Determine why drug is being taken. Consider implications of condition on dental treatment.
• *For patients taking this drug on a long-term basis:* Monitor vital signs. Blood dyscrasias rarely reported; anticipate increased bleeding, infection, and poor healing.
• If GI side effects occur, consider semisupine chair position.
• *Photophobia:* Direct dental light out of patient's eyes and offer dark glasses for comfort.

---

chloroquine HCl — see chloroquine
chloroquine phosphate — see chloroquine

---

chlorothiazide (klor-oh-THIGH-uh-zide)
Diurigen, Diuril
Drug Class: Thiazide diuretic

PHARMACOLOGY

Action
Enhances excretion of sodium, chloride, and water by interfering with transport of sodium ions across renal tubular epithelium.

Uses
Adjunctive treatment in edema associated with CHF, cirrhosis, and corticosteroid and estrogen therapy; edema caused by various forms of renal dysfunction such as nephrotic syndrome, acute glomerulonephritis, and chronic renal failure (oral and IV); management of hypertension (oral).

➔← DRUG INTERACTIONS RELATED TO DENTAL THERAPEUTICS

COX-1 inhibitors: Decreased antihypertensive effect (decreased prostaglandin synthesis)
• Monitor blood pressure.
Sympathomimetic amines: Hypokalemia (increased Intracellular uptake of potassium)
• Use local anesthetic agents containing a vasoconstrictor with caution.
• Monitor blood pressure and pulse rate.

ADVERSE EFFECTS

⚠ **ORAL:** Sialoadenitis.
CNS: Vertigo; paresthesia; dizziness; headache; restlessness.
CVS: Hypotension, orthostatic hypotension.
MISC: Photosensitivity; blood dyscrasia (leukopenia, thrombocytopenia, agranulocytosis, aplastic anemia, hemolytic anemia).
GI: Pancreatitis; diarrhea; vomiting; cramping; constipation; gastric irritation; nausea; anorexia.
RESP: Respiratory distress (e.g., pneumonitis, pulmonary edema).

CLINICAL IMPLICATIONS

General
- Determine why drug is being taken. Consider implications of condition on dental treatment.
- Monitor vital signs (e.g., BP, pulse pressure, rate, and rhythm) at each appointment to assess disease control. Do not provide elective dental treatment when BP is ≥180/110 or in the presence of other high-risk CV conditions. Refer to the section entitled "The Patient Taking Cardiovascular Drugs" in Chapter 6: *Clinical Medicine*.
- Use local anesthetic agents with vasoconstrictor with caution based on functional capacity of the patient and use aspirating technique to prevent intravascular injection.
- Monitor pulse rhythm to assess for electrolyte imbalance.
- Determine ability to adapt to stress of dental treatment. Consider short appointments.
- *Postural hypotension:* Monitor BP at the beginning and end of each appointment; anticipate syncope. Have patient sit upright for several min at the end of the dental appointment before dismissing.
- If GI side effects occur, consider semisupine chair position.
- Blood dyscrasias rarely reported; anticipate increased bleeding, infection, and poor healing.

Oral Health Education
- Encourage daily plaque control procedures for effective self-care in patients at risk for cardiovascular disease.

---

chlorpheniramine maleate (klor-fen-AIR-uh-meen MAL-ee-ate)

Aller-Chlor, Allergy, Chlo-Amine, Chlor-Trimeton Allergy 12 Hour, Chlor-Trimeton Allergy 8 Hour, Efidac 24

❚✦❚ Chlor-Tripolon

Drug Class: Alkylamine; Antihistamine

PHARMACOLOGY

Action
Competitively antagonizes histamine at H_1 receptor sites.

Uses
Temporary relief of sneezing; itchy, watery eyes; itchy nose or throat; and runny nose caused by hay fever (allergic) rhinitis or other respiratory allergies.

➜✦ DRUG INTERACTIONS RELATED TO DENTAL THERAPEUTICS
No documented drug-drug interactions. The absence of evidence is not evidence of safety.

ADVERSE EFFECTS
⚠ **ORAL:** Dry mouth.
CNS: Drowsiness (often transient); sedation; dizziness; faintness; disturbed coordination; nervousness; restlessness.
GI: Epigastric distress; anorexia; nausea; vomiting; diarrhea; constipation; change in bowel habits.
RESP: Thickening of bronchial secretions; chest tightness; wheezing; nasal stuffiness; dry nose and throat; sore throat; respiratory depression.
MISC: Hypersensitivity reactions; photosensitivity.

CLINICAL IMPLICATIONS

General
- Determine why drug is being taken. Consider implications of condition on dental treatment.
- Chronic dry mouth is possible; anticipate increased caries and candidiasis.
- Consider semisupine chair position to control effects of postnasal drainage.

- Be aware that patients with multiple allergies are at increased risk for allergy to dental drugs.
- If GI side effects occur, consider semisupine chair position.

Oral Health Education
- If chronic dry mouth occurs, recommend home fluoride therapy and use of nonalcoholic oral health care products.

---

chlorpromazine HCl (klor-PRO-muh-zeen HIGH-droe-KLOR-ide)
Chlorpromazine Hydrochloride, Thorazine
■✦■ Largactil

Drug Class: Antipsychotic, Phenothiazine; Antiemetic

PHARMACOLOGY
Action
Effects apparently caused by dopamine receptor blockade in CNS.

Uses
Management of manic phase of manic-depressive disorder; treatment of schizophrenia; relief of anxiety and restlessness prior to surgery; adjunct in treatment of tetanus; management of acute intermittent porphyria and severe behavioral and conduct disorders in children 1 to 12 yr of age; control of nausea and vomiting; relief of intractable hiccups.

Unlabeled Uses
Treatment of migraine headaches (IM or IV forms).

✦ DRUG INTERACTIONS RELATED TO DENTAL THERAPEUTICS
No documented drug-drug interactions. The absence of evidence is not evidence of safety.

ADVERSE EFFECTS
⚠ **ORAL:** Dry mouth, tardive dyskinesia, angioneurotic edema.
CNS: Faintness; drowsiness; dystonias; dizziness; extrapyramidal side effects (e.g., pseudo-parkinsonism); muscle spasms; motor restlessness; headache; weakness; tremor; fatigue; slurring; insomnia; vertigo; seizures; sedation; neuroleptic malignant syndrome; cerebral edema.
CVS: Postural hypotension; tachycardia.
GI: Dyspepsia; constipation; adynamic ileus (with possible complications resulting in death); nausea; atonic colon; obstipation.
RESP: Laryngospasm; bronchospasm; dyspnea; aspiration pneumonia; asthma; laryngeal edema.
MISC: Increased appetite and weight; polydipsia; heat stroke/hyperpyrexia; sudden death; anaphylactoid reactions; systemic lupus erythematosus–like syndrome; increased prolactin levels; photosensitivity; leukopenia; anemia; agranulocytosis.

CLINICAL IMPLICATIONS
General
- Determine why drug is being taken. Consider implications of condition on dental treatment.
- Extrapyramidal behaviors can complicate performance of oral procedures. If present, consult with MD to consider medication changes.
- *Geriatric patients:* Use lower dose.
- Chronic dry mouth is possible; anticipate increased caries and candidiasis.
- *Postural hypotension:* Monitor BP at the beginning and end of each appointment; anticipate syncope. Have patient sit upright for several min at the end of the dental appointment before dismissing.
- Blood dyscrasias rarely reported; anticipate increased bleeding, infection, and poor healing.
- Monitor vital signs.

Oral Health Education
- If chronic dry mouth occurs, recommend home fluoride therapy and use of nonalcoholic oral health care products.
- Evaluate manual dexterity; consider need for power toothbrush.

chlorpropamide (klor-PRO-puh-mide)

Diabinese

■✦■ APO-Chlorpropamide

■◆■ Deavynfar, Insogen

Drug Class: Antidiabetic, sulfonylurea

PHARMACOLOGY

Action
Decreases blood glucose by stimulating insulin release from pancreas.

Uses
Adjunct to diet to lower blood glucose in patients with type 2 diabetes mellitus whose hyperglycemia cannot be controlled by diet alone.

Unlabeled Uses
Control of neurogenic diabetes insipidus.

➡◀ DRUG INTERACTIONS RELATED TO DENTAL THERAPEUTICS
No documented drug-drug interactions. The absence of evidence is not evidence of safety.

ADVERSE EFFECTS
⚠ **ORAL:** Taste alteration; lichenoid reactions; thirst.
CNS: Dizziness; vertigo.
CVS: Arrhythmia; hypertension.
GI: GI disturbances (e.g., nausea, epigastric fullness, heartburn).
RESP: Rhinitis; dyspnea; pharyngitis.
MISC: Disulfiram-like reaction; weakness; paresthesia; fatigue; malaise; photosensitivity; blood dyscrasias (e.g., leukopenia, agranulocytosis, anemia, thrombocytopenia).

CLINICAL IMPLICATIONS

General
- Determine degree of disease control and current blood sugar levels. Goals should be <120 mg/dL and A1C <7%. A1C levels ≥8% indicate significant uncontrolled diabetes.
- The routine use of antibiotics in the dental management of diabetic patients is not indicated; however, antibiotic therapy in patients with poorly controlled diabetes has been shown to improve disease control and improve response following periodontal debridement.
- Monitor blood pressure because hypertension and dyslipidemia (CAD) are prevalent in diabetes mellitus.
- *Loss of blood sugar control:* Certain medical conditions (e.g., surgery, fever, infection, trauma) and drugs (e.g., corticosteroids) affect glucose control. In these situations, it may be necessary to seek medical consultation before surgical procedures.
- Obtain patient history regarding diabetic ketoacidosis or hypoglycemia with current drug regimen.
- Observe for signs of hypoglycemia (e.g., confusion, argumentativeness, perspiration, altered consciousness). Be prepared to treat hypoglycemic reactions with oral glucose or sucrose.
- Ensure patient has taken medication and eaten meal.
- Monitor vital signs (e.g., BP, pulse pressure, rate, and rhythm) at each appointment to assess disease control. Do not provide elective dental treatment when BP is ≥180/110 or

in the presence of other high-risk CV conditions. Refer to the section entitled "The Patient Taking Cardiovascular Drugs" in Chapter 6: *Clinical Medicine*.
- Determine ability to adapt to stress of dental treatment. Consider short, morning appointments.
- Medical consult advised if fasting blood glucose (FBG) is <70 mg/dL (hypoglycemic risk) or >200 mg/dL (hyperglycemic crisis risk).
- If insulin is used, consider time of peak hypoglycemic effect.
- If GI side effects occur, consider semisupine chair position.
- Blood dyscrasias rarely reported; anticipate increased bleeding, infection, and poor healing.

Oral Health Education
- Encourage daily plaque control procedures for effective self-care in patients at risk for cardiovascular disease.
- Explain role of diabetes in periodontal disease and the need to maintain effective plaque control and disease control.
- Advise patient to bring data on blood sugar values and A1C levels to dental appointments.

chlorthalidone (klor-THAL-ih-dohn)

Hygroton, Thalitone

■✦■ **Apo-Chlorthalidone**

■✦■ **Higroton**

Drug Class: Thiazide diuretic

PHARMACOLOGY

Action
Inhibits reabsorption of sodium and chloride in proximal portion of distal convoluted tubules.

Uses
Reduction of edema associated with CHF, cirrhosis, renal dysfunction, and corticosteroid and estrogen therapy; management of hypertension.

Unlabeled Uses
Treatment of calcium nephrolithiasis, osteoporosis, diabetes insipidus.

➡◀ DRUG INTERACTIONS RELATED TO DENTAL THERAPEUTICS

COX-1 inhibitors: Decrease antihypertensive effects (decreased prostaglandin synthesis)
- Monitor blood pressure.

ADVERSE EFFECTS

CNS: Dizziness; lightheadedness; vertigo; headache; paresthesias; weakness; restlessness; insomnia.
GI: Anorexia; gastric irritation; nausea; vomiting; abdominal pain or cramping; bloating; diarrhea; constipation; pancreatitis.
MISC: Muscle cramps or spasms; photosensitivity; blood dyscrasias (aplastic anemia, agranulocytosis, thrombocytopenia, leukopenia).

CLINICAL IMPLICATIONS

General
- Monitor vital signs (e.g., BP, pulse pressure, rate, and rhythm) at each appointment to assess disease control. Do not provide elective dental treatment when BP is ≥180/110 or in the presence of other high-risk CV conditions. Refer to the section entitled "The Patient Taking Cardiovascular Drugs" in Chapter 6: *Clinical Medicine*.
- Use local anesthetic agents with vasoconstrictor with caution based on functional capacity of the patient and use aspirating technique to prevent intravascular injection.

- Monitor pulse rhythm to assess for electrolyte imbalance.
- Determine ability to adapt to stress of dental treatment. Consider short appointments.
- Blood dyscrasias rarely reported; anticipate increased bleeding, infection, and poor healing.
- If GI side effects occur, consider semisupine chair position.

Oral Health Education

- Encourage daily plaque control procedures for effective self-care in patients at risk for cardiovascular disease.

Chlor-Trimeton Allergy 8 Hour — see chlorpheniramine maleate
Chlor-Trimeton Allergy 12 Hour — see chlorpheniramine maleate
Chlor-Tripolon — see chlorpheniramine maleate

---

cholestyramine (koe-less-TIE-ruh-meen)

LoCHOLEST, LoCHOLEST Light, Prevalite, Questran, Questran Light
■✦■ **Novo-Cholamine, Novo-Cholamine Light**
Drug Class: Antihyperlipidemic, bile acid sequestrant

PHARMACOLOGY

Action

Increases removal of bile acids from body by forming insoluble complexes in intestine, which are then excreted in feces. As body loses bile acids, it converts cholesterol from blood to bile acid, thus lowering serum cholesterol.

Uses

Reduction of serum cholesterol in patients with primary hypercholesterolemia; relief of pruritus associated with partial biliary obstruction.

Unlabeled Uses

Treatment of antibiotic-induced pseudomembranous colitis, bile salt-mediated diarrhea, and digitalis toxicity.

✦← DRUG INTERACTIONS RELATED TO DENTAL THERAPEUTICS

Acetaminophen: Decreased acetaminophen effect (decreased metabolism)
- Instruct patient to take acetaminophen 1 hr before cholestyramine.
- Monitor clinical status.

Metronidazole: Possible decreased metronidazole effect (decreased absorption)
- Avoid concurrent use.

Ibuprofen or naproxen: Possible decreased ibuprofen or naproxen effect
- Instruct patient to take ibuprofen 2 hr before or 6 hr after cholestyramine.
- Monitor clinical status.

ADVERSE EFFECTS

⚠ **ORAL:** Bleeding tendency (due to hypoprothrombinemia); dental caries; taste disturbance.
GI: Constipation (can be severe and at times accompanied by fecal impaction); aggravation of hemorrhoids; abdominal pain and distention; bleeding; belching; flatulence; nausea; vomiting; diarrhea; heartburn; anorexia; steatorrhea.
CVS: Tachycardia (infrequent).
MISC: Prolonged PT time; ecchymosis.

CLINICAL IMPLICATIONS

General

- High LDL cholesterol concentration is the major cause of atherosclerosis, which leads to CAD (e.g., angina, MI); determine degree of CV health and ability to withstand stress of dental treatment.

- Monitor vital signs (e.g., BP, pulse pressure, rate, and rhythm) at each appointment to assess disease control. Do not provide elective dental treatment when BP is ≥180/110 or in the presence of other high-risk CV conditions. Refer to the section entitled "The Patient Taking Cardiovascular Drugs" in Chapter 6: *Clinical Medicine*.
- If GI side effects occur, consider semisupine chair position.
- Monitor frequently to ensure adequate clotting during treatment that involves bleeding.

Oral Health Education

- Encourage daily plaque control procedures for effective self-care in patients at risk for cardiovascular disease.

Chronovera — see verapamil HCl

Cialis — see tadalafil

Cicloferon — see acyclovir

Cilag — see acetaminophen

Ciloxan — see ciprofloxacin

Cilpen — see dicloxacillin sodium

Cimetase — see cimetidine

---

cimetidine (sigh-MET-ih-deen)

Tagamet, Tagamet HB

■✦■ Apo-Cimetidine, Gen-Cimetidine, Novo-Cimetine, Nu-Cimet

■⛭■ Blocan, Cimetase, Cimetigal, Columina, Ulcedine, Zymerol

Drug Class: Histamine H₂ antagonist

PHARMACOLOGY

Action

Reversibly and competitively blocks histamine at H_2 receptors, particularly those in gastric parietal cells, leading to inhibition of gastric acid secretion.

Uses

Management of duodenal ulcer; treatment of gastroesophageal reflux disease (GERD), including erosive esophagitis; therapy for benign gastric ulcer; treatment of pathological hypersecretory conditions; prevention of upper GI bleeding.

Unlabeled Uses

Prevention of aspiration pneumonia and stress ulcers; herpes virus infection; chronic idiopathic urticaria; anaphylaxis (relieves dermatological symptoms only); dyspepsia; used before anesthesia to prevent aspiration pneumonitis; treatment of hyperparathyroidism and control of secary hyperparathyroidism in chronic hemodialysis patient; treatment of chronic viral warts in children.

➡◆ DRUG INTERACTIONS RELATED TO DENTAL THERAPEUTICS

Ketoconazole or itraconazole: Decreased ketoconazole or itraconazole effect (decreased absorption)
- Avoid concurrent use.

Aspirin: Possible aspirin toxicity (decreased metabolism)
- Avoid concurrent use.

Benzodiazepines: Possible benzodiazepine toxicity (decreased metabolism)
- Monitor clinical status.

Bupivacaine: Possible bupivacaine toxicity (decreased metabolism)
- Avoid concurrent use.

ADVERSE EFFECTS

CNS: Headache; somnolence; fatigue; dizziness; confusional states; hallucinations.
GI: Diarrhea.
RESP: Bronchospasm.
MISC: Gynecomastia; hypersensitivity reactions; transient pain at injection site; reversible exacerbation of joint symptoms with preexisting arthritis, including gouty arthritis.

CLINICAL IMPLICATIONS

General

• Determine why drug is being taken. Consider implications of condition on dental treatment.
• If patient has GI disease, consider semisupine chair position.
• Drugs that lower acidity in intestinal tract may interfere with absorption of some antibiotics (e.g., penicillin, tetracyclines).
• Use COX inhibitors with caution, they may exacerbate PUD and GERD.

Cimetigal — see cimetidine
Cimogal — see ciprofloxacin
Cinacort — see triamcinolone
Cipro — see ciprofloxacin
Cipro IV — see ciprofloxacin
Cipro XR — see ciprofloxacin
Ciprobiotic — see ciprofloxacin
Ciproflox — see ciprofloxacin

---

ciprofloxacin (sip-ROW-FLOX-uh-sin)

Ci'oxan, Cipro, Cipro IV, Cipro XR, Proquin XR

■◆■ Cimogal, Ciprobiotic, Ciproflox, Ciprofur, Ciproxina, Italnik, Kanzoflex, Microrgan, Mitroken, Nivoflox, Novoquin, Quinoflox, Sophixin, Suiflox, Zipra

Drug Class: Antibiotic, fluoroquinolone

PHARMACOLOGY

Action

Interferes with microbial DNA synthesis.

Uses

Treatment of infections of lower respiratory tract, skin and skin structure, bones and joints, and urinary tract; gonorrhea, chancroid, and infectious diarrhea caused by susceptible strains of specific organisms; typhoid fever; uncomplicated cervical and urethral gonorrhea; women with acute uncomplicated cystitis; acute sinusitis; nosocomial pneumonia; chronic bacterial prostatitis; complicated intra-abdominal infections; reduction of incidence or progression of inhalational anthrax following exposure to aerosolized *Bacillus anthracis*.
CIPRO IV: Empirical therapy for febrile neutropenic patients.
CIPRO XR: Uncomplicated and complicated UTIs; acute uncomplicated pyelonephritis.
OPHTHALMIC USE: Treatment of corneal ulcers and conjunctivitis caused by susceptible organisms.

Unlabeled Uses

Treatment of pulmonary exacerbations associated with cystic fibrosis; management of malignant external otitis, traveler's diarrhea, mycobacterial infections.

➡◀ DRUG INTERACTIONS RELATED TO DENTAL THERAPEUTICS

Diazepam: Possible diazepam toxicity (decreased metabolism)
• Monitor clinical status.

ADVERSE EFFECTS

⚠ **ORAL:** Dry, painful mouth (<1%); dysphagia.
CNS: Headache, restlessness (1%); agitation, confusion, delirium, toxic psychosis.
CVS: Hypertension, palpitations, syncope (<1%).
GI: Nausea (5%); diarrhea, vomiting, abdominal pain/discomfort (2%); constipation, flatulence, dyspepsia, pseudomembranous colitis.
MISC: Anaphylactic reactions, pancreatitis, vasculitis, photosensitivity (<1%).

CLINICAL IMPLICATIONS

General

• Determine why drug is being taken. Take precautions to avoid cross-contamination of microorganisms.
• If oral infection occurs that requires antibiotic therapy, select an appropriate product from a different class of anti-infectives.
• If prescribed by the DDS, ensure patient knows how to take the drug, how long it should be taken, and to report adverse effects (e.g., rash, difficult breathing, diarrhea, GI upset) immediately. See Chapter 4: *Medical Management of Odontogenic Infections.*
• Antibiotic-associated diarrhea can occur. Have patient contact DDS immediately if signs develop.
• Prolonged use of antibiotics may result in bacterial or fungal overgrowth of nonsusceptible microorganisms; anticipate candidiasis.

Ciprofur — see ciprofloxacin

Ciproxina — see ciprofloxacin

---

citalopram (sye-TAL-oh-pram)

Celexa

■▪■ Seropram

Drug Class: Antidepressant, selective serotonin reuptake inhibitor

PHARMACOLOGY

Action

Inhibits the CNS neuronal uptake of serotonin, potentiating serotonergic activity.

Uses

Treatment of major depression.

➡◀ DRUG INTERACTIONS RELATED TO DENTAL THERAPEUTICS

Tramadol: Increased risk of seizure (additive)
• Avoid concurrent use.

ADVERSE EFFECTS

⚠ **ORAL:** Dry mouth (20%); dental caries; taste perversion (>1%).
CNS: Dizziness; insomnia; somnolence; agitation; anxiety; anorexia; decreased libido; yawning; tremor.
CVS: Postural hypotension, tachycardia (>1%).
GI: Nausea; vomiting; diarrhea; dyspepsia.

RESP: Rhinitis, URI (5%); sinusitis (3%); cough (>1%).

MISC: Asthenia; arthralgia; fatigue; fever; myalgia; sweating.

CLINICAL IMPLICATIONS

General

- Determine why drug is being taken. Consider implications of condition on dental treatment.
- Determine ability to adapt to stress of dental treatment. Consider short appointments.
- Depressed or anxious patients may neglect self-care. Monitor for plaque control effectiveness.
- Chronic dry mouth is possible; anticipate increased caries and candidiasis.
- If GI or respiratory side effects occur, consider semisupine chair position.
- Monitor vital signs.
- *Postural hypotension:* Monitor BP at the beginning and end of each appointment; anticipate syncope. Have patient sit upright for several min at the end of the dental appointment before dismissing.

Oral Health Education

- If chronic dry mouth occurs, recommend home fluoride therapy and use of nonalcoholic oral health care products.

Citanest Forte with Epinephrine — see prilocaine HCl

Citanest Plain 4% Injection — see prilocaine HCl

Citoken — see piroxicam

Claravis — see isotretinoin

Clarinex — see desloratadine

Clarinex RediTabs — see desloratadine

---

clarithromycin (kluh-RITH-row-MY-sin)

Biaxin, Biaxin XL

I✦I Biaxin BID

▓▒▓ Adel, Klaricid, Mabicrol

Drug Class: Antibiotic, macrolide

PHARMACOLOGY

Action

Inhibits microbial protein synthesis.

Uses

Treatment of infections of respiratory tract, skin and skin structure; treatment of disseminated atypical mycobacterial infections caused by susceptible strains of specific microorganisms. Prevention of disseminated *Mycobacterium avium* complex disease in patients with advanced HIV infection. Clarithromycin in combination with omeprazole is indicated for the treatment of patients with an active duodenal ulcer associated with *Helicobacter pylori* infection.

CHILDREN: Acute otitis media.

➡← DRUG INTERACTIONS RELATED TO DENTAL THERAPEUTICS

Triazolam or midazolam: Possible triazolam or midazolam toxicity (decreased metabolism)
- Avoid concurrent use.

ADVERSE EFFECTS

⚠ **ORAL:** Abnormal taste (3%); glossitis; stomatitis; candidiasis.

CNS: Headache; dizziness; insomnia; nightmares; vertigo.

GI: Diarrhea; nausea; vomiting; dyspepsia; abdominal pain/discomfort.

RESP: Dyspnea; increased cough.

MISC: Urticaria; hypersensitivity; anaphylaxis; Stevens-Johnson syndrome.

CLINICAL IMPLICATIONS

General

- Determine why drug is being taken. Take precautions to avoid cross-contamination of microorganisms.
- If oral infection occurs that requires antibiotic therapy, select an appropriate product from a different class of anti-infectives.
- If prescribed by the DDS, ensure patient knows how to take the drug, how long it should be taken, and to report adverse effects (e.g., rash, difficult breathing, diarrhea, GI upset) immediately. See Chapter 4: *Medical Management of Odontogenic Infections*.
- Antibiotic-associated diarrhea can occur. Have patient contact DDS immediately if signs develop.
- Prolonged use of antibiotics may result in bacterial or fungal overgrowth of nonsusceptible microorganisms; anticipate candidiasis.
- If GI side effects occur, consider semisupine chair position.

Claritin — see loratadine

Claritin Hives Relief — see loratadine

Claritin Kids — see loratadine

Claritin Non-Drowsy Allergy — see loratadine

Claritin RediTabs — see loratadine

Claritin Skin Itch Relief — see hydrocortisone

Clarityne — see loratadine

clavulanate potassium/amoxicillin — see amoxicillin/clavulanate potassium

Clavulin — see amoxicillin/clavulanate potassium

---

clemastine fumarate (KLEM-ass-teen FEW-muh-rate)

Clemastine Fumarate, Dayhist-1, Tavist Allergy

◼◼◼ **Tavist**

Drug Class: Antihistamine, Ethanolamine

PHARMACOLOGY

Action

Competitively antagonizes histamine at H_1 receptor sites.

Uses

Relief of symptoms associated with allergic rhinitis or other upper respiratory allergies, such as sneezing, rhinorrhea, pruritus, and lacrimation; relief of mild, uncomplicated allergic skin manifestation of urticaria and angioedema.

➡◀ DRUG INTERACTIONS RELATED TO DENTAL THERAPEUTICS

No documented drug-drug interactions. The absence of evidence is not evidence of safety.

ADVERSE EFFECTS

⚠ **ORAL:** Stomatitis, dry mouth; (nasal spray) aphthous stomatitis, bitter, taste, taste loss.

CNS: Acute labyrinthitis; confusion; convulsions; disturbed coordination; dizziness; euphoria; excitation; fatigue; hysteria; insomnia; irritability; nervousness; neuritis; paresthesias; restlessness; sedation; sleepiness; tremor; vertigo.

CVS: Postural hypotension; bradycardia or tachycardia; palpitation.

GI: Epigastric distress; nausea; vomiting; diarrhea; constipation.

RESP: Thickening of bronchial secretions; chest tightness; wheezing; nasal stuffiness; dry nose and throat; sore throat; respiratory depression.

MISC: Hypersensitivity reactions; photosensitivity.

CLINICAL IMPLICATIONS

General
- Determine why drug is being taken. Consider implications of condition on dental treatment.
- Consider semisupine chair position to control effects of postnasal drainage.
- Be aware that patients with multiple allergies are at increased risk for allergy to dental drugs.
- Monitor vital signs.
- *Postural hypotension:* Monitor BP at the beginning and end of each appointment; anticipate syncope. Have patient sit upright for several min at the end of the dental appointment before dismissing.
- If GI side effects occur, consider semisupine chair position.
- Chronic dry mouth is possible; anticipate increased caries and candidiasis.

Oral Health Education
- If chronic dry mouth occurs, recommend home fluoride therapy and use of nonalcoholic oral health care products.

Cleocin — see clindamycin
Cleocin Pediatric — see clindamycin
Cleocin Phosphate — see clindamycin
Cleocin T — see clindamycin
Clexane — see enoxaparin sodium
Climaderm — see estradiol
Climara — see estradiol
Clindagel — see clindamycin
ClindaMax — see clindamycin
ClindaMax Lotion — see clindamycin

---

 clindamycin (KLIN-duh-MY-sin)
(clindamycin HCl, clindamycin palmitate HCl, clindamycin phosphate)

Cleocin: Capsules: 75, 150, 300 mg (as HCl)
Cleocin Pediatric: Granules for Oral Solution: 75 mg per 5 mL (as palmitate)
Cleocin, Cleocin Phosphate, Cleocin T, Clindets, Clindagel, ClindaMax, ClindaMax Lotion

■✦■ **Dalacin C Phosphate, Dalacin T Topical, Dalacin C, ratio-Clindamycin**

Drug Class: Antibiotic, lincosamide

PHARMACOLOGY

Action
Suppresses bacterial protein synthesis.

Uses
Treatment of serious infections caused by susceptible strains of specific microorganisms; treatment of acne vulgaris (topical use); treatment of bacterial vaginosis (vaginal use).

Contraindications
Hypersensitivity to lincosamides or any product component; history of regional enteritis, ulcerative colitis, or antibiotic-associated colitis.

Usual Dosage
Orodental Infection
ADULTS: *PO:* 150 to 300 mg q 6 hr. *IM/IV:* 0.6 to 2.7 g/day divided into 2 to 4 equal doses. For more serious infections, these doses may need to be increased. Do not use more than 600 mg in single IM injection.
CHILDREN: CLINDAMYCIN HCL: *PO:* 8 to 20 mg/kg/day divided into 3 to 4 doses.
CLINDAMYCIN PALMITATE HCL: *PO:* 8 to 25 mg/kg/day divided into 3 to 4 doses.

Pharmacokinetics
ABSORP: *Oral:* Rapidly absorbed. C_{max} is 2.5 mcg/mL. T_{max} is 45 min. Bioavailability is 90%. *IM:* T_{max} is 3 hr (adults) and 1 hr (children). *IV:* C_{max} is 7 to 14 mcg/mL. *Vaginal:* About 5% is absorbed.

DIST: Widely distributed (including bones); no significant levels attained in CSF. Excreted in breast milk.

METAB: Rapidly converted to active clindamycin.

EXCRET: The $t_{1/2}$ is 2.4 to 3.2 hr. About 10% of bioactivity is excreted in the urine and 3.6% in the feces; the remainder is excreted as inactive metabolites.

SPECIAL POP: *Renal failure:* The $t_{1/2}$ is increased slightly. Dosage adjustment is not usually needed.
Hepatic failure: The $t_{1/2}$ is increased slightly. Dosage adjustment is not usually needed.
Elderly: The $t_{1/2}$ is increased slightly. Dosage adjustment is not usually needed.

➡⬅ DRUG INTERACTIONS
Cyclosporine: Possible decreased cyclosporine effect (mechanism unknown)
 • Avoid concurrent use or monitor cyclosporine concentration.

ADVERSE EFFECTS
⚠ **ORAL:** Unpleasant taste, esophagitis.

CVS: Hypotension; cardiopulmonary arrest.

GI: Colitis, including pseudomembranous colitis (0.01% to 10%, more frequent with oral administration); diarrhea; nausea; vomiting; abdominal pain; esophagitis; anorexia.

HEMA: Neutropenia; leukopenia; agranulocytosis; thrombocytopenic purpura.

MISC: Pain after injection; induration and sterile abscess after IM injection; thrombophlebitis after IV infusion; anaphylaxis; transient eosinophilia, polyarthritis (rare); hypersensitivity (skin rash, urticaria, erythema multiforme, anaphylaxis); jaundice, liver function abnormalities. Topical or vaginal use may theoretically produce adverse effects seen with systemic use as a result of absorption.

CLINICAL IMPLICATIONS

General
When prescribed by DDS:
 • *Lactation:* Excreted in breast milk.
 • *Elderly:* May not tolerate diarrhea well (dehydration).

- *Hypersensitivity:* Use drug with caution in patients with asthma or significant allergies or in those who are atopic.
- *Renal failure:* Use drug with caution in patients with severe renal disease with severe metabolic aberrations. Dosage modifications may be necessary.
- *Hepatic failure:* Use drug with caution in patients with severe hepatic disease with severe metabolic aberrations.
- *Superinfection:* May result in bacterial or fungal overgrowth of nonsusceptible organisms.
- *Tartrazine sensitivity:* Some products contain tartrazine, which may cause allergic-type reactions in susceptible individuals.
- Monitor for signs of infection, especially fever, and for positive response to antibiotic therapy.
- Monitor patient for GI, dermatological, and general body side effects, and signs of superinfection. Report to health care provider if noted and significant. Immediately report severe diarrhea, diarrhea containing blood or pus, or severe abdominal cramping.

Pregnancy Risk Category: Category B.

Oral Health Education
When prescribed by DDS:

- Explain name, dose, action, and potential side effects of drug.
- Instruct patient to take exactly as prescribed and not to change the dosage or discontinue therapy unless advised by health care provider.
- Instruct patient to complete entire course of therapy, even if symptoms of infection have disappeared.
- Instruct patient to notify health care provider if infection does not appear to be improving or appears to be getting worse.
- Advise patient to report the following signs of superinfection to health care provider: black "furry tongue," white patches in mouth, foul-smelling stools, or vaginal itching or discharge.
- Warn patient that diarrhea containing blood or pus may be a sign of a serious disorder and to seek medical care if noted and not treat at home. Caution patient that this may occur even wk after completing therapy.
- Advise patient to report any other bothersome side effect to health care provider.
- Advise women to notify health care provider if pregnant, planning to become pregnant, or breast feeding.
- Instruct patient not to take any prescription or OTC medications, dietary supplements, or herbal preparations unless advised by health care provider.
- Advise patient that follow-up examinations and laboratory tests may be required to monitor therapy and to keep appointments.

Capsules and Oral Solution

- Advise patient or caregiver that capsules and oral solution can be taken without regard to meals but to take with food if stomach upset occurs.
- Advise patient to take capsules with a full glass of water.
- Advise patient or caregiver that oral solution should be administered using a dosing spoon or syringe.

---

clindamycin HCl — see clindamycin

clindamycin palmitate HCl — see clindamycin

clindamycin phosphate — see clindamycin

Clindets — see clindamycin

Clinoril — see sulindac

---

 clobetasol propionate (kloe-BEE-tah-sahl PRO-pee-oh-nate)

Cormax: Ointment: 0.05%
Embeline: Cream: 0.05%; Gel: 0.05%; Ointment: 0.05%

Embeline E: Cream: 0.05%
Temovate: Cream: 0.05%; Gel: 0.05%; Ointment: 0.05%
Clobex, Olux, Temovate Emollient
∎✳∎ **Dermovate, Gen-Clobetasol Cream/Ointment, Gen-Clobetasol Scalp Application, Novo-Clobetasol**

Drug Class: Corticosteroid, topical

PHARMACOLOGY

Action
Topical glucocorticoid with anti-inflammatory, antipruritic, and vasoconstrictive properties. Thought to act by inducing phospholipase A_2 inhibitory proteins, thus controlling biosynthesis of potent mediators of inflammation.

Uses
Relief of inflammatory and ulcerative conditions (Temovate); pruritic manifestations of corticosteroid-responsive dermatoses; moderate to severe plaque-type psoriasis.

Contraindications
Primary scalp infections (scalp application formulation). Standard considerations.

Usual Dosage
Oral inflammatory ulceration
Topical: Apply thin film to affected area qid.

➔✚ DRUG INTERACTIONS
No documented drug-drug interactions. The absence of evidence is not evidence of safety.

ADVERSE EFFECTS
MISC: Burning; itching; erythema; cracking of skin.

CLINICAL IMPLICATIONS

General
When prescribed by DDS:
* *Lactation:* Undetermined.
* *Children:* Not recommended in children younger than 12 yr of age. Children are at higher risk than adults of hypothalamic-pituitary-adrenal (HPA) axis suppression and Cushing syndrome when they are treated with topical corticosteroids.
* *Systemic:* Systemic absorption may produce HPA axis suppression and systemic side effects; HPA axis suppression shown at doses as low as 2 g/day.
* Therapy should be discontinued when control has been achieved. If no improvement is seen within 2 wk, reassessment of the diagnosis may be necessary.
* Obtain patient history, including drug history and any known allergies.

Pregnancy Risk Category: Category C.

Oral Health Education
When prescribed by DDS:
* Explain name, action, and potential side effects of drug.
* Teach patient or caregiver proper technique for applying cream, ointment, lotion, or gel: wash hands; apply sufficient cream or ointment to cover affected areas sparingly and gently massage into skin; wash hands after applying cream or ointment.
* Advise patient to apply medication as directed by health care provider.
* Advise patient that if a dose is missed to apply it as soon as remembered and then continue on regular schedule. If it is almost time for the next application, instruct patient to skip the dose and continue on regular schedule. Caution patient not to apply double doses.
* Caution patient to avoid contact with the eyes. Advise patient that if medication does come into contact with the eyes, to wash eyes with large amounts of cool water and contact health care provider if eye irritation occurs.

- Advise patient that symptoms should begin to improve fairly soon after starting treatment and to notify health care provider if condition does not improve, worsens, or if application site reactions (e.g., burning, stinging, redness, itching) develop.
- Advise patient that therapy is usually discontinued when control has been achieved.
- Advise women to notify health care provider if pregnant, planning to become pregnant, or breast feeding.
- Caution patient not to take any prescription or OTC drugs, dietary supplements, or herbal preparations without consulting health care provider.
- Advise patient that follow-up visits to monitor response to treatment may be required and to keep appointments.

Clobex — see clobetasol propionate

 # clocortolone pivalate (kloe-CORE-toe-lone PIH-vah-late)

Cloderm: Cream: Clocortolone pivalate 0.1%

Drug Class: Corticosteroid, topical (group III medium potency)

PHARMACOLOGY

Action

Topically applied corticosteroids diffuse across cell membranes to interact with cytoplasmic receptors located in both the dermal and intradermal cells similar to effects caused by systemic corticosteroids. Primary effect is due to an anti-inflammatory activity that is nonspecific.

Uses

Relief of inflammatory and pruritic manifestations of corticosteroid-responsive dermatoses: Some of the conditions in which topical corticosteroids have been proven effective include contact dermatitis, atopic dermatitis, nummular eczema, stasis eczema, asteatotic eczema, lichen planus, lichen simplex chronicus, insect and arthropod bite reactions, first- and second-degree localized burns, and sunburn.

Alternative/adjunctive treatment: Psoriasis, seborrheic dermatitis, severe diaper rash, dysidrosis, nodular prurigo, chronic discoid lupus erythematosus, alopecia areata, lymphocytic infiltration of the skin, mycosis fungoides, and familial benign pemphigus of Hailey-Hailey.

Possibly effective in the following conditions: Bullous pemphigoid, cutaneous mastocytosis, lichen sclerosus et atrophicus, and vitiligo.

Nonprescription hydrocortisone preparations: Temporary relief of itching associated with minor skin irritations, inflammation and rashes due to eczema, insect bites, poison ivy, poison oak, poison sumac, soaps, detergents, cosmetics, jewelry, seborrheic dermatitis, psoriasis, and external genital and anal itching.

Contraindications

Hypersensitivity to any component; monotherapy in primary bacterial infections such as impetigo, paronychia, erysipelas, cellulitis, angular cheilitis, erythrasma (clobetasol), treatment of rosacea, perioral dermatitis, or acne; use on the face, groin, or axilla (very high or high-potency agents); ophthalmic use (prolonged ocular exposure may cause steroid-induced glaucoma and cataracts). When applied to the eyelids or skin near the eyes, the drug may enter the eyes.

Usual Dosage

Mucous membrane inflammation or ulceration

CREAM 0.1%

ADULTS: Apply sparingly to affected areas 2 to 4 times daily.
CHILDREN: Limit to smallest amount compatible with therapy.

Pharmacokinetics

ABSORP: Absorbed systemically, especially when applied over large surface area.

➡️⬅ DRUG INTERACTIONS

No documented drug-drug interactions significant to dentistry. The absence of evidence is not evidence of safety.

ADVERSE EFFECTS

⚠️ **ORAL:** Perioral dermatitis; thinning of mucosa.
MISC: Burning; dryness; itching.

CLINICAL IMPLICATIONS

General

• Anticipate oral candidiasis when steroids are used.

Pregnancy Risk Category: Category C.

Oral Health Education

If prescribed by DDS:

• Ensure patient understands how to use product, amount to apply, method of application, and signs of adverse effects.
• Apply ointments, creams, or gels sparingly in a light film; rub in gently. Washing or soaking the area before application may increase drug penetration.
• Use only as directed. Do not put bandages, dressing, cosmetics, or other skin products over the treated area unless directed by your physician.
• Notify dentist if the condition being treated gets worse, or if burning, swelling, or redness develops.
• Avoid prolonged use on the face and in skin creases unless directed by dentist. Avoid contact with the eyes.
• If you forget a dose, apply it as soon as you remember and continue on your regular schedule. If it is almost time for the next application, wait and continue on your regular schedule. Do not apply double doses.
• *For parents of pediatric patients:* Do not use tight-fitting diapers or plastic pants on a child treated in the diaper area; these garments may work like occlusive dressings and cause more of the drug to be absorbed into your child's body.

Cloderm — see clocortolone pivalate

---

clomipramine HCl (kloe-MIH-pruh-meen HIGH-droe-KLOR-ide)

Anafranil

■✦■ **Apo-Clomipramine, Gen-Clomipramine, Novo-Clopamine**

Drug Class: Tricyclic antidepressant

PHARMACOLOGY

Action

Inhibits reuptake of serotonin in CNS.

Uses

Relief of obsessive-compulsive disorder.

Unlabeled Uses

Treatment of panic disorder or chronic pain (e.g., migraine, chronic tension headache, diabetic neuropathy, tic douloureux, cancer pain, peripheral neuropathy, postherpetic neuralgia, arthritic pain).

➡️⬅ DRUG INTERACTIONS RELATED TO DENTAL THERAPEUTICS

Tramadol: Increased risk of seizure (additive)
• Avoid concurrent use.

Sympathomimetic amines: Increased risk of hypertension and hypertensive crisis
- Use local anesthetic agents containing a vasoconstrictor with caution.
- Monitor blood pressure.

ADVERSE EFFECTS

⚠ **ORAL:** Dry mouth; halitosis.

CNS: Hyperthermia; confusion; hallucinations; delusions; nervousness; restlessness; agitation; panic; insomnia; nightmares; mania; exacerbation of psychosis; drowsiness; dizziness; weakness; fatigue; emotional lability; aggressive reaction; seizures.

CVS: Atrial flutter, bradycardia, ventricular tachycardia, postural hypotension.

GI: Nausea; vomiting; anorexia; GI distress; diarrhea; flatulence; constipation.

RESP: Pharyngitis; rhinitis; sinusitis; laryngitis; cough.

MISC: Numbness; tremors; breast enlargement; nonpuerperal lactation; extrapyramidal symptoms (e.g., pseudoparkinsonism, movement disorders, akathisia); vestibular disorder; muscle weakness; significant weight gain; hypothyroidism.

CLINICAL IMPLICATIONS

General
- Determine why drug is being taken. Consider implications of condition on dental treatment.
- Depressed or anxious patients may neglect self-care. Monitor for plaque control effectiveness.
- Determine ability to adapt to stress of dental treatment. Consider short appointments.
- Chronic dry mouth is possible; anticipate increased caries and candidiasis.
- Monitor vital signs.
- If GI side effects occur, consider semisupine chair position.
- *Postural hypotension:* Monitor BP at the beginning and end of each appointment; anticipate syncope. Have patient sit upright for several min at the end of the dental appointment before dismissing.
- Extrapyramidal behaviors can complicate performance of oral procedures. If present consult with MD to consider medication changes.

Oral Health Education
- If chronic dry mouth occurs, recommend home fluoride therapy and use of nonalcoholic oral health care products.
- Evaluate manual dexterity; consider need for power toothbrush.

---

 clonazepam (kloe-NAY-ze-pam)

Klonopin, Klonopin Wafers: Tablets: 0.5, 1, 2 mg; Tablets, orally disintegrating: 0.125, 0.25, 0.5, 1, 2 mg

■✢■ Apo-Clonazepam, Gen-Clonazepam, Novo-Clonazepam, Nu-Clonazepam, PMS-Clonazepam, ratio-Clonazepam, Rivotril, Rhoxal-clonazepam

■✦■ Kenoket, Rivotril

Drug Class: Anticonvulsant; Benzodiazepine
DEA Schedule: Schedule IV

PHARMACOLOGY

Action
Potentiates action of GABA, inhibitory neurotransmitter, resulting in increased neuronal inhibition and CNS depression, especially in limbic system and reticular formation.

Uses
Treatment of Lennox-Gastaut syndrome; management of akinetic and myoclonic seizures and absence seizures unresponsive to succinimides; panic disorders.

Unlabeled Uses

Treatment of restless leg syndrome, parkinsonian dysarthria, acute manic episodes of bipolar affective disorder, multifocal tic disorders, and neuralgias; adjunctive therapy for schizophrenia.

Contraindications

Hypersensitivity to benzodiazepines; psychoses; acute narrow-angle glaucoma; significant liver disease; shock; coma; acute alcohol intoxication.

➜← DRUG INTERACTIONS

No documented drug-drug interactions significant to dentistry. The absence of evidence is not evidence of safety.

ADVERSE EFFECTS

⚠ **ORAL:** Dry mouth, coated tongue, thirst (infrequent); excess salivation (rare).

CVS: SEIZURE DISORDERS: CV collapse; hypotension; phlebitis or thrombosis at IV sites.

CNS: PANIC DISORDER: Somnolence (50%); dizziness (12%); abnormal coordination (9%); ataxia, depression (8%); memory disturbance (5%); nervousness, reduced intellectual ability, dysarthria (4%); decreased libido (3%); emotional lability, confusion (2%).
SEIZURE DISORDERS: Drowsiness (50%); ataxia (30%); confusion; dizziness; lethargy; fatigue; apathy; memory impairment; disorientation; anterograde amnesia; restlessness; headache; slurred speech; aphonia; stupor; coma; euphoria; irritability; vivid dreams; psychomotor retardation; paradoxic reactions (e.g., anger, hostility, mania, insomnia, muscle spasms).

GI: PANIC DISORDER: Constipation (5%); decreased appetite (3%); abdominal pain (2%).
SEIZURE DISORDERS: Constipation; diarrhea; nausea; anorexia; vomiting.

RESP: PANIC DISORDER: Upper respiratory tract infection (10%); sinusitis (8%); rhinitis, coughing (4%); bronchitis (2%).

MISC: PANIC DISORDER: Fatigue (9%); influenza (5%); allergic reaction, myalgia (4%).
SEIZURE DISORDERS: Dependence/withdrawal syndrome (e.g., confusion, abnormal perception of movement, depersonalization, muscle twitching, psychosis, paranoid delusions, seizures).

CLINICAL IMPLICATIONS

General

- Determine why drug is being taken. Consider implications of condition on dental treatment.
- Determine ability to adapt to stress of dental treatment. Consider short appointments.
- Consider medical consult to determine disease control and influence on dental treatment.
- Determine level of disease control, type and frequency of seizure, and compliance with medication regimen.
- Chronic dry mouth is possible; anticipate increased caries and candidiasis.
- Geriatric, debilitated, and pediatric patients are more sensitive to the CNS effects of benzodiazepines.
- Monitor vital signs.

Pregnancy Risk Category: Category D.

Oral Health Education

- If chronic dry mouth occurs, recommend home fluoride therapy and use of nonalcoholic oral health care products.
- Evaluate manual dexterity; consider need for power toothbrush.

clonidine HCl (KLOE-nih-DEEN HIGH-droe-KLOR-ide)
Catapres, Catapres-TTS-1, Catapres-TTS-2, Catapres-TTS-3, Duraclon

■✦■ **APO-Clonidine, Dixarit, Novo-Clonidine, Nu-Clonidine**

■▨■ **Catapresan-100**

Drug Class: Antihypertensive; Antiadrenergic; Analgesic, centrally acting

PHARMACOLOGY
Action
Stimulates central alpha-adrenergic receptors to inhibit sympathetic cardioaccelerator and vasoconstrictor centers.

Uses
Management of hypertension. Used in combination with opiates for epidural use for relief of cancer pain.

Unlabeled Uses
Treatment of constitutional growth delay in children; diabetic diarrhea; Tourette syndrome; hypertensive urgencies; menopausal flushing; postherpetic neuralgia; diagnosis of pheochromocytoma; ulcerative colitis; reduction of allergen-induced inflammatory reactions in patients with extrinsic asthma; facilitation of smoking cessation; alcohol withdrawal; methadone/opiate detoxification.

➡◀ DRUG INTERACTIONS RELATED TO DENTAL THERAPEUTICS
No documented drug-drug interactions. The absence of evidence is not evidence of safety.

ADVERSE EFFECTS
⚠ **ORAL:** Dry mouth (40%); taste disturbances; angioedema of face and tongue.

CNS: Drowsiness; dizziness; sedation; nightmares; insomnia; nervousness or agitation; headache; fatigue.

CVS: Syncope; postural hypotension; tachycardia or bradycardia; palpitations.

GI: Constipation; anorexia; nausea; vomiting.

MISC: Increased sensitivity to alcohol; pallor; muscle weakness; muscle or joint pain; cramps of lower limbs; weakly positive Coombs test result; thrombocytopenia (rare).

CLINICAL IMPLICATIONS
General
* Determine why drug is being taken. Consider implications of condition on dental treatment.
* *Postural hypotension:* Monitor BP at the beginning and end of each appointment; anticipate syncope. Have patient sit upright for several min at the end of the dental appointment before dismissing.
* Chronic dry mouth is possible; anticipate increased caries and candidiasis.
* Monitor vital signs (e.g., BP, pulse pressure, rate, and rhythm) at each appointment to assess disease control. Do not provide elective dental treatment when BP is ≥180/110 or in the presence of other high-risk CV conditions. Refer to the section entitled "The Patient Taking Cardiovascular Drugs" in Chapter 6: *Clinical Medicine.*
* Use local anesthetic agents with vasoconstrictor with caution based on functional capacity of the patient and use aspirating technique to prevent intravascular injection.
* Determine ability to adapt to stress of dental treatment. Consider short appointments.
* Thrombocytopenia rarely reported; anticipate increased bleeding.

Oral Health Education
* If chronic dry mouth occurs, recommend home fluoride therapy and use of nonalcoholic oral health care products.
* Encourage daily plaque control procedures for effective self-care in patients at risk for cardiovascular disease.

Clonodifen — see diclofenac

clopidogrel (kloh-PID-oh-grel)
Plavix
Drug Class: Antiplatelet, aggregation inhibitor

PHARMACOLOGY
Action
Clopidogrel is a thienopyridine derivative, chemically related to ticlopidine, which inhibits platelet aggregation. It acts by irreversibly modifying the platelet adenosine diphosphate (ADP) receptor. Therefore, platelet aggregation is inhibited for both ADP-mediated and ADP-amplified (by other agonists) platelet activation. Consequently, platelets exposed to clopidogrel are affected for the remainder of their lifespan.

Uses
Reduction of atherosclerotic events (e.g., MI, stroke, vascular death) in patients with atherosclerosis documented by recent stroke, recent MI, or established peripheral arterial disease. Treatment of acute coronary syndrome (i.e., unstable angina/non-Q-wave MI), including patients managed medically and those managed with percutaneous coronary intervention (with or without stent) or coronary artery bypass graft.

➡◀ DRUG INTERACTIONS RELATED TO DENTAL THERAPEUTICS
COX-1 inhibitors: Possible increased bleeding (additive)
* Avoid concurrent use.

ADVERSE EFFECTS
⚠ **ORAL:** Taste disorder.
CNS: Headache (8%); dizziness (6%); depression (4%); confusion; hallucinations.
CVS: Chest pain; edema, hypertension (4%).
GI: Abdominal pain (6%); dyspepsia, diarrhea (5%); nausea (3%); colitis (including ulcerative or lymphocytic).
RESP: URI (9%); dyspnea (5%); rhinitis, bronchitis (4%); coughing (3%); influenza-like syndrome (8%); bronchospasm.
MISC: Accidental injury, pain (6%); fatigue (3%); hypersensitivity reactions; anaphylactoid reactions; thrombocytopenia.

CLINICAL IMPLICATIONS
General
* Ensure that clopidogrel is discontinued 5 days prior to elective surgery in patients in whom an antiplatelet effect is not desired.
* Determine why drug is being taken. Consider implications of condition on dental treatment.
* Determine bleeding time before completing procedures that may result in significant bleeding. Safe levels are <20 min.
* If uncontrolled bleeding develops, use hemostatic agents and positive pressure to induce hemostasis. Do not dismiss patient until bleeding is controlled.
* Thrombocytopenia rarely reported; anticipate increased bleeding.

Oral Health Education
* Encourage daily plaque control procedures for effective, nontraumatic self-care.

Clopsine — see clozapine

clorazepate dipotassium (klor-AZE-uh-PATE DIE-poe-TASS-ee-uhm)
Tranxene-SD, Tranxene-SD Half Strength, Tranxene T-tab

▮✦▮ Apo-Clorazepate, Novo-Clopate
▮✦▮ Tranxene

Drug Class: Antianxiety; Benzodiazepine
DEA Schedule: Schedule IV

PHARMACOLOGY

Action

Potentiates action of GABA, an inhibitory neurotransmitter, resulting in increased neuronal inhibition and CNS depression, especially in limbic system and reticular formation.

Uses

Management of anxiety disorders; relief of acute alcohol withdrawal symptoms; adjunctive therapy in management of partial seizures.

Unlabeled Uses

Treatment of irritable bowel syndrome.

➡◆ DRUG INTERACTIONS RELATED TO DENTAL THERAPEUTICS

No documented drug-drug interactions. The absence of evidence is not evidence of safety.

ADVERSE EFFECTS

⚠ **ORAL:** Dry mouth; coated tongue.

CNS: Drowsiness; confusion; ataxia; dizziness; lethargy; fatigue; apathy; memory impairment; disorientation; anterograde amnesia; restlessness; nervousness; headache; slurred speech; loss of voice; stupor; coma; euphoria; irritability; vivid dreams; psychomotor retardation; paradoxical reactions (e.g., anger, hostility, mania, insomnia, muscle spasms); depression; tremor.

CVS: Bradycardia or tachycardia; hypotension or hypertension; palpitations.

GI: Constipation; diarrhea; nausea; anorexia; vomiting.

MISC: Dependence/withdrawal syndrome; blood dyscrasias (e.g., leukopenia, agranulocytosis, thrombocytopenia).

CLINICAL IMPLICATIONS

General

- Determine why drug is being taken. Consider implications of condition on dental treatment.
- Chronic dry mouth is possible; anticipate increased caries and candidiasis.
- Determine ability to adapt to stress of dental treatment. Consider short appointments.
- Depressed or anxious patients may neglect self-care. Monitor for plaque control effectiveness.
- Monitor vital signs.
- If GI side effects occur, consider semisupine chair position.
- Blood dyscrasias rarely reported; anticipate increased bleeding, infection, and poor healing.
- *When prescribed by DDS:* May produce sedation, interfere with eye-hand coordination, and the ability to operate mechanical equipment. Inform patient not to drive, sign important papers, or operate mechanical equipment.

Oral Health Education

- If chronic dry mouth occurs, recommend home fluoride therapy and use of nonalcoholic oral health care products.
- Encourage daily plaque control procedures for effective, nontraumatic self-care.
- *When prescribed by DDS:* Warn patient not to drink alcoholic products while taking the drug.

Clorimet — see metoclopramide
Clostedal — see carbamazepine

clotrimazole (kloe-TRIM-uh-zole)

Mycelex: Troches: 10 mg
Cruex, Desenex, Gyne-Lotrimin 3, Gyne-Lotrimin 3 Combination Pack, Gyne-Lotrimin 7, Lotrimin AF, Mycelex-7, Mycelex-7 Combination Pack

■✦■ Canesten

■■■ Candimon, Lotrimin

Drug Class: Topical, antifungal

PHARMACOLOGY

Action
Inhibits yeast growth by increasing cell membrane permeability in susceptible fungi.

Uses
TOPICAL USE: Treatment of tinea pedis (athlete's foot), tinea cruris (jock itch), tinea corporis (ringworm), candidiasis, and tinea versicolor.
ORAL USE (TROCHE): Treatment of oropharyngeal candidiasis; prophylaxis of oropharyngeal candidiasis in specific groups of immunocompromised patients.
VAGINAL USE: Treatment of vulvovaginal candidiasis.

Contraindications
Standard considerations.

Usual Dosage
Oropharyngeal candidiasis
ADULTS AND CHILDREN OVER 3 YR: *PO:* One 10-mg troche (lozenge) dissolved slowly in the mouth 5 times/day for 14 days.
Prophylaxis
PO: One 10-mg troche dissolved slowly in the mouth tid.

Pharmacokinetics
ABSORP: After oral administration, the mean serum concentrations were about 4.98 and 3.23 mg/mL at 30 and 60 min, respectively. Minimally absorbed following topical administration.

➡✦ DRUG INTERACTIONS
No documented drug-drug interactions. The absence of evidence is not evidence of safety.

ADVERSE EFFECTS
GI: Nausea, vomiting (troche).

CLINICAL IMPLICATIONS

General
When prescribed by DDS:
- *Lactation:* Undetermined.
- Obtain patient history, including drug history and any known allergies. Note condition(s) that may predispose to recurrent infection (e.g., diabetes, concurrent antibiotic therapy, immunosuppression, HIV, AIDS) or liver disease (oral troche).
- Ensure that transaminases are determined periodically during prolonged therapy with oral troches, especially in patient with preexisting hepatic impairment.
- Monitor patient's response to therapy. Notify health care provider if symptoms do not improve or worsen.

Children
- *Oral (troches):* Safety not established in children younger than 3 yr.
- *Topical:* Safety and efficacy not established in children younger than 2 yr.
- *Recurrent infections:* May indicate underlying medical cause, including diabetes or HIV infection.

Pregnancy Risk Category: Category C (troches).

Oral Health Education
When prescribed by DDS:
- Explain name, dose, action, and potential side effects of drug.
- Instruct patient using OTC products to carefully read and follow the instructions that come with each package.
- Advise patient or caregiver that follow-up visits may be necessary and to keep appointments.

Oral Troche
- Teach patient proper technique for using oral troche as follows: slowly dissolve troche in mouth and retain saliva as long as possible before swallowing. Caution patient not to chew or swallow the troche.
- Advise patient to notify health care provider if any of the following occur: nausea, vomiting, abdominal cramps or discomfort, unpleasant mouth sensations, symptoms do not improve or worsen.

---

clozapine (KLOE-zuh-PEEN)

Clozapine, Clozaril, FazaClo

▌✦▌ Rhoxal-clozapine

▌✦▌ Clopsine, Leponex

Drug Class: Antipsychotic

PHARMACOLOGY
Action
Interferes with dopamine binding at D_1, D_2, D_3, and D_5 receptors in CNS; antagonizes adrenergic, cholinergic, histaminergic, and serotonergic neurotransmission.

Uses
Management of severely and chronically mentally ill schizophrenic patients who have not responded to or cannot tolerate standard antipsychotic drug treatment; to reduce risk of recurrent suicidal behavior in patients with schizophrenia or schizoaffective disorder who are judged to be at chronic risk for reexperiencing suicidal behavior (except orally disintegrating tablets).

➡◆ DRUG INTERACTIONS RELATED TO DENTAL THERAPEUTICS
Benzodiazepines: Syncope and respiratory arrest (mechanism unknown)
- Avoid concurrent use.

ADVERSE EFFECTS
⚠ **ORAL:** Salivation (31%); dry mouth (6%); salivary gland swelling, tongue numb/sore (1%).

CNS: Drowsiness/sedation (39%); dizziness/vertigo (19%); headache (7%); tremor, syncope (6%); disturbed sleep/nightmares, restlessness, hypokinesia/akinesia, agitation (4%); seizures, rigidity, akathisia, confusion (3%); fatigue, insomnia (2%); hyperkinesia, weakness, lethargy, ataxia, slurred speech, epileptiform movements/myoclonic jerks (high dose), depression, anxiety (1%); delirium; abnormal EEG; exacerbation of psychosis; myoclonus; paresthesia; mild cataplexy; status epilepticus.

CVS: Postural hypotension; syncope.

GI: Constipation (14%); nausea (5%); abdominal discomfort/heartburn (4%); nausea/vomiting (3%); diarrhea (2%); liver test abnormality, anorexia (1%); acute pancreatitis; dysphagia; fecal impaction; intestinal obstruction/paralytic ileus.

RESP: Dyspnea (1%); aspiration; pleural effusion.

MISC: Sweating (6%); fever (5%); muscle weakness; pain (back, neck, legs); muscle spasm; muscle pain/ache; hypersensitivity reactions; photosensitivity; vasculitis; myasthenic syndrome; rhabdomyolysis; creatine phosphokinase elevation; agranulocytosis (high risk).

CLINICAL IMPLICATIONS

General
- *General anesthesia:* Because of the CNS effects of clozapine, caution is advised in patients receiving general anesthesia.
- *Tardive dyskinesia:* This syndrome of potentially irreversible, involuntary dyskinetic movements has occurred with other antipsychotic agents. Incidence is highest among elderly, especially women.
- Due to the high risk for agranulocytosis, this drug is available only through a distribution system that ensures daily monitoring of WBC.
- Blood dyscrasias reported; anticipate increased bleeding, infection, and poor healing.
- Determine why drug is being taken. Consider implications of condition on dental treatment.
- Determine ability to adapt to stress of dental treatment. Consider short appointments.
- *Postural hypotension:* Monitor BP at the beginning and end of each appointment; anticipate syncope. Have patient sit upright for several min at the end of the dental appointment before dismissing.
- Depressed or anxious patients may neglect self-care. Monitor for plaque control effectiveness.
- Chronic dry mouth is possible; anticipate increased caries and candidiasis.
- Extrapyramidal behaviors can complicate performance of oral procedures. If present, consult with MD to consider medication changes.
- If GI side effects occur, consider semisupine chair position.

Oral Health Education
- If chronic dry mouth occurs, recommend home fluoride therapy and use of nonalcoholic oral health care products.
- Evaluate manual dexterity; consider need for power toothbrush.
- Encourage daily plaque control procedures for effective, nontraumatic self-care.

Clozaril — see clozapine
Codeine Contin — see codeine phosphate

---

codeine phosphate (KOE-deen FOS-fate)

■✦■ **Codeine Contin, ratio-Codeine**

Drug Class: Narcotic analgesic; Antitussive
DEA Schedule: Schedule II

PHARMACOLOGY

Action
Stimulates opiate receptors in the CNS; also causes respiratory depression, peripheral vasodilation, inhibition of intestinal peristalsis, stimulation of the chemoreceptors that cause vomiting, increased bladder tone, and suppression of cough reflex.

Uses
Relief of mild to moderate pain; cough suppression.

➜✦ DRUG INTERACTIONS RELATED TO DENTAL THERAPEUTICS

Bupivacaine: Possible respiratory depression (mechanism unknown)
- Use bupivacaine with caution.

ADVERSE EFFECTS
⚠ **ORAL:** Taste alterations; dry mouth; dysphagia.
CNS: Lightheadedness; dizziness; sedation; disorientation; incoordination; euphoria; delirium.
CVS: Bradycardia (common); tachycardia; postural hypotension; arrhythmia.
GI: Nausea; vomiting; constipation; abdominal pain; anorexia; biliary tract spasm.
RESP: Laryngospasm; depression of cough reflex; respiratory depression.
MISC: Tolerance; psychological and physical dependence with long-term use.

CLINICAL IMPLICATIONS
General
- Determine why drug is being taken. Consider implications of condition on dental treatment.
- If oral pain requires additional analgesics, consider nonopioid products.
- Chronic dry mouth is possible; anticipate increased caries and candidiasis.
- If GI side effects occur, consider semisupine chair position.
- *Postural hypotension:* Monitor BP at the beginning and end of each appointment; anticipate syncope. Have patient sit upright for several min at the end of the dental appointment before dismissing.

Oral Health Education
- If chronic dry mouth occurs, recommend home fluoride therapy and use of nonalcoholic oral health care products.
- *If prescribed by DDS:* Warn patient not to drive, sign important papers, or operate mechanical equipment.

---

codeine phosphate/acetaminophen — see acetaminophen/codeine phosphate
codeine phosphate/ASA — see aspirin/codeine phosphate
codeine phosphate/aspirin — see aspirin/codeine phosphate
CO Fluoxetine — see fluoxetine HCl
Co-Gesic — see acetaminophen/hydrocodone bitartrate
Cognex — see tacrine HCl

---

colesevelam HCl (koe-leh-SEV-eh-lam HIGH-droe-KLOR-ide)
Welchol
Drug Class: Antihyperlipidemic, bile acid sequestrant

PHARMACOLOGY
Action
Increases removal of bile acids from the body by binding bile acids in the intestine, impeding their reabsorption. As the bile acid pool becomes depleted, the conversion of cholesterol to bile acids is increased, which decreases serum cholesterol.

Uses
Adjunctive therapy to diet and exercise given alone or with an HMG-CoA reductase inhibitor for the reduction of elevated LDL cholesterol in patients with primary hypercholesterolemia (Fredrickson type IIa).

➭← DRUG INTERACTIONS RELATED TO DENTAL THERAPEUTICS
No documented drug-drug interactions. The absence of evidence is not evidence of safety.

ADVERSE EFFECTS
⚠ **ORAL:** Dental caries; bleeding; unpleasant taste; dysphagia.
GI: Constipation; dyspepsia; GI pain; nausea.

RESP: Pharyngitis.
CNS: Dizziness; lightheadedness; syncope.
CVS: Chest pain, tachycardia (infrequent).
MISC: Accidental injury; asthenia; myalgia.

CLINICAL IMPLICATIONS

General

- High LDL cholesterol concentration is the major cause of atherosclerosis, which leads to CAD (e.g., angina, MI); determine degree of CV health and ability to withstand stress of dental treatment.
- Monitor vital signs (e.g., BP, pulse pressure, rate, and rhythm) at each appointment to assess disease control. Do not provide elective dental treatment when BP ≥180/110 or in presence of other high-risk CV conditions. Refer to the section entitled "The Patient Taking Cardiovascular Drugs" in Chapter 6: *Clinical Medicine*.
- If GI side effects occur, consider semisupine chair position.

Oral Health Education

- Encourage daily plaque control procedures for effective self-care in patients at risk for cardiovascular disease.

Colestid — see colestipol HCl

---

colestipol HCl (koe-LESS-tih-pole HIGH-droe-KLOR-ide)

Colestid

Drug Class: Antihyperlipidemic, bile acid sequestrant

PHARMACOLOGY

Action

Increases removal of bile acids from body by forming insoluble complexes in the intestine, which are then excreted in feces. As body loses bile acids, it converts cholesterol from blood to bile acids, thus lowering serum cholesterol.

Uses

Reduction of cholesterol in patients with primary hypercholesterolemia who do not respond adequately to diet.

Unlabeled Uses

Treatment of digitalis toxicity.

➡◆ DRUG INTERACTIONS RELATED TO DENTAL THERAPEUTICS

No documented drug-drug interactions. The absence of evidence is not evidence of safety.

ADVERSE EFFECTS

⚠ **ORAL:** Dysphagia; dental bleeding; dental caries; taste disturbance.
GI: Constipation; abdominal pain and cramping; intestinal bloating; flatulence; indigestion; heartburn; diarrhea; nausea; vomiting; bloody hemorrhoids and stools; esophageal obstruction.
CVS: Chest pain, tachycardia (infrequent).
MISC: Increased PT; ecchymosis.

CLINICAL IMPLICATIONS

General

- High LDL cholesterol concentration is the major cause of atherosclerosis, which leads to CAD (e.g., angina, MI); determine degree of CV health and ability to withstand stress of dental treatment.

- Monitor vital signs (e.g., BP, pulse pressure, rate, and rhythm) at each appointment to assess disease control. Do not provide elective dental treatment when BP is ≥180/110 or in the presence of other high-risk CV conditions. Refer to the section entitled "The Patient Taking Cardiovascular Drugs" in Chapter 6: *Clinical Medicine*.
- If GI side effects occur, consider semisupine chair position.
- Increased PT, anemia are rarely reported; anticipate increased bleeding and poor healing.

Oral Health Education

- Encourage daily plaque control procedures for effective self-care in patients at risk for cardiovascular disease.

---

collagen — see microfibrillar collagen hemostat

Columina — see cimetidine

Combivent — see ipratropium bromide/albuterol sulfate

Combivent Inhalation Solution — see ipratropium bromide

Combivir — see lamivudine/zidovudine

Combunox — see ibuprofen/oxycodone

Commit — see nicotine

compound S — see zidovudine

Compoz Gel Caps — see diphenhydramine HCl

Compoz Nighttime Sleep Aid — see diphenhydramine HCl

Comtan — see entacapone

Conazol — see ketoconazole

Concerta — see methylphenidate HCl

Congest — see estrogens, conjugated or esterified

Congestion Relief — see pseudoephedrine

conjugated estrogen — see estrogens, conjugated or esterified

conjugated estrogens/medroxyprogesterone acetate — see estrogens, conjugated/medroxyprogesterone acetate

Consupren — see cyclosporine

Contac Cold 12 Hour Non-Drowsy — see pseudoephedrine

Controlip — see fenofibrate

Copal — see sulindac

Copegus — see ribavirin

Cordarone — see amiodarone

Cordran — see flurandrenolide

Cordran SP — see flurandrenolide

Cordran V — see flurandrenolide

Coreg — see carvedilol

Corgard — see nadolol

Cormax — see clobetasol propionate

Corogal — see nifedipine

Corotrend — see nifedipine

CortaGel — see hydrocortisone

Cortaid — see hydrocortisone
Cortaid Topical Spray — see hydrocortisone
Cortaid with Aloe — see hydrocortisone
Cort-Dome — see hydrocortisone
Cortef — see hydrocortisone
Cortenema — see hydrocortisone
cortisol — see hydrocortisone

cortisone (CORE-tih-sone)

Synonym: cortisone acetate

Cortone Acetate

Drug Class: Corticosteroid

PHARMACOLOGY

Action

As short-acting glucocorticoid; depresses formation, release, and activity of endogenous mediators of inflammation; has some salt-retaining properties.

Uses

Treatment of primary or secary adrenal cortex insufficiency; rheumatic disorders; collagen diseases; dermatological diseases; allergic states; allergic and inflammatory ophthalmic processes; respiratory diseases; hematological disorders; neoplastic diseases; edematous states (caused by nephrotic syndrome); GI diseases; multiple sclerosis; tuberculous meningitis; trichinosis with neurological or myocardial involvement.

➤← DRUG INTERACTIONS RELATED TO DENTAL THERAPEUTICS

COX-1 inhibitors: Increased risk of peptic ulcer disease (additive)
* Avoid concurrent use.

ADVERSE EFFECTS

⚠ **ORAL:** Impaired wound healing; petechia; oral candidiasis.

CNS: Convulsions; increased intracranial pressure with papilledema; vertigo; headache; neuritis/paresthesias; psychosis; fatigue; insomnia.

CVS: Arrhythmia; syncope; hypertension.

GI: Pancreatitis; abdominal distention; ulcerative esophagitis; nausea; vomiting; increased appetite and weight gain; peptic ulcer; small bowel and large bowel perforation, especially in inflammatory bowel disease.

MISC: Musculoskeletal effects (e.g., muscle weakness, myopathy, tendon rupture, osteoporosis, aseptic necrosis of femoral and humeral heads, spontaneous fractures); anaphylactoid reactions; aggravation or masking of infections; malaise; adrenal suppression.

CLINICAL IMPLICATIONS

General

* Determine why drug is being taken. Consider implications of condition on dental treatment.
* Be aware that signs of bacterial oral infection may be masked and anticipate oral candidiasis.
* Monitor blood pressure and pulse.
* Anticipate oral candidiasis when steroids are used.
* Anticipate addisonian or cushingoid complications affecting the head and neck area.
* The anticipated perioperative physiological stress in patients undergoing dental care (minor surgical stress) under local anesthesia should take only their usual daily glucocorticoid dose before dental intervention. No supplementation is justified.

Oral Health Education

- *Topical:* If prescribed by DDS, ensure patient understands how to use product, amount to apply, method of application, and signs of adverse effects.

---

cortisone acetate — see cortisone

Cortizone-5 — see hydrocortisone

Cortizone-10 — see hydrocortisone

Cortizone-10 Plus Maximum Strength — see hydrocortisone

Cortizone-10 Quickshot Spray — see hydrocortisone

Cortizone for Kids — see hydrocortisone

Cortoderm — see hydrocortisone

Cortone Acetate — see cortisone

Cotrim — see trimethoprim/sulfamethoxazole

Cotrim D.S. — see trimethoprim/sulfamethoxazole

co-trimoxazole — see trimethoprim/sulfamethoxazole

Cotrim Pediatric — see trimethoprim/sulfamethoxazole

Coumadin — see warfarin

Covera-HS — see verapamil HCl

Coversyl — see perindopril erbumine

Cozaar — see losartan potassium

Cremosan — see ketoconazole

Creo-Terpin — see dextromethorphan HBr

Crestor — see rosuvastatin calcium

Crixivan — see indinavir sulfate

Crolom — see cromolyn sodium

---

cromolyn sodium (KROE-moe-lin SO-dee-uhm)

Synonym: disodium cromoglycate

Crolom, Gastrocrom, Intal, NasalCrom

■✚■ Apo-Cromolyn Nasal Spray, Apo-Cromolyn Sterules, Nalcrom, Nu-Cromolyn

Drug Class: Respiratory inhalant

PHARMACOLOGY

Action

Stabilizes mast cells, which release histamine and other mediators of allergic reactions.

Uses

INHALATION: Prophylaxis of severe bronchial asthma; prevention of exercise-induced asthma; prevention of acute bronchospasm induced by environmental pollutants and known antigens.

NASAL SOLUTION: Prevention and treatment of allergic rhinitis.

ORAL: Treatment of mastocytosis.

OPHTHALMIC: Treatment of vernal keratoconjunctivitis, vernal conjunctivitis, and vernal keratitis.

Unlabeled Uses

ORAL: Symptoms of food allergies; eczema; dermatitis; ulceration; urticaria pigmentosa; chronic urticaria; hay fever; and postexercise bronchospasm.

➡◀ DRUG INTERACTIONS RELATED TO DENTAL THERAPEUTICS

No documented drug-drug interactions. The absence of evidence is not evidence of safety.

ADVERSE EFFECTS

⚠ **ORAL:** Dry mouth, throat; taste disturbance (common); stomatitis.
CNS: Dizziness; headache.
CVS: Tachycardia.
GI: Nausea; substernal burning; diarrhea (oral form).
RESP: Cough; wheezing; bronchospasm.
MISC: Joint pain and swelling.

CLINICAL IMPLICATIONS

General

- Determine why drug is being taken. Consider implications of condition on dental treatment.
- Monitor vital signs (e.g., BP, pulse rate, respiratory rate, and function); uncontrolled disease characterized by wheezing and coughing.
- Acute bronchoconstriction can occur during dental treatment; have bronchodilator inhaler available.
- Be aware that sulfites in local anesthetic with a vasoconstrictor can precipitate acute asthma attack in susceptible individuals.
- Inhalants can dry oral mucosa; anticipate candidiasis, increased calculus and plaque levels, and increased caries.

Oral Health Education

- If chronic dry mouth occurs, recommend home fluoride therapy and use of nonalcoholic oral health care products.
- Instruct to ensure that bronchodilator inhaler is present at each dental appointment.

Cruex — see clotrimazole

Cryocriptina — see bromocriptine mesylate

Cryoperacid — see loperamide HCl

Cryopril — see captopril

Cryosolona — see methylprednisolone

Cryoval — see valproic acid and derivatives

Cryoxifeno — see tamoxifen citrate

Curretab — see medroxyprogesterone acetate

---

cyclobenzaprine HCl (SIGH-kloe-BEN-zuh-preen HIGH-droe-KLOR-ide)

Flexeril

■✚■ Apo-Cyclobenzaprine, Gen-Cyclobenzaprine, Novo-Cycloprine, Nu-Cyclobenzaprine, ratio-Cyclobenzaprine

Drug Class: Skeletal muscle relaxant, centrally acting

PHARMACOLOGY

Action

Relieves skeletal muscle spasms of local origin without interfering with muscle function by acting within CNS at brainstem. Structurally and pharmacologically related to tricyclic antidepressants.

Uses

Relief of muscle spasms associated with acute painful musculoskeletal conditions.

Unlabeled Uses

Treatment of fibrositis.

DRUG INTERACTIONS RELATED TO DENTAL THERAPEUTICS

No documented drug-drug interactions. The absence of evidence is not evidence of safety.

ADVERSE EFFECTS

⚠ **ORAL:** Dry mouth (27%); unpleasant taste (3%); tongue swelling, discoloration (<1%), thirst.

CNS: Drowsiness; dizziness; fatigue; asthenia; headache; nervousness; convulsions; confusion.

CVS: Tachycardia, hypotension, palpitations, syncope (<1%); arrhythmia.

MISC: Photosensitization; extrapyramidal behaviors.

GI: Nausea; constipation; dyspepsia.

CLINICAL IMPLICATIONS

General

- Determine why drug is being taken. Consider implications of condition on dental treatment.
- Extrapyramidal behaviors can complicate performance of oral procedures. If present, consult with MD to consider medication changes.
- Chronic dry mouth is possible; anticipate increased caries and candidiasis.
- Monitor blood pressure and pulse.
- If GI side effects occur, consider semisupine chair position.
- *For back pain:* Consider semisupine chair position for patient comfort.

Oral Health Education

- If chronic dry mouth occurs, recommend home fluoride therapy and use of nonalcoholic oral health care products.

---

cycloserine (sigh-kloe-SER-een)

Seromycin Pulvules

Drug Class: Anti-infective; Antitubercular

PHARMACOLOGY

Action

Inhibits cell wall synthesis in susceptible strains of certain microorganisms.

Uses

Treatment of active pulmonary and extrapulmonary tuberculosis when organisms are susceptible (after failure of adequate treatment with primary medications); treatment of UTIs caused by susceptible bacteria when conventional therapy has failed; treatment of Gaucher disease.

DRUG INTERACTIONS RELATED TO DENTAL THERAPEUTICS

No documented drug-drug interactions. The absence of evidence is not evidence of safety.

ADVERSE EFFECTS

CNS: Convulsions; drowsiness; somnolence; headache; tremor; dysarthria; vertigo; confusion; loss of memory; psychoses with suicidal tendencies, behavior changes, hyperirritability, aggression, paresis; hyperreflexia; paresthesias; major and minor clonic seizures; coma; dizziness.

CVS: Arrhythmia.

MISC: Tremors.

CLINICAL IMPLICATIONS

General

- Determine why drug is being taken (prevention or treatment). Consider implications of condition on dental treatment.
- Complete medical consult to ensure noninfectious state exists before providing dental treatment.
- *For dental emergencies:* Follow special precautions to minimize disease transmission (particulate respirators) or refer patient to a hospital-based dental facility.
- Question patient about CNS side effects and use of alcoholic beverages; anticipate seizure activity if alcohol is used.

---

cyclosporin A — see cyclosporine

---

cyclosporine (SIGH-kloe-spore-EEN)

Synonym: cyclosporin A

Gengraf, Neoral, Restasis, Sandimmune

■ ✦ ■ **Rhoxal-cyclosporine, Sandimmune**

■ ■ **Consupren**

Drug Class: Immunosuppressant

PHARMACOLOGY

Action

Suppresses cell-mediated immune reactions and some humoral immunity, but exact mechanism is not known.

Uses

Prophylaxis of organ rejection in kidney, liver, and heart allogeneic transplants in conjunction with adrenal corticosteroid therapy; treatment of chronic rejection in patients previously treated with other immunosuppressive agents; increase tear production in patients whose tear production is presumed to be suppressed because of ocular inflammation associated with keratoconjunctivitis sicca (ophthalmic emulsion).
GENGRAF, NEORAL: Treatment of severe active rheumatoid arthritis (RA) where disease is not adequately responsive to methotrexate; treatment of adult, nonimmunocompromised patients with severe, recalcitrant, plaque psoriasis who have failed to respond to a least one systemic therapy or in patients for whom other systemic therapies are contraindicated or cannot be tolerated.

➔✦ DRUG INTERACTIONS RELATED TO DENTAL THERAPEUTICS

Fluconazole, ketoconazole, or itraconazole: Renal toxicity (decreased cyclosporine metabolism)
- Avoid concurrent use.

Metronidazole: Possible cyclosporine toxicity (decreased metabolism)
- Avoid concurrent use.

ADVERSE EFFECTS

⚠ **ORAL:** Gingival hyperplasia (16%); gingivitis, stomatitis, glossitis, salivary gland enlargement, tongue disorder (nonspecified), tooth disorder (nonspecified) (3%); gingival bleeding (1%); herpes simplex; candidiasis.

CNS: Tremor (55%); headache (15%); convulsions (5%); confusion, depression, dizziness, insomnia, migraine, paresthesia ($\geq$3%); anxiety, decreased or increased libido, nervousness, emotional lability, hypoesthesia, vertigo, impaired concentration, neuropathy, paranoia, somnolence, asthenia ($\leq$3%); encephalopathy.

CVS: Hypertension; chest pain.

GI: Nausea, vomiting (10%); diarrhea (8%); abdominal discomfort (≤7%); anorexia, dyspepsia, flatulence, rectal hemorrhage (≥3%); dysphagia, enanthema, eructation, esophagitis, gastric ulcer, gastroenteritis, gastritis, peptic ulcer (≤3%); hiccups (≤2%); constipation (≥1%).

RESP: Sinusitis (7%); bronchitis, coughing, dyspnea, respiratory tract infection, pneumonia (≥3%); abnormal chest sounds, tonsillitis, bronchospasm (≤3%).

MISC: Cramps (4%); accidental trauma, fever, flu-like symptoms, pain, purpura (≥3%); abscess, bacterial infection, cellulitis, fungal infection, herpes zoster, moniliasis, viral infection, tumor, malaise (≤3%); allergic reaction, edema, fever (≤2%); increased appetite (≥1%).

CLINICAL IMPLICATIONS

General
- Determine why drug is being taken. Consider implications of condition on dental treatment.
- Consider medical consult to determine disease control and influence on dental treatment.
- Be aware that signs of bacterial oral infection may be masked and anticipate oral candidiasis.
- Immunosuppressant therapy reduces host response to infection.
- Monitor vital signs.
- If GI or respiratory side effects occur, consider semisupine chair position.

Oral Health Education
- Evaluate manual dexterity; consider need for power toothbrush.
- Encourage daily plaque control procedures for effective self-care.

Cycrin — see medroxyprogesterone acetate

Cyklokapron — see tranexamic acid

Cymbalta — see duloxetine HCl

Cystospaz — see hyoscyamine sulfate

Cytomel — see liothyronine sodium

Cytotec — see misoprostol

Dabex — see metformin HCl

---

daclizumab (da-KLIZ-uh-mab)
Zenapax

Drug Class: Immunosuppressive

PHARMACOLOGY

Action
Binds with high-affinity to the Tac subunit of the high-affinity interleukin-2 (IL-2) complex and inhibits IL-2 binding, thereby impairing the response of the immune system to antigenic challenges.

Uses
Prophylaxis of acute organ rejection in patients receiving renal transplants.

➜← DRUG INTERACTIONS RELATED TO DENTAL THERAPEUTICS
No documented drug-drug interactions. The absence of evidence is not evidence of safety.

ADVERSE EFFECTS
⚠ **ORAL:** Impaired wound healing; increased bleeding.
CNS: Tremor, headache, dizziness, insomnia (≥5%); depression, anxiety (2% to <5%).

CVS: Hypertension or hypotension; tachycardia; bleeding.

GI: Constipation, nausea, diarrhea, vomiting, abdominal pain, pyrosis, dyspepsia, abdominal distention, epigastric pain (≥5%); flatulence, gastritis, hemorrhoids (2% to <5%).

RESP: Dyspnea, pulmonary edema, coughing (≥5%); atelectasis, congestion, hypoxia, rales, abnormal breath sounds, pleural effusion (2% to <5%).

MISC: Posttraumatic pain, chest pain, fever, pain, fatigue (≥5%); shivering, generalized weakness, prickly sensation (2% to <5%). The safety of daclizumab was determined in patients receiving concomitant cyclosporine and corticosteroids.

CLINICAL IMPLICATIONS

General

- Determine why drug is being taken. Consider implications of condition on dental treatment.
- Consider medical consult to determine physical status and influence on dental treatment.
- Monitor vital signs.
- If GI or respiratory side effects occur, consider semisupine chair position.

Oral Health Education

- Encourage daily plaque control procedures for effective, nontraumatic self-care.

Dafloxen — see naproxen

Dalacin C — see clindamycin

Dalacin C Phosphate — see clindamycin

Dalacin T Topical — see clindamycin

Dalalone — see dexamethasone

Dalalone DP — see dexamethasone

Dalalone LA — see dexamethasone

Dalmane — see flurazepam HCl

d'ALPHA E Softgels — see vitamin E

D-alpha tocopherol — see vitamin E

D-alpha tocopheryl acetate — see vitamin E

Daonil — see glyburide

Dapacin — see acetaminophen

Dapsoderm-X — see dapsone

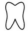 **dapsone** (DAP-sone)

Aczone: Gel: 5%
Dapsone: Tablets: 25, 100 mg

■▬■ **Dapsoderm-X**

Drug Class: Anti-infective; Leprostatic

PHARMACOLOGY

Action

Mechanism of action is unknown; however, dapsone is bactericidal and bacteriostatic against *Mycobacterium leprae*.

Uses
TABLETS: Treatment of dermatitis herpetiformis; leprosy.
GEL: Acne vulgaris.

➡◆ DRUG INTERACTIONS
No documented drug-drug interactions. The absence of evidence is not evidence of safety.

ADVERSE EFFECTS
CVS: Tachycardia.
CNS: Peripheral neuropathy; motor loss; muscle weakness; insomnia; headache; psychosis.
GI: Nausea; vomiting; abdominal pains; pancreatitis; vertigo.
RESP: Pulmonary eosinophilia.
MISC: Fever; phototoxicity; hypoalbuminemia; lupus erythematosus; infectious mononucleosis–like syndrome; hemolytic anemia (high doses), methemoglobinemia.

CLINICAL IMPLICATIONS
General
- Determine why drug is being taken. Consider implications of condition on dental treatment.
- If GI side effects occur, consider semisupine chair position.
- Monitor vital signs.
- Blood dyscrasias rarely reported; anticipate increased infection and poor healing.

Pregnancy Risk Category: Category C.

Oral Health Education
When prescribed by DDS:
- Explain name, dose, action, and potential side effects of drug.
- Review dosing schedule and prescribed length of therapy with patient.
- Advise patient that medication may be started at a low dose and then gradually increased to provide maximum benefit.
- Instruct patient to continue to take other prescribed medications while taking dapsone.
- Emphasize to patient that treatment will be lengthy and that the entire course of treatment must be completed to avoid relapse or development of resistance.
- Advise patient to take each dose with food if GI upset occurs.
- Instruct patient to stop using and notify health care provider immediately if any of the following symptoms occur: skin rash, sore throat, fever, paleness, purple discoloration of skin, yellowing of skin or eyes, muscle weakness.
- Advise women to notify health care provider if pregnant, planning to become pregnant, or breast feeding.
- Advise patient that drug may cause blurred vision or dizziness and to use caution while driving or performing other tasks requiring mental alertness until tolerance is determined.
- Instruct patient to not take any prescription or OTC medications or dietary supplements unless advised by health care provider.
- Advise patient that follow-up visits and laboratory tests will be required to monitor therapy and to keep appointments.

---

darifenacin (dar-ih-FEN-ah-sin)
Enablex
Drug Class: Anticholinergic

PHARMACOLOGY
Action
Competitive muscarinic receptor antagonist.

Uses

Treatment of overactive bladder with symptoms of urge urinary incontinence, urgency, and frequency.

➜← DRUG INTERACTIONS RELATED TO DENTAL THERAPEUTICS

Clarithromycin: Possible increased darifenacin toxicity (decreased metabolism)
• Avoid concurrent use.
Ketoconazole or itraconazole: Possible increased darifenacin toxicity (decreased metabolism)
• Avoid concurrent use.

ADVERSE EFFECTS

⚠ **ORAL:** Dry mouth (20% to 35%).
CVS: Hypertension (≥1%).
CNS: Headache (7%); asthenia (3%); dizziness (2%).
GI: Constipation (21%); dyspepsia (8%); abdominal pain, nausea (4%); diarrhea (2%); vomiting (≥1%).
RESP: Bronchitis, sinusitis (≥1%).
MISC: Accidental injury, flu-like syndrome (3%); pain, peripheral edema (≥1%).

CLINICAL IMPLICATIONS

General

• Determine why drug is being taken. Consider implications of condition on dental treatment.
• Chronic dry mouth is possible; anticipate increased caries and candidiasis.
• If GI side effects occur, consider semisupine chair position.

Oral Health Education

• If chronic dry mouth occurs, recommend home fluoride therapy and use of nonalcoholic oral health care products.

Darvocet A500 — see acetaminophen/propoxyphene
Darvocet-N 50 — see acetaminophen/propoxyphene
Darvocet-N 100 — see acetaminophen/propoxyphene
Darvon Compound-32 Pulvules — see narcotic analgesic combinations
Darvon Compound-65 Pulvules — see narcotic analgesic combinations
Darvon Pulvules — see propoxyphene HCl
Darvon-N — see propoxyphene HCl
Datril — see acetaminophen
Dayhist-1 — see clemastine fumarate
Daypro — see oxaprozin
ddC — see zalcitabine
Deavynfar — see chlorpropamide
Decadron — see dexamethasone
Decadronal — see dexamethasone
Decadron-LA — see dexamethasone
Decadron Phosphate — see dexamethasone
Decaject — see dexamethasone
Decaject-L.A. — see dexamethasone

Decaspray — see dexamethasone
Decofed Syrup — see pseudoephedrine
Decorex — see dexamethasone
Defed-6o — see pseudoephedrine
Deflox — see diclofenac

delavirdine mesylate (dell-ah-VER-deen MEH-sih-late)

Rescriptor

Drug Class: Antiretroviral, non-nucleoside reverse transcriptase inhibitor

PHARMACOLOGY

Action
Inhibits replication of HIV-1 infection by interfering with DNA synthesis.

Uses
Treatment of HIV-1 infection in combination with appropriate antiretroviral agents when therapy is warranted.

✦← DRUG INTERACTIONS RELATED TO DENTAL THERAPEUTICS

Ketoconazole: Possible delavirdine toxicity (decreased metabolism)
 • Avoid concurrent use.
Benzodiazepines: Increased benzodiazepine toxicity (decreased metabolism)
 • Monitor clinical status.

ADVERSE EFFECTS

⚠ **ORAL:** Lip edema; aphthous stomatitis; dry mouth; dysphagia; gingivitis; gingival bleeding; gagging; increased salivation; thirst; stomatitis; sialadenitis; tongue edema; taste perversion.

CNS: Lethargy; headache; migraine; abnormal coordination; agitation; amnesia; anxiety; change in dreams; cognitive impairment; confusion; depression; disorientation; dizziness; emotional lability; hallucination; hyperesthesia; impaired concentration; insomnia; manic symptoms; nervousness; neuropathy; nightmares; paranoid symptoms; paresthesia; restlessness; somnolence; tingling; tremor; vertigo.

CVS: Bradycardia or tachycardia; syncope; postural hypotension; palpitations.

GI: Nausea; diarrhea; vomiting; abdominal cramps; distention; pain; anorexia; bloody stool; colitis; constipation; decreased appetite; diverticulitis; duodenitis; dyspepsia; enteritis; fecal incontinence; flatulence; gastritis; gastroesophageal reflux; GI bleeding; increased appetite; pancreatitis; rectal disorder.

RESP: URI; bronchitis; chest congestion; cough; dyspnea.

MISC: Asthenia; back pain; chest pain; flank pain; chills; edema; fever; flu-like syndrome; lethargy; weakness; malaise; neck rigidity; sebaceous and epidermal cysts; muscle cramps; paralysis; weight increase or decrease; arthralgia; arthritis; bone disorder; bone pain; myalgia; tendon disorder; tenosynovitis; tetany; photophobia; blood dyscrasias (e.g., thrombocytopenia, leukopenia, anemia, others).

CLINICAL IMPLICATIONS

General
 • Determine why drug is being taken. Consider implications of condition on dental treatment.
 • Consider medical consult to determine disease control and influence on dental treatment.
 • Anticipate oral candidiasis when HIV disease is reported.
 • Chronic dry mouth is possible; anticipate increased caries and candidiasis.
 • *Photophobia:* Direct dental light out of patient's eyes and offer dark glasses for comfort.
 • If GI side effects occur, consider semisupine chair position.

- Monitor vital signs.
- This drug is frequently prescribed in combination with one or more other antiviral agents. Side effects of all agents must be considered during the drug review process.
- Antibiotic prophylaxis should be considered when <500 PMN/mm³ are reported; elective dental treatment should be delayed until blood values improve above this level.
- Blood dyscrasias rarely reported; anticipate increased bleeding, infection, and poor healing.

Oral Health Education
- If chronic dry mouth occurs, recommend home fluoride therapy and use of nonalcoholic oral health care products.
- Encourage daily plaque control procedures for effective self-care since HIV infection reduces host resistance.
- Recommend frequent maintenance prophylaxis when immunosuppression is evident.

Delestrogen — see estradiol

Del-Mycin — see erythromycin

Delsym — see dextromethorphan HBr

Delta-Cortef — see prednisolone

Deltasone — see prednisone

Demadex — see torsemide

Demerol — see meperidine HCl

Denavir — see penciclovir

DentaGel 1.1% — see sodium fluoride

Denta 5000 Plus — see sodium fluoride

DentiPatch — see lidocaine HCl

Denvar — see cefixime

Depacon — see valproic acid and derivatives

Depakene — see valproic acid and derivatives

Depakote — see valproic acid and derivatives

Depakote ER — see valproic acid and derivatives

depMedalone 40 — see methylprednisolone

depMedalone 80 — see methylprednisolone

Depo-Estradiol — see estradiol

Depo-Medrol — see methylprednisolone

Deponit — see nitroglycerin

Depopred-40 — see methylprednisolone

Depopred-80 — see methylprednisolone

Depo-Provera — see medroxyprogesterone acetate

Dermacort — see hydrocortisone

DermaFlex — see lidocaine HCl

Dermalog — see halcinonide

Dermol HC — see hydrocortisone

Dermovate — see clobetasol propionate

Dermtex HC Maximum Strength Spray — see hydrocortisone

Desenex — see clotrimazole

desipramine HCl (dess-IPP-ruh-meen HIGH-droe-KLOR-ide)

Norpramin: Tablets: 10, 25, 50, 75, 100, 150 mg

■✦■ **Apo-Desipramine, Novo-Desipramine, Nu-Desipramine, PMS-Desipramine, ratio-Desipramine**

Drug Class: Tricyclic antidepressant

PHARMACOLOGY

Action
Inhibits reuptake of norepinephrine and serotonin in CNS.

Uses
Relief of symptoms of depression.

Unlabeled Uses
Facilitation of cocaine withdrawal; treatment of panic and eating disorders (e.g., bulimia nervosa).

Contraindications
Hypersensitivity to any tricyclic antidepressant. Not to be given in combination with or within 14 days of treatment with an MAO inhibitor; cross-sensitivity may occur across the dibenzazepines. Do not give during acute recovery phases of MI.

Usual Dosage
ADULTS: *PO:* 100 to 300 mg/day. May be given in divided doses or once daily at bedtime. ELDERLY AND ADOLESCENT PATIENTS: *PO:* 25 to 150 mg/day.

Pharmacokinetics
ABSORP: Rapidly absorbed.
METAB: Metabolized in the liver.
EXCRET: Approximately 70% excreted in the urine; $t_{1/2}$ is 12 to 24 hr.
ONSET: 2 to 5 days.
PEAK: 2 to 3 wk.
SPECIAL POP: *Elderly:* Rate of metabolism is slower. Dosage adjustment recommended.

➜✦ DRUG INTERACTIONS

Tramadol: Increased risk of seizures (additive)
• Avoid concurrent use.
Ibuprofen: Possible desipramine toxicity (mechanism unknown)
• Avoid concurrent use.
Sympathomimetic amines: Hypertension and hypertensive crisis (inhibition of epinephrine uptake)
• Use local anesthetic agents containing a vasoconstrictor with caution.
• Monitor blood pressure.

ADVERSE EFFECTS
⚠ **ORAL:** Dry mouth; aphthous stomatitis; stomatitis; taste disturbance; tardive dyskinesia.
CVS: Orthostatic hypotension; hypertension; tachycardia; palpitations; arrhythmias; ECG changes; hypertensive episodes during surgery; stroke; heart block; CHF.
CNS: Confusion; disturbed concentration; hallucinations; delusions; nervousness; numbness; tremors; extrapyramidal symptoms (pseudoparkinsonism, movement disorders, akathisia); restlessness; agitation; panic; insomnia; nightmares; mania; exacerbation of psychosis; drowsiness; dizziness; weakness; fatigue; emotional lability; seizures.
GI: Nausea; vomiting; anorexia; GI distress; diarrhea; flatulence; constipation.
RESP: Pharyngitis; rhinitis; sinusitis; bronchospasm; cough.

CLINICAL IMPLICATIONS

General

- Determine why drug is being taken. Consider implications of condition on dental treatment.
- Extrapyramidal behaviors can complicate performance of oral procedures. If conditions present, consult with MD to consider medication changes.
- *Postural hypotension:* Monitor BP at the beginning and end of each appointment; anticipate syncope. Have patient sit upright for several min at the end of the dental appointment before dismissing.
- Blood dyscrasias rarely reported; anticipate increased bleeding, infection, and poor healing.
- Chronic dry mouth is possible; anticipate increased caries and candidiasis.
- Monitor vital signs.
- If GI side effects occur, consider semisupine chair position.
- Depressed or anxious patients may neglect self-care. Monitor for plaque control effectiveness.
- Determine ability to adapt to stress of dental treatment. Consider short appointments.

When prescribed by DDS:

- *Lactation:* Excreted in breast milk.
- *Children:* Not recommended in children younger than 12 yr.
- *Special Risk:* Use drug with caution in patients with history of seizures, urinary retention, urethral or ureteral spasm, angle-closure glaucoma, increased intraocular pressure, or cardiovascular disorders; in patients receiving thyroid medication and in patients who have hepatic or renal impairment, schizophrenia, or paranoia.
- *Overdosage:* Confusion, agitation, hallucinations, seizures, status epilepticus, clonus, choreoathetosis, hyperactive reflexes, positive Babinski signs, coma, cardiac arrhythmias, renal failure, flushing, dry mouth, dilated pupils, hyperpyrexia.

Pregnancy Risk Category: Category C.

Oral Health Education

- If chronic dry mouth occurs, recommend home fluoride therapy and use of nonalcoholic oral health care products.
- Encourage daily plaque control procedures for effective, nontraumatic self-care.

When prescribed by DDS:

- Warn patient of risk of seizure.
- Instruct patient to keep wkly record of weight.
- Teach patient how to take BP and heart rate.
- Explain missed medication procedure: 2 hr, wait until next scheduled dose. Do not double doses.
- Teach proper techniques for oral hygiene to help prevent/treat dry mucous membranes.
- Tell patient to increase fluid intake.
- Inform male patients of possible sexual dysfunction.
- Tell patient of possible difficulty urinating.
- Instruct patient to avoid intake of alcoholic beverages or other CNS depressants.
- Advise patient that drug may cause drowsiness and to use caution while driving or performing other tasks requiring mental alertness.
- Advise patient to complete full course of therapy; may take 4 to 6 wk to see full benefits.

---

desloratadine (dess-lore-AT-ah-deen)

Clarinex, Clarinex RediTabs

■✦■ Aerius

Drug Class: Antihistamine

PHARMACOLOGY

Action

Long-acting histamine antagonist with selective H_1-receptor histamine antagonist activity.

Uses

Relief of nasal and nonnasal symptoms of seasonal and perennial allergic rhinitis; in chronic idiopathic urticaria, for relief of symptoms of pruritus and reduction in number and size of hives.

➜← DRUG INTERACTIONS RELATED TO DENTAL THERAPEUTICS

Ketoconazole: Possible desloratadine toxicity (decreased metabolism)
• Avoid concurrent use.

ADVERSE EFFECTS

⚠ **ORAL:** Dry mouth, nose, throat; (nasal spray) bitter taste.
CNS: Headache (14%); fatigue (5%); dizziness (4%); somnolence (2%).
CVS: Tachycardia.
GI: Nausea (5%); dyspepsia (3%).
MISC: Myalgia (3%); photosensitivity; hypersensitivity (e.g., rash, pruritus, urticaria, edema, dyspnea, anaphylaxis).

CLINICAL IMPLICATIONS

General

• Determine why drug is being taken. Consider implications of condition on dental treatment.
• Consider semisupine chair position to control effects of postnasal drainage.
• Be aware that patients with multiple allergies are at increased risk for allergy to dental drugs.
• Chronic dry mouth is possible; anticipate increased caries and candidiasis.

Oral Health Education

• If chronic dry mouth occurs, recommend home fluoride therapy and use of nonalcoholic oral health care products.

Desocort — see desonide

---

desonide (DESS-oh-nide)

DesOwen, Tridesilon

■✦■ **Desocort**

■✦■ **DesOwen**

Drug Class: Corticosteroid, topical

PHARMACOLOGY

Action

Low-potency topical corticosteroid that depresses formation, release, and activity of endogenous mediators of inflammation including prostaglandins, kinins, histamine, liposomal enzymes, and complement system; modifies body's immune response.

Uses

Relief of inflammatory and pruritic manifestations of corticosteroid-responsive dermatoses.

➜← DRUG INTERACTIONS RELATED TO DENTAL THERAPEUTICS

No documented drug-drug interactions. The absence of evidence is not evidence of safety.

ADVERSE EFFECTS

⚠ **ORAL:** Burning; itching; erythema; perioral dermatitis.

CLINICAL IMPLICATIONS

General
- Determine why drug is being taken. Consider implications of condition on dental treatment.
- Because of the anticipated perioperative physiological stress in undergoing dental care (minor surgical stress) under local anesthesia, patients should take only their usual daily glucocorticoid dose before dental intervention. No supplementation is justified.
- Anticipate oral candidiasis when steroids are used.

Oral Health Education
- *If prescribed by DDS:* Ensure patient understands how to use product, amount to apply, method of application, and signs of adverse effects.

DesOwen — see desonide

Desoxi — see desoximetasone

desoximetasone (dess-OX-ee-MET-ah-sone)
Topicort, Topicort LP

■✦■ Desoxi

Drug Class: Corticosteroid, topical

PHARMACOLOGY

Action
High-potency topical corticosteroid that depresses formation, release, and activity of endogenous mediators of inflammation including prostaglandins, kinins, histamine, liposomal enzymes, and complement system; modifies the body's immune response.

Uses
Relief of inflammation and pruritic manifestations of corticosteroid-responsive dermatoses.

➠✦ DRUG INTERACTIONS RELATED TO DENTAL THERAPEUTICS
No documented drug-drug interactions. The absence of evidence is not evidence of safety.

ADVERSE EFFECTS
⚠ ORAL: Burning; itching; erythema; perioral dermatitis.

CLINICAL IMPLICATIONS

General
- Determine why drug is being taken. Consider implications of condition on dental treatment.
- The anticipated perioperative physiological stress in patients undergoing dental care (minor surgical stress) under local anesthesia should take only their usual daily glucocorticoid dose before dental intervention. No supplementation is justified.
- Anticipate oral candidiasis when steroids are used.

Oral Health Education
- *If prescribed by DDS:* Ensure patient understands how to use product, amount to apply, method of application, and signs of adverse effects.

Desyrel — see trazodone HCl

Desyrel Dividose — see trazodone HCl

Detensol — see propranolol HCl

Detrol — see tolterodine tartrate

Detrol LA — see tolterodine tartrate

Detrusitol — see tolterodine tartrate
Dexagrin — see dexamethasone
Dexair — see dexamethasone
Dexameth — see dexamethasone

---

 dexamethasone (DEX-uh-METH-uh-sone)
(dexamethasone acetate, dexamethasone sodium phosphate)

Aeroseb-Dex: Aerosol: 0.01%
AK-Dex: Solution: 0.1%
Dalalone DP: Injection: 16 mg/mL suspension
Dalalone LA: Injection: 8 mg/mL suspension
Decadron: Tablets: 0.5, 0.75, 4 mg; Elixir: 0.5 mg/5 mL
Dalalone, Decaject, Dexasone, Dexone, Solurex: Injection: 4 mg/mL
Decadron-LA, Decaject-L.A., Dexasone-L.A., Dexone LA, Solurex LA: Injection: 8-mg/mL suspension
Decadron Phosphate: Cream: 0.1%; Injection: 4 mg/mL, 24 mg/mL; Ointment: 0.05%; Solution: 0.1%
Decaspray: Aerosol: 0.04%
Dexameth, Dexone: Tablets: 0.5, 0.75, 1.5, 4 mg
Hexadrol: Tablets: 1.5 mg, 4 mg, Therapeutic Pack; Elixir: 0.5 mg/5 mL
Maxidex: Suspension: 0.1%
Hexadrol Phosphate: Injection: 4 mg/mL, 10 mg/mL, 20 mg/mL

■✦■ Dexair, PMS-Dexamethasone, ratio-Dexamethasone

■✦■ Alin, Alin Depot, Decadronal, Decorex, Dexagrin, Dibasona, Indarzona

Drug Class: Corticosteroid

PHARMACOLOGY

Action

Synthetic long-acting glucocorticoid that depresses formation, release, and activity of endogenous mediators of inflammation including prostaglandins, kinins, histamine, liposomal enzymes, and complement system. Also modifies body's immune response.

Uses

Testing of adrenal cortical hyperfunction; management of primary or secary adrenal cortex insufficiency, rheumatic disorders, collagen diseases, dermatological diseases, allergic states, allergic and inflammatory ophthalmic processes, respiratory diseases, hematological disorders, neoplastic diseases, cerebral edema associated with primary or metastatic brain tumor, craniotomy or head injury, edematous states (caused by nephrotic syndrome), GI diseases, multiple sclerosis, tuberculous meningitis, trichinosis with neurological or myocardial involvement.
INTRALESIONAL ADMINISTRATION: Treatment for keloids, psoriatic plaques, discoid lupus erythematosus, alopecia areata.
INTRA-ARTICULAR OR SOFT TISSUE ADMINISTRATION: Short-term adjunctive treatment synovitis of osteoarthritis, rheumatoid arthritis, acute gouty arthritis, posttraumatic osteoarthritis.
TOPICAL: Treatment of inflammatory and pruritic manifestations of corticosteroid-responsive dermatoses.
ORAL INHALATION: Treatment of corticosteroid-responsive and bronchial asthma bronchospastic states.

INTRANASAL: Treatment of allergic or inflammatory nasal conditions, nasal polyps (excluding those originating within sinuses).

OPHTHALMIC: Treatment of steroid-responsive inflammatory conditions of palpebral and bulbar conjunctiva, lid, cornea, and anterior segment of globe.

Unlabeled Uses

Treatment of acute mountain sickness, bacterial meningitis, bronchopulmonary dysplasia in preterm infants; diagnosis of depression; treatment of hirsutism; and use as antiemetic.

Contraindications

Systemic fungal infections; IM use in idiopathic thrombocytopenic purpura; administration of live virus vaccines; topical monotherapy in primary bacterial infections; intranasal use in untreated localized infections involving nasal mucosa; ophthalmic use in acute superficial herpes simplex keratitis, fungal diseases of ocular structures, vaccinia, varicella, and ocular tuberculosis.

Usual Dosage

All dosages shown are for adults unless indicated otherwise.

DEXAMETHASONE

INITIAL DOSE: *PO:* 0.75 to 9 mg/day.

TOPICAL: Apply sparingly to affected areas qid.

Pharmacokinetics

METAB: Metabolized in the liver by CYP3A4.

EXCRET: The $t_{1/2}$ is 1.8 to 3.5 hr.

ONSET: Rapid (injection).

DURATION: Short (injection).

➜◄ DRUG INTERACTIONS

Ketoconazole or itraconazole: Possible dexamethasone toxicity (decreased metabolism)
- Avoid concurrent use.

Aspirin: Decreased aspirin effect (mechanism unknown)
- Monitor clinical status.

Midazolam: Possible decreased midazolam effect (increased metabolism)
- Monitor clinical status.

COX-1 inhibitors: Increased risk of peptic ulcer disease (additive)
- Avoid concurrent use.

ADVERSE EFFECTS

CVS: Impaired wound healing; ulcerative esophagitis.

CVS: Thromboembolism or fat embolism; thrombophlebitis; necrotizing angiitis; cardiac arrhythmias or ECG changes; syncopal episodes; hypertension; myocardial rupture; CHF.

CNS: Convulsions; increased intracranial pressure with papilledema (pseudotumor cerebri); vertigo; headache; neuritis; paresthesias; psychosis.

GI: Pancreatitis; abdominal distension; ulcerative esophagitis; nausea; vomiting; increased appetite and weight gain; peptic ulcer with perforation and hemorrhage; bowel perforation.

RESP: Wheezing (oral inhalation).

MISC: Musculoskeletal effects (e.g., weakness, myopathy, muscle mass loss, osteoporosis, spontaneous fractures); endocrine abnormalities (e.g., menstrual irregularities, cushingoid state, growth suppression in children, sweating, decreased carbohydrate tolerance, hyperglycemia, glycosuria, increased insulin or sulfonylurea requirements in patients with diabetes, anaphylactoid or hypersensitivity reactions); aggravation or masking of infections; malaise; leukocytosis; fatigue; insomnia. Osteonecrosis; tendon rupture; infection; skin atrophy; postinjection flare; hypersensitivity; facial flushing (intra-articular). Topical use may theoretically produce adverse reactions seen with systemic use because of absorption.

CLINICAL IMPLICATIONS
General
- Determine why drug is being taken. Consider implications of condition on dental treatment.
- Be aware that signs of bacterial oral infection may be masked and anticipate oral candidiasis.
- If GI side effects occur, consider semisupine chair position.
- Prophylactic antibiotics may be indicated to prevent infection if surgery or periodontal debridement is planned.
- Due to the anticipated perioperative physiological stress, patients undergoing dental care (minor surgical stress) under local anesthesia should take only their usual daily glucocorticoid dose before dental intervention. No supplementation is justified.

When used or prescribed by DDS:
- *Lactation:* Excreted in breast milk.
- *Children:* May be more susceptible to adverse reactions from topical use than are adults. Observe growth and development of infants and children on prolonged therapy.
- *Elderly:* May require lower doses.
- *Renal failure:* Use cautiously; monitor renal function.
- *Sulfite sensitivity:* Some products may contain sodium bisulfite, which may cause allergic-type reactions in some individuals.
- *Adrenal suppression:* Prolonged therapy may lead to hypothalamic-pituitary-adrenal suppression.
- *Fluid and electrolyte balance:* Can cause elevated BP, salt and water retention, and increased potassium and calcium excretion. Dietary salt restriction and potassium supplementation may be needed.
- *Hepatitis:* May be harmful in chronic active hepatitis positive for hepatitis B surface antigen.
- *Infections:* May mask signs of infection. May decrease host-defense mechanisms to prevent dissemination of infection.
- *Ocular effects:* Use systemically with caution in ocular herpes simplex because of possible corneal perforation.
- *Ophthalmic use:* Prolonged use may result in glaucoma or other complications.
- *Peptic ulcer:* May contribute to peptic ulceration, especially in large doses.
- *Stress:* Increased dosage of rapidly acting corticosteroid may be needed before, during, and after stressful situations.
- *Withdrawal:* Abrupt discontinuation may result in adrenal insufficiency. Discontinue gradually.
- *Overdosage:* Fever, myalgia, arthralgia, malaise, anorexia, nausea, skin desquamation, orthostatic hypotension, dizziness, fainting, dyspnea, hypoglycemia (acute overdose); moon face, central obesity, striae, hirsutism, acne, ecchymoses, hypertension, osteoporosis, myopathy, sexual dysfunction, diabetes, hyperlipidemia, peptic ulcer, infection, electrolyte and fluid imbalance (chronic cushingoid changes).

Pregnancy Risk Category: Pregnancy category undetermined (systemic use); Category C (topical uses).

Oral Health Education
When used or prescribed by DDS:
- Caution patient that stopping drug abruptly is dangerous and may cause adrenal insufficiency.
- Explain rationale for tapering off medication when that time comes.
- Teach patient or family procedures for correctly administering specific form of drug (e.g., ophthalmic, inhalation, topical).
- Caution patient against receiving immunizations while drug is being taken.
- Advise patient on long-term therapy to carry medication identification card or to wear bracelet. In case of emergency, this information is important for treatment.
- Instruct patient to avoid people with infections, particularly respiratory.
- If patient is receiving intranasal form, instruct patient to clear nasal passages of secretions before administering drug.
- If topical, advise patient not to use occlusive dressings such as plastic wrap ~12 hr a

day. Occlusion may lead to sweat retention and to bacterial and fungal infections. Remember that tight-fitting plastic diapers on infants may also be occlusive.
- Teach patient to take oral forms with meals or snacks if GI irritation occurs.
- Review guidelines for missed doses of particular product with patient.
- Teach patient on long-term therapy how to keep a weight record.
- Instruct patient to inform other health care providers if taking a steroid.
- Review signs of infection and remind patient that fever, swelling, and redness may be masked in infection.
- Review possible side effects of dexamethasone with patient and to report these to health care provider.

---

dexamethasone acetate — see dexamethasone

dexamethasone sodium phosphate — see dexamethasone

Dexasone — see dexamethasone

Dexasone-L.A. — see dexamethasone

Dexedrine — see dextroamphetamine sulfate

Dexedrine Spansules — see dextroamphetamine sulfate

DexFerrum — see ferrous salts

---

dexmethylphenidate HCl (DEX-meth-ill-FEN-ih-date HIGH-droe-KLOR-ide)

Focalin, Focalin XR

Drug Class: CNS stimulant, psychotherapeutic
DEA Schedule: Schedule II

PHARMACOLOGY

Action
Exact mechanism of action is unknown; however, may block the reuptake of norepinephrine and dopamine into presynaptic neurons and increase release of these monoamines into extraneuronal spaces.

Uses
Treatment of attention deficit hyperactivity disorder (ADHD).

➤← DRUG INTERACTIONS RELATED TO DENTAL THERAPEUTICS

Pilocarpine: Increased myopia (mechanism unknown)
- Monitor clinical status.

ADVERSE EFFECTS

CNS: Twitching; insomnia; nervousness; dizziness; drowsiness; dyskinesia; headache; Tourette syndrome; toxic psychosis; depressed mood; neuroleptic malignant syndrome.
CVS: Arrhythmia, angina, palpitation, tachycardia; (less common) bradycardia; hypotension or hypertension.
GI: Anorexia; abdominal pain; nausea; loss of appetite.
MISC: Fever; arthralgia; leukopenia, anemia.

CLINICAL IMPLICATIONS

General
- Determine why drug is being taken. Consider implications of condition on dental treatment.
- Patients with ADHD may have short attention spans; consider short appointment.
- Monitor vital signs.
- If GI side effects occur, consider semisupine chair position.
- Blood dyscrasias rarely reported; anticipate increased bleeding, infection, and poor healing.

Oral Health Education
- Encourage daily plaque control procedures for effective, nontraumatic self-care.

Dexone — see dexamethasone
Dexone LA — see dexamethasone
dextroamphetamine — see dextroamphetamine sulfate
dextroamphetamine and amphetamine — see amphetamine and dextroamphetamine

---

dextroamphetamine sulfate (DEX-troe-am-FET-uh-meen SULL-fate)

Synonym: dextroamphetamine

Dexedrine, Dexedrine Spansules, Dextrostat
Drug Class: CNS stimulant, amphetamine
DEA Schedule: Schedule II

PHARMACOLOGY

Action
Activates noradrenergic neurons causing CNS and respiratory stimulation; stimulates satiety center in brain causing appetite suppression.

Uses
Treatment of narcolepsy, attention deficit hyperactivity disorder; adjunct therapy for short-term (i.e., no longer than a few weeks) exogenous obesity when alternative therapy has been ineffective.

➡◀ DRUG INTERACTIONS RELATED TO DENTAL THERAPEUTICS
Pilocarpine: Increased myopia (mechanism unknown)
- Monitor clinical status.

ADVERSE EFFECTS
⚠ **ORAL:** Dry mouth; unpleasant taste.
CNS: Nervousness; tremors; dizziness; insomnia; euphoria; headache.
CVS: Arrhythmia; tachycardia; palpitation; hypertension.
MISC: Accidental injury; asthenia; fever; infection; viral infection; allergy.
GI: Diarrhea; constipation; anorexia.

CLINICAL IMPLICATIONS

General
- Determine why drug is being taken. Consider implications of condition on dental treatment.
- Patients with ADHD may have short attention spans; consider short appointment.
- Monitor vital signs.
- Chronic dry mouth is possible; anticipate increased caries and candidiasis.

Oral Health Education
- If chronic dry mouth occurs, recommend home fluoride therapy and use of nonalcoholic oral health care products.

---

dextromethorphan HBr (DEX-troe-meth-OR-fan HIGH-droe-BROE-mide)

Benylin Adult, Benylin DM, Benylin Pediatric, Creo-Terpin, Delsym, Diabetes CF, Drixoral Cough Liquid Caps, Hold DM, Pediatric Vicks 44d Dry Hacking Cough

and Head Congestion, Pertussin CS, Pertussin ES, Robitussin Cough Calmers, Robitussin Pediatric, Scot-Tussin DM Cough Chasers, Silphen DM, St. Joseph Cough Suppressant, Sucrets 4-hr Cough, Sucrets Cough Control, Suppress, Trocal, Vicks Dry Hacking Cough

■✦■ Balminil DM, Balminil DM Children, Benylin DM, Benylin DM 12 Hour, Benylin DM for Children, Benylin DM for Children 12 Hour, Koffex DM, Robitussin Children's, Robitussin Honey Cough DM

■✦■ Athos, Bekidiba Dex, Neopulmonier, Romilar

Drug Class: Antitussive, Nonnarcotic

PHARMACOLOGY

Action
Suppresses cough by central action on cough center in medulla.

Uses
Management of nonproductive cough.

✦✦ DRUG INTERACTIONS RELATED TO DENTAL THERAPEUTICS
No documented drug-drug interactions. The absence of evidence is not evidence of safety.

ADVERSE EFFECTS
GI: Nausea.
CNS: Dizziness; drowsiness.

CLINICAL IMPLICATIONS

General
• Determine why drug is being taken. Consider implications of condition on dental treatment.
• Consider semisupine chair position to assist respiratory function.

Oral Health Education
• Inform patient that syrup has sugar and to use fluoride products to prevent dental caries.

Dextrostat — see dextroamphetamine sulfate

DiaBeta — see glyburide

Diabetes CF — see dextromethorphan HBr

Diabetic Tussin EX — see guaifenesin

Diabinese — see chlorpropamide

Diar-aid — see loperamide HCl

Diastat — see diazepam

Diatex — see diazepam

Diaval — see tolbutamide

Diazemuls — see diazepam

---

 diazepam (DIE-aze-uh-pam)

Diastat: Gel, rectal: 2.5 mg (pediatric), 10, 15, 20 mg (adult)
Diazepam: Solution, oral: 1 mg/mL; Injection: 1, 5 mg/mL
Diazepam Intensol: Solution (intensol): 5 mg/mL
Valium: Tablets: 2, 5, 10 mg

▮✦▮ Apo-Diazepam, Diazemuls, Valium Roche Oral

▮✦▮ Alboral, Diatex, Ortopsique, Pacitran, Valium

Drug Class: Antianxiety; Benzodiazepine; Anticonvulsant

DEA Schedule: Schedule IV

PHARMACOLOGY

Action

Potentiates action of GABA, an inhibitory neurotransmitter, resulting in increased neural inhibition and CNS depression, especially in limbic system and reticular formation.

Uses

Management of anxiety disorders; relief of acute alcohol withdrawal symptoms; relief of preoperative apprehension and anxiety and reduction of memory recall; treatment of muscle spasms, convulsive disorders (used adjunctively), and status epilepticus.

Unlabeled Uses

Treatment of irritable bowel syndrome; relief from panic attack.

Usual Dosage

Individualize dosage; increase cautiously.

Anxiety

ADULTS: *PO:* 2 to 10 mg bid to qid. *IM/IV:* 2 to 10 mg; repeat in 3 to 4 hr if needed.

Preoperative (anxiety and tension)

ADULTS: *IM:* 10 mg before surgery.

Status epilepticus and severe recurrent convulsive disorders

ADULTS: *IM/IV:* (IV preferred) 5 to 10 mg initially; then 5 to 10 mg at 10-to-15 min intervals (max total dose, 30 mg). If needed, repeat in 2 to 4 hr.

CHILDREN 5 YR AND OLDER: *IM/IV:* 1 mg q 2 to 5 min (max total dose, 10 mg). If needed, repeat in 2 to 4 hr.

INFANTS AND CHILDREN 1 MO TO 5 YR: *IM/IV:* 0.2 to 0.5 mg slowly q 2 to 5 min (max total dose, 5 mg).

Pharmacokinetics

ABSORP: *IM:* Slow and erratic absorption unless administered in the deltoid muscle; C_{max} is lower than oral or IV administration.

ORAL: T_{max} is 0.5 to 2 hr.

DIST: 95% to 98% protein bound. Highly lipophilic. Crosses the placenta and is excreted in breast milk.

METAB: Metabolized in the liver (involving CYP2C19 and CYP3A4) to desmethyldiazepam (active) and two minor active metabolites.

EXCRET: The $t_{1/2}$ is 20 to 80 hr.

ONSET: Rapid.

SPECIAL POP: *Hepatic failure:* The $t_{1/2}$ is prolonged and Cl decreased in those with alcoholic cirrhosis.

Elderly: The $t_{1/2}$ is increased and Cl is decreased.

Children: The $t_{1/2}$ is longer in neonates and children under 2 yr; $t_{1/2}$ is shorter in children 2 to 16 yr.

➡✦ DRUG INTERACTIONS

Acetaminophen: Possible diazepam toxicity (mechanism unknown)
 • Monitor clinical status.

Itraconazole: Possible increased diazepam effect (decreased metabolism)
 • Monitor clinical status.

Naproxen: Possible delayed onset of action of naproxen (delayed absorption)
 • Prescribe a loading dose.

ADVERSE EFFECTS

⚠ **ORAL:** Dry mouth; coated tongue.

CNS: Drowsiness; confusion; ataxia; dizziness; lethargy; fatigue; apathy; memory impairment; disorientation; anterograde amnesia; restlessness; headache; slurred speech; loss of voice; stupor; coma; euphoria; irritability; vivid dreams; psychomotor retardation; paradoxical reactions (e.g., anger, hostility, mania, insomnia, muscle spasms); depression; dysarthria; hypoactivity; tremor; vertigo.

CVS: Hypotension or hypertension; bradycardia or tachycardia; palpitations.

GI: Constipation; diarrhea; nausea; anorexia; vomiting.

MISC: Dependency/withdrawal symptoms; blood dyscrasias (leukopenia, thrombocytopenia, agranulocytosis).

CLINICAL IMPLICATIONS

General
- Determine why drug is being taken. Consider implications of condition on dental treatment.
- Determine ability to adapt to stress of dental treatment. Consider short appointments.
- Depressed or anxious patients may neglect self-care. Monitor for plaque control effectiveness.
- Monitor vital signs.
- Chronic dry mouth is possible; anticipate increased caries and candidiasis.
- Blood dyscrasias rarely reported; anticipate increased bleeding, infection and poor healing.

Pregnancy Risk Category: Category D. Avoid drug especially during first trimester because of possible increased risk of congenital malformations.

Oral Health Education
- If chronic dry mouth occurs, recommend home fluoride therapy and use of nonalcoholic oral health care products.
- Encourage daily plaque control procedures for effective, nontraumatic self-care.

Diazepam Intensol — see diazepam

Dibacilina — see ampicillin

Dibasona — see dexamethasone

Dibent — see dicyclomine HCl

---

diclofenac (die-KLOE-fen-ak)

Cataflam, Solaraze, Voltaren, Voltaren-XR

■✦■ **Apo-Diclo, Apo-Diclo Rapide, Apo-Diclo SR, Novo-Difenac, Novo-Difenac K, Novo-Difenac SR, Nu-Diclo, Nu-Diclo-SR, PMS-Diclofenac, PMS-Diclofenac SR, Voltaren Ophtha, Voltaren Rapide**

■◉■ **3-A Ofteno, Artrenac, Cataflam, Clonodifen, Deflox, Dicloran, Dolaren, Dolflam, Dolo Pangavit-D, Fustaren, Galedol, Lifenac, Lifenal, Liroken, Logesic, Merxil, Selectofen, Volfenac Gel, Volfenac Retard, Voltaren**

Drug Class: Analgesic; NSAID

PHARMACOLOGY

Action
Decreases inflammation, pain, and fever, probably through inhibition of COX activity and prostaglandin synthesis.

Uses
Treatment of rheumatoid arthritis, ankylosing spondylitis, and osteoarthritis. Potassium salt is approved for management of mild to moderate pain and primary dysmenorrhea when prompt pain relief is needed.

OPHTHALMIC: Treatment of postoperative inflammation after cataract removal; temporary relief of pain and photophobia following corneal refractive surgery.

TOPICAL: Treatment of actinic keratosis.

Unlabeled Uses

Treatment of biliary colic, enuresis, glomerular disease, gout, migraine headache, and renal colic.

➡◆ DRUG INTERACTIONS RELATED TO DENTAL THERAPEUTICS

No documented drug-drug interactions. The absence of evidence is not evidence of safety.

ADVERSE EFFECTS

⚠ **ORAL:** Taste disorder, dry mouth, aphthous stomatitis, esophageal ulceration (<1%).

CNS: ORAL TABLET: Dizziness, headache (1% to 10%).
OPHTHALMIC: Dizziness, headache, insomnia (≤3%).
TOPICAL: Headache, anxiety, dizziness, hypokinesia (>1%).

CVS: ORAL TABLET: Palpitations; tachycardia; hypotension; hypertension.

GI: ORAL TABLET: Abdominal pain, constipation, diarrhea, dyspepsia, flatulence, gross bleeding/perforation, heartburn, nausea, GI ulcers (gastric/duodenal), vomiting (1% to 10%).
OPHTHALMIC: Abdominal pain, nausea, vomiting (≤3%).
TOPICAL: Abdominal pain, constipation, diarrhea, dyspepsia (>1%).

RESP: TOPICAL: Asthma, dyspnea, pneumonia, sinusitis (>1%).

MISC: OPHTHALMIC: Asthenia, chills, fever, pain, viral infection, facial edema (≤3%).
TOPICAL: Accidental injury, allergic reaction, asthenia, back pain, chest pain, chills, flu-like syndrome, neck pain, pain (>1%).

CLINICAL IMPLICATIONS

General

- Determine why drug is being taken. Consider implications of condition on dental treatment.
- Chronic dry mouth is possible; anticipate increased caries, candidiasis, and lichenoid mucositis.
- Use COX inhibitors with caution; they may exacerbate PUD and GERD.
- *Arthritis:* Consider patient comfort and need for semisupine chair position.
- If GI side effects occur, consider semisupine chair position.
- Monitor vital signs.

Oral Health Education

- Evaluate manual dexterity; consider need for power toothbrush.

Dicloran — see diclofenac
Diclotride — see hydrochlorothiazide

---

dicloxacillin sodium (DIE-klox-uh-SILL-in SO-dee-uhm)

Dicloxacillin Sodium

■▨■ Brispen, Cilpen, Ditterolina, Posipen

Drug Class: Antibiotic, penicillin

PHARMACOLOGY

Action

Inhibits bacterial cell wall mucopeptide synthesis.

Uses

Treatment of infections caused by penicillinase-producing staphylococcal infection; initial therapy of suspected staphylococcal infection.

➡️⬅️ DRUG INTERACTIONS RELATED TO DENTAL THERAPEUTICS
No documented drug-drug interactions. The absence of evidence is not evidence of safety.

ADVERSE EFFECTS
⚠️ **ORAL:** Glossitis; stomatitis; sore mouth or tongue; dry mouth; furry tongue; black hairy tongue; taste perversion
CNS: Dizziness; fatigue; insomnia; reversible hyperactivity; seizures.
CVS: Tachycardia; hypotension; palpitations.
GI: Gastritis; anorexia; nausea; vomiting; abdominal pain or cramps; diarrhea or bloody diarrhea; rectal bleeding; flatulence; enterocolitis; pseudomembranous colitis.
MISC: Hypersensitivity reactions that may lead to death; vaginitis; hyperthermia; blood dyscrasias (e.g., thrombocytopenia, hemolytic anemia, leukopenia, others).

CLINICAL IMPLICATIONS
General
- Determine why drug is being taken. Take precautions to avoid cross-contamination of microorganisms.
- If oral infection that requires antibiotic therapy occurs, select an appropriate product from a different class of anti-infectives.
- Antibiotic-associated diarrhea may occur. Have patient contact DDS immediately if signs develop.
- Prolonged use of antibiotics may result in bacterial or fungal overgrowth of nonsusceptible microorganisms; anticipate candidiasis.
- Monitor vital signs.
- If GI side effects occur, consider semisupine chair position.
- Blood dyscrasias rarely reported; anticipate increased bleeding, infection, and poor healing.

Oral Health Education
- Encourage daily plaque control procedures for effective, nontraumatic self-care.

---

dicyclomine HCl (die-SIGH-kloe-meen HIGH-droe-KLOR-ide)
Antispas, Bemote, Bentyl, Byclomine, Dibent, Dilomine, Di-Spaz, Or-Tyl
■✦■ Bentylol, Lomine
Drug Class: Anticholinergic; Antispasmodic

PHARMACOLOGY
Action
Relieves smooth muscle spasm of GI tract through anticholinergic effects and direct action on GI smooth muscle.

Uses
Treatment of functional bowel/irritable bowel syndrome (e.g., irritable colon, spastic colon, mucous colitis).

Unlabeled Uses
Intestinal colic in children older than 6 mo.

➡️⬅️ DRUG INTERACTIONS RELATED TO DENTAL THERAPEUTICS
No documented drug-drug interactions. The absence of evidence is not evidence of safety.

ADVERSE EFFECTS
⚠️ **ORAL:** Dry mouth; taste disturbance.
CNS: Headache; flushing; nervousness; drowsiness; weakness; dizziness; confusion; insomnia; fever (especially in children); mental confusion or excitement (especially in elderly, even with small doses); CNS stimulation (restlessness, tremor); light-headedness.
CVS: Palpitations.

GI: Nausea; vomiting; dysphagia; heartburn; constipation; bloated feeling; paralytic ileus.
RESP: Nasal congestion.
MISC: Suppression of lactation; decreased sweating; photophobia.

CLINICAL IMPLICATIONS

General

- Anticholinergics have strong xerostomic effects. Anticipate increased caries activity and candidiasis.
- *Photophobia:* Direct dental light out of patient's eyes and offer dark glasses for comfort.

Oral Health Education

- If chronic dry mouth occurs, recommend home fluoride therapy and use of nonalcoholic oral health care products.

---

dideoxycytidine — see zalcitabine

---

 diflorasone diacetate (die-FLORE-ah-sone die-ASS-eh-tate)

Psorcon E: Cream: 0.05%; Ointment: 0.05%
Drug Class: Anti-inflammatory agent; Corticosteroid, topical

PHARMACOLOGY

Action

Therapeutic effects are caused by anti-inflammatory activity that is nonspecific (i.e., that act against most causes of inflammation including mechanical, chemical, microbiological, and immunological).

Uses

Relief of the anti-inflammatory and pruritic manifestations of corticosteroid responsive dermatoses.

Contraindications

Standard considerations.

Usual Dosage

Occlusive dressings may be used for certain conditions.
CREAM
ADULTS: *Topical:* Apply sparingly to affected area 1 to 3 times/day.
OINTMENT
ADULTS: *Topical:* Apply sparingly to affected area 1 to 4 times/day.

➡◀ DRUG INTERACTIONS

No documented drug-drug interactions. The absence of evidence is not evidence of safety.

ADVERSE EFFECTS

MISC: Systemic absorption may produce reversible hypothalamic pituitary adrenal (HPA) axis suppression, manifestations of Cushing syndrome, hyperglycemia, and glycosuria.

CLINICAL IMPLICATIONS

General

When prescribed by DDS:

- *Lactation:* Use with caution. It is not known whether topical corticosteroids could result in sufficient systemic absorption to produce adverse effects in infants.
- *Children:* Children may be more susceptible to topical corticosteroid-induced HPA axis suppression and Cushing syndrome than adults because of larger skin surface area to body weight ratio.
- *Systemic effects:* Systemic absorption of topical corticosteroids has produced reversible

HPA axis suppression, Cushing syndrome, hyperglycemia, and glycosuria. Conditions that may augment systemic absorption include use over large body surface areas, prolonged use, and occlusive dressings.

Pregnancy Risk Category: Category C.

Oral Health Education
When prescribed by DDS:
- Explain name, action, and potential side effects of drug.
- Advise patient to apply medication bid as directed by health care provider.
- Caution patient not to bandage, cover, or wrap treated skin areas or use cosmetics or other skin products over treated areas unless advised by health care provider.
- Caution patient to avoid contact with the eyes. Advise patient that if medication does come into contact with the eyes, to wash eyes with large amounts of cool water and contact health care provider if eye irritation occurs.
- Advise patient that symptoms should begin to improve fairly soon after starting treatment and to notify health care provider if condition does not improve, worsens, or if application site reactions (e.g., burning, stinging, redness, itching) develop.
- Advise patient that therapy is usually discontinued when control has been achieved.
- Advise patient that follow-up visits to monitor response to treatment may be required and to keep appointments.

Diflucan — see fluconazole

Diflucan-150 — see fluconazole

---

diflunisal (die-FLOO-nih-sal)

Dolobid

■✦■ **Apo-Diflunisal, Novo-Diflunisal, Nu-Diflunisal**

Drug Class: Analgesic; Salicylate

PHARMACOLOGY
Action
Decreases inflammation and relieves pain by inhibiting prostaglandin synthesis and release.

Uses
Relief of mild to moderate pain, rheumatoid arthritis, and osteoarthritis.

➡◆ DRUG INTERACTIONS RELATED TO DENTAL THERAPEUTICS
No documented drug-drug interactions. The absence of evidence is not evidence of safety.

ADVERSE EFFECTS
CNS: Headache; somnolence; insomnia; dizziness.
CVS: Palpitations; chest pain.
GI: Nausea; dyspepsia; GI pain; diarrhea; GI bleeding.
RESP: Bronchospasm.
MISC: Anaphylaxis; hypersensitivity syndrome (e.g., fever, chills, rash, liver or kidney dysfunction, leukopenia, thrombocytopenia, eosinophilia, DIC).

CLINICAL IMPLICATIONS
General
- Determine why drug is being taken. Consider implications of condition on dental treatment.
- Use COX inhibitors with caution, they may exacerbate PUD and GERD.
- *Arthritis:* Consider patient comfort and need for semisupine chair position.
- If GI side effects occur, consider semisupine chair position.
- Blood dyscrasias rarely reported; anticipate increased bleeding, infection, and poor healing.

Oral Health Education
• Evaluate manual dexterity; consider need for power toothbrush.

Difoxacil — see norfloxacin
Digitek — see digoxin

digoxin (dih-JOX-in)
Digitek, Lanoxicaps, Lanoxin

■🍁■ **Mapluxin**

Drug Class: Cardiac glycoside

PHARMACOLOGY
Action
Increases force and velocity of myocardial systolic contraction (i.e., positive inotropic action), slows heart rate, and decreases conduction through atrioventricular node.

Uses
Treatment of CHF, atrial fibrillation, atrial flutter, paroxysmal atrial tachycardia, cardiogenic shock.

➡◀ DRUG INTERACTIONS RELATED TO DENTAL THERAPEUTICS
Itraconazole: Digoxin toxicity (decreased clearance)
• Avoid concurrent use.
Diazepam: Possible digoxin toxicity (decreased metabolism)
• Monitor clinical status.
Sympathomimetic amines: Increased incidence of cardiac arrhythmias (additive)
• Use local anesthetic agents containing a vasoconstrictor with caution.
• Monitor pulse rate and character.
Tetracyclines: Increased digoxin toxicity (increased absorption)
• Avoid concurrent use.

ADVERSE EFFECTS
⚠ **ORAL:** Increased gag reflex.
CNS: Headache; weakness; apathy; drowsiness; mental depression; confusion; disorientation.
CVS: Palpitation; tachycardia.
MISC: Thrombocytopenia (rare).
GI: Anorexia; nausea; vomiting; diarrhea.

CLINICAL IMPLICATIONS
General
• Determine why drug is being taken. Consider implications of condition on dental treatment.
• Digoxin adverse effects are dose dependent and occur at doses higher than needed for therapeutic efficacy; however, doses must be titrated regularly to ensure accuracy.
• Monitor vital signs (e.g., BP, pulse pressure, rate, and rhythm) at each appointment to assess disease control. Do not provide elective dental treatment when BP is ≥180/11c or in the presence of other high-risk CV conditions. Refer to the section entitled "The Patient Taking Cardiovascular Drugs" in Chapter 6: *Clinical Medicine.*
• Use local anesthetic agents with vasoconstrictor with caution based on functional capacity of the patient and use aspirating technique to prevent intravascular injection.
• Determine ability to adapt to stress of dental treatment. Consider short appointments.
• Blood dyscrasias rarely reported; anticipate increased bleeding.

Oral Health Education
• Encourage daily plaque control procedures for effective self-care in patients at risk for cardiovascular disease.

Dilacoran — see verapamil HCl
Dilacor XR — see diltiazem HCl
Dilantin — see phenytoin
Dilantin-125 — see phenytoin
Dilantin Infatab — see phenytoin
Dilantin Kapseals — see phenytoin
Dilantin-30 Pediatric — see phenytoin
Dilatrate-SR — see isosorbide dinitrate
Dilatrend — see carvedilol
Dilaudid — see hydromorphone HCl
Dilaudid-HP — see hydromorphone HCl
Dilaudid-HP Plus — see hydromorphone HCl
Dilaudid Sterile Powder — see hydromorphone HCl
Dilaudid-XP — see hydromorphone HCl
Dilocaine — see lidocaine HCl
Dilomine — see dicyclomine HCl
Diltia XT — see diltiazem HCl

diltiazem HCl (dill-TIE-uh-zem HIGH-droe-KLOR-ide)

Cardizem, Cardizem CD, Cardizem LA, Cartia XT, Dilacor XR, Diltia XT, Diltiazem Hydrochloride Extended Release, Taztia XT, Tiazac

■✦■ **Apo-Diltiaz, Apo-Diltiaz CD, Apo-Diltiaz Injectable, Apo-Diltiaz SR, Gen-Diltiazem, Novo-Diltiazem, Novo-Diltiazem SR, Nu-Diltiaz, Nu-Diltiaz-CD, ratio-Diltiazem CD, Rhoxal-diltiazem CD**

■●■ **Angiotrofin, Angiotrofin AP, Angiotrofin Retard, Presoken, Presoquim, Tilazem**

Drug Class: Calcium channel blocker

PHARMACOLOGY

Action
Inhibits movement of calcium ions across cell membrane in systemic and coronary vascular smooth muscle; slows calcium ion movement across cell membranes in both cardiac muscle and cardiac pacemaker cells, decreasing sinuatrial and atrioventricular (AV) conduction.

Uses
ORAL: Treatment of angina pectoris caused by coronary artery spasm; chronic stable angina (classic effort-associated angina); essential hypertension (extended- and sustained-release forms only).
PARENTERAL: Treatment of atrial fibrillation or flutter; paroxysmal supraventricular tachycardia.

➡◀ DRUG INTERACTIONS RELATED TO DENTAL THERAPEUTICS

Midazolam or triazolam: Increased sedation after oral administration (decreased metabolism)
• Avoid concurrent use.

ADVERSE EFFECTS
⚠ **ORAL:** Dry mouth, dysgeusia, thirst, gingival hyperplasia (2%).

CNS: Dizziness (6%); headache, fatigue (5%); asthenia (3%); abnormal dreams, amnesia, depression, gait abnormalities, hallucinations, insomnia, nervousness, paresthesia, personality change, somnolence, tremor (<2%); lightheadedness; weakness; shakiness; extrapyramidal symptoms.

CVS: Bradycardia (6%); tachycardia, syncope, hypotension, postural hypotension, arrhythmia, chest pain, palpitations (≤2%).

GI: Nausea (1%); anorexia, constipation, diarrhea, vomiting (<2%); abdominal discomfort; cramps; dyspepsia.

RESP: Cough (2%); dyspnea (<2%).

MISC: Lower limb edema (7%); edema (5%); flushing (1%); allergic reactions, pain (<2%); angioedema; photosensitivity.

CLINICAL IMPLICATIONS
General
- Determine why drug is being taken. Consider implications of condition on dental treatment.
- Monitor vital signs (e.g., BP, pulse pressure, rate, and rhythm) at each appointment to assess disease control. Do not provide elective dental treatment when BP ≥180/110 or in presence of other high-risk CV conditions. Refer to the section entitled "The Patient Taking Cardiovascular Drugs" in Chapter 6: *Clinical Medicine*.
- Use local anesthetic agents with vasoconstrictor with caution based on functional capacity of the patient and use aspirating technique to prevent intravascular injection.
- Anticipate gingival hyperplasia; consider MD consult to recommend different drug regimen if periodontal health is compromised.
- Determine ability to adapt to stress of dental treatment. Consider short appointments.
- Chronic dry mouth is possible; anticipate increased caries and candidiasis.
- *Postural hypotension:* Monitor BP at the beginning and end of each appointment; anticipate syncope. Have patient sit upright for several min at the end of the dental appointment before dismissing.
- If GI side effects occur, consider semisupine chair position.

Oral Health Education
- If chronic dry mouth occurs, recommend home fluoride therapy and use of nonalcoholic oral health care products.
- Encourage daily plaque control procedures for effective self-care in patients at risk for cardiovascular disease.

Diltiazem Hydrochloride Extended Release — see diltiazem HCl
Dimantil — see warfarin
Dimefor — see metformin HCl
Dimelor — see acetohexamide

---

dimenhydrinate (die-men-HIGH-drih-nate)
Calm-X, Children's Dramamine, Dimetabs, Dinate, Dramamine, Dramanate, Dymenate, Hydrate, Triptone

■✦■ Apo-Dimenhydrinate, Gravol

■✦■ Vomisin

Drug Class: Antiemetic; Antivertigo; Anticholinergic

PHARMACOLOGY
Action
Directly inhibits labyrinthine stimulation for up to 3 hr.
Uses
Prevention and treatment of motion sickness, dizziness, nausea, vomiting.

Unlabeled Uses

Treatment of Ménière disease, nausea and vomiting of pregnancy, postoperative nausea, and vomiting.

✦ DRUG INTERACTIONS RELATED TO DENTAL THERAPEUTICS

No documented drug-drug interactions. The absence of evidence is not evidence of safety.

ADVERSE EFFECTS

⚠ **ORAL:** Dry mouth, nose, throat.

CNS: Sedation; hallucinations; delirium; drowsiness; confusion, nervousness; restlessness; headache; insomnia; tingling, heaviness and weakness of hands; vertigo; dizziness; lassitude; excitation.

CVS: Palpitations; hypotension; tachycardia.

GI: Nausea; vomiting; diarrhea; GI distress; constipation; anorexia.

RESP: Tightness of chest; wheezing; thickening of bronchial secretions.

MISC: Anaphylaxis; photosensitivity.

CLINICAL IMPLICATIONS

General

- Determine why drug is being taken. Consider implications of condition on dental treatment.
- Chronic dry mouth is possible; anticipate increased caries and candidiasis.
- Monitor vital signs, including respiration rate and qualities.
- Be aware that patients with multiple allergies are at increased risk for allergy to dental drugs.
- Consider semisupine chair position to control effects of postnasal drainage.
- If GI or respiratory side effects occur, consider semisupine chair position.

Oral Health Education

- If chronic dry mouth occurs, recommend home fluoride therapy and use of nonalcoholic oral health care products.

Dimetabs — see dimenhydrinate

Dimodan — see disopyramide phosphate

Dinate — see dimenhydrinate

Diovan — see valsartan

Diovan HCT — see valsartan/hydrochlorothiazide

Dipedyne — see zidovudine

Diphen AF — see diphenhydramine HCl

Diphenhist — see diphenhydramine HCl

Diphenhist Captabs — see diphenhydramine HCl

Diphenhydramine — see diphenhydramine HCl

---

 diphenhydramine HCl (die-fen-HIGH-druh-meen HIGH-droe-KLOR-ide)

40 Winks, AllerMax Maximum Strength, Compoz Nighttime Sleep Aid, Maximum Strength Nytol, Midol PM, Snoozefast, Twilite: Tablets: 50 mg
AllerMax, Banophen Allergy, Benadryl Children's Allergy, Benadryl Children's Dye Free, Diphen AF, Scot-Tussin Allergy, Siladryl: Elixir, liquid: 12.5 mg per 5 mL
Banophen, Dormin: Tablets: 25 mg; Capsules: 25 mg
Benadryl Allergy: Capsules, soft-gels: 25 mg; Tablets: 25 mg; Tablets, chewable: 12.5 mg

Benadryl Dye Free Allergy Liqui Gels, Compoz Gel Caps: Capsules, soft gels: 25 mg
Diphenhist: Solution: 12.5 mg per 5 mL
Diphenhist Captabs, Miles Nervine, Nytol, Simply Sleep, Sleep-Eze 3, Sleepwell 2-nite: Tablets: 25 mg
Diphenhydramine, Hyrexin-50: Injection: 50 mg/mL
Genahist: Tablets: 25 mg; Capsules: 25 mg; Liquid: 12.5 mg per 5 mL
Hydramine Cough, Sylphen Cough, Tusstat: Syrup: 12.5 mg per 5 mL
Maximum Strength Sleepinal Capsules and Soft Gels, Maximum Strength Unisom SleepGels: Capsules: 50 mg
Sominex: Tablets: 25, 50 mg
Theraflu Thin Strips Multisymptom: Strips, orally disintegrating: 25 mg
Triaminic Thin Strips Cough and Runny Nose: Strips, orally disintegrating: 12.5 mg

■✦■ **Allerdryl, Allernix, Nytol Extra Strength, PMS-Diphenhydramine, Simply Sleep, Unisom Extra Strength, Unisom Extra Strength Sleepgels**

Drug Class: Antihistamine, ethanolamine

PHARMACOLOGY
Action
Competitively antagonizes histamine at H_1 receptor sites.

Uses
Symptomatic relief of perennial and seasonal allergic rhinitis, vasomotor rhinitis, and allergic conjunctivitis; temporary relief of runny nose and sneezing caused by common cold; dermatographism; treatment of urticaria and angioedema; amelioration of allergic reactions to blood or plasma; adjunct to epinephrine and other standard measures in anaphylaxis; relief of uncomplicated allergic conditions of immediate type when oral therapy is impossible or contraindicated (parenteral form); treatment and prophylactic treatment of motion sickness (injection only); nighttime sleep aid; management of parkinsonism (including drug-induced) in elderly who are intolerant of more potent agents, in mild cases in other age groups, and in combination with centrally acting anticholinergics; control of cough, due to colds or allergy (syrup formulations).

Contraindications
Hypersensitivity to antihistamines; asthma attack; MAO inhibitor therapy; history of sleep apnea; use in newborn or premature infants and in nursing women; use as a local anesthetic.

Usual Dosage
Hypersensitivity Reactions, Type 1/Antiparkinsonism/Motion Sickness
ADULTS: *PO:* 25 to 50 mg q 4 to 6 hr (max, 300 mg/day). *IV/IM:* 10 to 50 mg IV at a rate not exceeding 25 mg/min or 100 mg deep IM if required (max, 400 mg/day).
CHILDREN (6 TO YOUNGER THAN 12 YR OF AGE): *PO:* 12.5 to 25 mg q 4 to 6 hr (max, 150 mg). *IV/IM:* 5 mg/kg/day or 150 mg/m²/day (max, 300 mg divided into 4 doses at a rate not exceeding 25 mg/min or deep IM).
Nighttime Sleep Aid
ADULTS: *PO:* 50 mg at bedtime.

Pharmacokinetics
ABSORP: T_{max} is 1 to 4 hr (oral).
DIST: Widely distributed, including the CNS. Excreted in breast milk. 98% to 99% protein bound.
METAB: Metabolized in the liver.
EXCRET: A portion of the drug excreted unchanged in the urine. The $t_{1/2}$ is 1 to 4 hr.

ONSET: Rapid onset (IV or IM).

DURATION: 6 to 8 hr.

➡◀ DRUG INTERACTIONS

Acetaminophen: Delayed absorption of acetaminophen (delayed gastric emptying)
• Monitor clinical status.

Metoprolol: Possible metoprolol toxicity (decreased metabolism)
• Monitor clinical status.

Venlafaxine: Possible venlafaxine toxicity (decreased metabolism)
• Monitor clinical status.

ADVERSE EFFECTS

⚠ **ORAL:** Stomatitis; aphthous stomatitis, taste disturbance (nasal spray).

CVS: Orthostatic hypotension; palpitations; bradycardia; tachycardia; reflex tachycardia; extrasystoles; faintness.

CNS: Drowsiness (often transient); sedation; dizziness; faintness; disturbed coordination.

GI: Epigastric distress; nausea; vomiting; diarrhea; constipation; change in bowel habits.

RESP: Thickening of bronchial secretions; chest tightness; wheezing; respiratory depression.

MISC: Hypersensitivity reactions; photosensitivity.

CLINICAL IMPLICATIONS

General

• Determine why drug is being taken. Consider implications of condition on dental treatment.
• Consider semisupine chair position to control effects of postnasal drainage.
• Be aware that patients with multiple allergies are at increased risk for allergy to dental drugs.
• If GI or respiratory side effects occur, consider semisupine chair position.
• *Postural hypotension:* Monitor BP at the beginning and end of each appointment; anticipate syncope. Have patient sit upright for several min at the end of the dental appointment before dismissing.
• Monitor vital signs.

When prescribed by DDS:

• *Lactation:* Excreted in breast milk.
• *Children:* Overdosage may cause hallucinations, convulsions, and death. Antihistamines may diminish mental alertness. In young children, drug may produce paradoxical excitation. Use with caution in children younger than 2 yr of age.
• *Elderly:* Greater risk of dizziness, excessive sedation, syncope, toxic confusional states, and hypotension in patients older than 60 yr of age. Dosage reduction may be required.
• *Hypersensitivity:* May occur. Have epinephrine 1:1,000 immediately available.
• *Hepatic failure:* Use with caution in patients with cirrhosis or other liver diseases.
• *Special risk:* Use with caution in patients predisposed to urinary retention, prostatic hypertrophy, history of bronchial asthma, increased intraocular pressure, hyperthyroidism, CV disease, or hypertension. Use with considerable caution in patients with narrow-angle glaucoma, stenosing peptic ulcer, pyloroduodenal obstruction, symptomatic prostatic hypertrophy, or bladder neck obstruction.
• *Sulfite sensitivity:* Some diphenhydramine products may contain sulfites as preservatives and aspartame as sweetener. Avoid in sulfite-allergic patients and in patients with phenylketonuria, respectively.
• *Respiratory disease:* Generally not recommended to treat lower respiratory tract symptoms, including asthma.
• *Overdosage:* Circulatory collapse; cardiac arrest; respiratory depression or arrest; toxic psychosis; coma; stupor; seizures; ataxia; anxiety; incoherence; hyperactivity; combativeness; anhidrosis; fever; hot, dry, or flushed skin; dry mucous membranes; dysphagia; decreased bowel sounds; dilated and sluggish pupils.

Pregnancy Risk Category: Category B.

Oral Health Education
When prescribed by DDS:

- Explain name, dose, action, and potential side effects of drug.
- Caution patient using OTC product to read package label before using and not to exceed dose or frequency of administration instructions.
- Advise patient to take each dose without regard to meals but to take with food if stomach upset occurs.
- Advise patient using diphenhydramine to prevent motion sickness to take first dose at least 30 min before exposure to motion and take subsequent doses after each meal and at bedtime for duration of journey.
- Advise patient using diphenhydramine as a sleep aid to take dose at least 30 min before bedtime and not to use for more than 2 wk. Caution patient that if insomnia persists for more than 2 wk, it may be a symptom of a serious underlying illness and to inform health care provider.
- Advise patient or caregiver using liquid, oral solution, elixir, or syrup to measure and administer prescribed dose using dosing syringe, dosing spoon, or dosing cup.
- Advise patient that if a dose is missed to take it as soon as possible unless it is nearing time for the next scheduled dose, then advise patient to skip the missed dose and take the next dose at the regularly scheduled time. Caution patient not to double the dose to catch up.
- Advise patient that if allergy symptoms are not controlled not to increase the dose of medication or frequency of use but to inform his or her health care provider. Caution patient that larger doses or more frequent dosing does not increase effectiveness and may cause excessive drowsiness or other side effects.
- Instruct patient to stop taking drug and immediately report any of the following symptoms to health care provider: persistent dizziness; excessive drowsiness; severe dry mouth, nose, or throat; flushing; unexplained shortness of breath or difficulty breathing; unusual tiredness or weakness; sore throat, fever, or other signs of infection; bleeding or unusual bruising; fast or irregular heartbeat; excitability, confusion, or changes in thinking or behavior; chest tightness; difficulty urinating.
- Advise patient that medication may cause drowsiness or dizziness and not to drive or perform other activities requiring mental alertness until tolerance is determined.
- Advise patient to take sips of water, suck on ice chips or sugarless hard candy, or chew sugarless gum if dry mouth occurs.
- Caution patient that alcohol and other CNS depressants (e.g., sedatives) will have additional sedative effects if taken with diphenhydramine.
- Caution patient not to take any OTC antihistamines or any other product containing diphenhydramine, including topical products, while taking this medication unless advised by health care provider.
- Caution patient that medication may cause sensitivity to sunlight and to avoid excessive exposure to the sun or UV light (e.g., tanning booths) and to wear protective clothing and use sunscreens until tolerance is determined.
- If patient is to have allergy skin testing, advise patient not to take the medication for at least 4 days before the skin testing.
- Advise women to notify health care provider if pregnant, planning to become pregnant, or breast feeding.
- Caution patient not to take any prescription or OTC medications, herbal preparations, or dietary supplements unless advised by health care provider.

Diprivan — see propofol

Diprolene — see betamethasone

Diprolene AF — see betamethasone

Diprolene Glycol — see betamethasone

Diprosone — see betamethasone

dipyridamole (DIE-pih-RID-uh-mole)

Dipyridamole, Persantine

■❖■ **Dirinol, Lodimol, Trompersantin**

Drug Class: Antiplatelet; Diagnostic agent

PHARMACOLOGY

Action

Lengthens abnormally shortened platelet survival time in a dose-dependent manner by inhibiting platelet aggregation in response to various stimuli, such as platelet activating factor, collagen, and adenosine diphosphate. Vasodilation may result from inhibition of adenosine uptake, which is an important mediator of coronary vasodilation.

Uses

Adjunct to coumarin anticoagulants in prevention of postoperative thromboembolic complication of cardiac valve replacement (oral). Alternative to exercise in thallium myocardial perfusion imaging for evaluating coronary artery disease in patients who cannot exercise adequately (IV).

➡◀ DRUG INTERACTIONS RELATED TO DENTAL THERAPEUTICS

No documented drug-drug interactions. The absence of evidence is not evidence of safety.

ADVERSE EFFECTS

CNS: ORAL: Dizziness (14%); headache (2%); fatigue; malaise.
IV: Headache, dizziness (12%); paresthesia, fatigue (1%).
GI: ORAL: Abdominal distress (6%); diarrhea; vomiting; nausea, dyspepsia.
IV: Nausea (5%); dyspepsia (1%).
RESP: IV: Dyspnea (3%).
MISC: ORAL: Flushing; hypersensitivity (e.g., rash, urticaria, severe bronchospasm, angioedema); arthritis; paresthesia.
IV: Flushing, unspecific pain (3%).

CLINICAL IMPLICATIONS

General

- Determine why drug is being taken. Consider implications of condition on dental treatment.
- Determine bleeding time before completing procedures that may result in significant bleeding. Safe levels are <20 min.
- Monitor vital signs (BP, pulse pressure, rate, and rhythm) at each appointment to assess disease control. Do not provide elective dental treatment when BP is ≥180/110 or in the presence of other high-risk CV conditions. Refer to the section entitled "The Patient Taking Cardiovascular Drugs" in Chapter 6: *Clinical Medicine*.
- If GI side effects occur, consider semisupine chair position.

Oral Health Education

- Encourage daily plaque control procedures for effective self-care in patients at risk for cardiovascular disease.

---

dipyridamole/aspirin — see aspirin/dipyridamole
Dirinol — see dipyridamole
disodium cromoglycate — see cromolyn sodium
D-isoephedrine — see pseudoephedrine

disopyramide phosphate (DIE-so-PIR-uh-mide)

Norpace, Norpace CR

❚✦❚ Rythmodan, Rythmodan-LA

❚❚ Dimodan

Drug Class: Antiarrhythmic

PHARMACOLOGY

Action

Decreases rate of diastolic depolarization; decreases upstroke velocity; increases action potential duration; prolongs refractory period.

Uses

Suppression and documented prevention of ventricular arrhythmias considered to be life threatening.

Unlabeled Uses

Treatment of paroxysmal supraventricular tachycardia.

➡◆ DRUG INTERACTIONS RELATED TO DENTAL THERAPEUTICS

No documented drug-drug interactions. The absence of evidence is not evidence of safety.

ADVERSE EFFECTS

⚠ **ORAL:** Dry mouth (32%).

CNS: Dizziness, fatigue, headache, malaise (3% to 9%); nervousness (1% to 3%).

CVS: Hypotension, arrhythmia, syncope, chest pain, CHF signs.

GI: Constipation (11%); nausea, pain/bloating/gas (3% to 9%); anorexia, diarrhea, vomiting (1% to 3%).

RESP: Shortness of breath (1% to 3%).

MISC: Aches, pain (3% to 9%); thrombocytopenia, agranulocytosis (rare).

CLINICAL IMPLICATIONS

General

- Determine why drug is being taken. Consider implications of condition on dental treatment.
- Monitor vital signs (e.g., BP, pulse pressure, rate, and rhythm) at each appointment to assess disease control. Do not provide elective dental treatment when BP is ≥180/110 or in the presence of other high-risk CV conditions. Refer to the section entitled "The Patient Taking Cardiovascular Drugs" in Chapter 6: *Clinical Medicine*.
- Use local anesthetic agents with vasoconstrictor with caution based on functional capacity of the patient and use aspirating technique to prevent intravascular injection.
- Determine ability to adapt to stress of dental treatment. Consider short appointments.
- Chronic dry mouth is possible; anticipate increased caries and candidiasis.
- If GI side effects occur, consider semisupine chair position.
- Blood dyscrasias rarely reported; anticipate increased bleeding, infection, and poor healing.

Oral Health Education

- If chronic dry mouth occurs, recommend home fluoride therapy and use of nonalcoholic oral health care products.
- Encourage daily plaque control procedures for effective self-care in patients at risk for cardiovascular disease.

Di-Spaz — see dicyclomine HCl

disulfiram (die-SULL-fih-ram)

Antabuse

Drug Class: Antialcoholic agent

PHARMACOLOGY

Action

Produces intolerance to alcohol by blocking oxidation of acetaldehyde by enzyme aldehyde dehydrogenase, resulting in high blood levels of acetaldehyde and unpleasant physical symptoms.

Uses

Aid in management of alcoholism in selected patients who want to remain in state of enforced sobriety.

➜← DRUG INTERACTIONS RELATED TO DENTAL THERAPEUTICS

Benzodiazepines: Possible benzodiazepine toxicity (decreased metabolism)
- Monitor clinical status.

Metronidazole: Organic brain syndrome (mechanism unknown)
- Avoid concurrent use.

ADVERSE EFFECTS

⚠ **ORAL:** Taste disturbances.

CNS: Drowsiness; fatigue; headache; psychotic reactions.

GI: Nausea, vomiting (if alcohol ingested).

MISC: Peripheral neuropathy; polyneuritis; optic or peripheral neuritis; impotence.

CLINICAL IMPLICATIONS

General

- Determine why drug is being taken. Consider implications of condition on dental treatment.
- Determine whether patient is in a professional treatment program.
- Avoid prescribing opioids for dental pain. Acetaminophen is appropriate if GI bleeding is present.
- Do not recommend or prescribe alcohol-containing mouth rinses.
- Be aware that patient may be taking opioid antagonists and CNS depressant drugs.
- Liver disease may be present resulting in increased bleeding due to a deficiency of vitamin K–dependent clotting factors.
- Alcohol and tobacco use and abuse predispose to oral squamous cell carcinoma; perform oral cancer exam routinely.

Oral Health Education

- Most patients with alcoholism have poor oral health due to neglect. Encourage daily self-care to prevent periodontal disease.

Ditropan — see oxybutynin Cl

Ditropan XL — see oxybutynin Cl

Ditterolina — see dicloxacillin sodium

Diurigen — see chlorothiazide

Diuril — see chlorothiazide

divalproex sodium — see valproic acid and derivatives

Dixarit — see clonidine HCl

Dixonal — see piroxicam

docosanol (doe-KOE-sah-nole)

Abreva

Drug Class: Antiviral, topical

PHARMACOLOGY

Action

Prevents fusion of herpes simplex virus with cell membrane, thereby blocking entry and viral replication.

Uses

Cold sores, fever blisters.

Contraindications

Age 11 yr and younger.

➡◀ DRUG INTERACTIONS RELATED TO DENTAL THERAPEUTICS

No documented drug-drug interactions. The absence of evidence is not evidence of safety.

ADVERSE EFFECTS

⚠ **ORAL:** Tingling at application site.

CLINICAL IMPLICATIONS

General

- Topical OTC cream to be applied by cotton bud 5 times a day during prodromal period of herpes labialis outbreak to shorten healing time and duration of symptoms.
- FDA approved for children older than age 12 yr and adults.

Oral Health Education

- Warn patient to wash hands after use and to apply agent with cotton bud, not fingers, because herpes virus in contagious.
- Instruct patient to apply at first sign of extraoral herpes outbreak; not intended for use inside mouth.

dofetilide (doe-FEH-till-ide)

Tikosyn

Drug Class: Antiarrhythmic

PHARMACOLOGY

Action

Blockade of the cardiac ion channel carrying the rapid component of the delayed rectifier potassium currents.

Uses

Maintenance of normal sinus rhythm (delay in time to recurrence of atrial fibrillation/atrial flutter [AF/AFl]) in patients with AF/AFl of more than 1 wk duration who have been converted to normal sinus rhythm; conversion of AF/AFl to normal sinus rhythm.

Unlabeled Uses

Ventricular arrhythmias.

➡◀ DRUG INTERACTIONS RELATED TO DENTAL THERAPEUTICS

Ketoconazole or itraconazole: Increased cardiac arrhythmias (decreased metabolism)
- Avoid concurrent use.

ADVERSE EFFECTS

CNS: Headache; dizziness; insomnia; migraine.
CVS: Bradycardia, syncope, cerebral stroke (≤2%).

GI: Diarrhea; abdominal pain.
RESP: Respiratory tract infection; dyspnea.
MISC: Flu-like syndrome; back pain; edema; facial paralysis; paralysis; paresthesia; sudden death.

CLINICAL IMPLICATIONS

General

• Determine why drug is being taken. Consider implications of condition on dental treatment.
• Monitor vital signs (e.g., BP, pulse pressure, rate, and rhythm) at each appointment to assess disease control. Do not provide elective dental treatment when BP is ≥180/110 or in the presence of other high-risk CV conditions. Refer to the section entitled "The Patient Taking Cardiovascular Drugs" in Chapter 6: *Clinical Medicine.*
• Use local anesthetic agents with vasoconstrictor with caution based on functional capacity of the patient and use aspirating technique to prevent intravascular injection.
• Determine ability to adapt to stress of dental treatment. Consider short appointments.

Oral Health Education

• Encourage daily plaque control procedures for effective self-care in patients at risk for cardiovascular disease.

Dola — see ketorolac tromethamine

Dolac — see ketorolac tromethamine

Dolacet — see acetaminophen/hydrocodone bitartrate

Dolaren — see diclofenac

Dolflam — see diclofenac

Dolobid — see diflunisal

Dolo Pangavit-D — see diclofenac

Dolophine HCl — see methadone HCl

Dolorac — see capsaicin

Dolotor — see ketorolac tromethamine

Dolzycam — see piroxicam

---

donepezil (dawn-EPP-uh-zill)

Aricept

■◆■ **Eranz**

Drug Class: Reversible cholinesterase inhibitor

PHARMACOLOGY

Action

Increases acetylcholine by inhibiting acetylcholinesterase, thereby increasing cholinergic function.

Uses

Treatment of mild to moderate dementia of the Alzheimer type.

➡◆ DRUG INTERACTIONS RELATED TO DENTAL THERAPEUTICS

Ketoconazole: Possible donepezil toxicity (mechanism unknown)
• Avoid concurrent use.

ADVERSE EFFECTS

⚠ **ORAL:** Tooth pain (unspecified).
CNS: Depression; abnormal dreams; somnolence; insomnia; fatigue; dizziness.

CVS: Postural hypotension, syncope (2%); hypotension or hypertension; bradycardia; tachycardia.

GI: Nausea (11%); diarrhea; vomiting; anorexia; fecal incontinence; GI bleeding; bloating; epigastric pain.

RESP: Dyspnea; sore throat; bronchitis.

MISC: Muscle cramps; arthritis; ecchymoses (4%); thrombocytopenia, eosinophilia (<1%).

CLINICAL IMPLICATIONS

General

- Patient may experience hypotension or hypertension. Monitor vital signs at each appointment; anticipate syncope.
- Ensure that caregiver is present at every dental appointment and understands informed consent.
- *Postural hypotension:* Monitor BP at the beginning and end of each appointment; anticipate syncope. Have patient sit upright for several min at the end of the dental appointment before dismissing.
- If GI side effects occur, consider semisupine chair position.
- Blood dyscrasias rarely reported; anticipate increased bleeding, infection, and poor healing.

Oral Health Education

- Teach caregiver to assist patient with oral self-care practices.

Donnamar — see hyoscyamine sulfate

Donnatal — see hyoscyamine sulfate

Dorcol Children's Decongestant — see pseudoephedrine

Dormicum — see midazolam HCl

Dormin — see diphenhydramine HCl

Doryx — see doxycycline hyclate

---

doxazosin mesylate (DOX-uh-ZOE-sin MEH-suh-late)

Cardura

■✚■ Apo-Doxazosin, Cardura-1, Cardura-2, Cardura-4, Gen-Doxazosin, Novo-Doxazosin, ratio-Doxazosin

Drug Class: Antihypertensive; Antiadrenergic, peripherally acting

PHARMACOLOGY

Action

Selectively blocks postsynaptic alpha$_1$-adrenergic receptors, resulting in dilation of arterioles and veins.

Uses

Treatment of hypertension, alone or in combination with other agents; treatment of benign prostatic hyperplasia (BPH).

➔← DRUG INTERACTIONS RELATED TO DENTAL THERAPEUTICS

No documented drug-drug interactions. The absence of evidence is not evidence of safety.

ADVERSE EFFECTS

⚠ **ORAL:** Dry mouth (2%), taste perversion (<0.5%).

CNS: Dizziness (19%); headache (14%); fatigue/malaise (12%); somnolence (5%); vertigo, nervousness (2%); anxiety, kinetic disorders, ataxia, hypertonia, muscle cramps, insomnia, depression (1%).

CVS: Postural hypotension (<2%); palpitation, chest pain, arrhythmia, syncope (1%).

GI: Nausea (3%); diarrhea (2%); constipation, dyspepsia, flatulence (1%).
RESP: Dyspnea, rhinitis (3%); respiratory disorder (1%).
MISC: Pain, chest pain (2%); flushing, rash, pruritus (1%); leukopenia, thrombocytopenia (<0.5%).

CLINICAL IMPLICATIONS

General

- Determine why drug is being taken. Consider implications of condition on dental treatment.
- Monitor vital signs (e.g., BP, pulse pressure, rate, and rhythm) at each appointment to assess disease control. Do not provide elective dental treatment when BP is ≥180/110 or in the presence of other high-risk CV conditions. Refer to the section entitled "The Patient Taking Cardiovascular Drugs" in Chapter 6: *Clinical Medicine.*
- Use local anesthetic agents with vasoconstrictor with caution based on functional capacity of the patient and use aspirating technique to prevent intravascular injection.
- Determine ability to adapt to stress of dental treatment. Consider short appointments.
- *Postural hypotension:* Monitor BP at the beginning and end of each appointment; anticipate syncope. Have patient sit upright for several min at the end of the dental appointment before dismissing.
- Chronic dry mouth is possible; anticipate increased caries activity and candidiasis.
- If GI side effects occur, consider semisupine chair position.
- Blood dyscrasias rarely reported; anticipate increased bleeding, infection, and poor healing.

Oral Health Education

- If chronic dry mouth occurs, recommend home fluoride therapy and use of nonalcoholic oral health care products.
- Encourage daily plaque control procedures for effective self-care in patients at risk for cardiovascular disease.

---

doxepin HCl (DOX-uh-pin HIGH-droe-KLOR-ide)

Sinequan, Zonalon
■✚■ Apo-Doxepin, Novo-Doxepin

Drug Class: Antianxiety; Antidepressant, tricyclic

PHARMACOLOGY

Action

Moderately blocks reuptake of norepinephrine and weakly blocks reuptake of serotonin; also produces antihistaminic and anticholinergic activity.

Uses

Treatment of psychoneurotic patients with depression and/or anxiety; depression and/or anxiety associated with alcoholism (not to be taken concomitantly with alcohol); depression and/or anxiety associated with organic disease (the possibility of drug interaction should be considered if the patient is receiving other drugs concomitantly); psychotic depressive disorders with associated anxiety including involutional depression and manic-depressive disorders; moderate pruritus with atopic dermatitis or lichen simplex chronicus (topical).

Unlabeled Uses

Neurogenic pain, peptic ulcer disease.

➡◀ DRUG INTERACTIONS RELATED TO DENTAL THERAPEUTICS

Sympathomimetic amines: Hypertension and hypertensive crisis with epinephrine (inhibition of epinephrine uptake)
- Use local anesthetic agents containing a vasoconstrictor with caution.
- Monitor blood pressure.

ADVERSE EFFECTS

⚠ **ORAL:** Dry mouth; taste perversion; aphthous stomatitis.
CNS: Dizziness; drowsiness; headache; confusion; weakness; tremors; convulsions; fatigue; disorientation; hallucinations; numbness; paresthesias; ataxia; extrapyramidal symptoms; tardive dyskinesia.
CVS: Tachycardia; palpitations; arrhythmia; postural hypotension; hypotension; hypertension.
GI: Nausea; constipation; paralytic ileus; vomiting; indigestion; diarrhea; anorexia.
RESP: Exacerbation of asthma.
MISC: Hyperthermia; alopecia; sweating; chills.

CLINICAL IMPLICATIONS

General

* Determine why drug is being taken. Consider implications of condition on dental treatment.
* Depressed or anxious patients may neglect self-care. Monitor for plaque control effectiveness.
* Determine ability to adapt to stress of dental treatment. Consider short appointments.
* Chronic dry mouth is possible; anticipate increased caries activity and candidiasis.
* *Postural hypotension:* Monitor BP at the beginning and end of each appointment; anticipate syncope. Have patient sit upright for several min at the end of the dental appointment before dismissing.
* Extrapyramidal behaviors can complicate performance of oral procedures. If present, consult with MD to consider medication changes.
* Monitor vital signs.
* *When prescribed by DDS:* May produce sedation, interfere with eye-hand coordination, and the ability to operate mechanical equipment. Inform patient not to drive, sign important papers, or operate mechanical equipment.

Oral Health Education

* If chronic dry mouth occurs, recommend home fluoride therapy and use of nonalcoholic oral health care products.
* Evaluate manual dexterity; consider need for power toothbrush.

When prescribed by DDS:

* Warn patient not to drink alcoholic products while taking the drug.
* Warn patient not to drive, sign important papers, or operate mechanical equipment.

Doxy 100 — see doxycycline hyclate
Doxy 200 — see doxycycline hyclate
Doxycin — see doxycycline hyclate

---

 doxycycline hyclate (DOX-ee-SIGH-kleen)

Atridox: Local application: 42.5 mg (as hyclate, 10%)
Doryx: Capsules, coated pellets: 75, 100 mg (as hyclate)
Monodox: Capsules: 50, 100 mg (as monohydrate)
Periostat: Tablets: 20 mg (as hyclate)
Vibramycin: Capsules: 50, 100 mg (as hyclate); Powder for Oral Suspension: 25 mg (as monohydrate) per 5 mL when reconstituted; Syrup: 50 mg per 5 mL (as calcium)
Vibra-Tabs: Tablets: 100 mg (as hyclate)
Adoxa, Doxy 100, Doxy 200

■✦■ Apo-Doxy, Apo-Doxy-Tabs, Doxycin, Novo-Doxylin, Nu-Doxycycline, ratio-Doxycycline

■▶■ **Vibramicina**

Drug Class: Antibiotic, tetracycline

PHARMACOLOGY

Action

Inhibits bacterial protein synthesis.

Uses

Treatment of infections caused by susceptible strains of gram-positive and gram-negative bacteria (e.g., *Rickettsia*, *Mycoplasma pneumoniae*); treatment of trachoma and susceptible infections when penicillins are contraindicated; treatment of acute intestinal amebiasis; uncomplicated gonorrhea in adults; prophylaxis of malaria caused by *Plasmodium falciparum*; anthrax (including inhalational anthrax); severe acne.

Periodontitis

TABLET: Adjunct treatment to scaling and root planing to promote attachment level gain and reduce pocket depth.

SUBGINGIVAL APPLICATION: For chronic adult periodontitis for a gain in clinical attachment, reduction in probing depth, and reduction in bleeding on probing.

Contraindications

Hypersensitivity to tetracyclines; nursing mothers, infants, and children (Periostat).

Usual Dosage

Infection

ADULTS AND CHILDREN OLDER THAN 8 YR AND WEIGHING MORE THAN 45 KG: *PO:* 200 mg on the first day (100 mg q 12 hr) then 100 mg/day.

CHILDREN OLDER THAN 8 YR AND WEIGHING 45 KG OR LESS: *PO:* 4.4 mg/kg divided into two doses on day 1 followed by 2.2 mg/kg/day as a single dose or divided into two doses on subsequent days. For more severe infections, 4.4 mg/kg may be used.

Periodontitis (Periostat, Atridox)

ADULTS: *PO:* 20 mg bid as an adjunct following scaling and root planing for up to 9 mo. Administer tablets at least 2 hr before or after meals.

ADULTS: *Subgingival Application:* Variable dose, depending on the size, shape, and number of pockets being treated (see product information for preparation and administration).

Pharmacokinetics

ABSORP: Well absorbed. T_{max} is 2 hr (oral). C_{max} is 2.6 mcg/mL (200-mg oral dose), 2.5 to 3.6 mcg/mL (100- to 200-mg IV dose). Absorption may be decreased by 20% when given with food or milk.

DIST: Bound to plasma proteins. Crosses the placenta; excreted in breast milk.

EXCRET: Approximately 40% excreted by the kidneys in 72 hr. The $t_{1/2}$ is 18 to 22 hr.

SPECIAL POP: *Renal failure:* Excretion by the kidneys may fall as low as 1% to 5% in 72 hr in those with Ccr less than 10 mL/min.

➡◀ DRUG INTERACTIONS

Anticoagulants, oral: Increased anticoagulant effect (mechanism unknown)
- Avoid concurrent use or monitor prothrombin time.

Barbiturates: Decreased doxycycline effect (increased metabolism)
- Avoid concurrent use.

Carbamazepine: Decreased doxycycline effect (increased metabolism)
- Avoid concurrent use.

Digoxin: Possible digoxin toxicity (decreased metabolism)
- Avoid concurrent use.

Methotrexate: Possible methotrexate toxicity (mechanism unknown)
- Avoid concurrent use.

Phenytoin: Decreased doxycycline effect (increased metabolism)
- Avoid concurrent use.

Rifampin: Possible decreased doxycycline effect (increased metabolism)
- Avoid concurrent use.

Theophylline: Possible theophylline toxicity (mechanism unknown)
- Avoid concurrent use.

Zinc: Decreased doxycycline effect (decreased absorption)
- Avoid concurrent use.

ADVERSE EFFECTS

⚠ **ORAL:** Glossitis; dysphagia; candidiasis; sore throat; black hairy tongue.

CNS: Dizziness; headache; pseudotumor cerebri (manifested by headache and blurred vision).

GI: Anorexia; nausea; vomiting; diarrhea; enterocolitis; inflammatory lesions (with monilial overgrowth) in anogenital area; abdominal pain or discomfort; bulky loose stools; sore throat.

MISC: Bulging fontanelle (infants); benign intracranial hypertension (adults); photosensitivity.

CLINICAL IMPLICATIONS

General

When prescribed by DDS:
- *Lactation:* Excreted in breast milk.
- *Children:* Not recommended in children younger than 8 yr of age; abnormal bone formation and tooth discoloration may result.
- *Renal failure:* Dosage reduction may be required.
- *Hepatic failure:* Doses greater than 2 g/day associated with liver failure; monitor function and avoid other hepatotoxic drugs.
- *Superinfection:* Prolonged use may result in bacterial or fungal overgrowth.
- *Photosensitivity:* Photosensitivity may occur; avoid exposure to sunlight or ultraviolet light.
- *Special considerations:* Doxycycline periodontal local application has not been clinically evaluated for use in the regeneration of alveolar bone, use in immunocompromised patients, or for use in patients with conditions involving extremely severe periodontal defects with very little remaining periodontium.
- Obtain patient history, including drug history and any known allergies. Note renal or hepatic impairment, sulfite sensitivity (oral syrup only), or history of allergy or intolerance to other tetracycline antibiotics.
- Ensure that women are not pregnant or breast feeding.

Pregnancy Risk Category: Category D.

Oral Health Education

When prescribed by DDS:
- Explain name, dose, action, and potential side effects of drug.
- Review dosing schedule and prescribed length of therapy with patient. Advise patient that dose and duration of therapy are dependent on site and cause of infection.
- Instruct patient using tablets or capsules to take prescribed dose with a full glass of water.
- Advise patient to take without regard to meals but to take with food if GI upset occurs.
- Advise patient using other oral doxycycline products to take 1 hr before or 2 hr after antacids containing aluminum, calcium, or magnesium, or preparations containing iron or zinc.
- Instruct patient to complete entire course of therapy, even if symptoms of infection have disappeared.
- Advise patient to discontinue therapy and contact health care provider immediately if skin rash, hives, itching, shortness of breath, headache, or blurred vision occurs.
- Advise patient that medication may cause photosensitivity (i.e., sensitivity to sunlight) and to avoid unnecessary exposure to sunlight or tanning lamps and to use sunscreens and wear protective clothing to avoid photosensitivity reactions.

- Caution women taking oral contraceptives that doxycycline may make birth control pills less effective and to use nonhormonal forms of contraception during treatment.
- Advise women to notify health care provider if pregnant, planning to become pregnant, or breastfeeding.
- Caution patient that drug may cause dizziness, light-headedness, or blurred vision and to use caution while driving or performing other hazardous tasks until tolerance is determined.
- Advise patient to report the following signs of superinfection to health care provider: black "furry" tongue, white patches in mouth, foul-smelling stools, or vaginal itching or discharge.
- Warn patient that diarrhea containing blood or pus may be a sign of a serious disorder and to seek medical care if noted and not treat at home.
- Caution patient not to take any prescription or OTC medications, dietary supplements, or herbal preparations unless advised by health care provider.
- Advise patient to discard any unused doxycycline by the expiration date noted on the label.
- Advise patient that follow-up examinations and laboratory tests may be required to monitor therapy and to keep appointments.

Periostat
- Inform patient that this antibiotic will be taken daily for up to 9 mo to help treat periodontitis.
- Warn patient that although this is a tetracycline antibiotic, the dose is too small to treat infections and should not be used for that purpose.
- Instruct patient to take 1 hr before or 2 hr after meals with a full glass of water.
- Advise patient to take either 2 hr before or 2 hr after antacids containing aluminum, calcium, or magnesium, preparations containing iron or zinc, or dairy products (e.g., milk, cheese, ice cream).

Subgingival application
- Caution patient to avoid any mechanical oral hygiene procedure (e.g., tooth brushing, flossing) on any treated areas for 7 days after application.

Drafilyn — see aminophylline

Dramamine — see dimenhydrinate

Dramamine Less Drowsy — see meclizine

Dramanate — see dimenhydrinate

Drenural — see bumetanide

Drixoral Cough Liquid Caps — see dextromethorphan HBr

Dry E 400 — see vitamin E

---

duloxetine HCl (doo-LOX-eh-teen HIGH-droe-KLOR-ide)
Cymbalta

Drug Class: Antidepressant

PHARMACOLOGY
Action
Unknown; however, potentiation of serotonergic and noradrenergic activity in the CNS is suspected.

Uses
Treatment of major depressive disorder.

➡◀ DRUG INTERACTIONS RELATED TO DENTAL THERAPEUTICS
No documented drug-drug interactions. The absence of evidence is not evidence of safety.

ADVERSE EFFECTS

⚠️ **ORAL:** Dry mouth (15%).

CNS: Insomnia (11%); dizziness (9%); fatigue (8%); somnolence (7%); tremor, anxiety, decreased libido, abnormal orgasm (3%); initial insomnia, irritability, lethargy, nervousness, nightmare, restlessness, sleep disorder (≥1%).

CVS: Hot flushes; palpitations; hypertension.

MISC: Back pain; arthralgia.

GI: Nausea (20%); constipation (11%); diarrhea (8%); vomiting (5%); gastritis (≥1%).

RESP: URI; cough.

CLINICAL IMPLICATIONS

General

• Determine why drug is being taken. Consider implications of condition on dental treatment.
• Depressed or anxious patients may neglect self-care. Monitor for plaque control effectiveness.
• Determine ability to adapt to stress of dental treatment. Consider short appointments.
• Prescribe CNS depressants in small quantities for limited amounts of time.
• Chronic dry mouth is possible; anticipate increased caries and candidiasis.
• If GI side effects occur, consider semisupine chair position.
• Monitor vital signs.

Oral Health Education

• If chronic dry mouth occurs, recommend home fluoride therapy and use of nonalcoholic oral health care products.

Duocet — see acetaminophen/hydrocodone bitartrate

DuoNeb — see ipratropium bromide/albuterol sulfate

Duo-Trach Kit — see lidocaine HCl

Duracef — see cefadroxil

Duraclon — see clonidine HCl

Duradyne DHC — see acetaminophen/hydrocodone bitartrate

Duragesic — see fentanyl transdermal system

Duragesic-25 — see fentanyl transdermal system

Duragesic-50 — see fentanyl transdermal system

Duragesic-75 — see fentanyl transdermal system

Duragesic-100 — see fentanyl transdermal system

Duralith — see lithium

Duralmor LP — see morphine sulfate

Duralone-40 — see methylprednisolone

Duralone-80 — see methylprednisolone

Duramorph — see morphine sulfate

Durater — see famotidine

Duratuss-G — see guaifenesin

Duricef — see cefadroxil

Durogesic — see fentanyl transdermal system

Duvoid — see bethanechol chloride

Dymelor — see acetohexamide

Dymenate — see dimenhydrinate
Dynacin — see minocycline HCl
DynaCirc — see isradipine
DynaCirc CR — see isradipine
Dynafed Pseudo — see pseudoephedrine
Dyrenium — see triamterene
E.E.S. 200 — see erythromycin
E.E.S. 400 — see erythromycin
E.E.S. Granules — see erythromycin
Easprin — see aspirin
E-Base — see erythromycin
Ecapresan — see captopril
Ecaten — see captopril
EC Naprosyn — see naproxen
Econopred — see prednisolone
Econopred Plus — see prednisolone
Ecotrin — see aspirin
Ecotrin Adult Low Strength — see aspirin
Ecotrin Maximum Strength — see aspirin
Edecrin — see ethacrynic acid
Edecrin Sodium — see ethacrynic acid
Edenol — see furosemide
ED-IN-SOL — see ferrous salts
ED-SPAZ — see hyoscyamine sulfate
E.E.S. 600 — see erythromycin

---

efavirenz (EH-fah-VIE-renz)

Sustiva

Drug Class: Antiretroviral, non-nucleoside reverse transcriptase inhibitor

PHARMACOLOGY

Action

Noncompetitive inhibition of HIV-1 reverse transcriptase.

Uses

Treatment of HIV-1 infection in combination with other antiretroviral agents.

➤← DRUG INTERACTIONS RELATED TO DENTAL THERAPEUTICS

Midazolam or triazolam: Prolonged sedation following oral administration (decreased metabolism)
 • Monitor clinical status.

ADVERSE EFFECTS

⚠ **ORAL:** Mucosal ulceration.
CNS: Dizziness (28.1%); fatigue, headache, hypesthesia, impaired concentration (8.3%); insomnia (16.3%); abnormal dreams (6.2%); somnolence (7%); depression; anorexia; ner-

vousness; ataxia; confusion; impaired coordination; paresthesia; neuropathy; tremor; agitation; emotional lability; hallucination; psychosis.
CVS: Flushing; palpitations.
GI: Nausea; vomiting; diarrhea; dyspepsia; abdominal pain.
RESP: Cough; dyspnea.
MISC: Arthralgia; myalgia; asthenia; fever; pain.

CLINICAL IMPLICATIONS
General
- Determine why drug is being taken. Consider implications of condition on dental treatment.
- Consider medical consult to determine disease control and influence on dental treatment.
- If GI side effects occur, consider semisupine chair position.
- Anticipate oral candidiasis when HIV disease is reported.
- This drug is frequently prescribed in combination with one or more other antiviral agents. Side effects of all agents must be considered during the drug review process.
- Antibiotic prophylaxis should be considered when <500 PMN/mm³ are reported; elective dental treatment should be delayed until blood values improve above this level.

Oral Health Education
- Evaluate manual dexterity; consider need for power toothbrush.
- Recommend frequent maintenance prophylaxis when immunosuppression is evident.
- Encourage daily plaque control procedures for effective self-care since HIV infection reduces host resistance.

Efexor — see venlafaxine
Effer-K — see potassium products
Effexor — see venlafaxine
Effexor XR — see venlafaxine
Efidac 24 — see chlorpheniramine maleate
Efudex — see fluorouracil
Efudix — see fluorouracil
ELA-Max — see lidocaine HCl
Elantan — see isosorbide mononitrate
Elavil — see amitriptyline HCl
Eldepryl — see selegiline HCl
Elequine — see levofloxacin

---

eletriptan hydrobromide (ell-eh-TRIP-tan HIGH-droe-BROE-mide)
Relpax
Drug Class: Analgesic, migraine

PHARMACOLOGY
Action
Selective agonist for vascular serotonin (5-HT₁) receptor subtype, causing vasoconstriction of cranial arteries.

Uses
Acute treatment of migraine with or without aura.

➡➡◄ DRUG INTERACTIONS RELATED TO DENTAL THERAPEUTICS

Ketoconazole or itraconazole: Increased vasospastic effect of eletriptan (decreased metabolism)
- Avoid concurrent use.

ADVERSE EFFECTS

⚠ **ORAL:** Dry mouth (4%); dysphagia (e.g., throat tightness, difficulty swallowing) (2%).
CNS: Dizziness, somnolence (7%); headache (4%); hypertonia, hypesthesia, paresthesia, vertigo (≥1%).
GI: Nausea (8%); dyspepsia.
RESP: Pharyngitis (≥1%).
MISC: Asthenia (10%); pain, tightness, or pressure in chest (4%); stomach pain, cramps, or pressure, abdominal pain or discomfort (2%); back pain, chills (≥1%).

CLINICAL IMPLICATIONS

General

- Monitor vital signs (e.g., BP, pulse). Drugs for prevention are sympatholytic; drugs for treatment of acute attack are sympathomimetic.
- If GI side effects occur, consider semisupine chair position.
- This drug is for acute use during migraine attack. Patient is unlikely to present for oral health care appointment.

Elidel — see pimecrolimus

Elixomin — see theophylline

Elixophyllin — see theophylline

Elocom — see mometasone furoate

Elocon — see mometasone furoate

Eltor 120 — see pseudoephedrine

Embeline — see clobetasol propionate

Embeline E — see clobetasol propionate

Emgel — see erythromycin

EMLA — see lidocaine HCl/prilocaine

EMLA Patch — see lidocaine HCl/prilocaine

Emo-Cort — see hydrocortisone

Empirin — see aspirin

Empirin with Codeine #2 — see aspirin/codeine phosphate

Empirin with Codeine #3 — see aspirin/codeine phosphate

Empirin with Codeine #4 — see aspirin/codeine phosphate

---

emtricitabine (em-try-SIGH-tah-bean)

Emtriva

Drug Class: Antiviral

PHARMACOLOGY

Action

Inhibits activity of HIV-1 reverse transcriptase by competing with the natural substrate deoxycytidine 5'-triphosphate and by being incorporated into nascent viral DNA, resulting in chain termination.

Uses

In combination with other antiretroviral agents for the treatment of HIV-1 infections in adults.

➜← DRUG INTERACTIONS RELATED TO DENTAL THERAPEUTICS

No documented drug-drug interactions. The absence of evidence is not evidence of safety.

ADVERSE EFFECTS

CNS: Headache (13%); insomnia (7%); depressive disorders (6%); paresthesia (5%); dizziness, neuropathy/peripheral neuritis (4%); abnormal dreams (2%).

GI: Diarrhea (23%); nausea (18%); vomiting (9%); dyspepsia (4%), abdominal pain (8%).

RESP: Increased cough (14%).

MISC: Asthenia (16%); arthralgia (3%); myalgia (4%).

CLINICAL IMPLICATIONS

General

- Determine why drug is being taken. Consider implications of condition on dental treatment.
- Consider medical consult to determine disease control and influence on dental treatment.
- Anticipate oral candidiasis when HIV disease is reported.
- If GI side effects occur, consider semisupine chair position.
- This drug is frequently prescribed in combination with one or more other antiviral agents. Side effects of all agents must be considered during the drug review process.
- Antibiotic prophylaxis should be considered when <500 PMN/mm³ are reported; elective dental treatment should be delayed until blood values improve above this level.

Oral Health Education

- Recommend frequent maintenance prophylaxis when immunosuppression is evident.
- Encourage daily plaque control procedures for effective self-care since HIV infection reduces host resistance.

Emtriva — see emtricitabine

E-Mycin — see erythromycin

Enablex — see darifenacin

Enaladil — see enalapril maleate

---

enalapril maleate (EH-NAL-uh-prill MAL-ee-ate)

Vasotec, Vasotec IV

■▄■ **Enaladil, Feliberal, Glioten, Kenopril, Norpril, Palane, Pulsol, Renitec**

Drug Class: Antihypertensive; ACE inhibitor

PHARMACOLOGY

Action

Competitively inhibits angiotensin I–converting enzyme, preventing conversion of angiotensin I to angiotensin II, a potent vasoconstrictor that also stimulates release of aldosterone. Results in decrease in BP, reduced sodium absorption, and potassium retention.

Uses

Treatment of hypertension and symptomatic CHF in combination with diuretics and digitalis and asymptomatic left ventricular dysfunction.

Unlabeled Uses

Treatment of diabetic nephropathy, childhood hypertension, hypertension related to scleroderma, and renal crisis scleroderma.

➡◀ DRUG INTERACTIONS RELATED TO DENTAL THERAPEUTICS

COX-1 inhibitors: Decreased hypertensive effect (decreased prostaglandin synthesis)
• Monitor blood pressure.

ADVERSE EFFECTS

⚠ **ORAL:** Stomatitis, taste alterations, glossitis, dry mouth (1%).
CNS: Headache (5%); dizziness (4%); fatigue (3%); vertigo (2%); asthenia (1%).
CVS: Chest pain; hypotension; orthostatic hypotension.
GI: Abdominal pain, diarrhea (2%); nausea, vomiting (1%).
RESP: Bronchitis, cough, dyspnea (1%).
MISC: Neutropenia, thrombocytopenia, bone marrow suppression (0.5% to 1%).

CLINICAL IMPLICATIONS

General
• Monitor vital signs (e.g., BP, pulse pressure, rate, and rhythm) at each appointment to assess disease control. Do not provide elective dental treatment when BP is ≥180/110 or in the presence of other high-risk CV conditions. Refer to the section entitled "The Patient Taking Cardiovascular Drugs" in Chapter 6: *Clinical Medicine*.
• Use local anesthetic agents with vasoconstrictor with caution based on functional capacity of the patient and use aspirating technique to prevent intravascular injection.
• If coughing is problematic, consider semisupine chair position for treatment.
• Chronic dry mouth is possible; anticipate increased caries, candidiasis, and lichenoid mucositis.
• *Postural hypotension:* Monitor BP at the beginning and end of each appointment; anticipate syncope. Have patient sit upright for several min at the end of the dental appointment before dismissing.
• Determine ability to adapt to stress of dental treatment. Consider short appointments.
• Blood dyscrasias rarely reported; anticipate increased bleeding, infection, and poor healing.
• If GI side effects occur, consider semisupine chair position.

Oral Health Education
• If chronic dry mouth occurs, recommend home fluoride therapy and use of nonalcoholic oral health care products.
• Encourage daily plaque control procedures for effective self-care in patients at risk for cardiovascular disease.

Enbrel — see etanercept
Endantadine — see amantadine HCl
Endocodone — see oxycodone HCl

---

enfuvirtide (en-FYOO-veer-tide)

Fuzeon

Drug Class: Antiretroviral, fusion inhibitor

PHARMACOLOGY

Action
Interferes with entry of HIV-1 into cells by inhibiting fusion of viral and cellular membranes.

Uses
In combination with other antiretroviral agents for the treatment of HIV-1 infection in treatment-experienced patients with evidence of HIV-1 replication despite ongoing antiretroviral therapy.

➡◀ DRUG INTERACTIONS RELATED TO DENTAL THERAPEUTICS

No documented drug-drug interactions. The absence of evidence is not evidence of safety.

ADVERSE EFFECTS

⚠ **ORAL:** Herpes simplex; taste disturbance.

CNS: Fatigue; peripheral neuropathy; insomnia; depression; anxiety; decreased appetite; Guillain-Barré syndrome; sixth cranial nerve palsy.

GI: Diarrhea; nausea; anorexia; constipation; upper abdominal pain (3%); pancreatitis.

RESP: Cough; sinusitis; pneumonia.

MISC: Influenza; flu-like symptoms; myalgia; fever.

CLINICAL IMPLICATIONS

General

- Determine why drug is being taken. Consider implications of condition on dental treatment.
- Consider medical consult to determine disease control and influence on dental treatment.
- Anticipate oral candidiasis when HIV disease is reported.
- If GI side effects occur, consider semisupine chair position.
- This drug is frequently prescribed in combination with one or more other antiviral agents. Side effects of all agents must be considered during the drug review process.
- Antibiotic prophylaxis should be considered when <500 PMN/mm^3 are reported; elective dental treatment should be delayed until blood values improve above this level.

Oral Health Education

- Recommend frequent maintenance prophylaxis when immunosuppression is evident.
- Encourage daily plaque control procedures for effective self-care since HIV infection reduces host resistance.

Enjuvia — see estrogens, synthetic conjugated, a or b

---

enoxaparin sodium (eh-NOX-uh-par-in SO-dee-uhm)

Lovenox

■✦■ **Lovenox HP**

■✦■ **Clexane**

Drug Class: Anticoagulant; Low molecular weight heparin

PHARMACOLOGY

Action

Causes higher anti-factor Xa to antithrombin activities (anti-factor IIa) ratio than heparin, which may prevent thrombosis.

Uses

Prevention of deep vein thrombosis (DVT), which may lead to pulmonary embolism (PE) in patients undergoing hip or knee replacement surgery or abdominal surgery; in conjunction with warfarin sodium for inpatient treatment of acute DVT with and without PE or outpatient treatment of acute DVT without PE; prevention of ischemic complications of unstable and non-Q-wave MI when coadministered with aspirin in medical patients who are at risk for thromboembolic complications due to severely restricted mobility during acute illness.

➡◀ DRUG INTERACTIONS RELATED TO DENTAL THERAPEUTICS

COX-1 inhibitors: Increased risk of bleeding (additive)
- Avoid concurrent use.

ADVERSE EFFECTS

GI: Nausea (3%); diarrhea.

RESP: Dyspnea (3.3%).

MISC: Local irritation and pain; hematoma, hemorrhage (4% to 13 %); thrombocytopenia; nausea; confusion; fever; edema; peripheral edema; injection site hemorrhage; epidural or spinal hematoma; systemic allergic reactions (i.e., pruritus, urticaria, anaphylactoid reactions); vesiculobullous rash; purpura; thrombocytosis; hyperlipidemia.

CLINICAL IMPLICATIONS

General

• Determine why drug is being taken. Consider implications of condition on dental treatment.
• Determine prothrombin time or INR before completing procedures that may result in significant bleeding. Safe level of INR for invasive dental procedures is 2-3. INR is calculated from PT.
• If uncontrolled bleeding develops, use hemostatic agents and positive pressure to induce hemostasis. Do not dismiss patient until bleeding is controlled.
• Blood dyscrasias rarely reported; anticipate increased bleeding, infection, and poor healing.
• Monitor frequently to ensure adequate clotting during treatment that involves bleeding.

Oral Health Education

• Encourage daily plaque control procedures for effective, nontraumatic self-care.

---

entacapone (en-TACK-ah-pone)

Comtan
Drug Class: Antiparkinson

PHARMACOLOGY

Action

The exact mechanism of action is unknown. Inhibits catechol-*O*-methyl transferase (COMT), thus blocking the degradation of catechols including dopamine and levodopa. This may lead to more sustained levels of dopamine and consequently a more prolonged antiparkinson effect.

Uses

As an adjunct to levodopa/carbidopa for the treatment of idiopathic Parkinson disease in patients who experience signs and symptoms of end-of-dose "wearing-off."

➜← DRUG INTERACTIONS RELATED TO DENTAL THERAPEUTICS

Sympathomimetic amines: Tachycardia (mechanism unknown)
• Use local anesthetic agents containing a vasoconstrictor with caution.
• Monitor pulse rate and character.

ADVERSE EFFECTS

⚠ **ORAL:** Dry mouth (3%); taste disturbance (1%).

CNS: Dyskinesia; hyperkinesia; hypokinesia; dizziness; anxiety; somnolence; agitation; hallucinations.

GI: Nausea; diarrhea; abdominal pain; constipation; vomiting; dyspepsia; flatulence; gastritis.

RESP: Dyspnea.

MISC: Sweating; back pain; fatigue; asthenia.

CLINICAL IMPLICATIONS

General

• Determine why drug is being taken. Consider implications of condition on dental treatment.

- Extrapyramidal behaviors associated with Parkinson disease can complicate access to oral cavity and complicate oral procedures.
- Chronic dry mouth is possible; anticipate increased caries and candidiasis.
- If GI side effects occur, consider semisupine chair position.

Oral Health Education
- If chronic dry mouth occurs, recommend home fluoride therapy and use of nonalcoholic oral health care products.
- Evaluate manual dexterity; consider need for power toothbrush.

Entocort Capsules — see budesonide
Entocort EC — see budesonide
Entocort Enema — see budesonide
Entrophen — see aspirin
Epamin — see phenytoin
Epiject — see valproic acid and derivatives

---

 epinephrine (epp-ih-NEFF-rin)

Adrenalin Chloride: Solution for injection: 1 mg/mL (1:1,000), 10 mg/mL (1:100) as hydrochloride
EpiPen: Solution: 1 mg/mL (1:1,000)
EpiPen Jr.: Solution: 0.5 mg/mL (1:2,000)
microNefrin, S2: Solution for inhalation: 2.25% racepinephrine hydrochloride
Primatene Mist: Aerosol: 0.22 mg epinephrine per spray

▮✦▮ Adrenalin, Vaponefrin

Drug Class: Alpha agonist; Beta agonist

PHARMACOLOGY
Action
Stimulates alpha- and beta-receptors (alpha-receptors at high doses; beta$_1$- and beta$_2$-receptors at moderate doses) within sympathetic nervous system. Relaxes smooth muscle of bronchi and iris and is antagonist of histamine.

Uses
Treatment and prophylaxis of cardiac arrest and attacks of transitory AV heart block; treatment of Adams-Stokes syndrome; treatment of hay fever; relief of bronchial asthma; treatment of syncope caused by heart block or carotid sinus hypersensitivity; symptomatic relief of serum sickness, urticaria, and angioedema; relaxation of uterine musculature; anaphylaxis; allergic reactions (e.g., bronchospasm, urticaria, pruritus, angioneurotic edema, swelling of the lips, eyelids, tongue, and nasal mucosa) because of anaphylactic shock caused by stinging insects (primarily of the order *Hymenoptera*, which includes bees, wasps, hornets, yellow jackets, bumble bees, and fire ants); severe allergic or anaphylactoid reactions caused by allergy injections; exposures to pollens, dusts, molds, foods, drugs; exercise; unknown substances (so-called idiopathic anaphylaxis); severe, life-threatening asthma attacks characterized by wheezing, dyspnea, and inability to breathe.
NASAL SOLUTION: Treatment of nasal congestion; relief of eustachian tube congestion.
INHALATION: Temporary relief from acute paroxysms of bronchial asthma and other states; treatment of postintubation and infectious croup.

Contraindications
Hypersensitivity to epinephrine; narrow-angle glaucoma; concomitant use during general anesthesia with halogenated hydrocarbons or cyclopropane; cerebral arteriosclerosis or or-

ganic brain damage; use with anesthesia for fingers and toes; use during labor; phenothi-azine-induced circulatory collapse; MAO inhibitor therapy; nonanaphylactic shock during general anesthesia with halogenated hydrocarbons or cyclopropane; organic heart disease; cardiac dilation and coronary insufficiency.

Usual Dosage

Allergic Emergencies
ADULTS: *IM:* (Epipen) Usual dose is 0.3 mg.
CHILDREN: *IM:* (Epipen or Epipen Jr) 0.01 mg/kg is recommended.

Pharmacokinetics
ABSORP: Depends on dose form.
DIST: Depends on dose form.
METAB: Inactivated by enzymatic transformation to metanephrine or normetanephrine; these are subsequently conjugated and excreted in the urine.
EXCRET: Mostly excreted in urine as inactive metabolites; remainder excreted as un-changed drug or conjugated.
ONSET: 5 to 10 min (SC), 1 to 5 min (inhalation).
DURATION: 4 to 6 hr (SC), 1 to 4 hr (IM), 1 to 3 hr (inhalation).

➜← DRUG INTERACTIONS

Antidepressants, tricyclic: Hypertension or hypertensive crisis (inhibition of norepinephrine uptake)
• Monitor clinical status.
Beta-adrenergic blockers: Decreased antianaphylactic effect (beta-blockade)
• Increased epinephrine may be required in anaphylaxis.
Cocaine: Ventricular arrhythmias (additive)
• Monitor clinical status.
Cyclopropane: Cardiac arrhythmias (mechanism unknown)
• Monitor clinical status.
Digoxin: Increased tendency to cardiac arrhythmias (additive)
• Monitor clinical status.
Entacapone: Tachycardia (mechanism unknown)
• Monitor clinical status.
Guanadrel: Decreased antihypertensive effect (blockade of guanadrel uptake at target site)
• Monitor clinical status.
Halothane: Possible fatal arrhythmias (additive)
• Monitor clinical status.
Midodrine: Risk of severe hypertension (additive)
• Monitor clinical status.
Pilocarpine: Increased myopia (mechanism unknown)
• Monitor clinical status.

ADVERSE EFFECTS
⚠ **ORAL:** Dry mucosa, taste disturbance (inhalation).
CVS: Cardiac arrhythmias and excessive hypertension; palpitations (especially in hyperthy-roid and hypertensive patients); tachycardia; anginal pain in predisposed patients; cerebral and subarachnoid hemorrhage; flushing.
CNS: Anxiety; headache; restlessness; tremor; weakness; hemiplegia; dizziness; insomnia.
GI: Nausea; vomiting.
RESP: Shortness of breath.
MISC: Severe metabolic acidosis; pallor; urticaria; wheal and hemorrhage at site of injec-tion; necrosis at injection site following repeated injections; sweating; transient elevations of blood glucose; elevated serum lactic acid.

CLINICAL IMPLICATIONS
General
• Determine why drug is being taken. Consider implications of condition on dental treat-ment.

- Monitor vital signs (e.g., BP, pulse rate, respiratory rate and function); uncontrolled respiratory disease is characterized by wheezing and coughing.
- *Asthma:* Acute bronchoconstriction can occur during dental treatment; have bronchodilator inhaler available.
- Inhalants can dry oral mucosa; anticipate candidiasis, increased calculus and plaque levels, and increased caries.

When used by DDS:
- *Lactation:* Excreted in breast milk.
- *Children:* Administer drug with caution. Syncope has occurred in asthmatic children.
- *Special risk:* Use drug with caution in elderly patients and patients with CV disease, pulmonary edema, hypertension, hyperthyroidism, diabetes, psychoneurotic illness, asthma, prefibrillatory rhythm, or anesthetic cardiac accidents.
- *Sulfite sensitivity:* Some products contain sulfites; use drug with caution in sulfite-sensitive individuals.
- *Bronchial asthma/emphysema:* Administer with extreme caution to patients with long-standing bronchial asthma and emphysema who develop degenerative heart disease.
- *Cerebrovascular hemorrhage:* May result from overdosage or inadvertent IV injection.
- *Fatalities:* Death may result from pulmonary edema because of peripheral constriction and cardiac stimulation produced.
- *Pulmonary edema:* May cause fatalities because of peripheral constriction or cardiac stimulation.
- *Overdosage:* Precordial distress, vomiting, headache, shortness of breath, unusually elevated BP, cerebrovascular hemorrhage, pulmonary arterial hypertension, pulmonary edema, ventricular hyperirritability, bradycardia, tachycardia, arrhythmias, extreme pallor, cold skin, metabolic acidosis, kidney failure.

Pregnancy Risk Category: Category C.

Oral Health Education
- If chronic dry mouth occurs, recommend home fluoride therapy and use of nonalcoholic oral health care products.

When used by DDS:
- In a life-threatening medical emergency, the use of epinephrine takes precedence over all other considerations.

EpiPen — see epinephrine

EpiPen Jr. — see epinephrine

Epitol — see carbamazepine

Epival — see valproic acid and derivatives

Epivir — see lamivudine

Epivir-HBV — see lamivudine

EPO — see epoetin alfa

---

epoetin alfa (eh-POE-eh-tin AL-fuh)
Synonym: erythropoietin; EPO

Epogen, Procrit
█✦█ **Eprex**

Drug Class: Recombinant human erythropoietin

PHARMACOLOGY
Action
Stimulates red blood cell (RBC) production.

Uses
Treatment of anemia related to chronic renal failure, zidovudine therapy in HIV-infected patients and nonmyeloid malignancies. Reduction of allogeneic blood transfusions in surgery patients.

➥⬅ DRUG INTERACTIONS RELATED TO DENTAL THERAPEUTICS

No documented drug-drug interactions. The absence of evidence is not evidence of safety.

ADVERSE EFFECTS

CNS: Headache; seizures; insomnia.
CVS: Hypertension (24%).
GI: Nausea (11%); vomiting; diarrhea; constipation; dyspepsia.
RESP: Shortness of breath; cough.
MISC: Allergy, including anaphylaxis, skin rashes, and urticaria; fever; paresthesia; arthralgia (11%); edema; pruritus; antibody-induced pure red cell aplasia (postmarketing).

CLINICAL IMPLICATIONS

General
- Drug used for variety of reasons. Determine why drug is being taken. Consider implications of condition on dental treatment.
- *Malignancy:* Medical consultation to determine WBC and platelet count before invasive dental procedures, including periodontal debridement.
- Blood dyscrasias rarely reported; anticipate increased bleeding, infection, and poor healing.
- Monitor vital signs.
- If GI side effects occur, consider semisupine chair position.

Oral Health Education
- Recommend frequent maintenance prophylaxis when immunosuppression is evident.

Epogen — see epoetin alfa
Eprex — see epoetin alfa

---

eprosartan mesylate (eh-pro-SAHR-tan MES-il-ayt)

Teveten

Drug Class: Antihypertensive; Angiotensin II antagonist

PHARMACOLOGY

Action
Antagonizes the effect of angiotensin II (vasoconstriction and aldosterone secretion) by blocking the angiotensin II receptor (AT_1 receptor) in vascular smooth muscle and the adrenal gland, producing decreased BP.

Uses
Treatment of hypertension.

➥⬅ DRUG INTERACTIONS RELATED TO DENTAL THERAPEUTICS

No documented drug-drug interactions. The absence of evidence is not evidence of safety.

ADVERSE EFFECTS

⚠ **ORAL:** Dry mouth, gingivitis, periodontitis, toothache (<1%).
CNS: Fatigue; depression.
CVS: Chest pain; bradycardia; palpitations; hypotension; orthostatic hypotension.
GI: Abdominal pain.
RESP: URI; rhinitis; pharyngitis; coughing.
MISC: Arthralgia.

CLINICAL IMPLICATIONS

General
- Monitor vital signs (e.g., BP, pulse pressure, rate, and rhythm) at each appointment to assess disease control. Do not provide elective dental treatment when BP is ≥180/110 or

in the presence of other high-risk CV conditions. Refer to the section entitled "The Patient Taking Cardiovascular Drugs" in Chapter 6: *Clinical Medicine*.
- Determine ability to adapt to stress of dental treatment. Consider short appointments.
- Use local anesthetic agents with vasoconstrictor with caution based on functional capacity of the patient and use aspirating technique to prevent intravascular injection.
- If coughing is problematic, consider semisupine chair position for treatment.
- Chronic dry mouth is possible; anticipate increased caries, candidiasis, and lichenoid mucositis.
- *Postural hypotension:* Monitor BP at the beginning a\nd end of each appointment; anticipate syncope. Have patient sit upright for several min at the end of the dental appointment before dismissing.

Oral Health Education
- If chronic dry mouth occurs, recommend home fluoride therapy and use of nonalcoholic oral health care products.
- Encourage daily plaque control procedures for effective self-care in patients at risk for cardiovascular disease.

Eranz — see donepezil

Ergocaf — see ergotamine tartrate

Ergomar — see ergotamine tartrate

---

ergotamine tartrate (ehr-GOT-ah-meen TAR-trate)
Ergomar

■▧■ **Ergocaf, Sydolil**

Drug Class: Ergotamine derivatives

PHARMACOLOGY
Action
Reduces extracranial blood flow, causes decline in amplitude of pulsation in the cranial arteries, and decreases hyperperfusion of the territory of the basilar artery; produces constriction of both arteries and veins.

Uses
Abort or prevent vascular headache (e.g., migraine).

➡◆ DRUG INTERACTIONS RELATED TO DENTAL THERAPEUTICS
Ketoconazole or itraconazole: Increased vasospastic effects (decreased metabolism)
- Avoid concurrent use.

Drug Interactions

ADVERSE EFFECTS
CVS: Tachycardia or bradycardia; pulselessness.
GI: Nausea; vomiting.
MISC: Weakness of legs; limb muscle pain; numbness and tingling of the fingers and toes; precordial pain; localized edema; itching.

CLINICAL IMPLICATIONS
General
- Determine why drug is being taken. Consider implications of condition on dental treatment.
- Monitor vital signs (e.g., BP, pulse). Drugs for prevention are sympatholytic; drugs for treatment of acute attack are sympathomimetic.
- If GI side effects occur, consider semisupine chair position.

Oral Health Education
• Evaluate manual dexterity; consider need for power toothbrush.

Eritroquim — see erythromycin

Erybid — see erythromycin

Eryc — see erythromycin

Erycette — see erythromycin

Eryderm — see erythromycin

Erymax — see erythromycin

EryPed — see erythromycin

EryPed 200 — see erythromycin

EryPed 400 — see erythromycin

EryPed Drops — see erythromycin

Ery-Tab — see erythromycin

Erythra-Derm — see erythromycin

Erythrocin Stearate — see erythromycin

---

erythromycin (eh-RITH-row-MY-sin)

A/T/S, Akne-mycin, Del-Mycin, E.E.S. 200, E.E.S. 400, E.E.S. Granules, E-Base, Emgel, E-Mycin, Eryc, Erycette, Eryderm, Erymax, EryPed, EryPed 200, EryPed 400, EryPed Drops, Ery-Tab, Erythra-Derm, Erythrocin Stearate, Ilosone, Ilotycin, Ilotycin Gluceptate, PCE Dispertab, Theramycin Z

█✦█ Apo-Erythro Base, Apo-Erythro E-C, Apo-Erythro-ES, Apo-Erythro-S, E.E.S. 600, Erybid, Novorythro Encap, Nu-Erythromycin-S, PMS-Erythromycin

█✦█ Eritroquim, Ilosone, Latotryd, Lauricin, Lauritran, Lederpax, Luritran, Optomicin, Pantomicina, Procephal, Tromigal

Drug Class: Antibiotic, macrolide

PHARMACOLOGY

Action
Interferes with microbial protein synthesis.

Uses
ORAL/IV: Treatment of infections of respiratory tract, skin and skin structure, and sexually transmitted diseases caused by susceptible organisms; treatment of pertussis, diphtheria, erythrasma, intestinal amebiasis, conjunctivitis of newborn, and Legionnaire disease; prevention of attacks of rheumatic fever; prevention of bacterial endocarditis.
OPHTHALMIC: Treatment of superficial ocular infections caused by strains of susceptible organism.
TOPICAL: Treatment of acne vulgaris.

Unlabeled Uses
Treatment of *Neisseria gonorrhoeae* in pregnancy; treatment of diarrhea caused by *Campylobacter jejuni*; as alternative to penicillin in selected infections, *Treponema pallidum, Lymphogranuloma venereum, Granuloma inguinale, Haemophilus ducreyi* (chancroid). Other uses as alternative to penicillins include the following: anthrax, Vincent gingivitis, erysipeloid, tetanus, actinomycosis, *Nocardia* infections (with a sulfonamide), *Eikenella corrodens* infections, *Borrelia* infections (including early Lyme disease).

➡️⬅️ DRUG INTERACTIONS RELATED TO DENTAL THERAPEUTICS

Midazolam or triazolam: Increased midazolam or triazolam toxicity (decreased metabolism)
• Monitor clinical status.

ADVERSE EFFECTS

⚠️ **ORAL:** Candidiasis (high dosage, prolonged use).
CVS: Arrhythmia (rare).
GI: Diarrhea; nausea; vomiting abdominal pain/cramping.
RESP: Cough; dyspnea.
MISC: Venous irritation or phlebitis with IV administration; pseudomembranous colitis (rare).

CLINICAL IMPLICATIONS

General

• Determine why drug is being taken. Take precautions to avoid cross-contamination of microorganisms.
• If oral infection occurs that requires antibiotic therapy, select an appropriate product from a different class of anti-infectives.
• This drug lacks the spectrum to manage odontogenic infection and has a strong risk of causing antibiotic-resistant microbes to develop. See Chapter 4: *Medical Management of Odontogenic Infections.*
• Antibiotic-associated diarrhea can occur. If prescribed by DDS, have patient contact DDS immediately if signs develop.
• Prolonged use of antibiotics may result in bacterial or fungal overgrowth of nonsusceptible microorganisms; anticipate candidiasis.

Oral Health Education

• Inform patient that antibacterial drug regimens must be followed to completion.

---

erythropoietin — see epoetin alfa

---

escitalopram oxalate (ESS-sigh-TAL-oh-pram OX-ah-late)

Lexapro

Drug Class: Antidepressant, selective serotonin reuptake inhibitor

PHARMACOLOGY

Action

Inhibits the CNS neuronal uptake of serotonin, potentiating serotonergic activity.

Uses

Treatment of major depressive disorders and generalized anxiety.

➡️⬅️ DRUG INTERACTIONS RELATED TO DENTAL THERAPEUTICS

Tramadol: Increased risk of seizure (additive)
• Avoid concurrent use.

ADVERSE EFFECTS

⚠️ **ORAL:** Dry mouth (9%); caries (3%); taste disturbance.
CNS: Headache (24%); insomnia (14%); somnolence (13%); decreased libido, dizziness (7%); decreased appetite, abnormal dreaming, lethargy (3%); paresthesia, yawning (2%); light-headedness, migraine, increased appetite, irritability, impaired concentration ($\geq$1%); grand mal seizures.
CVS: Hot flushes, chest pain ($\geq$1%); hypertension, palpitations.
GI: Nausea (18%); diarrhea (14%); constipation, indigestion (6%); vomiting (3%); abdominal pain, flatulence; heartburn, abdominal cramps, gastroenteritis ($\geq$1%); GI hemorrhage, pancreatitis.

RESP: Sinusitis (2%); rhinitis (5%); bronchitis, congestion, coughing, sinus headache (≥1%).

MISC: Increased sweating (8%); influenza-like symptoms, fatigue (5%); allergy, fever; angioedema, neuroleptic malignant syndrome, serotonin syndrome.

CLINICAL IMPLICATIONS

General
- Determine why drug is being taken. Consider implications of condition on dental treatment.
- Determine ability to adapt to stress of dental treatment. Consider short appointments.
- Depressed or anxious patients may neglect self-care. Monitor for plaque control effectiveness.
- Monitor vital signs (e.g., BP, pulse rate) and respiratory function.
- If GI side effects occur, consider semisupine chair position.

Oral Health Education
- If chronic dry mouth occurs, recommend home fluoride therapy and use of nonalcoholic oral health care products.
- Encourage daily plaque control procedures for effective self-care.

Esclim — see estradiol

Esidrix — see hydrochlorothiazide

Eskalith — see lithium

Eskalith CR — see lithium

---

esomeprazole magnesium (es-om-ME-pray-zol mag-NEE-zhum)

Nexium

Drug Class: Gastrointestinal; Proton pump inhibitor

PHARMACOLOGY

Action
Suppresses gastric acid secretion by blocking proton pump within gastric parietal cells.

Uses
Treatment of heartburn and other symptoms of gastroesophageal reflux disease (GERD); short-term treatment in healing and symptomatic resolution of erosive esophagitis; maintain symptom resolution and healing of erosive esophagitis; in combination with amoxicillin and clarithromycin for treatment of *Helicobacter pylori* infection and duodenal ulcer disease to eradicate *H. pylori*; reduction in occurrence of gastric ulcers associated with continuous NSAID therapy in patients at risk of developing gastric ulcers.

➡◀ DRUG INTERACTIONS RELATED TO DENTAL THERAPEUTICS

Ketoconazole or itraconazole: Possible decreased ketoconazole or itraconazole effect (decreased absorption)
- Avoid concurrent use.

ADVERSE EFFECTS
⚠ **ORAL:** Ulcerative stomatitis, tongue edema (<1%).
CNS: Headache (6%).
CVS: Hypertension, tachycardia (1%).
GI: Diarrhea (≥1%); nausea; flatulence; abdominal pain; constipation; pancreatitis.
MISC: Anaphylactic reaction.

CLINICAL IMPLICATIONS
General
- Determine why drug is being taken. Consider implications of condition on dental treatment.
- If patient has GI disease, consider semisupine chair position.
- Anticipate chemical erosion of teeth.
- Substernal pain (heartburn) may mimic pain of cardiac origin.
- Monitor vital signs.

Oral Health Education
- Inform patient that toothbrushing should not be completed after reflux, but to only rinse with water, then use home fluoride product to minimize chemical erosion–related caries.

---

esterified estrogen — see estrogens, conjugated or esterified

Estrace — see estradiol

Estraderm — see estradiol

Estraderm 25 — see estradiol

Estraderm TTS — see estradiol

---

estradiol (ESS-truh-DIE-ole)
(stradiol cypionate, estradiol valerate)

Alora, Climara, Delestrogen, Depo-Estradiol, Esclim, Estrace, Estraderm, Estrasorb, Estring, Gynodiol, Vivelle, Vivelle-Dot

■✦■ **Estraderm 25, Estradot**

■◆■ **Climaderm, Estraderm TTS, Ginedisc, Oestrogel, Systen**

Drug Class: Estrogens

PHARMACOLOGY
Action
Promotes growth and development of female reproductive system and secary sex characteristics; affects release of pituitary gonadotropins; inhibits ovulation and prevents postpartum breast engorgement; conserves calcium and phosphorous and encourages bone formation; overrides stimulatory effects of testosterone.

Uses
Management of moderate to severe vasomotor symptoms associated with menopause, female hypogonadism, female castration, primary ovarian failure, postpartum breast engorgement, and atrophic conditions caused by deficient endogenous estrogen production; atrophic urethritis; palliative treatment of metastatic breast or prostate cancer in selected women and men; prevention and treatment of osteoporosis; abnormal uterine bleeding caused by hormonal imbalance in the absence of organic pathology and only when associated with a hypoplastic or atrophic endometrium.

➜◆ DRUG INTERACTIONS RELATED TO DENTAL THERAPEUTICS
No documented drug-drug interactions. The absence of evidence is not evidence of safety.

ADVERSE EFFECTS
⚠ **ORAL:** Toothache; tooth disorder (unspecified).
CNS: Headache; migraine; dizziness; depression; insomnia; anxiety; emotional lability; chorea; nervousness; mood disturbance; irritability; somnolence; exacerbation of epilepsy.
CVS: Thromboembolism; syncope; hypertension.
GI: Nausea; vomiting; abdominal cramps; bloating; colitis; acute pancreatitis; diarrhea; dyspepsia; flatulence; gastritis; gastroenteritis; enlarged abdomen; hemorrhoids; increased incidence of gallbladder disease.

RESP: URI; sinusitis; rhinitis; pharyngitis; flu-like symptoms; allergy; bronchitis; chest pain.
MISC: Pain at injection site; redness and irritation at site of transdermal system; increase or decrease in weight; reduced carbohydrate tolerance; edema; breast tenderness; acute intermittent porphyria; vaginal bleeding; hypersensitivity reactions; back pain; arthritis; arthralgia; hot flushes; leg edema; otitis media; breast enlargement and pain; nipple discharge; galactorrhea; fibrocystic breast changes; increased triglycerides.

CLINICAL IMPLICATIONS

General
- Determine why drug is being taken. Consider implications of condition on dental treatment.
- Monitor vital signs.
- If GI side effects occur, consider semisupine chair position.

Oral Health Education
- Inform patient who smokes about the risks of using tobacco products with estrogens.

---

estradiol cypionate/medroxyprogesterone acetate (ESS-truh-DIE-ole SIP-ee-oh-nate/meh-DROX-ee-pro-JESS-tuh-rone ASS-uh-TATE)

Synonym: medroxyprogesterone acetate/estradiol cypionate

Lunelle

Drug Class: Estrogen; Progestin

PHARMACOLOGY

Action
ESTRADIOL: Inhibits ovulation.
MEDROXYPROGESTERONE: Inhibits secretion of pituitary gonadotropins, thereby preventing follicular maturation and ovulation.

Uses
Prevention of pregnancy.

➡◀ DRUG INTERACTIONS RELATED TO DENTAL THERAPEUTICS
No documented drug-drug interactions. The absence of evidence is not evidence of safety.

ADVERSE EFFECTS

CNS: Depression; headache; dizziness; nervousness; migraine; emotional lability; change in appetite; asthenia.
GI: Nausea; colitis; abdominal pain; enlarged abdomen.
MISC: Hypersensitivity (e.g., anaphylactic reactions, rash); persistent melasma.

CLINICAL IMPLICATIONS

General
- *Women:* If anti-infective therapy is needed for oral infection, recommend additional birth control method.

Oral Health Education
- Inform patient who smokes about the risks of using tobacco products with estrogens.

---

estradiol valerate — see estradiol

Estradot — see estradiol

Estrasorb — see estradiol

Estring — see estradiol

estrogens, conjugated or esterified (ESS-truh-janz)
(conjugated estrogen, esterified estrogen)
Menest, Premarin, Premarin IV
◼✢◼ **C.E.S., Congest**

Drug Class: Estrogens

PHARMACOLOGY
Action
Promotes growth and development of female reproductive system and secary sex characteristics; affects release of pituitary gonadotropins; inhibits ovulation and prevents postpartum breast engorgement; conserves calcium and phosphorous and encourages bone formation; overrides stimulatory effects of testosterone.

Uses
Management of moderate to severe vasomotor symptoms associated with menopause; treatment of atrophic vaginitis, kraurosis vulvae, female hypogonadism, symptoms of female castration, and primary ovarian failure; prevention and treatment of osteoporosis (conjugated estrogens); palliative treatment of metastatic breast or prostate cancer in selected women and men; treatment of postpartum breast engorgement and abnormal uterine bleeding (parenteral form).

➡◀ DRUG INTERACTIONS RELATED TO DENTAL THERAPEUTICS
No documented drug-drug interactions. The absence of evidence is not evidence of safety.

ADVERSE EFFECTS
⚠ **ORAL:** Toothache (unspecified).
CNS: Headache; migraine; dizziness; depression; anxiety; emotional lability.
CVS: Thromboembolism, syncope, hypertension.
GI: Nausea; vomiting; abdominal cramps; bloating; colitis; acute pancreatitis; diarrhea; dyspepsia; flatulence; gastritis; gastroenteritis; enlarged abdomen; hemorrhoids.
RESP: URI; sinusitis; rhinitis; pharyngitis; flu-like symptoms; allergy; bronchitis; chest pain.
MISC: Increase or decrease in weight; reduced glucose tolerance; edema; changes in libido; breast tenderness; acute intermittent porphyria; vaginal bleeding; hypersensitivity reactions; back pain; arthritis; arthralgia; hot flushes; leg edema; otitis media.

CLINICAL IMPLICATIONS
General
• Monitor vital signs.
• If GI side effects occur, consider semisupine chair position.

Oral Health Education
• Inform patient about the risks of using tobacco products during estrogen therapy.

estrogens, conjugated/medroxyprogesterone acetate (ESS-truh-janz, KAHN-juh-gay-tuhd/meh-DROX-ee-pro-JESS-tuh-rone ASS-uh-TATE)
Synonym: conjugated estrogens/medroxyprogesterone acetate; medroxyprogesterone acetate/conjugated estrogens

Premphase, Prempro

Drug Class: Sex hormones

PHARMACOLOGY

Action

Conjugated estrogens: promotes growth and development of female reproductive system and secary sex characteristics; affects release of pituitary gonadotropins; inhibits ovulation and prevents postpartum breast engorgement; conserves calcium and phosphorous and encourages bone formation; overrides stimulatory effects of testosterone; progesterone: inhibits secretion of pituitary gonadotropins, thereby preventing follicular maturation and ovulation (contraceptive effect); inhibits spontaneous uterine contraction; transforms proliferative endometrium into secretory endometrium.

Uses

Treatment of moderate to severe vasomotor symptoms associated with menopause; treatment of vulval and vaginal atrophy; osteoporosis prevention.

Unlabeled Uses

Treatment of hypercholesterolemia in postmenopausal women.

➡️⬅️ DRUG INTERACTIONS RELATED TO DENTAL THERAPEUTICS

No documented drug-drug interactions. The absence of evidence is not evidence of safety.

ADVERSE EFFECTS

⚠️ **ORAL:** Tooth disorder (unspecified).

CNS: Headache; depression; dizziness; hypertonia; nervousness; migraine; chorea; insomnia; somnolence; change in libido.

CVS: Thromboembolism, hypertension.

GI: Abdominal pain and cramps; diarrhea; dyspepsia; flatulence; nausea; changes in appetite; vomiting; bloating.

MISC: Accidental injury; back pain; flu-like syndrome; infection; pain; pelvic pain; arthralgia; leg cramps; gallbladder disease; pancreatitis; fatigue; aggravation of porphyria; anaphylactoid reaction; anaphylaxis.

CLINICAL IMPLICATIONS

General

- Monitor vital signs.
- If GI side effects occur, consider semisupine chair position.

Oral Health Education

- Inform patient about the risks of using tobacco products during estrogen therapy.

---

estrogens, synthetic conjugated, a or b (ESS-truh-janz, sin-THE-tik KAHN-juh-gay-tuhd)

Synonym: synthetic conjugated estrogens

Cenestin, Enjuvia

Drug Class: Estrogens

PHARMACOLOGY

Action

Estrogens are responsible for the development and maintenance of the female reproductive system and secary sexual characteristics. Circulating estrogens modulate the pituitary secretion of the gonadotropins luteinizing hormone (LH) and follicle-stimulating hormone (FSH) through a negative feedback mechanism and estrogen-replacement therapy acts to reduce the elevated levels of these hormones seen in postmenopausal women.

Uses
Treatment of moderate to severe symptoms associated with menopause (synthetic conjugated estrogens, A or B); vulvar and vaginal atrophy (synthetic conjugated estrogens, A only).

➔← DRUG INTERACTIONS RELATED TO DENTAL THERAPEUTICS
No documented drug-drug interactions. The absence of evidence is not evidence of safety.

ADVERSE EFFECTS
⚠ **ORAL:** Tooth disorder (unspecified).

CNS: Depression; dizziness; hypertonia; insomnia; nervousness; paresthesia; vertigo; headache; asthenia.

CVS: Thromboembolism; increased blood pressure.

GI: Abdominal pain; constipation; diarrhea; dyspepsia; flatulence; nausea; vomiting.

RESP: Cough; pharyngitis; rhinitis; bronchitis; sinusitis.

MISC: Back pain; fever; infection; pain; accidental injury; flu-like syndrome; leg cramps.

CLINICAL IMPLICATIONS
General
- Monitor vital signs.
- If GI side effects occur, consider semisupine chair position.

Oral Health Education
- Inform patient about the risks of using tobacco products during estrogen therapy.

---

estropipate (ESS-troe-PIH-pate)
Synonym: piperazine estrone sulfate

Ogen, Ortho-Est

Drug Class: Estrogens

PHARMACOLOGY
Action
Promotes growth and development of female reproductive system and secary sex characteristics; affects release of ovulation and prevents postpartum breast engorgement; conserves calcium and phosphorous and encourages bone formation; overrides stimulatory effects of testosterone.

Uses
Management of moderate to severe vasomotor symptoms associated with menopause; female hypogonadism, female castration, primary ovarian failure, and atrophic conditions caused by deficient endogenous estrogen production; prevention and treatment of osteoporosis.

➔← DRUG INTERACTIONS RELATED TO DENTAL THERAPEUTICS
No documented drug-drug interactions. The absence of evidence is not evidence of safety.

ADVERSE EFFECTS
⚠ **ORAL:** Toothache (unspecified).

CNS: Headache; migraine; dizziness; depression; insomnia; anxiety; emotional lability.

CVS: Thromboembolism; hypertension.

GI: Nausea; vomiting; abdominal cramps; bloating; colitis; acute pancreatitis; diarrhea; dyspepsia; flatulence; gastritis; gastroenteritis; enlarged abdomen; hemorrhoids.

RESP: URI; sinusitis; rhinitis; pharyngitis; flu-like symptoms; allergy; bronchitis; chest pain.

MISC: Increase or decrease in weight; edema; changes in libido; breast tenderness; acute intermittent porphyria; vaginal bleeding; hypersensitivity reactions; back pain; arthritis; arthralgia; hot flushes; otitis media.

CLINICAL IMPLICATIONS

General
- Determine why drug is being taken. Consider implications of condition on dental treatment.
- Monitor vital signs.
- If GI side effects occur, consider semisupine chair position.

Oral Health Education
- Inform patient about the risks of using tobacco products during estrogen therapy.

---

eszopiclone (es-zoe-PIK-lone)

Lunesta

Drug Class: Sedative; Hypnotic

PHARMACOLOGY

Action
Precise mechanism is unknown; however, binding with GABA-receptor complexes located close to or allosterically coupled to benzodiazepine receptors is suspected.

Uses
Treatment of insomnia.

➥← DRUG INTERACTIONS RELATED TO DENTAL THERAPEUTICS

Clarithromycin: Possible increased eszopiclone toxicity (decreased metabolism)
- Avoid concurrent use.

Ketoconazole or itraconazole: Possible increased eszopiclone toxicity (decreased metabolism)
- Avoid concurrent use.

ADVERSE EFFECTS

⚠ **ORAL:** Dry mouth (7%); unpleasant taste (34%).

CNS: Headache (21%); somnolence (10%); dizziness (7%); nervousness (5%); depression (4%); anxiety, confusion, hallucinations, decreased libido, abnormal dreams, neuralgia (3%); migraine (≥1%).

GI: Dyspepsia, nausea (5%); diarrhea (4%); vomiting (3%).

RESP: Respiratory infection (10%).

MISC: Pain (5%); accidental injury, viral infection (3%); chest pain, peripheral edema (≥1%).

CLINICAL IMPLICATIONS

General
- Determine why drug is being taken. Consider implications of condition on dental treatment.
- Use benzodiazepines with caution; risk of drug abuse and dependence.
- Chronic dry mouth is possible; anticipate increased caries activity and candidiasis.
- If GI side effects occur, consider semisupine chair position.

Oral Health Education
- If chronic dry mouth occurs, recommend home fluoride therapy and use of nonalcoholic oral health care products.

---

etanercept (EE-tan-err-sept)

Enbrel

Drug Class: Immunomodulator

PHARMACOLOGY

Action

Binds specifically to tumor necrosis factor (TNF), blocks its interaction with cell surface TNF receptors, and modulates biological responses that are induced or regulated by TNF.

Uses

Reducing signs and symptoms and inhibiting the progression of structural damage in moderately to severely active rheumatoid arthritis; reducing signs and symptoms of moderately to severely active polyarticular-course juvenile rheumatoid arthritis (JRA) in patients responding inadequately to one or more disease-modifying antirheumatic drugs; reducing signs and symptoms of psoriatic arthritis; reducing signs and symptoms in patients with active ankylosing spondylitis. May be used in combination with methotrexate (MTX) in patients who do not respond adequately to MTX alone in the treatment of rheumatoid or psoriatic arthritis.

Unlabeled Uses

Psoriasis; treatment of Wegener granulomatosis (orphan status).

➡️⬅️ DRUG INTERACTIONS RELATED TO DENTAL THERAPEUTICS

No documented drug-drug interactions. The absence of evidence is not evidence of safety.

ADVERSE EFFECTS

⚠ **ORAL:** Mouth ulcers (6%); altered taste, dry mouth.

CNS: Headache (24%); dizziness (8%); hydrocephalus; seizure; stroke; cerebral ischemia; multiple sclerosis; depression.
JRA PATIENTS: Personality disorder; aseptic meningitis; paresthesias; isolated demyelinating conditions (e.g., transverse myelitis, optic neuritis).

CVS: Thrombophlebitis; hypertension; hypotension.

GI: Nausea (15%); dyspepsia (11%); abdominal pain (10%); vomiting (5%); GI bleeding; cholecystitis; pancreatitis; GI hemorrhage.
JRA PATIENTS: Gastroenteritis; esophagitis/gastritis.
POSTMARKETING: Anorexia; diarrhea; intestinal perforation.

RESP: Upper respiratory tract infections (31%); cough (6%); respiratory disorder (5%); pulmonary embolism; dyspnea.
POSTMARKETING: Interstitial lung disease; pulmonary disease; worsening of prior lung disorder.

MISC: Non–upper respiratory tract infections (51%); asthenia (11%); peripheral edema (8%).
JRA PATIENTS: Group A streptococcal septic shock; soft tissue and postoperative wound infection; varicella infection.
POSTMARKETING IN PEDIATRIC PATIENTS: Abscess with bacteremia; tuberculous arthritis.
POSTMARKETING: Angioedema; fatigue; fever; flu-like symptoms; generalized pain; sepsis; death.

CLINICAL IMPLICATIONS

General

- Determine why drug is being taken. Consider implications of condition on dental treatment.
- Monitor vital signs.
- If GI side effects occur, consider semisupine chair position.

Oral Health Education

- If hands are affected, consider recommendation of powered devices for plaque control.
- Recommend frequent maintenance prophylaxis when immunosuppression is evident.

---

ethacrynate — see ethacrynic acid

ethacrynic acid (eth-uh-KRIN-ik ASS-id)
Synonym: ethacrynate

Edecrin, Edecrin Sodium

Drug Class: Loop diuretic

PHARMACOLOGY

Action
Inhibits reabsorption of sodium and chloride in proximal and distal tubules and in loop of Henle.

Uses
Treatment of edema associated with CHF, cirrhosis, or renal disease; treatment of ascites, congenital heart disease, nephrotic syndrome.

Unlabeled Uses
Treatment of glaucoma; treatment of nephrogenic diabetes insipidus, hypercalcemia.

➜← DRUG INTERACTIONS RELATED TO DENTAL THERAPEUTICS
No documented drug-drug interactions. The absence of evidence is not evidence of safety.

ADVERSE EFFECTS
CNS: Apprehension; confusion; fatigue; malaise; vertigo; headache; dysphagia.
GI: Anorexia; nausea; vomiting; diarrhea; pancreatitis; discomfort; pain; sudden watery, profuse diarrhea; bleeding.
MISC: Fever; chills; severe neutropenia, thrombocytopenia, agranulocytosis.

CLINICAL IMPLICATIONS

General
- Monitor vital signs (e.g., BP, pulse pressure, rate, and rhythm) at each appointment to assess disease control. Do not provide elective dental treatment when BP is ≥180/110 or in the presence of other high-risk CV conditions. Refer to the section entitled "The Patient Taking Cardiovascular Drugs" in Chapter 6: *Clinical Medicine.*
- Use local anesthetic agents with vasoconstrictor with caution based on functional capacity of the patient and use aspirating technique to prevent intravascular injection.
- Monitor pulse rhythm to assess for electrolyte imbalance.
- Determine ability to adapt to stress of dental treatment. Consider short appointments.
- Blood dyscrasias rarely reported; anticipate increased bleeding, infection, and poor healing.

Oral Health Education
- Encourage daily plaque control procedures for effective self-care in patients at risk for cardiovascular disease.

ethambutol HCl (eth-AM-byoo-tahl HIGH-droe-KLOR-ide)
Myambutol

Drug Class: Anti-infective; Antitubercular

PHARMACOLOGY

Action
Inhibits synthesis of one or more metabolites, causing impairment of cell metabolism, arrest of multiplication, and cell death.

Uses
Treatment of pulmonary tuberculosis in combination with one or more other antituberculous agents.

→← DRUG INTERACTIONS RELATED TO DENTAL THERAPEUTICS

No documented drug-drug interactions. The absence of evidence is not evidence of safety.

ADVERSE EFFECTS

CNS: Malaise; headache; dizziness; mental confusion; disorientation; possible hallucinations; numbness and tingling of extremities.

GI: Anorexia; nausea; vomiting; GI upset; abdominal pain.

RESP: Pulmonary infiltrates.

MISC: Hypersensitivity (e.g., anaphylactoid reactions, dermatitis, pruritus); fever; joint pain.

CLINICAL IMPLICATIONS

General

• Determine why drug is being taken (prevention or treatment). Consider implications of condition on dental treatment.

• Complete medical consult to ensure noninfectious state exists before providing dental treatment.

• *For dental emergencies:* Follow special precautions to minimize disease transmission (particulate respirators) or refer patient to a hospital-based dental facility.

• If GI side effects occur, consider semisupine chair position.

Oral Health Education

• Evaluate manual dexterity; consider need for power toothbrush.

EtheDent — see sodium fluoride

---

ethionamide (eh-THIGH-ohn-ah-mide)

Trecator-SC, Trecator

Drug Class: Anti-infective; Antitubercular

PHARMACOLOGY

Action

Inhibition of peptide synthesis in susceptible organisms is suspected.

Uses

Treatment of tuberculosis, in combination with other agents, in patients with *Mycobacterium tuberculosis* resistant to isoniazid or rifampin, or when there is intolerance to other antituberculous agents.

→← DRUG INTERACTIONS RELATED TO DENTAL THERAPEUTICS

No documented drug-drug interactions. The absence of evidence is not evidence of safety.

ADVERSE EFFECTS

⚠ **ORAL:** Excessive salivation; metallic taste; stomatitis.

CNS: Psychotic disturbances; depression; drowsiness; dizziness; headache; restlessness; peripheral neuritis.

CVS: Postural hypotension.

GI: Nausea; vomiting; diarrhea; abdominal pain; anorexia.

MISC: Photosensitivity; pellagra-like syndrome.

CLINICAL IMPLICATIONS

General

• Determine why drug is being taken (prevention or treatment). Consider implications of condition on dental treatment.

• Complete medical consult to ensure noninfectious state exists before providing dental treatment.

• *For dental emergencies:* Follow special precautions to minimize disease transmission (particulate respirators) or refer patient to a hospital-based dental facility.

- If GI side effects occur, consider semisupine chair position.
- *Postural hypotension:* Monitor BP at the beginning and end of each appointment; anticipate syncope. Have patient sit upright for several min at the end of the dental appointment before dismissing.

ethosuximide (ETH-oh-SUX-ih-mide)
Zarontin
Drug Class: Anticonvulsant, succinimide
PHARMACOLOGY
Action
Elevates seizure threshold and suppresses paroxysmal spike and wave activity associated with lapses of consciousness common in absence (petit mal) seizures.

Uses
Control of absence (petit mal) seizures.

➡️⬅ DRUG INTERACTIONS RELATED TO DENTAL THERAPEUTICS
No documented drug-drug interactions. The absence of evidence is not evidence of safety.
ADVERSE EFFECTS
⚠ **ORAL:** Gingival enlargement; tongue swelling.
CNS: Drowsiness; headache; dizziness; euphoria; hiccups; irritability; hyperactivity; lethargy; fatigue; ataxia; psychological disturbances (e.g., sleep disorders, night terrors, poor concentration, aggressiveness).
MISC: Blood dyscrasias (e.g., leukopenia, agranulocytosis, eosinophilia); erythema multiforme, Stevens-Johnson syndrome, photophobia.
GI: Anorexia; GI upset; nausea; vomiting; cramps; epigastric and abdominal pain; weight loss (common).
CLINICAL IMPLICATIONS
General
- Determine why drug is being taken. Consider implications of condition on dental treatment.
- Determine level of disease control, type and frequency of seizure, and compliance with medication regimen.
- Determine ability to adapt to stress of dental treatment. Consider short appointments.
- If GI side effects occur, consider semisupine chair position.
- *Photophobia:* Direct dental light out of patient's eyes and offer dark glasses for comfort.
- Blood dyscrasias rarely reported; anticipate increased bleeding, infection, and poor healing.

Oral Health Education
- Encourage daily plaque control procedures for effective, nontraumatic self-care.

Etodine — see povidone iodine

---

etodolac (EE-toe-DOE-lak)
Lodine, Lodine XL
■✚■ **Apo-Etodolac, Ultradol**
■❖■ **Retard**
Drug Class: Analgesic; NSAID
PHARMACOLOGY
Action
Decreases inflammation, pain, and fever, probably through inhibition of COX activity and prostaglandin synthesis.

Uses

Management of pain (Lodine only); management of signs and symptoms of osteoarthritis and rheumatoid arthritis.

Unlabeled Uses

Control of symptoms of rheumatoid arthritis; treatment of temporal arteritis.

➡◆ DRUG INTERACTIONS RELATED TO DENTAL THERAPEUTICS

No documented drug-drug interactions. The absence of evidence is not evidence of safety.

ADVERSE EFFECTS

⚠ **ORAL:** Dry mouth, stomatitis, taste disturbance (1%).

CNS: Dizziness; headaches; drowsiness; insomnia; asthenia; malaise; depression; nervousness.

GI: Dyspepsia; nausea; vomiting; diarrhea; indigestion; heartburn; abdominal pain; constipation; flatulence; gastritis; melena; anorexia; peptic ulcers.

RESP: Asthma.

MISC: Chills; fever.

CLINICAL IMPLICATIONS

General

- Determine why drug is being taken. Consider implications of condition on dental treatment.
- *Arthritis:* Consider patient comfort and need for semisupine chair position.
- If GI side effects occur, consider semisupine chair position.

Oral Health Education

- Evaluate manual dexterity; consider need for power toothbrush.

Euglucon — see glyburide

Eumetinex — see amoxicillin

Eutirox — see levothyroxine sodium

Evista — see raloxifene hydrochloride

Evoxac — see cevimeline HCl

Exelon — see rivastigmine tartrate

Extended Release Bayer 8-Hour — see aspirin

Extra Strength Bayer Enteric 500 Aspirin — see aspirin

Extra Strength Dynafed E.X. — see acetaminophen

---

ezetimibe (Ezz-ET-ih-mibe)

Zetia

Drug Class: Antihyperlipidemic

PHARMACOLOGY

Action

Inhibits absorption of cholesterol by the small intestine.

Uses

Administration alone or with HMG-CoA reductase inhibitors as adjunctive therapy to diet for reduction of elevated total cholesterol, LDL, and apolipoprotein in patients with primary hypercholesterolemia; with atorvastatin or simvastatin for the reduction of elevated total cholesterol and LDL levels in patients with homozygous familial hypercholesterolemia as an adjunct to other lipid-lowering treatments or if such treatments are unavailable; as adjunctive therapy to diet for the reduction of elevated sitosterol and campesterol levels in patients with homozygous familial sitosterolemia.

➪◀ DRUG INTERACTIONS RELATED TO DENTAL THERAPEUTICS
No documented drug-drug interactions. The absence of evidence is not evidence of safety.

ADVERSE EFFECTS
CNS: Fatigue; headache; dizziness.
GI: Diarrhea; abdominal pain.
RESP: Coughing; URI.
MISC: Back pain; arthralgia; viral infection; myalgia; chest pain.

CLINICAL IMPLICATIONS

General
- High LDL cholesterol concentration is the major cause of atherosclerosis, which leads to CAD (angina, MI); determine degree of CV health and ability to withstand stress of dental treatment.
- Monitor vital signs (e.g., BP, pulse pressure, rate, and rhythm) at each appointment to assess disease control. Do not provide elective dental treatment when BP is ≥180/110 or in the presence of other high-risk CV conditions. Refer to the section entitled "The Patient Taking Cardiovascular Drugs" in Chapter 6: *Clinical Medicine*.
- Consider semisupine chair position for patient comfort.

Oral Health Education
- Encourage daily plaque control procedures for effective self-care in patients at risk for cardiovascular disease.

Ezide — see hydrochlorothiazide

Facicam — see piroxicam

Factive — see gemifloxacin mesylate

---

 famciclovir (fam-SYE-kloe-veer)

Famvir: Tablets: 125, 250, 500 mg

Drug Class: Anti-infective; Antiviral

PHARMACOLOGY

Action
Converts to penciclovir, which inhibits viral DNA replication by interfering with viral DNA polymerase.

Uses
Treatment of acute herpes zoster infection; treatment or suppression of recurrent genital herpes infection in immunocompetent patients; treatment of recurrent mucocutaneous herpes simplex infections in HIV-infected patients.

Contraindications
Hypersensitivity to famciclovir, other components of the formulation, or penciclovir cream.

Usual Dosage
Herpes Zoster
Adults: *PO:* 500 mg q 8 hr for 7 days. Initiate treatment immediately after diagnosis.
HIV-Infected Patients
Adults: Recurrent Orolabial or Genital Herpes: *PO:* 500 mg bid for 7 days.

Pharmacokinetics

ABSORP: Bioavailability is about 77%. T_{max} is 0.9 hr. $AUC_{0 \cdot \check{z}}$ is 2.24 to 8.95 depending on dose. C_{max} is 0.8 to 3.3 mcg/mL depending on the dose.

DIST: Vd is about 1.08 L/kg; 20% bound to plasma proteins.

METAB: Hepatic route; deacetylated and oxidized to form inactive penciclovir metabolites.

EXCRET: Cl is about 36.6 L/hr; about 75% is renally cleared. The $t_{1/2}$ is about 2 to 3 hr.

SPECIAL POP: *Renal failure:* With Ccr 40 to 59 mL/min, Cl_R is about 13 L/hr and $t_{1/2}$ is about 3.4 hr. With Ccr 20 to 39 mL/min, Cl_R is about 4.24 L/hr and $t_{1/2}$ is about 6.2 hr. With Ccr less than 20 mL/min, Cl_R is about 1.64 L/hr and $t_{1/2}$ is about 13.4 hr. *Hepatic failure:* Penciclovir C_{max} decreased 44%; T_{max} increased by 0.75 hr.

➔◀ DRUG INTERACTIONS

No documented drug-drug interactions. The absence of evidence is not evidence of safety.

ADVERSE EFFECTS

CNS: Headache (39%); paresthesia, migraine (3%); confusion; delirium; disorientation; confusional state.

GI: Nausea (13%); diarrhea (9%); abdominal pain (8%); vomiting, flatulence (5%).

MISC: Fatigue (5%).

CLINICAL IMPLICATIONS

General

- Determine why drug is being taken. Consider implications of condition on dental treatment.
- Consider medical consult to determine disease control and influence on dental treatment.
- If GI side effects occur, consider semisupine chair position.

When used or prescribed by DDS:

- Ensure patient knows how to take the drug, how long it should be taken, and to report adverse effects (e.g., rash, difficult breathing, diarrhea, GI upset immediately). See Chapter 4: *Medical Management of Odontogenic Infections.*
- *Lactation:* Undetermined.
- *Children:* Safety and efficacy not established.
- *Renal failure:* Dosage adjustment is recommended when Ccr is 60 mL/min or less.

Pregnancy Risk Category: Category B.

Oral Health Education

When prescribed by DDS:

- Explain name, dose, action, and potential side effects of drug.
- Review dose and appropriate dosing schedule depending on condition being treated (e.g., shingles, cold sores, recurrent herpes). Instruct patient to take medication exactly as prescribed and not to stop taking or change the dose unless advised by health care provider.
- Advise patient that medication can be taken without regard to meals but to take with food if stomach upset occurs.
- Remind patient using medication for recurrent episodes of herpes to initiate therapy at the first sign or symptom or recurrence and that medication may not be effective if started more than 6 hr after onset of signs or symptoms of recurrence.
- Advise patient with herpes that this drug is not a cure for herpes and does not prevent transmission of virus.
- Advise patient to contact health care provider if medication does not seem to be controlling lesions and/or symptoms or if intolerable side effects develop.
- Advise women to notify health care provider if pregnant, planning to become pregnant, or breast feeding.
- Instruct patient to not take any prescription or OTC medications or dietary supplements unless advised by health care provider.
- Advise patient that follow-up visits may be necessary to monitor therapy and to keep appointments.

famotidine (fuh-MOE-tih-deen)

Pepcid, Pepcid AC, Pepcid AC, Pepcid AC, Pepcid RPD

■✚■ **Apo-Famotidine, Gen-Famotidine, Novo-Famotidine, Nu-Famotidine, Pepcid IV, ratio-Famotidine, Rhoxal-famotidine**

■❧■ **Durater, Famoxal, Farmotex, Pepcidine, Sigafam**

Drug Class: Histamine H_2 antagonist

PHARMACOLOGY

Action

Reversibly and competitively blocks histamine at H_2 receptors, particularly those in gastric parietal cells, leading to inhibition of gastric acid secretion.

Uses

Short-term treatment and maintenance therapy for duodenal ulcer, GERD (including erosive or ulcerative disease), benign gastric ulcer, treatment of pathological hypersecretory conditions.

Unlabeled Uses

Treatment of upper GI bleeding; prevention of stress ulcers; before anesthesia for prevention of pulmonary aspiration of gastric acid.

➡✚ DRUG INTERACTIONS RELATED TO DENTAL THERAPEUTICS

Naproxen: Possible decreased naproxen effect (decreased absorption)
• Monitor clinical status.

ADVERSE EFFECTS

⚠ **ORAL:** Dry mouth; taste disorder.

CNS: Headache; somnolence; fatigue; dizziness; confusion; hallucinations; agitation or anxiety; depression; insomnia; paresthesias.

CVS: Palpitations.

GI: Diarrhea; constipation; nausea; vomiting; abdominal discomfort; anorexia.

RESP: Bronchospasm.

MISC: Arthralgia; thrombocytopenia.

CLINICAL IMPLICATIONS

General

• Determine why drug is being taken. Consider implications of condition on dental treatment.
• If patient has GI disease, consider semisupine chair position.
• Use COX inhibitors with caution, they may exacerbate PUD and GERD.
• Chronic dry mouth is possible; anticipate increased caries activity and candidiasis.
• Blood dyscrasias rarely reported; anticipate increased bleeding.

Oral Health Education

• If chronic dry mouth occurs, recommend home fluoride therapy and use of nonalcoholic oral health care products.

Famoxal — see famotidine

Famvir — see famciclovir

Faraxen — see naproxen

Farmotex — see famotidine

FazaClo — see clozapine

Fe⁵⁰ — see ferrous salts

Febrin — see acetaminophen

felbamate (FELL-buh-mate)
Felbatol

Drug Class: Anticonvulsant

PHARMACOLOGY
Action
May reduce seizure spread in generalized tonic-clonic or partial seizures and may increase seizure threshold in absence seizures.

Uses
Monotherapy or adjunctive therapy in treatment of partial seizures with and without generalization in epileptic adults. Adjunctive therapy in treatment of partial and generalized seizures associated with Lennox-Gastaut syndrome in children.

➡️◀ DRUG INTERACTIONS RELATED TO DENTAL THERAPEUTICS
No documented drug-drug interactions. The absence of evidence is not evidence of safety.

ADVERSE EFFECTS
⚠️ **ORAL:** Dry mouth (2.6%); taste perversion.

CNS: Insomnia; headache; anxiety; somnolence; dizziness; nervousness; tremor; abnormal gait; depression; paresthesia; ataxia; stupor; thinking abnormalities; emotional lability.

CVS: Chest pain, tachycardia, palpitations (1%).

GI: Dyspepsia; vomiting; constipation; diarrhea; nausea; anorexia; abdominal pain; hiccups.

RESP: URI; coughing.

MISC: Fatigue; weight decrease; facial edema; fever; pain; hypophosphatemia; myalgia.

CLINICAL IMPLICATIONS
General
- Determine why drug is being taken. Consider implications of condition on dental treatment.
- Determine level of disease control, type and frequency of seizure, and compliance with medication regimen.
- Determine ability to adapt to stress of dental treatment. Consider short appointments.
- Chronic dry mouth is possible; anticipate increased caries activity and candidiasis.
- Monitor vital signs.
- If GI side effects occur, consider semisupine chair position.

Felbatol — see felbamate

Feldene — see piroxicam

Feliberal — see enalapril maleate

---

felodipine (feh-LOW-dih-peen)
Plendil

🔳🍁🔳 **Renedil**

🔳🔳 **Logimax, Munobal**

Drug Class: Calcium channel blocker

PHARMACOLOGY
Action
Inhibits movement of calcium ions across cell membrane in systemic and coronary vascular smooth muscle, altering contractile process.

Uses

Treatment of hypertension.

➡◆ DRUG INTERACTIONS RELATED TO DENTAL THERAPEUTICS

Itraconazole: Possible felodipine toxicity (decreased metabolism)
- Avoid concurrent use.

ADVERSE EFFECTS

⚠ **ORAL:** Dry mouth; thirst; gingival hyperplasia.

CNS: Headache; dizziness; lightheadedness; nervousness; psychiatric disturbances; paresthesias; somnolence; asthenia; insomnia; anxiety; irritability.

CVS: Arrhythmia, chest pain, hypotension, tachycardia, palpitations, syncope.

GI: Nausea; diarrhea; constipation; abdominal discomfort; cramps; dyspepsia; vomiting; flatulence.

RESP: Nasal or chest congestion; sinusitis; rhinitis; pharyngitis; shortness of breath; wheezing; cough; sneezing; respiratory infections.

MISC: Muscle cramps, pain, or inflammation.

CLINICAL IMPLICATIONS

General

- Monitor vital signs (e.g., BP, pulse pressure, rate and rhythm) at each appointment to assess disease control. Do not provide elective dental treatment when BP is ≥180/110 or in presence of other high-risk CV conditions. Refer to the section entitled "The Patient Taking Cardiovascular Drugs" in Chapter 6: *Clinical Medicine*.
- Use local anesthetic agents with vasoconstrictor with caution based on functional capacity of the patient and use aspirating technique to prevent intravascular injection.
- Determine ability to adapt to stress of dental treatment. Consider short appointments.
- Consider semisupine chair position to assist respiratory function.
- Anticipate gingival hyperplasia; consider MD consult to recommend different drug regimen if periodontal health is compromised.
- Chronic dry mouth is possible; anticipate increased caries, candidiasis, and lichenoid mucositis.
- If GI side effects occur, consider semisupine chair position.

Oral Health Education

- Encourage daily plaque control procedures for effective self-care in patient at risk for cardiovascular disease.

Femiron — see ferrous salts

Fenesin — see guaifenesin

Fenidantoin — see phenytoin

Fenitron — see phenytoin

---

fenofibrate (FEN-oh-fih-brate)

Lofibra, Tricor, Triglide

■✦■ **Apo-Fenofibrate, Apo-Feno-Micro, Gen-Fenofibrate Micro, Lipidil Micro, Lipidil Supra, Nu-Fenofibrate, PMS-Fenofibrate Micro**

■▪■ **Controlip, Lipidil**

Drug Class: Antihyperlipidemic

PHARMACOLOGY

Action

Mechanism not well established. Apparently decreases plasma levels of triglycerides by decreasing their synthesis. Also reduces plasma levels of VLDL cholesterol by reducing their release into the circulation and increasing catabolism. Reduces serum uric acid levels by increasing urinary excretion of uric acid.

Uses

Adjunctive therapy to diet for treatment of hypertriglyceridemia in adult patients with type 4 or 5 hyperlipidemia who are at risk of pancreatitis; adjunctive therapy to diet for the reduction of LDL cholesterol, total cholesterol, triglycerides, and apo B, and to increase HDL cholesterol in adults with primary hypercholesterolemia or mixed dyslipidemia (Fredrickson types IIa and IIb).

➜← DRUG INTERACTIONS RELATED TO DENTAL THERAPEUTICS

No documented drug-drug interactions. The absence of evidence is not evidence of safety.

ADVERSE EFFECTS

⚠ **ORAL:** Tooth disorder (unspecified).

CNS: Dizziness; insomnia; paresthesia; headache; fatigue; asthenia.

CVS: Angina; hypertension or hypotension; palpitations; tachycardia; arrhythmia.

GI: Dyspepsia; nausea; vomiting; diarrhea; constipation; abdominal pain; flatulence; eructation; increased appetite; pancreatitis.

RESP: Rhinitis; sinusitis; cough; respiratory disorder.

MISC: Flu syndrome; arthralgia; back pain; hypersensitivity reactions (including severe skin rashes, Stevens-Johnson syndrome, toxic epidermal necrolysis); myositis; myopathy; rhabdomyolysis; photosensitivity disorder.

CLINICAL IMPLICATIONS

General

- High LDL cholesterol concentration is the major cause of atherosclerosis, which leads to CAD (angina, MI); determine degree of CV health and ability to withstand stress of dental treatment.
- Monitor vital signs (e.g., BP, pulse pressure, rate and rhythm) at each appointment to assess disease control. Do not provide elective dental treatment when BP is ≥180/110 or in presence of other high-risk CV conditions. Refer to the section entitled "The Patient Taking Cardiovascular Drugs" in Chapter 6: *Clinical Medicine*.
- If GI side effects occur, consider semisupine chair position.

Oral Health Education

- Encourage daily plaque control procedures for effective self-care in patient at risk for cardiovascular disease.

---

fenoprofen calcium (FEN-oh-PRO-fen KAL-see-uhm)

Nalfon Pulvules

Drug Class: Analgesic; NSAID

PHARMACOLOGY

Action

Decreases inflammation, pain and fever, probably through inhibition of cyclooxygenase activity and prostaglandin synthesis.

Uses

Symptomatic relief for rheumatoid arthritis, osteoarthritis, mild to moderate pain.

Unlabeled Uses

Symptomatic relief for juvenile rheumatoid arthritis; migraine prophylaxis and treatment.

➜← DRUG INTERACTIONS RELATED TO DENTAL THERAPEUTICS

No documented drug-drug interactions significant to dentistry. The absence of evidence is not evidence of safety.

ADVERSE EFFECTS

⚠ **ORAL:** Dry mouth (1%).
CNS: Dizziness; drowsiness; headaches; nervousness; anxiety; confusion; somnolence.
CVS: Palpitations; tachycardia.
GI: Heartburn; dyspepsia; nausea; vomiting; diarrhea; constipation; increased or decreased appetite; indigestion; GI bleeding; ulceration; abdominal distress/cramps/pain; flatulence; occult blood in stool.
RESP: Bronchospasm; laryngeal edema; hemoptysis; shortness of breath.
MISC: Agranulocytosis, thrombocytopenia, hemolytic anemia, aplastic anemia (<1%).

CLINICAL IMPLICATIONS

General
- Determine why drug is being taken. Consider implications of condition on dental treatment.
- *Arthritis:* Consider patient comfort and need for semisupine chair position.
- Monitor vital signs.
- Blood dyscrasias rarely reported; anticipate increased bleeding, infection, and poor healing.
- Chronic dry mouth is possible; anticipate increased caries and candidiasis.
- If GI side effects occur, consider semisupine chair position.

Oral Health Education
- Encourage daily plaque control procedures for effective, nontraumatic self-care.
- If chronic dry mouth occurs, recommend home fluoride therapy and use of nonalcoholic oral health care products.

Fentanest — see fentanyl transdermal system

---

fentanyl transdermal system (FEN-tuh-nill)

Duragesic-25, Duragesic-50, Duragesic-75, Duragesic-100

▌✦▌ Duragesic

▌✦▌ Durogesic, Fentanest

Drug Class: Narcotic analgesic

PHARMACOLOGY

Action
A potent, short-acting, rapid-onset opiate agonist that relieves pain by stimulating opiate receptors in CNS.

Uses
Management of chronic pain refractory to less potent agents.

➔← DRUG INTERACTIONS RELATED TO DENTAL THERAPEUTICS

Fluconazole: Fentanyl toxicity (decreased metabolism)
- Monitor clinical status.

Midazoleme: Hypoxemia and apnea (decreased sympathetic tone)
- Monitor clinical status.

Lidocaine: Possible CNS and respiratory depression (additive)
- Monitor clinical status.

ADVERSE EFFECTS

⚠ **ORAL:** Dry mouth.
CNS: Lightheadedness; dizziness; sedation; disorientation; incoordination; headache; hallucinations; euphoria; depression; seizures.
CVS: Orthostatic hypotension.
GI: Nausea; vomiting; constipation; abdominal pain; diarrhea; dyspepsia.

RESP: Laryngospasm; depression of cough reflex; dyspnea; hypoventilation.
MISC: Tolerance; psychological and physical dependence with long-term use.

CLINICAL IMPLICATIONS
General
- Determine why drug is being taken. Consider implications of condition on dental treatment.
- If oral pain requires additional analgesics, consider nonopioid products.
- Chronic dry mouth is possible; anticipate increased caries and candidiasis.
- *Postural hypotension:* Monitor BP at the beginning and end of each appointment; anticipate syncope. Have patient sit upright for several min at the end of the dental appointment before dismissing.
- If GI side effects occur, consider semisupine chair position.
- Monitor vital signs (e.g., BP, pulse rate) and respiratory function.

Oral Health Education
- If chronic dry mouth occurs, recommend home fluoride therapy and use of nonalcoholic oral health care products.

Feosol — see ferrous salts
Feostat — see ferrous salts
Feratab — see ferrous salts
Fer-gen-sol — see ferrous salts
Fergon — see ferrous salts
Fer-In-Sol — see ferrous salts
Fer-Iron — see ferrous salts
Ferodan — see ferrous salts
Ferrex 150 — see ferrous salts
Ferro-Sequels — see ferrous salts

---

ferrous salts (FER-uhs salts)

Fe^{50}, Femiron, Feosol, Feostat, Feratab, Fer-gen-sol, Fergon, Fer-In-Sol, Fer-Iron, Ferrex 150, Ferro-Sequels, Hemocyte, Hytinic, Icar, Ircon, Nephro-Fer, Niferex, Niferex-150, Nu-Iron, Nu-Iron 150, Slow-FE, Vitron-C, ED-IN-SOL, DexFerrum

■✦■ Apo-Ferrous Sulfate, Ferodan, Palafer

■◗■ Ferval

Drug Class: Iron product

PHARMACOLOGY
Action
Iron is a major factor in oxygen transport and an essential mineral component of hemoglobin, myoglobin, and several enzymes.

Uses
Prevention and treatment of iron-deficiency anemia.

Unlabeled Uses
Use with epoetin to ensure hematological response to epoetin.

� DRUG INTERACTIONS RELATED TO DENTAL THERAPEUTICS
Tetracyclines: Decreased tetracycline effect and decreased iron effect (decreased absorption)

- Give iron 3 hr before or 2 hr after tetracycline.
- Doxycycline does not appear to interact.

ADVERSE EFFECTS
⚠ **ORAL:** Teeth staining with liquid formulation.
GI: Irritation; anorexia; nausea; vomiting; diarrhea; constipation; dark stool.

CLINICAL IMPLICATIONS
General
- Determine why drug is being taken. Consider implications of condition on dental treatment.
- Anemia can result in poor wound healing.

Ferval — see ferrous salts
Feverall — see acetaminophen
Feverall Junior Strength — see acetaminophen

---

fexofenadine HCl (fex-oh-FEN-ah-deen HIGH-droe-KLOR-ide)
Allegra
█✦█ **Allegra 12 Hour, Allegra 24 Hour**
Drug Class: Antihistamine

PHARMACOLOGY
Action
Competitively antagonizes histamine at the H_1-receptor site.

Uses
Symptomatic relief of symptoms (nasal and nonnasal) associated with seasonal allergic rhinitis; treatment of uncomplicated skin manifestations of chronic idiopathic urticaria.

➡◀ DRUG INTERACTIONS RELATED TO DENTAL THERAPEUTICS
No documented drug-drug interactions. The absence of evidence is not evidence of safety.

ADVERSE EFFECTS
CNS: Headache (11%); drowsiness, dizziness (2%); fatigue (1%).
GI: Nausea (2%); dyspepsia (1%).
RESP: URI (4%).
MISC: Viral infection (cold, flu); accidental injury, back pain (3%); fever, pain (2%).

CLINICAL IMPLICATIONS
General
- Determine why drug is being taken. Consider implications of condition on dental treatment.
- Consider semisupine chair position to control effects of postnasal drainage.
- Be aware that patients with multiple allergies are at increased risk for allergy to dental drugs.
- Chronic dry mouth is possible; anticipate increased caries and candidiasis.

Oral Health Education
- If chronic dry mouth occurs, recommend home fluoride therapy and use of nonalcoholic oral health care products.

---

fexofenadine HCl/pseudoephedrine HCl (fex-oh-FEN-ah-deen HIGH-droe-KLOR-ide/SUE-doe-eh-FED-rin HIGH-droe-KLOR-ide)
Synonym: pseudoephedrine HCl/fexofenadine HCl

Allegra-D

Drug Class: Antihistamine, decongestant

PHARMACOLOGY

Action

FEXOFENADINE: Competitively antagonizes histamine at the H₁-receptor site.

PSEUDOEPHEDRINE: Causes vasoconstriction and subsequent shrinkage of nasal mucous membranes by alpha-adrenergic stimulation, promoting nasal drainage.

Uses

Relief of symptoms associated with seasonal allergic rhinitis.

➡◀ DRUG INTERACTIONS RELATED TO DENTAL THERAPEUTICS

No documented drug-drug interactions. The absence of evidence is not evidence of safety.

ADVERSE EFFECTS

⚠ **ORAL:** Dry mouth.

CNS: Headache; insomnia; dizziness; agitation; nervousness; anxiety; excitability, restlessness, weakness, drowsiness, fear, tenseness, hallucinations, seizures (pseudoephedrine).

GI: Nausea; dyspepsia; abdominal pain.

RESP: URI; respiratory difficulties.

MISC: Back pain.

CLINICAL IMPLICATIONS

General

- Determine why drug is being taken. Consider implications of condition on dental treatment.
- Consider semisupine chair position to control effects of postnasal drainage.
- Be aware that patients with multiple allergies are at increased risk for allergy to dental drugs.
- Chronic dry mouth is possible; anticipate increased caries and candidiasis.

Oral Health Education

- If chronic dry mouth occurs, recommend home fluoride therapy and use of nonalcoholic oral health care products.

---

finasteride (fih-NASS-teer-IDE)

Propecia, Proscar

🔳 Propeshia

Drug Class: Androgen hormone inhibitor

PHARMACOLOGY

Action

Inhibits conversion of testosterone into 5-alpha-dihydrotestosterone, a potent androgen.

Uses

PROPECIA: Treatment of male pattern hair loss (androgenic alopecia) in men only.

PROSCAR: Treatment of symptomatic BPH in men with enlarged prostate; in combination with doxazosin to reduce the risk of symptomatic progression of BPH.

➡◀ DRUG INTERACTIONS RELATED TO DENTAL THERAPEUTICS

No documented drug-drug interactions. The absence of evidence is not evidence of safety.

ADVERSE EFFECTS

CNS: PROPECIA: Decreased libido (2%).
PROSCAR: Decreased libido (10%); dizziness (7%); headache, somnolence (2%).
CVS: PROSCAR: Postural hypotension (9%); hypotension.
RESP: PROSCAR: Rhinitis (1%).
MISC: PROSCAR: Asthenia (5%).

CLINICAL IMPLICATIONS

General
- Determine why drug is being taken. Consider implications of condition on dental treatment.
- *Postural hypotension:* Monitor BP at the beginning and end of each appointment; anticipate syncope. Have patient sit upright for several min at the end of the dental appointment before dismissing.

Findol — see ketorolac tromethamine

Fisopred — see prednisolone

FK506 — see tacrolimus

Flagenase — see metronidazole

Flagyl — see metronidazole

Flagyl 375 — see metronidazole

Flagyl ER — see metronidazole

Flagyl I.V. — see metronidazole

Flagyl I.V. RTU — see metronidazole

Flamicina — see ampicillin

Flanax — see naproxen

---

flavoxate (flay-voke-sate)

Urispas

███ Bladuril

Drug Class: Urinary tract antispasmodic; Alkalinizer

PHARMACOLOGY

Action
Counteracts smooth muscle spasms of urinary tract.

Uses
Symptomatic relief of dysuria, urgency, nocturia, suprapubic pain, frequency, and incontinence associated with cystitis, prostatitis, urethritis, and urethrocystitis/urethrotrigonitis.

➡◀ DRUG INTERACTIONS RELATED TO DENTAL THERAPEUTICS
No documented drug-drug interactions. The absence of evidence is not evidence of safety.

ADVERSE EFFECTS
⚠ **ORAL:** Dry mouth.
CNS: Nervousness; headache; drowsiness; mental confusion.
CVS: Tachycardia; palpitations.
GI: Nausea; vomiting.
MISC: High fever; leukopenia.

CLINICAL IMPLICATIONS

General

- Monitor vital signs.
- Chronic dry mouth is possible; anticipate increased caries and candidiasis.
- If GI side effects occur, consider semisupine chair position.

Oral Health Education

- If chronic dry mouth occurs, recommend home fluoride therapy and use of nonalcoholic oral health care products.

---

flecainide acetate (fleh-CANE-ide ASS-uh-TATE)

Tambocor

Drug Class: Antiarrhythmic

PHARMACOLOGY

Action

Produces a dose-related decrease in intracardiac conduction in all parts of the heart; also has local anesthetic activity.

Uses

Prevention of PAF associated with disabling symptoms; PSVTs, including AV nodal reentrant tachycardia and AV reentrant tachycardia; prevention of documented life-threatening ventricular arrhythmias, such as sustained VT.

DRUG INTERACTIONS RELATED TO DENTAL THERAPEUTICS

No documented drug-drug interactions. The absence of evidence is not evidence of safety.

ADVERSE EFFECTS

⚠ **ORAL:** Dry mouth; taste changes; swollen lips, tongue, mouth (unspecified).

CNS: Dizziness including lightheadedness, faintness, unsteadiness, and near syncope (19%); headache (10%); fatigue (8%); asthenia, tremor (5%); hypoesthesia, paresthesia, paresis, ataxia, flushing, increased sweating, vertigo, syncope, somnolence, anxiety, insomnia, depression, malaise (1% to <3%).

CVS: Sinus bradycardia; tachycardia; arrhythmia; hypertension or hypotension.

GI: Nausea (9%); constipation (4%); abdominal pain (3%); vomiting, diarrhea, dyspepsia, anorexia (1% to <3%).

RESP: Dyspnea (10%).

MISC: Edema (4%); fever (1% to <3%); photophobia.

CLINICAL IMPLICATIONS

General

- Monitor vital signs (e.g., BP, pulse pressure, rate, and rhythm) at each appointment to assess disease control. Do not provide elective dental treatment when BP is ≥180/110 or in presence of other high-risk CV conditions. Refer to the section entitled "The Patient Taking Cardiovascular Drugs" in Chapter 6: *Clinical Medicine*.
- Determine ability to adapt to stress of dental treatment. Consider short appointments.
- Use local anesthetic agents with vasoconstrictor with caution based on functional capacity of the patient and use aspirating technique to prevent intravascular injection.
- Chronic dry mouth is possible; anticipate increased caries and candidiasis.
- *Photophobia:* Direct dental light out of patient's eyes and offer dark glasses for comfort.
- If GI side effects occur, consider semisupine chair position.

Oral Health Education

- If chronic dry mouth occurs, recommend home fluoride therapy and use of nonalcoholic oral health care products.
- Encourage daily plaque control procedures for effective self-care in patient at risk for cardiovascular disease.

Flemoxon — see amoxicillin
Flexen — see naproxen
Flexeril — see cyclobenzaprine HCl
Flogen — see naproxen
Flogosan — see piroxicam
Flomax — see tamsulosin HCl
Flonase — see fluticasone propionate
Florazole ER — see metronidazole
Florinef — see fluticasone propionate
Florinef Acetate — see fludrocortisone acetate
Floven HF — see fluticasone propionate
Flovent — see fluticasone propionate
Flovent Diskus — see fluticasone propionate
Flovent Rotadisk — see fluticasone propionate
Floxacin — see norfloxacin
Floxin — see ofloxacin

 fluconazole (flew-KOE-nuh-zole)

Diflucan: Tablets: 50, 100, 150, 200 mg; Powder for Oral Suspension: 10, 40 mg/mL when reconstituted; Injection: 2 mg/mL

■✦■ Apo-Fluconazole, Apo-Fluconazole-150, Diflucan-150

■▨■ Afungil, Neofomiral, Oxifungol, Zonal

Drug Class: Anti-infective; Antifungal

PHARMACOLOGY

Action
Interferes with the formation of fungal cell membrane, causing leakage of cellular contents and cell death.

Uses
Oropharyngeal and esophageal candidiasis; vaginal candidiasis; prevention of candidiasis in bone marrow transplant; *Cryptococcal meningitis.*

Contraindications
Coadministration of cisapride; hypersensitivity to any component of the product.

Usual Dosage
Oropharyngeal or esophageal candidiasis
ADULTS: *PO/IV:* 200 mg first day, followed by 100 mg once a day thereafter for a minimum of 2 wk for oropharyngeal candidiasis, or for 3 wk and at least 2 wk following resolution of symptoms for esophageal candidiasis.
CHILDREN: *PO/IV:* 6 mg/kg on first day, followed by 3 mg/kg once a day thereafter for minimum of 2 wk for oropharyngeal candidiasis or 3 wk (at least 2 wk after symptom resolution) for esophageal candidiasis.

Pharmacokinetics
ABSORP: Bioavailability is more than 90%. T_{max} is 1 to 2 hr.
DIST: Apparent Vd is 0.65 L/kg, and it is 11% to 12% protein bound. Ratio of tissue (fluid)

concentrations to concurrent plasma concentrations is as follows: CSF 0.5 to 0.9, saliva 1, sputum 1, blister fluid 1, urine 10, normal skin 10, nails 1, blister skin 2, vaginal tissue 1, and vaginal fluid 0.4 to 0.7.
EXCRET: Mean body Cl is 0.23 mL/min/kg; $t_{1/2}$ is 20 to 50 hr. The drug is cleared primarily by renal excretion, about 80% in urine as unchanged drug and 11% excreted in urine as metabolites.
HEMODIALYSIS: A 3-hr session decreases plasma concentrations about 50%.
SPECIAL POP: *Renal failure:* Pharmacokinetics are markedly affected; there is an inverse relationship between $t_{1/2}$ and Ccr.

➤◀ DRUG INTERACTIONS

Alfentanil: Alfentanil toxicity (decreased metabolism)
• Monitor clinical status.
Anticoagulants, oral: Increased anticoagulant effect (decreased metabolism)
• Use with caution.
Antidepressants, tricyclic: Possible nortriptyline or amitriptyline toxicity (decreased metabolism)
• Monitor clinical status.
Caffeine: Possible caffeine toxicity (decreased metabolism)
• Monitor clinical status.
Carbamazepine: Possible carbamazepine toxicity (decreased metabolism)
• Monitor clinical status.
COX-2 inhibitors: Possible celecoxib toxicity (decreased metabolism)
• Avoid concurrent use.
Cyclosporine: Renal toxicity (decreased metabolism)
• Avoid concurrent use or monitor cyclosporine concentration.
Glimepiride: Possible increased risk of hypoglycemia (decreased metabolism)
• Monitor blood glucose.
Glipizide: Severe hypoglycemia (decreased metabolism)
• Monitor blood glucose.
Irbesartan: Possible irbesartan toxicity (decreased metabolism)
• Monitor clinical status.
Losartan: Possible losartan toxicity (decreased metabolism)
• Monitor clinical status.
Methadone: Possible methadone toxicity (decreased metabolism)
• Monitor clinical status.
Nifedipine: Possible nifedipine toxicity (decreased metabolism)
• Monitor blood pressure.
Phenytoin: Phenytoin toxicity (decreased metabolism)
• Avoid concurrent use or monitor phenytoin concentration.
Rifabutin: Uveitis (decreased metabolism)
• Monitor clinical status.
Rifampin: Decreased fluconazole effect (increased metabolism)
• Avoid concurrent use.
Saquinavir: Possible saquinavir toxicity (decreased metabolism)
• Monitor clinical status.
Tacrolimus: Possible tacrolimus toxicity (decreased metabolism)
• Avoid concurrent use or monitor tacrolimus concentration.
Theophylline: Possible theophylline toxicity (decreased metabolism)
• Monitor clinical status.
Verapamil: Possible verapamil toxicity (decreased metabolism)
• Monitor blood pressure.
Zidovudine: Possible zidovudine toxicity (decreased metabolism)
• Monitor clinical status.

ADVERSE EFFECTS

⚠ **ORAL:** Taste disturbance (1%).
CVS: QT prolongation (including torsades de pointes).
CNS: Headache (2%).
GI: Nausea (4% [children 2%]); vomiting (2% [children 5%]); abdominal pain (2% [children 3%]); diarrhea (2%).
MISC: Leukopenia; thrombocytopenia; hypokalemia.

CLINICAL IMPLICATIONS

General
- Determine why drug is being taken. Consider implications of condition on dental treatment.
- Blood dyscrasias rarely reported; anticipate increased bleeding, infection, and poor healing.
- If GI side effects occur, consider semisupine chair position.

If prescribed by DDS:
- Ensure patient knows how to take the drug, how long it should be taken, and to immediately report adverse effects (e.g., rash, difficult breathing, diarrhea, GI upset). See Chapter 4: *Medical Management of Odontogenic Infections*.
- Single-dose regimen is associated with more adverse effects.
- *Lactation:* Excreted in breast milk.
- *Children:* An open-label, randomized, controlled trial has shown fluconazole to be effective in children 6 mo to 13 yr old. Efficacy has not been established in infants younger than 6 mo.
- *Renal failure:* Dosage reduction based on Ccr may be necessary.
- *Anaphylaxis:* Anaphylaxis occurred rarely.
- *Dermatologic changes:* Exfoliative skin disorders reported.
- *Hepatic injury:* Monitor patients with abnormal LFT results for development of more severe hepatic injury.
- *Immunocompromised patients:* To prevent relapse, patients with AIDS and cryptococcal meningitis usually require maintenance therapy.
- *Overdosage:* Hallucinations, paranoid behavior.

Pregnancy Risk Category: Category C.

Oral Health Education

When prescribed by DDS:
- Explain name, dose, action, and potential side effects of drug.
- Advise patient to read *Patient Information* leaflet before starting therapy and with each refill.
- Review dosing schedule and prescribed length of therapy with patient. Advise patient that treatment may be prolonged (e.g., several wk or mo) and to continue medication until advised to stop using by health care provider.

Tablets and Suspension
- Advise patient that tablets can be taken with a full glass of water without regard to meals but to take with food if GI upset occurs.
- Advise patient using suspension that the suspension can be taken without regard to meals but to take with food if GI upset occurs.
- Advise patient or caregiver to shake suspension well before measuring dose and to measure prescribed dose of suspension using dosing cup, spoon, or syringe.
- Advise patient that if a dose is missed, to take as soon as remembered. However, if it is nearing the time for the next dose, to skip the dose and take the next dose at the regularly scheduled time.
- Remind patient to complete entire course of therapy, even if symptoms of infection have disappeared.
- Advise patient to inform health care provider if infection does not improve or worsens.
- Advise patient to contact health care provider immediately if skin rash, persistent nausea or vomiting, dark urine, or yellowing of skin or eyes occur.
- Advise women to notify health care provider if pregnant, planning to become pregnant, or breast feeding.

- Instruct patient not to take any prescription or OTC medications or dietary supplements unless advised by health care provider.
- Advise patient that follow-up examinations and lab tests may be required to monitor therapy and to keep appointments.

---

fludrocortisone acetate (flew-droe-CORE-tih-sone ASS-uh-TATE)

Florinef Acetate

Drug Class: Mineralocorticoid

PHARMACOLOGY

Action

Exerts salt-retaining (mineralocorticoid) activity by acting on renal distal tubules to enhance reabsorption of sodium and increasing urinary excretion of potassium, hydrogen, and magnesium ions.

Uses

Partial replacement therapy for primary and secary adrenocortical insufficiency in Addison disease; treatment of salt-losing adrenogenital syndrome.

Unlabeled Uses

Treatment of severe orthostatic hypotension.

➡️⬅️ DRUG INTERACTIONS RELATED TO DENTAL THERAPEUTICS

Aspirin: Reduced aspirin effect (mechanism unknown)
- Monitor clinical status.

Midazolam: Possible decreased midazolam effect (increased metabolism)
- Monitor clinical status.

COX-1 inhibitors: Increased risk of peptic ulcer disease (additive)
- Monitor clinical status.

ADVERSE EFFECTS

⚠ **ORAL:** Masking of infection.

CNS: Convulsions; vertigo; severe mental disturbance.

CVS: Hypertension; thrombophlebitis.

GI: Peptic ulcer; pancreatitis.

MISC: Hypokalemic alkalosis. May also cause adverse reactions associated with glucocorticoids (e.g., dexamethasone); impaired wound healing, petechia, ecchymoses; secary adrenocortical and pituitary unresponsiveness in times of stress (i.e., surgery, infection); osteoporosis.

CLINICAL IMPLICATIONS

General

- Determine why drug is being taken. Consider implications of condition on dental treatment.
- Due to the anticipated perioperative physiological stress, patients undergoing dental care (i.e., minor surgical stress) under local anesthesia should take only their usual daily glucocorticoid dose before dental intervention. No supplementation is justified.
- Anticipate addisonian or cushingoid complications affecting the head and neck area.
- Be aware that signs of bacterial oral infection may be masked and anticipate oral candidiasis.
- Monitor vital signs (e.g., BP pulse).

Oral Health Education

- Encourage daily plaque control procedures for effective self-care.

Flumadine — see rimantadine HCl

flumazenil (flew-MAZ-ah-nil)

Romazicon: Injection: 0.1 mg/mL

█✚█ **Anexate**

█▒█ **Lanexat**

Drug Class: Benzodiazepine antagonist

PHARMACOLOGY

Action
Antagonizes actions of benzodiazepines on CNS by blocking receptors.

Uses
Complete or partial reversal of sedative effects of benzodiazepines where general anesthesia is induced or maintained with benzodiazepines, where sedation produced with benzodiazepines for diagnostic or therapeutic procedures, and for the management of benzodiazepine overdose.

Usual Dosage
Reversal of conscious sedation or in general anesthesia
ADULTS: *IV:* 0.2 mg over 15 sec. If desired level of consciousness is not achieved in 45 sec, additional 0.2 mg doses can be administered at 60 sec intervals (max, 1 mg). In event of re-sedation, repeat doses (0.2 mg/min to max 1 mg) at 20 min intervals as needed (max, 3 mg/hr).
Management of suspected benzodiazepine overdose
ADULTS: *IV:* 0.2 mg over 30 sec. If desired level of consciousness is not achieved in 30 sec, an additional dose of 0.3 mg over 30 sec can be administered. Further doses of 0.5 mg over 30 sec can be administered at 1 min intervals as needed (max, 3 mg).

Pharmacokinetics
ABSORP: Mean C_{max} is 24 ng/mL (range, 11 to 43 ng/mL); mean AUC was 15 ng hr/mL (range, 10 to 22 ng hr/mL).
DIST: Initial distribution $t_{1/2}$ is 7 to 15 min. $Vd_{initial}$ is 0.5 L/kg; Vd_{ss} is 0.l77 to 1.60 L/kg. Protein binding is about 50%.
METAB: Primarily hepatically metabolized and dependent on hepatic blood flow (highly extracted).
EXCRET: Terminal $t_{1/2}$ is 41 to 79 min. Total clearance is 0.7 to 1.3 L/hr/kg (increases by 50% during ingestion of food). Less than 1% is excreted unchanged in the urine; 90% to 95% is excreted in urine and 5% to 10% in feces.
ONSET: 1 to 2 min.
PEAK: 6 to 10 min.
DURATION: Related to the plasma concentration of the benzodiazepine as well as the dose of flumazenil.
SPECIAL POP: *Hepatic failure:* MODERATE: Mean total clearance decreased 40% to 60%; $t_{1/2}$ increases to 1.3 hr. *Severe:* Mean total clearance decreased 75%; $t_{1/2}$ increases to 2.4 hr.
Children 1 to 17 yr: The $t_{1/2}$ is shorter and more variable, ranging 20 to 75 min.

➡◀ DRUG INTERACTIONS
No documented drug-drug interactions. The absence of evidence is not evidence of safety.

ADVERSE EFFECTS

⚠ **ORAL:** Dry mouth.

CNS: Convulsions; headache; dizziness; agitation; emotional lability; fatigue; paresthesia; insomnia; dyspnea; hypoesthesia.

GI: Nausea; vomiting.

RESP: Hyperventilation.

MISC: Injection site pain; injection site reaction.

CLINICAL IMPLICATIONS

General

- This is an acute use drug to reverse sedative effects of benzodiazepines used in general anesthesia. Patients would be very unlikely to report taking this drug.

Pregnancy Risk Category: Category C.

---

flunisolide (flew-NISS-oh-lide)

AeroBid, AeroBid-M, Nasarel

■✱■ Apo-Flunisolide, ratio-Flunisolide

Drug Class: Corticosteroid

PHARMACOLOGY

Action

Has local anti-inflammatory activity on lung or nasal mucosa with minimal systemic effect. May decrease number and activity of cells involved in inflammatory response and enhance effect of other drugs or endogenous substances that aid in bronchodilation.

Uses

INHALATION: Maintenance treatment of asthma for patients requiring long-term treatment with corticosteroids.

INTRANASAL: Symptoms of perennial or seasonal rhinitis.

➜← DRUG INTERACTIONS RELATED TO DENTAL THERAPEUTICS

No documented drug-drug interactions. The absence of evidence is not evidence of safety.

ADVERSE EFFECTS

⚠ **ORAL:** ORAL INHALATION: Unpleasant taste (10%); candidiasis (1% to 9%); mouth irritation (1 to 3%).
NASAL SPRAY: Aftertaste (17%).

CNS: ORAL INHALATION: Headache (25%); dizziness, irritability, nervousness, shakiness (3% to 9%); anxiety, depression, faintness, fatigue, hyperactivity, hypoactivity, insomnia, moodiness, numbness, vertigo (1% to 3%).

GI: ORAL INHALATION: Nausea/vomiting (25%); diarrhea; upset stomach; abdominal pain; heartburn; constipation; dyspepsia; gas.
NASAL SPRAY Aftertaste (17%); nausea (>1%).

RESP: ORAL INHALATION: Upper respiratory tract infection (25%); cold symptoms, nasal congestion (15%); chest congestion, cough, hoarseness, sneezing, sputum, wheezing (3% to 9%); bronchitis, chest tightness, dyspnea, epistaxis, head stuffiness, laryngitis, pleurisy, pneumonia (1% to 3%).
NASAL SPRAY: Increased cough (>1%).

MISC: ORAL INHALATION: Flu (10%); chest pain, decreased appetite, edema, fever (3% to 9%); chills, peripheral edema, sweating, weakness, malaise, increased appetite (1% to 3%).

CLINICAL IMPLICATIONS
General
- Monitor vital signs (e.g., BP, pulse rate, respiratory rate and function); uncontrolled disease characterized by wheezing and coughing.
- Acute bronchoconstriction can occur during dental treatment; have bronchodilator inhaler available.
- Anticipate oral candidiasis when steroids are used.
- Due to the anticipated perioperative physiological stress (minor surgical stress), patients undergoing dental care under local anesthesia should take only their usual daily glucocorticoid dose before dental intervention. No supplementation is justified.
- Be aware that sulfites in local anesthetic with vasoconstrictor can precipitate acute asthma attack in susceptible individuals.

Oral Health Education
- Teach patient to rinse mouth and gargle vigorously with water after inhaled steroid use to minimize the potential for candidiasis.
- Encourage daily plaque control procedures for effective self-care.

---

fluocinonide (flew-oh-SIN-oh-nide)

Lidex: Cream: 0.05%; Gel: 0.05%; Ointment: 0.05%; Topical Solution: 0.05%
Lidex-E: Cream: 0.05%
Vanos: Cream: 0.1%

▌✦▐ Tiamol, Topsyn

Drug Class: Corticosteroid

PHARMACOLOGY
Action
Depresses formation, release, and activity of endogenous mediators of inflammation such as prostaglandins, kinins, histamine, liposomal enzymes, and complement system.

Uses
Relief of inflammatory and pruritic manifestations of corticosteroid-responsive dermatoses.

Contraindications
Standard considerations.

Usual Dosage
Apply to the affected area as a thin film 4 qid.

➜✦ DRUG INTERACTIONS
Decreased doxycycline effect (increased metabolism)
- Avoid concurrent use.

ADVERSE EFFECTS
⚠ ORAL: Burning; stinging; cracking of mucosa; erythema.

CLINICAL IMPLICATIONS
General
When prescribed by DDS:
- *Lactation:* Unknown whether topical administration could result in sufficient systemic absorption to produce detectable quantities in human breast milk. Exercise caution when topical corticosteroids are administered to a nursing woman.
- *Children:* May demonstrate greater susceptibility to topical corticosteroid-induced hypothalaimic pituitary-adrenal (HPA) axis suppression and Cushing syndrome.

Pregnancy Risk Category: Category C.

Oral Health Education
When prescribed by DDS:
* Explain name, action, and potential side effects of drug.
* Advise patient to apply medication as directed by health care provider.
* Caution patient not to bandage, cover, or wrap treated skin areas or use cosmetics or other skin products over treated areas unless advised by health care provider.
* Caution patient to avoid contact with the eyes. Advise patient that if medication does come into contact with the eyes, to wash eyes with large amounts of cool water and contact health care provider if eye irritation occurs.
* Advise patient that symptoms should begin to improve fairly soon after starting treatment and to notify health care provider if condition does not improve, worsens, or if application site reactions (e.g., burning, stinging, redness, itching) develop.
* Advise patient that therapy is usually discontinued when control has been achieved.
* Advise patient that follow-up visits to monitor response to treatment may be required and to keep appointments.

Fluoride — see sodium fluoride
Fluoride Loz — see sodium fluoride
fluoride sodium — see sodium fluoride
Fluorigard — see sodium fluoride
Fluorinse — see sodium fluoride
Fluoritab — see sodium fluoride
Fluoroplex — see fluorouracil

---

fluorouracil (FLURE-oh-YOUR-uh-sill)
Adrucil, Carac, Efudex, Fluoroplex

■◆■ **Efudix**

Drug Class: Pyrimidine antimetabolite

PHARMACOLOGY
Action
The metabolism of fluorouracil in the anabolic pathway blocks the methylation reaction of deoxyuridylic acid to thymidylic acid. In this manner, fluorouracil interferes with the synthesis of DNA and to a lesser extent inhibits the formation of RNA.

Uses
Colon, rectum, breast, gastric, and pancreatic carcinoma (injection); multiple actinic or solar keratoses, superficial basal cell carcinoma (topical).

Unlabeled Uses
Ovarian, cervical, bladder, hepatic, islet cell, prostate, endometrial, esophageal, and head and neck carcinoma.

➡◀ DRUG INTERACTIONS RELATED TO DENTAL THERAPEUTICS
Metronidazole: Metronidazole toxicity (decreased metabolism)
* Avoid concurrent use.

ADVERSE EFFECTS
⚠ **ORAL:** Adrucil: Stomatitis; esophagopharyngitis (which may lead to sloughing and ulceration).
Efudex: Cases of miscarriage/birth defect (ventricular septal defect) when applied to mucous membranes; metallic taste; stomatitis.

CNS: ADRUCIL: Acute cerebellar syndrome (may persist after discontinuation of treatment); nystagmus; headache; disorientation; confusion; euphoria.
CARAC: Headache (3%).
GI: ADRUCIL: Diarrhea; anorexia; nausea; emesis (most common); GI ulceration; bleeding.
MISC: ADRUCIL: Thrombophlebitis; epistaxis; nail changes (including loss of nails).
CARAC: Edema (35%); common cold (2%); allergy (1%).

CLINICAL IMPLICATIONS

General
- Determine why drug is being taken. Consider implications of condition on dental treatment.
- Advise products for palliative relief of oral manifestations (e.g., stomatitis, mucositis, xerostomia, etc.).
- Medical consultation to determine WBC and platelet count before invasive dental procedures, including periodontal debridement.
- Anticipate recurrent herpes simplex and varicella zoster infections.

Oral Health Education
- Encourage daily plaque control procedures for effective, nontraumatic self-care.

Fluoxac — see fluoxetine HCl

---

fluoxetine HCl (flew-OX-uh-teen HIGH-droe-KLOR-ide)
Prozac, Prozac Weekly, Sarafem

█✚█ Apo-Fluoxetine, CO Fluoxetine, Gen-Fluoxetine, Novo-Fluoxetine, Nu-Fluoxetine, PMS-Fluoxetine, ratio-Fluoxetine, Rhoxal-fluoxetine, STCC-Fluoxetine

█▸█ Fluoxac, Siquial

Drug Class: Antidepressant

PHARMACOLOGY

Action
Blocks reuptake of serotonin, enhancing serotonergic function.

Uses
PROZAC: Depression; OCD; bulimia nervosa, panic disorder.
SARAFEM: PMDD.

Unlabeled Uses
Alcoholism; anorexia nervosa; attention deficit hyperactivity disorder; bipolar II disorder; borderline personality disorder; chronic rheumatoid pain; diabetic peripheral neuropathy; kleptomania; levodopa-induced dyskinesia; migraine, chronic daily headaches, and tension-type headache; narcolepsy; schizophrenia; social phobia; trichotillomania.

➡← DRUG INTERACTIONS RELATED TO DENTAL THERAPEUTICS

Itraconazole: Possible fluoxetine toxicity (decreased metabolism)
- Avoid concurrent use.

Diazepam or alprazolam: Possible impairment of skills related to driving (decreased metabolism)
- Warn patient.

Chloral hydrate: Prolonged drowsiness (mechanism unknown)
- Monitor clinical status.

Tramadol: Increased risk of seizure (additive)
- Avoid concurrent use.

ADVERSE EFFECTS

⚠ **ORAL:** Dry mouth; taste disturbance.

CNS: Agitation; anxiety; nervousness; headache; insomnia; abnormal dreams; drowsiness; dizziness; tremor; fatigue; decreased libido; decreased concentration; seizures; delusions; hallucinations; coma.

CVS: Chest pain, hypertension, palpitations, vasodilation (3%); postural hypotension (1%).

GI: Nausea; vomiting; diarrhea; anorexia; upset stomach; constipation; abdominal pain.

RESP: Flu-like symptoms; bronchitis; rhinitis; yawning; coughing; asthma; pneumonia; apnea; lung edema; pleural effusion.

MISC: Weakness; chills; joint or muscle pain; fever; hypersensitivity reaction; photophobia (1%).

CLINICAL IMPLICATIONS

General
- Determine why drug is being taken. Consider implications of condition on dental treatment.
- Determine ability to adapt to stress of dental treatment. Consider short appointments.
- Monitor vital signs.
- If GI side effects occur, consider semisupine chair position.
- Chronic dry mouth is possible; anticipate increased caries and candidiasis.
- *Photophobia:* Direct dental light out of patient's eyes and offer dark glasses for comfort.
- *Postural hypotension:* Monitor BP at the beginning and end of each appointment; anticipate syncope. Have patient sit upright for several min at the end of the dental appointment before dismissing.
- Depressed or anxious patients may neglect self care. Monitor for plaque control effectiveness.

Oral Health Education
- Encourage daily plaque control procedures for effective self-care.
- If chronic dry mouth occurs, recommend home fluoride therapy and use of nonalcoholic oral health care products.

---

fluphenazine decanoate — fluphenazine decanoate
fluphenazine HCl — see fluphenazine
Fluphenazine Hydrochloride — see fluphenazine
Fluphenazine Omega — see fluphenazine

---

fluphenazine (flew-FEN-uh-zeen)

(fluphenazine decanoate, fluphenazine HCl)

Fluphenazine Hydrochloride, Prolixin Decanoate

■✢■ **Apo-Fluphenazine, Apo-Fluphenazine Decanoate Injection, Fluphenazine Omega, Modecate, Modecate Concentrate, Moditen hydrochloride, PMS-Fluphenazine Decanoate**

Drug Class: Antipsychotic, phenothiazine

PHARMACOLOGY

Action
Blocks dopamine receptor in CNS.

Uses
FLUPHENAZINE HYDROCHLORIDE: Management of psychotic disorders.

Fluphenazine Decanoate: Long-acting parenteral depot products for long-term neuroleptic therapy.

Unlabeled Uses

Nausea/vomiting.

➔← DRUG INTERACTIONS RELATED TO DENTAL THERAPEUTICS

No documented drug-drug interactions. The absence of evidence is not evidence of safety.

ADVERSE EFFECTS

⚠ **ORAL:** Salivation; tardive dyskinesia; dry mouth.

CNS: Pseudoparkinsonism; dyskinesia; motor restlessness; oculogyric crises; opisthotonos; hyperreflexia; headache; weakness; tremor; fatigue; slurring; insomnia; vertigo; seizures; drowsiness; hallucinations; lethargy; increased libido; lightheadedness; faintness; dizziness.

CVS: Hypertension; tachycardia.

GI: Nausea; dyspepsia; constipation; fecal impaction; paralytic ileus; adynamic ileus (may result in death).

RESP: Laryngospasm; bronchospasm; dyspnea; acute fulminating pneumonia or pneumonitis.

MISC: Increases in appetite and weight; polydipsia; increased prolactin levels; neuroleptic malignant syndrome; loss of appetite; peripheral edema; sudden unexpected and unexplained death; photosensitivity; blood dyscrasias (e.g., agranulocytosis, eosinophilia, leukocytosis, leukopenia).

CLINICAL IMPLICATIONS

General

- Determine why drug is being taken. Consider implications of condition on dental treatment.
- Extrapyramidal behaviors can complicate performance of oral procedures. If present, consult with MD to consider medication changes.
- Depressed or anxious patients may neglect self-care. Monitor for plaque control effectiveness.
- Monitor vital signs.
- Blood dyscrasias rarely reported; anticipate increased bleeding, infection, and poor healing.
- If GI side effects occur, consider semisupine chair position.
- Chronic dry mouth is possible; anticipate increased caries and candidiasis.

Oral Health Education

- Encourage daily plaque control procedures for effective, nontraumatic self-care.
- If chronic dry mouth occurs, recommend home fluoride therapy and use of nonalcoholic oral health care products.

Flura — see sodium fluoride

Flura-Loz — see sodium fluoride

---

flurandrenolide (FLURE-an-DREEN-oh-lide)

Cordran V, Cordran SP, Cordran

Drug Class: Corticosteroid, topical

PHARMACOLOGY

Action

Decreases inflammation by suppression of PMN migration and reversal of increased capillary permeability

Uses

Inflammatory dermatoses.

➡◀ DRUG INTERACTIONS RELATED TO DENTAL THERAPEUTICS

No documented drug-drug interactions. The absence of evidence is not evidence of safety.

ADVERSE EFFECTS

⚠ **ORAL:** Perioral dermatitis; thinning of mucosa when applied to mucosa.
MISC: Numbness of fingers; thinning of skin.

CLINICAL IMPLICATIONS

General

- Determine why drug is being taken. Consider implications of condition on dental treatment.
- Be aware that signs of bacterial oral infection may be masked and anticipate oral candidiasis.

Oral Health Education

- *If prescribed by DDS:* Ensure patient understands how to use product, amount to apply, method of application, and signs of adverse effects.

---

flurazepam HCl (flure-AZE-uh-pam HIGH-droe-KLOR-ide)

Dalmane

■✦■ Apo-Flurazepam, Novo-Flupam

Drug Class: Sedative; Hypnotic; Benzodiazepine

PHARMACOLOGY

Action

Potentiates action of gamma-aminobutyric acid (GABA), an inhibitory neurotransmitter, resulting in increased neural inhibition and CNS depression, especially in limbic system and reticular formation.

Uses

Treatment of insomnia.

➡◀ DRUG INTERACTIONS RELATED TO DENTAL THERAPEUTICS

No documented drug-drug interactions. The absence of evidence is not evidence of safety.

ADVERSE EFFECTS

⚠ **ORAL:** Dry mouth; taste alterations.
CNS: Dizziness; drowsiness; lightheadedness; staggering; ataxia; falling; lethargy; confusion; impaired memory; headache; weakness; paradoxical excitement; talkativeness; euphoria; apprehension; irritability; hallucinations; slurred speech; depression.
CVS: Palpitations; chest pain; tachycardia.
GI: Heartburn; nausea and vomiting; diarrhea; constipation; anorexia; upset stomach; GI pain.
RESP: Shortness of breath.
MISC: Tolerance; physical and psychological dependence; body and joint pains; sweating; flushing; leukopenia granulocytopenia.

CLINICAL IMPLICATIONS

General

- Determine ability to adapt to stress of dental treatment. Consider short appointments.
- Depressed or anxious patients may neglect self-care. Monitor for plaque control effectiveness.

- Monitor vital signs.
- Chronic dry mouth is possible; anticipate increased caries and candidiasis.
- If GI side effects occur, consider semisupine chair position.
- Blood dyscrasias rarely reported; anticipate increased infection and poor healing.

Oral Health Education

- If chronic dry mouth occurs, recommend home fluoride therapy and use of nonalcoholic oral health care products.

---

flurbiprofen (FLURE-bih-PRO-fen)

(flurbiprofen sodium)

Ansaid, Ocufen

■✦■Apo-Flurbiprofen, Froben, Froben SR, Novo-Flurbiprofen, Novo-Flurprofen, Nu-Flurbiprofen, ratio-Flurbiprofen

Drug Class: Analgesic; NSAID

PHARMACOLOGY

Action

Decreases inflammation, pain, and fever, probably through inhibition of COX activity and prostaglandin synthesis.

Uses

SYSTEMIC: Treatment of rheumatoid arthritis and osteoarthritis.
OPHTHALMIC: Inhibition of intraoperative miosis.

Unlabeled Uses

Treatment of juvenile rheumatoid arthritis; migraine; dysmenorrhea; sunburn; mild to moderate pain; acute gout; ankylosing spondylitis; tendinitis; bursitis; inflammation after cataract surgery; uveitis.

➡◀ DRUG INTERACTIONS RELATED TO DENTAL THERAPEUTICS

No documented drug-drug interactions. The absence of evidence is not evidence of safety.

ADVERSE EFFECTS

⚠ **ORAL:** Dry mouth; stomatitis (1%).
CNS: Dizziness; drowsiness; vertigo; headaches; nervousness; migraine; anxiety; confusion.
CVS: Hypertension, arrhythmia (1%).
GI: Heartburn; dyspepsia; nausea; vomiting; anorexia; diarrhea; constipation; increased or decreased appetite; indigestion; GI bleeding; ulceration.
RESP: Bronchospasm; laryngeal edema; dyspnea; hemoptysis; shortness of breath.
MISC: Hyperglycemia; hypoglycemia; hyponatremia blood dyscrasias (e.g., leukopenia, thrombocytopenia) (<1%).

CLINICAL IMPLICATIONS

General

- Determine why drug is being taken. Consider implications of condition on dental treatment.
- Use COX inhibitors with caution; they may exacerbate PUD and GERD.
- *Arthritis:* Consider patient comfort and need for semisupine chair position.
- Chronic dry mouth is possible; anticipate increased caries, candidiasis, and lichenoid mucositis.
- Monitor vital signs.
- If GI side effects occur, consider semisupine chair position.

- Blood dyscrasias rarely reported; anticipate increased bleeding, infection, and poor healing.

Oral Health Education
- If chronic dry mouth occurs, recommend home fluoride therapy and use of nonalcoholic oral health care products.
- Encourage daily plaque control procedures for effective, nontraumatic self-care.

---

flurbiprofen sodium — see flurbiprofen

---

fluticasone propionate (flew-TICK-ah-SONE PRO-pee-oh-nate)
Flonase, Flovent, Flovent Diskus, Flovent Rotadisk
■✦■ **Florinef, Floven HF**
Drug Class: Corticosteroid

PHARMACOLOGY

Action
Exerts potent anti-inflammatory effect on nasal passages.

Uses
Management of the nasal symptoms of seasonal and perennial allergic and nonallergic rhinitis in adults and pediatric patients age 4 yr and older (Flonase); patients requiring oral corticosteroid therapy for asthma (Flovent, Flovent Rotadisk, Flovent Diskus); maintenance treatment of asthma as prophylactic therapy in patients age 4 yr and older (Flovent Diskus, Flovent Rotadisk) and 12 yr and older (Flovent).

➔← DRUG INTERACTIONS RELATED TO DENTAL THERAPEUTICS
No documented drug-drug interactions. The absence of evidence is not evidence of safety.

ADVERSE EFFECTS
⚠ **ORAL:** FLOVENT INHALATION POWDER: Oral ulcerations, dental discomfort and pain, oral erythema and rashes, mouth and tongue disorders, oral discomfort and pain, tooth decay (1% to 3%).
FLOVENT INHALATION AEROSOL: Candidiasis (2% to 5%).
CNS: FLONASE: Headache (16%); dizziness (1% to 3%).
FLOVENT INHALATION AEROSOL: Headache (22%); giddiness (1% to 3%); dizziness.
FLOVENT INHALATION POWDER: Headache (14%); dizziness, sleep disorders, migraines, paralysis of cranial nerves, mood disorders, malaise, fatigue (1% to 3%).
GI: FLONASE: Nausea, vomiting (5%); abdominal pain, diarrhea (1% to 3%).
FLOVENT INHALATION AEROSOL: Nausea, vomiting diarrhea, dyspepsia, stomach disorder (1% to 3%).
FLOVENT INHALATION POWDER: Nausea, vomiting (8%); viral infection (5%); discomfort/pain (4%); diarrhea, GI signs and symptoms, gastroenteritis, infection abdominal discomfort and pain (1% to 3%).
RESP: FLONASE: Asthma symptoms (7%); cough (4%); bronchitis (1% to 3%).
FLOVENT INHALATION AEROSOL: Upper respiratory tract infection (22%); influenza (8%); bronchitis, chest congestion (1% to 3%).
FLOVENT INHALATION POWDER: Upper respiratory tract infection (21%); bronchitis (8%); lower respiratory infection, cough (5%); upper respiratory inflammation (4%).
MISC: FLONASE: Fever, flu-like symptoms, aches and pains (1% to 3%); hypersensitivity (including angioedema, anaphylaxis/anaphylactoid reactions); growth suppression.
FLOVENT INHALATION AEROSOL: Fever; immediate and delayed hypersensitivity, including urticaria, rash, angioedema, and bronchospasm (≤2%).

FLOVENT INHALATION POWDER: Fever (7%); viral infection (5%); immediate and delayed hypersensitivity reactions, including rash, angioedema, and bronchospasm (<2%); soft-tissue injury, contusions, hematomas, wounds, lacerations, postoperative complications, burns, poisoning and toxicity, pressure-induced disorders, chest symptoms, pain, edema, swelling, bacterial infections, fungal infections, mobility disorders, cysts, lumps, masses (1% to 3%).

CLINICAL IMPLICATIONS

General

- Monitor vital signs (e.g., BP, pulse rate, respiratory rate and function); uncontrolled disease characterized by wheezing and coughing.
- Acute bronchoconstriction can occur during dental treatment; have bronchodilator inhaler available.
- Despite the anticipated perioperative physiological stress (i.e., minor surgical stress), patients undergoing dental care under local anesthesia should take only their usual daily glucocorticoid dose before dental intervention. No supplementation is justified.
- Anticipate oral candidiasis when steroids are used.
- Be aware that sulfites in local anesthetic with vasoconstrictor can precipitate acute asthma attack in susceptible individuals.
- Inhalants can dry oral mucosa; anticipate increased calculus, plaque levels, and caries.

Oral Health Education

- Teach patient to rinse mouth and gargle vigorously with water after inhaled steroid use to minimize the potential for candidiasis.
- Encourage daily plaque control procedures for effective self-care.
- If chronic dry mouth occurs, recommend home fluoride therapy and use of nonalcoholic oral health care products.

---

fluticasone propionate/salmeterol (flew-TICK-ah-SONE PRO-pee-oh-nate/sal-MEET-ah-rahl)

Synonym: salmeterol/fluticasone propionate

Advair Diskus

Drug Class: Respiratory inhalant combination

PHARMACOLOGY

Action

FLUTICASONE: Inhibits multiple cell types (e.g., mast cells) and mediator production or secretion (e.g., histamine) involved in the asthmatic response.

SALMETEROL: Produces bronchodilation by relaxing bronchial smooth muscle through beta-2-receptor stimulation.

Uses

Long-term maintenance treatment of asthma; COPD associated with chronic bronchitis.

✦← DRUG INTERACTIONS RELATED TO DENTAL THERAPEUTICS

No documented drug-drug interactions. The absence of evidence is not evidence of safety.

ADVERSE EFFECTS

The following adverse reactions occurred at a rate of at least 1% and were more common than in the placebo group.

⚠ **ORAL:** Candidiasis; dental discomfort and pain; oral ulcerations; taste disturbance.

CNS: Headache; sleep disorders; tremors; hypnagogical effects; compressed nerve symptoms.

CVS: Palpitations; tachycardia.

GI: Nausea; vomiting; GI discomfort and pain; diarrhea; GI infections (including viral); GI signs and symptoms; gastroenteritis; GI disorders; constipation; appendicitis.

RESP: Upper respiratory tract inflammation and infection; viral respiratory infections; bronchitis; cough; wheezing; chest symptoms; pneumonia; lower respiratory signs and symptoms; lower respiratory tract infections.

MISC: Muscle injuries; fractures; wounds; lacerations; contusions; hematoma; burns; arthralgia; articular rheumatism; muscle stiffness; tightness and rigidity; bone and cartilage disorders; allergies and allergic reactions; viral and bacterial infections; pain.

CLINICAL IMPLICATIONS

General

- Determine why drug is being taken. Consider implications of condition on dental treatment.
- Monitor vital signs (e.g., BP, pulse rate, respiratory rate and function); uncontrolled disease characterized by wheezing and coughing.
- Acute bronchoconstriction can occur during dental treatment; have bronchodilator inhaler available.
- Ensure that bronchodilator inhaler is present at each dental appointment.
- Due to the anticipated perioperative physiological stress (minor surgical stress), patients undergoing dental care under local anesthesia should take only their usual daily glucocorticoid dose before dental intervention. No supplementation is justified.
- Anticipate oral candidiasis when steroids are used.
- Be aware that sulfites in local anesthetic with vasoconstrictor can precipitate acute asthma attack in susceptible individuals.
- Inhalants can dry oral mucosa; anticipate candidiasis, increased calculus, plaque levels, and caries activity.

Oral Health Education

- Teach patient to rinse mouth and gargle vigorously with water after inhaled steroid use to minimize the potential for candidiasis.
- If chronic dry mouth occurs, recommend home fluoride therapy and use of nonalcoholic oral health care products.

---

fluvastatin (FLEW-vah-stat-in)

Lescol, Lescol XL

■▨■ Canef

Drug Class: Antihyperlipidemic, HMG-CoA reductase inhibitor

PHARMACOLOGY

Action

Increases rate at which body removes cholesterol from blood and reduces production of cholesterol in body by inhibiting enzyme that catalyzes early rate-limiting step in cholesterol synthesis; increases HDL; reduces LDL, VLDL, and triglycerides.

Uses

ATHEROSCLEROSIS: To slow the progression of coronary atherosclerosis.

HYPERCHOLESTEROLEMIA: To reduce elevated total cholesterol, LDL, apo-B, and triglyceride cholesterol levels and to increase HDL levels.

SECONDARY PREVENTION OF CORONARY EVENTS: To reduce the risk of undergoing coronary revascularization procedures in patients with coronary heart disease.

➡◆ DRUG INTERACTIONS RELATED TO DENTAL THERAPEUTICS

No documented drug-drug interactions. The absence of evidence is not evidence of safety.

ADVERSE EFFECTS

CNS: Headache (9%); fatigue, insomnia (3%).

GI: Dyspepsia (8%); diarrhea, abdominal pain (5%); nausea, flatulence (3%).

RESP: Bronchitis (7.6%), URI (16%).

MISC: Flu-like symptoms (7%); accidental trauma (5%); back pain, myalgia (5%).

CLINICAL IMPLICATIONS

General

- High LDL cholesterol concentration is the major cause of atherosclerosis, which leads to CAD (angina, MI); determine degree of CV health and ability to withstand stress of dental treatment.
- Monitor vital signs (e.g., BP, pulse pressure, rate and rhythm) at each appointment to assess disease control. Do not provide elective dental treatment when BP is ≥180/110 or in presence of other high-risk CV conditions. refer to the section entitled "The patient Taking Cardiovascular Drugs" in Chapter 6: *Clinical Medicine*.
- If GI or respiratory side effects occur, consider semisupine chair position.

Oral Health Education

- Encourage daily plaque control procedures for effective self-care in patient at risk for cardiovascular disease.

---

fluvoxamine maleate (flu-VOX-uh-meen MAL-ee-ate)

Luvox

■✚■ Apo-Fluvoxamine, Novo-Fluvoxamine, Nu-Fluvoxamine, PMS-Fluvoxamine, ratio-Fluvoxamine

Drug Class: Antidepressant, selective serotonin inhibitor

PHARMACOLOGY

Action

Inhibits neuronal reuptake of serotonin in brain.

Uses

Treatment of obsessive-compulsive disorder (OCD).

➡✚ DRUG INTERACTIONS RELATED TO DENTAL THERAPEUTICS

Tramadol: Increased risk of seizures (additive)
- Avoid concurrent use.

ADVERSE EFFECTS

⚠ ORAL: Dry mouth (14%); tooth discoloration, taste disturbances (3%); dysphagia (2%).
CNS: Headache, somnolence (22%); insomnia (21%); nervousness (12%); dizziness (11%); tremor, anxiety (5%); hypertonia, agitation, depression, stimulation (2%).
CVS: Palpitations, vasodilation (3%); postural hypotension, hypertension, tachycardia (≥1%).
GI: Nausea (40%); diarrhea (11%); constipation, dyspepsia (10%); anorexia (6%); vomiting (5%); flatulence (4%).
RESP: URI (9%); dyspnea, yawn (2%).
MISC: Asthenia (14%); flu-like syndrome (3%); chills (2%).

CLINICAL IMPLICATIONS

General

- Determine why drug is being taken. Consider implications of condition on dental treatment.
- Chronic dry mouth is possible; anticipate increased caries activity and candidiasis.
- Depressed or anxious patients may neglect self-care. Monitor for plaque control effectiveness.
- Determine ability to adapt to stress of dental treatment. Consider short appointments.
- Monitor vital signs.
- If GI side effects occur, consider semisupine chair position.
- *Postural hypotension:* Monitor BP at the beginning and end of each appointment; anticipate syncope. Have patient sit upright for several min at the end of the dental appointment before dismissing.

Oral Health Education
- Encourage daily plaque control procedures for effective self-care.
- If chronic dry mouth occurs, recommend home fluoride therapy and use of nonalcoholic oral health care products.

Flynoken — see folic acid
Focalin — see dexmethylphenidate HCl
Focalin XR — see dexmethylphenidate HCl

folic acid (FOE-lik ASS-id)
Folvite
■✦■ Apo-Folic
■✦■ AF Valdecasas, Flynoken, Folitab
Drug Class: Vitamin

PHARMACOLOGY
Action
Required for nucleoprotein synthesis and maintenance of normal erythropoiesis; precursor of tetrahydrofolic acid, which is necessary for transformylation reactions in the biosynthesis of purines and thymidylates of nucleic acids.

Uses
Megaloblastic anemia caused by folic acid deficiency as may be seen in tropical or nontropical sprue in anemias of nutritional origin, pregnancy, infancy, or childhood.

➜◆ DRUG INTERACTIONS RELATED TO DENTAL THERAPEUTICS
No documented drug-drug interactions. The absence of evidence is not evidence of safety.

ADVERSE EFFECTS
Adverse effects are rare.

CLINICAL IMPLICATIONS
General
- Determine why drug is being taken. Consider implications of condition on dental treatment.
- Anemias can reduce wound healing.

Folitab — see folic acid
Folvite — see folic acid
Foradil Aerolizer — see formoterol fumarate

formoterol fumarate (fore-MOE-ter-ole FEW-mah-rate)
Foradil Aerolizer
■✦■ Oxeze Turbuhaler
■✦■ Oxis
Drug Class: Selective beta-2 bronchodilator; Sympathomimetic

PHARMACOLOGY
Action
Relaxes bronchial smooth muscles.

Uses
Long-term maintenance treatment of asthma; prevention of bronchospasms; prevention of exercise-induced bronchospasm; concomitant therapy with short-acting beta$_2$-agonists, in-

haled or systemic corticosteroids, and theophylline therapy; long-term administration in the maintenance of bronchoconstriction in patients with COPD, including chronic bronchitis and emphysema.

➤◀ DRUG INTERACTIONS RELATED TO DENTAL THERAPEUTICS

No documented drug-drug interactions. The absence of evidence is not evidence of safety.

ADVERSE EFFECTS

⚠ **ORAL:** Dry mouth; taste disturbance.
CNS: Nervousness; headache; tremor; dizziness; fatigue; malaise; insomnia; dysphoria.
CVS: Palpitation, tachycardia (frequent).
GI: Nausea; gastroenteritis; abdominal pain; dyspepsia.
RESP: Bronchitis; URI; dyspnea; chest infection.
MISC: Muscle cramps; viral infection.

CLINICAL IMPLICATIONS

General

- Determine why drug is being taken. Consider implications of condition on dental treatment.
- Monitor vital signs (e.g., BP, pulse rate) and respiratory function. Uncontrolled disease characterized by wheezing, coughing.
- Acute bronchoconstriction can occur during dental treatment; have bronchodilator inhaler available.
- Ensure that bronchodilator inhaler is present at each dental appointment.
- Be aware that sulfites in local anesthetic with vasoconstrictor can precipitate acute asthma attack in susceptible individuals.
- Inhalants can dry oral mucosa; anticipate candidiasis, increased calculus, plaque levels, and increased caries.

Oral Health Education

- Rinse mouth with water after bronchodilator use to prevent dryness.
- If chronic dry mouth occurs, recommend home fluoride therapy and use of nonalcoholic oral health care products.

Formula E — see guaifenesin
Fortamet — see metformin HCl
Forteo — see teriparatide
Fortical — see calcitonin-salmon
Fortovase — see saquinavir mesylate
Fortovase Roche — see saquinavir mesylate
Fosamax — see alendronate sodium
Fosfocil — see fosfomycin tromethamine

---

fosfomycin tromethamine (foss-foe-MY-sin troe-METH-ah-meen)

Monurol

▌▬▌ **Fosfocil**

Drug Class: Antibiotic

PHARMACOLOGY

Action

Interferes with bacterial cell wall biosynthesis.

Uses

Treatment of uncomplicated UTI (acute cystitis) in women caused by susceptible strains of specific microorganisms.

➔← DRUG INTERACTIONS RELATED TO DENTAL THERAPEUTICS

No documented drug-drug interactions. The absence of evidence is not evidence of safety.

ADVERSE EFFECTS

⚠ **ORAL:** Dry mouth (1%).
CNS: Headache; dizziness.
GI: Diarrhea; nausea; dyspepsia; abdominal pain.
RESP: Rhinitis (4.5%).
MISC: Asthenia; back pain; pain.

CLINICAL IMPLICATIONS

General

• This drug is administered in a one-dose regimen; chronic dry mouth is unlikely to occur.
• If GI side effects occur, consider semisupine chair position.

---

fosinopril sodium (FAH-sin-oh-PRILL SO-dee-uhm)

Monopril

Drug Class: Antihypertensive; ACE inhibitor

PHARMACOLOGY

Action

Competitively inhibits angiotensin I-converting enzyme, preventing conversion of angiotensin I to angiotensin II, a potent vasoconstrictor that also stimulates release of aldosterone. Results in decrease in BP, reduced sodium reabsorption, and potassium retention.

Uses

Hypertension; heart failure.

➔← DRUG INTERACTIONS RELATED TO DENTAL THERAPEUTICS

COX-1 inhibitors: Decreased hypotensive effect of fosinopril (decreased prostaglandin synthesis)
• Monitor blood pressure.

ADVERSE EFFECTS

⚠ **ORAL:** Dry mouth (1%); taste disturbance.
CNS: Dizziness (12%); weakness (1%).
CVS: Chest pain (2%), hypotension (4%), orthostatic hypotension, syncope (1%).
GI: Diarrhea (2%); nausea, vomiting (1%).
RESP: Cough (10%); URI (2%).
MISC: Musculoskeletal pain (3.3%).

CLINICAL IMPLICATIONS

General

• Monitor vital signs (e.g., BP, pulse pressure, rate and rhythm) at each appointment to assess disease control. Do not provide elective dental treatment when BP is ≥180/110 or in presence of other high-risk CV conditions. Refer to the section entitled "The Patient Taking Cardiovascular Drugs" in Chapter 6: *Clinical Medicine.*
• Use local anesthetic agents with vasoconstrictor with caution based on functional capacity of the patient and use aspirating technique to prevent intravascular injection.
• Determine ability to adapt to stress of dental treatment. Consider short appointments.
• If coughing is problematic, consider semisupine chair position for treatment.
• Susceptible patient with DM may experience severe recurrent hypoglycemia.
• Chronic dry mouth is possible; anticipate increased caries, candidiasis, and lichenoid mucositis.
• *Postural hypotension:* Monitor BP at the beginning and end of each appointment; antici-

pate syncope. Have patient sit upright for several min at the end of the dental appointment before dismissing.
- If GI side effects occur, consider semisupine chair position.

Oral Health Education
- If chronic dry mouth occurs, recommend home fluoride therapy and use of nonalcoholic oral health care products.
- Encourage daily plaque control procedures for effective self-care in patient at risk for cardiovascular disease.

Fresenizol — see metronidazole
Fresofol — see propofol
Froben — see flurbiprofen
Froben SR — see flurbiprofen
Frova — see frovatriptan succinate

---

frovatriptan succinate (froe-va-TRIP-tan SUK-sin-AYT)
Frova

Drug Class: Analgesic, migraine

PHARMACOLOGY

Action
Selectively agonizes 5-hydroxy-tryptamine$_1$ (5-HT$_{1B/1D}$) receptor, inhibiting excessive dilation of extracerebral and intracranial arteries in migraine.

Uses
Acute treatment of migraine attacks with or without aura in adults.

➡️ DRUG INTERACTIONS RELATED TO DENTAL THERAPEUTICS
No documented drug-drug interactions. The absence of evidence is not evidence of safety.

ADVERSE EFFECTS
⚠️ **ORAL:** Dry mouth (3%).
CNS: Dizziness (8%); fatigue (5%); headache, paresthesia (4%); dysesthesia, hypoesthesia, insomnia, anxiety (≥1%).
CVS: Chest pain (2%).
GI: Dyspepsia (2%); vomiting, abdominal pain, diarrhea (≥1%).
RESP: Sinusitis, rhinitis (≥1%).
MISC: Hot or cold sensation (3%); pain (≥1%).

CLINICAL IMPLICATIONS

General
- Monitor vital signs (e.g., BP and pulse). Drugs for prevention are sympatholytic; drugs for treatment of acute attack are sympathomimetic.
- If GI side effects occur, consider semisupine chair position.
- This drug is for acute use during migraine attack. Patient is unlikely to present for oral health care appointment.

Froxal — see cefuroxime
Fungoral — see ketoconazole
Furadantin — see nitrofurantoin
Furadantina — see nitrofurantoin
Furosemide Special — see furosemide

furosemide (fyu-ROH-se-mide)

Lasix

■✦■ **Apo-Furosemide, Furosemide Special, Lasix Special,**

■✦■ **Edenol, Henexal, Selectofur, Zafimida**

Drug Class: Loop diuretic

PHARMACOLOGY

Action

Inhibits reabsorption of sodium and chloride in proximal and distal tubules and loop of Henle.

Uses

Treatment of edema associated with CHF, cirrhosis, and renal disease; hypertension.

➜✦ DRUG INTERACTIONS RELATED TO DENTAL THERAPEUTICS

Chloral hydrate: Vasomotor instability (mechanism unknown)
- Avoid concurrent use.

COX-1 inhibitors: Decreased antihypertensive effect (decreased prostaglandin synthesis)
- Monitor blood pressure.

Sympathomimetic amines:
- Use local anesthetic agents containing a vasoconstrictor with caution (hypokalemia with epinephrine).
- Monitor blood pressure, as well as pulse rate and character.

ADVERSE EFFECTS

⚠ **ORAL:** Oral irritation (unspecified); dry mouth, thirst.

CNS: Vertigo; headache; dizziness; paresthesia; restlessness; fever.

CVS: Orthostatic hypotension, thrombophlebitis; irregular heartbeat (hypokalemia).

GI: Anorexia; nausea; vomiting; diarrhea; gastric irritation; cramping; constipation; pancreatitis.

MISC: Muscle spasm; weakness; blood dyscrasias (leukopenia, agranulocytosis, thrombocytopenia, anemia); photosensitivity.

CLINICAL IMPLICATIONS

General

- Determine why drug is being taken. Consider implications of condition on dental treatment.
- Monitor vital signs (e.g., BP, pulse pressure, rate and rhythm) at each appointment to assess disease control. Do not provide elective dental treatment when BP is ≥180/110 or in presence of other high-risk CV conditions. Refer to the section entitled "The Patient Taking Cardiovascular Drugs" in Chapter 6: *Clinical Medicine.*
- Use local anesthetic agents with vasoconstrictor with caution based on functional capacity of the patient and use aspirating technique to prevent intravascular injection.
- This drug frequently used to manage symptoms of CHF; determine ability to adapt to stress of dental treatment. Consider short appointments.
- Monitor pulse rhythm to assess for electrolyte imbalance.
- *Postural hypotension:* Monitor BP at the beginning and end of each appointment; anticipate syncope. Have patient sit upright for several min at the end of the dental appointment before dismissing.
- Blood dyscrasias rarely reported; anticipate increased bleeding, infection, and poor healing.
- Chronic dry mouth is possible; anticipate increased caries, candidiasis, and lichenoid mucositis.

Oral Health Education
- Encourage daily plaque control procedures for effective self-care in patient at risk for cardiovascular disease.
- If chronic dry mouth occurs, recommend home fluoride therapy and use of nonalcoholic oral health care products.

Fustaren — see diclofenac

Fuxen — see naproxen

Fuzeon — see enfuvirtide

 gabapentin (GAB-uh-PEN-tin)

Neurontin: Capsules: 100, 300, 400 mg

▮✴▮ **Apo-Gabapentin, Novo-Gabapentin, PMS-Gabapentin**

Drug Class: Anticonvulsant

PHARMACOLOGY

Action
Mechanism unknown; gabapentin-binding sites have been found in neocortex and hippocampus areas of the brain.

Uses
Adjunctive therapy in treatment of partial seizures with or without secary generalization in patients older than 12 yr with epilepsy; adjunctive therapy for partial seizures in children 3 to 12 yr; management of postherpetic neuralgia in adults.

Contraindications
Standard considerations.

Usual Dosage
Postherpetic neuralgia
ADULTS: *PO:* Start with a single 300-mg dose on day 1, 600 mg on day 2 (divided bid), and 900 mg on day 3 (divided tid). Subsequently, titrate the dose upward as needed for pain relief to a daily dose of 1800 mg (divided tid).

Pharmacokinetics
ABSORP: Bioavailability is approximately 60%.
DIST: Less than 3% bound to plasma proteins. Vd is about 58 L.
METAB: Not significantly metabolized in humans.
EXCRET: Excreted unchanged in urine. $T_{1/2}$ is 5 to 7 hr.
SPECIAL POP: *Renal failure:* In Ccr less than 30 mL/min, $t_{1/2}$ is about 52 hr. *Hemodialysis:* $T_{1/2}$ is about 132 hr on nondialysis days; gabapentin is significantly removed by hemodialysis.

➡✚ DRUG INTERACTIONS
Antacids: Possible decreased gabapentin effect (decreased metabolism)
- Monitor clinical status.

Propranolol: Possible increased risk of dystonia (mechanism unknown)
- Monitor clinical status.

Phenytoin: Phenytoin toxicity (decreased metabolism)
- Avoid concurrent use.

ADVERSE EFFECTS
⚠ **ORAL:** Dry mouth (4.8%) or throat; dental abnormalities (unspecified).
CVS: Hypertension; vasodilation.
CNS: Somnolence; dizziness; ataxia; tremor; nervousness; dysarthria; amnesia; depression;

abnormal thinking; twitching; abnormal coordination; vertigo; hyperkinesia; paresthesia; reflex abnormality; hostility; anxiety.

GI: Dyspepsia; increased appetite; anorexia; flatulence.

RESP: Rhinitis; pharyngitis; coughing; pneumonia.

MISC: Fatigue; weight increase; back pain; peripheral edema; impotence; leukopenia; asthenia; malaise; facial edema; arthralgia.

CLINICAL IMPLICATIONS

General
- Determine why drug is being taken. Consider implications of condition on dental treatment.
- Determine ability to adapt to stress of dental treatment. Consider short appointments.
- Determine level of disease control, type and frequency of seizure, and compliance with medication regimen.
- Chronic dry mouth is possible; anticipate increased caries and candidiasis.
- Blood dyscrasias rarely reported; anticipate increased infection and poor healing.

When used or prescribed by DDS:
- *Lactation:* Secreted in breast milk.
- *Children:* Safety and efficacy in children below 3 yr not established; safety and efficacy in management of postherpetic neuralgia in pediatric patients not established.
- *Elderly:* Because of age-related renal impairment, dosage adjustment may be required.
- *Renal failure:* Dose reduction recommended.
- *Carcinogenic:* May have carcinogenic potential.
- *Serious adverse effects:* During clinical trials, some patients experienced status epilepticus, and 8 sudden, unexplained deaths occurred. The association of these events with gabapentin use is unclear.
- *Withdrawal:* Do not discontinue antiepileptic drugs abruptly because of possible increased seizure frequency from drug withdrawal.
- *Overdosage:* Ataxia, labored breathing, ptosis, sedation, hypoactivity or excitation, double vision, slurred speech, drowsiness, lethargy, diarrhea.

Pregnancy Risk Category: Category C.

Oral Health Education
- If chronic dry mouth occurs, recommend home fluoride therapy and use of nonalcoholic oral health care products.
- Evaluate manual dexterity; consider need for power toothbrush.

When used or prescribed by DDS:
- Instruct patient to take medication at least 2 hr after taking antacid.
- Explain that missed dose should be taken as soon as remembered but that two doses should not be taken together. Instruct patient to call health care provider if at least two doses are missed.
- Instruct patient to report the following symptoms to health care provider: excessive fatigue or weakness, dizziness, somnolence, incoordination, tremor or other symptoms of CNS depression, change in normal behavior, weight gain, back pain, alterations in GI system, alteration in skin or mucous membranes, fluid retention, general body discomfort, anorexia, visual disturbances, impotence.
- Advise patient that drug may cause drowsiness and to use caution while driving or performing other tasks requiring mental alertness.

Gabitril Filmtabs — see tiagabine HCl

---

galantamine HBr (gah-LAN-tah-meen HIGH-droe-BRO-mide)
Reminyl

Drug Class: Cholinesterase inhibitor

PHARMACOLOGY

Action

May enhance cholinergic function by increasing acetylcholine.

Uses

Treatment of mild to moderate dementia of the Alzheimer type.

✦✦ DRUG INTERACTIONS RELATED TO DENTAL THERAPEUTICS

No documented drug-drug interactions. The absence of evidence is not evidence of safety.

ADVERSE EFFECTS

CNS: Dizziness; fatigue; headache; tremor; depression; insomnia; somnolence; agitation; confusion; anxiety; hallucinations.
CVS: Bradycardia, syncope (2%).
GI: Nausea; vomiting; anorexia; diarrhea; abdominal pain; dyspepsia; constipation; flatulence.
RESP: Rhinitis; URI; bronchitis; coughing.
MISC: Injury; back pain; peripheral edema; asthenia; falling; thrombocytopenia.

CLINICAL IMPLICATIONS

General

- Patient may experience hypotension or hypertension. Monitor vital signs at each appointment; anticipate syncope.
- If GI side effects occur, consider semisupine chair position.
- Blood dyscrasias rarely reported; anticipate increased bleeding, infection, and poor healing.
- Ensure that caregiver is present at every dental appointment and understands informed consent.

Oral Health Education

- Encourage daily plaque control procedures for effective, nontraumatic self-care.

Galedol — see diclofenac
Gantrisin Pediatric — see sulfisoxazole
Gastrocrom — see cromolyn sodium
Gastrosed — see hyoscyamine sulfate

---

gatifloxacin (ga-ti-FLOKS-a-sin)

Tequin, Zymar

Drug Class: Antibiotic, fluoroquinolone

PHARMACOLOGY

Action

Treatment of infections caused by susceptible strains of the designated microorganism.

Uses

For treatment of bacterial infections, including chronic bronchitis; acute sinusitis; community-acquired pneumonia; uncomplicated and complicated UTIs; pyelonephritis; uncomplicated urethral and cervical gonorrhea; uncomplicated skin and skin structure infections; uncomplicated rectal infections in women; bacterial conjunctivitis (ophthalmic).

Unlabeled Uses

Atypical pneumonia; chronic prostatitis.

➡️⬅️ DRUG INTERACTIONS RELATED TO DENTAL THERAPEUTICS
No documented drug-drug interactions. The absence of evidence is not evidence of safety.

ADVERSE EFFECTS
⚠️ **ORAL:** Glossitis, candidiasis, stomatitis, mouth ulcer, taste perversion (<3%).

CNS: Abnormal dreams; insomnia; paresthesia; tremors; vasodilation; vertigo; agitation; anxiety; confusion; headache; dizziness; asthenia.

CVS: Palpitations (<3%).

GI: Abdominal pain; constipation; dyspepsia; vomiting; nausea; diarrhea; anorexia.

RESP: Dyspnea; pharyngitis.

MISC: Allergic reaction; chills; fever; back pain; chest pain.

CLINICAL IMPLICATIONS
General
- Determine why drug is being taken. Take precautions to avoid cross-contamination of microorganisms.
- If oral infection occurs that requires antibiotic therapy, select an appropriate product from a different class of anti-infectives.
- Prolonged use of antibiotics may result in bacterial or fungal overgrowth of nonsusceptible microorganisms; anticipate candidiasis.
- If GI side effects occur, consider semisupine chair position.

Gee-Gee — see guaifenesin

Gelfoam — see absorbable gelatin sponge

Gel-Kam — see sodium fluoride

Gel-Tin — see sodium fluoride

---

gemfibrozil (gem-FIE-broe-ZILL)
Lopid
■✚■ Apo-Gemfibrozil, Gen-Gemfibrozil, Novo-Gemfibrozil, Nu-Gemfibrozil, PMS-Gemfibrozil

Drug Class: Antihyperlipidemic

PHARMACOLOGY
Action
Decreases blood levels of triglycerides and VLDL by decreasing their production. Also decreases cholesterol and increases HDL.

Uses
Treatment of hypertriglyceridemia in adult patients with type IV or V hyperlipidemia that presents risk of pancreatitis and does not respond to diet; reduction of coronary heart disease risk in type IIb patients who have low HDL levels (in addition to elevated LDL and triglycerides) and have not responded to other measures.

➡️⬅️ DRUG INTERACTIONS RELATED TO DENTAL THERAPEUTICS
No documented drug-drug interactions. The absence of evidence is not evidence of safety.

ADVERSE EFFECTS
⚠️ **ORAL:** Taste perversion.

CNS: Fatigue; vertigo; headache.

GI: Dyspepsia; abdominal pain; diarrhea; nausea; vomiting; constipation; acute appendicitis.

MISC: Muscle pain or weakness; myositis; rhabdomyolysis; anemia, leukopenia, thrombocytopenia.

CLINICAL IMPLICATIONS

General
- High LDL cholesterol concentration is the major cause of atherosclerosis, which leads to CAD (angina, MI); determine degree of CV health and ability to withstand stress of dental treatment.
- Monitor vital signs (e.g., BP, pulse pressure, rate and rhythm) at each appointment to assess disease control. Do not provide elective dental treatment when BP is ≥180/110 or in presence of other high-risk CV conditions. Refer to the section entitled "The Patient Taking Cardiovascular Drugs" in Chapter 6: *Clinical Medicine*.
- If GI side effects occur, consider semisupine chair position.
- Blood dyscrasias rarely reported; anticipate increased bleeding, infection, and poor healing.

Oral Health Education
- Encourage daily plaque control procedures for effective self-care in patient at risk for cardiovascular disease.

---

gemifloxacin mesylate (jeh-mih-FLOKS-ah-sin MEH-sih-LATE)
Factive

Drug Class: Antibiotic, fluoroquinolone

PHARMACOLOGY

Action
Interferes with microbial DNA synthesis.

Uses
Treatment of acute bacterial exacerbation of chronic bronchitis and community-acquired pneumonia (mild to moderate) caused by susceptible strains of designated microorganisms.

➔← DRUG INTERACTIONS RELATED TO DENTAL THERAPEUTICS
No documented drug-drug interactions. The absence of evidence is not evidence of safety.

ADVERSE EFFECTS
⚠ **ORAL:** Taste disturbance; candidiasis, dry mouth (1%).
CNS: Headache, dizziness (1%).
CVS: Arrhythmias; syncope.
MISC: Leukopenia; thrombocytopenia.
GI: Diarrhea (4%); nausea (3%); vomiting, abdominal pain (1%).

CLINICAL IMPLICATIONS

General
- Determine why drug is being taken. Take precautions to avoid cross-contamination of microorganisms.
- If oral infection occurs that requires antibiotic therapy, select an appropriate product from a different class of anti-infectives.
- Prolonged use of antibiotics may result in bacterial or fungal overgrowth of nonsusceptible microorganisms; anticipate candidiasis.
- Monitor vital signs.
- If GI side effects occur, consider semisupine chair position.
- Blood dyscrasias rarely reported; anticipate increased bleeding, infection, and poor healing.

Oral Health Education
- Encourage daily plaque control procedures for effective, nontraumatic self-care.

Gen-Acebutolol — see acebutolol HCl
Gen-Acebutolol Type S — see acebutolol HCl
Gen-Acyclovir — see acyclovir
Genahist — see diphenhydramine HCl
Gen-Alprazolam — see alprazolam
Gen-Amantadine — see amantadine HCl
Gen-Amiodarone — see amiodarone
Gen-Amoxicillin — see amoxicillin
Genapap — see acetaminophen
Genapap Extra Strength — see acetaminophen
Genapap Infants' Drops — see acetaminophen
Genaphed — see pseudoephedrine
Gen-Atenolol — see atenolol
Genatuss — see guaifenesin
Gen-Azathioprine — see azathioprine
Gen-Beclo Aq. — see beclomethasone dipropionate
Gen-Budesonide AQ — see budesonide
Gen-Buspirone — see buspirone HCl
Gen-Captopril — see captopril
Gen-Carbamazepine CR — see carbamazepine
Gen-Cimetidine — see cimetidine
Gen-Clobetasol Cream/Ointment — see clobetasol propionate
Gen-Clobetasol Scalp Application — see clobetasol propionate
Gen-Clomipramine — see clomipramine HCl
Gen-Clonazepam — see clonazepam
Gen-Cyclobenzaprine — see cyclobenzaprine HCl
Gen-Diltiazem — see diltiazem HCl
Gen-Doxazosin — see doxazosin mesylate
Genebs — see acetaminophen
Genebs Extra Strength — see acetaminophen
Gen-Famotidine — see famotidine
Gen-Fenofibrate Micro — see fenofibrate
Gen-Fluoxetine — see fluoxetine HCl
Gen-Gemfibrozil — see gemfibrozil
Gen-Glybe — see glyburide
Gengraf — see cyclosporine
Gen-Indapamide — see indapamide
Gen-Ipratropium — see ipratropium bromide
Gen-K — see potassium products
Gen-Lovastatin — see lovastatin

Gen-Medroxy — see medroxyprogesterone acetate
Gen-Metformin — see metformin HCl
Gen-Metoprolol — see metoprolol
Gen-Minocycline — see minocycline HCl
Gen-Nabumetone — see nabumetone
Gen-Naproxen EC — see naproxen
Gen-Nitro — see nitroglycerin
Gen-Nortriptyline — see nortriptyline HCl
Gen-Oxybutynin — see oxybutynin Cl
Gen-Pindolol — see pindolol
Gen-Piroxicam — see piroxicam
Genpril — see ibuprofen
Genprin — see aspirin
Gen-Salbutamol Respirator Solution — see albuterol
Gen-Salbutamol Sterinebs P.F. — see albuterol
Gen-Selegiline — see selegiline HCl
Gen-Sotalol — see sotalol HCl
Gen-Tamoxifen — see tamoxifen citrate
Gen-Temazepam — see temazepam
Gen-Terbinafine — see terbinafine
Gen-Ticlopidine — see ticlopidine HCl
Gen-Timolol — see timolol maleate
Gen-Trazodone — see trazodone HCl
Gen-Triazolam — see triazolam
Genuine Bayer — see aspirin
Gen-Valproic — see valproic acid and derivatives
Gen-Verapamil — see verapamil HCl
Gen-Verapamil SR — see verapamil HCl
Gen-Warfarin — see warfarin
Geodon — see ziprasidone
GG-Cen — see guaifenesin
Gilbenil — see glyburide
Gimalxina — see amoxicillin
Ginedisc — see estradiol

---

glimepiride (GLIE-meh-pie-ride)

Amaryl

Drug Class: Antidiabetic, sulfonylurea

PHARMACOLOGY

Action

Decreases blood glucose by stimulating insulin release from pancreas. May also decrease hepatic glucose production as well as increase sensitivity to insulin.

Uses

Adjunct to diet and exercise in type 2 diabetic patients whose hyperglycemia cannot be controlled by diet and exercise alone; in combination with insulin for type 2 diabetic patients with secary failure to oral sulfonylureas.

➡◀ DRUG INTERACTIONS RELATED TO DENTAL THERAPEUTICS

Fluconazole: Possible increased risk of hypoglycemia (decreased metabolism)
- Monitor blood sugar.

ADVERSE EFFECTS

⚠ **ORAL:** Thirst; pharyngitis.

CNS: Headache; dizziness.

CVS: Arrhythmia; flushing; hypertension; syncope.

GI: Nausea; vomiting; GI pain; diarrhea.

RESP: Dyspnea.

MISC: Asthenia; hyponatremia with or without syndrome of inappropriate antidiuretic hormone (SIADH); hypoglycemia; photosensitivity; leukopenia; thrombocytopenia; agranulocytosis; aplastic and hemolytic anemia.

CLINICAL IMPLICATIONS

General

- Determine degree of disease control and current blood sugar levels. Goals should be <120 mg/dL and A1C <7%. A1C levels >8% indicate significant uncontrolled diabetes.
- The routine use of antibiotics in the dental management of diabetic patients is not indicated; however, antibiotic therapy in patients with poorly controlled diabetes has been shown to improve disease control and improve response after periodontal debridement.
- Monitor blood pressure because hypertension and dyslipidemia (CAD) are prevalent in DM.
- *Loss of blood sugar control:* certain medical conditions (e.g., surgery, fever, infection, trauma) and drugs (e.g., corticosteroids) affect glucose control. In these situations, it may be necessary to seek medical consultation before surgical procedures.
- Obtain patient history regarding diabetic ketoacidosis or hypoglycemia with current drug regimen.
- Observe for signs of hypoglycemia (e.g., confusion, argumentative, perspiration, altered consciousness). Be prepared to treat hypoglycemic reactions with oral glucose or sucrose.
- Ensure patient has taken medication and eaten meal.
- Monitor vital signs (e.g., BP, pulse pressure, rate and rhythm) at each appointment to assess disease control. Do not provide elective dental treatment when BP is ≥180/110 or in presence of other high-risk CV conditions. Refer to the section entitled "The Patient Taking Cardiovascular Drugs" in Chapter 6: *Clinical Medicine.*
- Determine ability to adapt to stress of dental treatment. Consider short, morning appointments.
- Medical consult advised if fasting blood glucose is <70 mg/dL (hypoglycemic risk) or >200 mg/dL (hyperglycemic crisis risk).
- *If insulin is used:* Consider time of peak hypoglycemic effect.
- Blood dyscrasias rarely reported; anticipate increased bleeding, infection, and poor healing.

Oral Health Education

- Explain role of diabetes in periodontal disease and the need to maintain effective plaque control and disease control.
- Advise patient to bring data on blood sugar values and A1C levels to dental appointments.
- Encourage daily plaque control procedures for effective self-care in patient at risk for cardiovascular disease.

Glioten — see enalapril maleate

glipizide (GLIP-ih-zide)

Glucotrol, Glucotrol XL

■**Glupitel, Minodiab**

Drug Class: Antidiabetic, sulfonylurea

PHARMACOLOGY

Action

Decreases blood glucose by stimulating insulin release from pancreas and by increasing tissue sensitivity to insulin.

Uses

Adjunct to diet to lower blood glucose in patients with type 2 diabetes mellitus whose hyperglycemia cannot be controlled by diet alone.

➡◀ DRUG INTERACTIONS RELATED TO DENTAL THERAPEUTICS

Fluconazole: Hypoglycemia (decreased metabolism of glipizide)
• Monitor blood sugar.

ADVERSE EFFECTS

⚠ **ORAL:** Thirst; pharyngitis.
CNS: Dizziness; vertigo.
CVS: Arrhythmia; flushing; hypertension; syncope.
GI: GI disturbances (e.g., nausea, epigastric fullness, heartburn); diarrhea.
RESP: Dyspnea.
MISC: Disulfiram-like reaction; weakness; paresthesia; fatigue; malaise; hypoglycemia; photosensitivity; leukopenia; thrombocytopenia; agranulocytosis; aplastic and hemolytic anemia.

CLINICAL IMPLICATIONS

General

• Determine degree of disease control and current blood sugar levels. Goals should be <120 mg/dL and A1C <7%. A1C levels ≥8% indicate significant uncontrolled diabetes.
• The routine use of antibiotics in the dental management of diabetic patients is not indicated; however, antibiotic therapy in patients with poorly controlled diabetes has been shown to improve disease control and improve response after periodontal debridement.
• Monitor blood pressure because hypertension and dyslipidemia (CAD) are prevalent in DM.
• *Loss of blood sugar control:* certain medical conditions (e.g., surgery, fever, infection, trauma) and drugs (e.g., corticosteroids) affect glucose control. In these situations, it may be necessary to seek medical consultation before surgical procedures.
• Obtain patient history regarding diabetic ketoacidosis or hypoglycemia with current drug regimen.
• Observe for signs of hypoglycemia (e.g., confusion, argumentativeness, perspiration, altered consciousness). Be prepared to treat hypoglycemic reactions with oral glucose or sucrose.
• Ensure patient has taken medication and eaten meal.
• Monitor vital signs (e.g., BP, pulse pressure, rate and rhythm) at each appointment to assess disease control. Do not provide elective dental treatment when BP is ≥180/110 or in presence of other high-risk CV conditions. Refer to the section entitled "The Patient Taking Cardiovascular Drugs" in Chapter 6: *Clinical Medicine.*
• Determine ability to adapt to stress of dental treatment. Consider short, morning appointments.
• Medical consult advised if fasting blood glucose is <70 mg/dL (hypoglycemic risk) or >200 mg/dL (hyperglycemic crisis risk).
• *If insulin is used:* Consider time of peak hypoglycemic effect.
• Blood dyscrasias rarely reported; anticipate increased bleeding, infection, and poor healing.

Oral Health Education

- Explain role of diabetes in periodontal disease and the need to maintain effective plaque control and disease control.
- Advise patient to bring data on blood sugar values and A1C levels to dental appointments.
- Encourage daily plaque control procedures for effective self-care in patient at risk for cardiovascular disease.

---

glipizide/metformin HCl (GLIP-ih-zide/met-FORE-min HIGH-droe-KLOR-ide)

Synonym: metformin HCl/glipizide

Metaglip

Drug Class: Antidiabetic combination, sulfonylurea and biguanide

PHARMACOLOGY

Action

GLIPIZIDE: Decreases blood glucose by stimulating insulin release from pancreas and by increasing tissue sensitivity to insulin.

METFORMIN: Decreases blood glucose by reducing hepatic glucose production and may decrease intestinal absorption of glucose and increase response to insulin.

Uses

Initial treatment as an adjunct to diet and exercise, to improve glycemic control in patients with type 2 diabetes whose hyperglycemia cannot be satisfactorily managed with diet and exercise alone; sec-line therapy when diet, exercise, and initial treatment with a sulfonylurea or metformin do not result in adequate glycemic control in patients with type 2 diabetes.

➔ DRUG INTERACTIONS RELATED TO DENTAL THERAPEUTICS

Fluconazole: Hypoglycemia (decreased metabolism of glipizide)
- Monitor clinical status.

ADVERSE EFFECTS

⚠ **ORAL:** Thirst; pharyngitis.
CVS: Hypertension (>5%).
CNS: Dizziness, headache (>5%).
GI: Diarrhea, nausea, vomiting, abdominal pain (>5%).
RESP: URI (>5%).
MISC: Musculoskeletal pain (>5%).

CLINICAL IMPLICATIONS

General

- Determine degree of disease control and current blood sugar levels. Goals should be <120 mg/dL and A1C <7%. A1C levels ≥8% indicate significant uncontrolled diabetes.
- The routine use of antibiotics in the dental management of diabetic patients is not indicated; however, antibiotic therapy in patients with poorly controlled diabetes has been shown to improve disease control and improve response after periodontal debridement.
- Monitor blood pressure because hypertension and dyslipidemia (CAD) are prevalent in diabetes mellitus.
- *Loss of blood sugar control:* Certain medical conditions (e.g., surgery, fever, infection, trauma) and drugs (e.g., corticosteroids) affect glucose control. In these situations, it may be necessary to seek medical consultation before surgical procedures.
- Obtain patient history regarding diabetic ketoacidosis or hypoglycemia with current drug regimen.
- Observe for signs of hypoglycemia (e.g., confusion, argumentativeness, perspiration, al-

tered consciousness). Be prepared to treat hypoglycemic reactions with oral glucose or sucrose.
- Ensure patient has taken medication and eaten meal.
- Monitor vital signs (e.g., BP, pulse pressure, rate and rhythm) at each appointment to assess disease control. Do not provide elective dental treatment when BP is ≥180/110 or in presence of other high-risk CV conditions. Refer to the section entitled "The Patient Taking Cardiovascular Drugs" in Chapter 6: *Clinical Medicine*.
- Determine ability to adapt to stress of dental treatment. Consider short morning appointments.
- Medical consult advised if fasting blood glucose (FBG) is <70 mg/dL (hypoglycemic risk) or >200 mg/dL (hyperglycemic crisis risk).
- *If insulin is used:* Consider time of peak hypoglycemic effect.
- Blood dyscrasias rarely reported; anticipate increased bleeding, infection, and poor healing.

Oral Health Education
- Explain role of diabetes in periodontal disease and the need to maintain effective plaque control and disease control.
- Advise patient to bring data on blood sugar values and A1C levels to dental appointments.
- Encourage daily plaque control procedures for effective self-care in patient at risk for cardiovascular disease.

GlucaGen — see glucagon

---

 glucagon (GLUE-kuh-gahn)

GlucaGen, Glucagon Emergency Kit, Glucagon Diagnostic Kit: Powder for injection: 1 mg (1 unit)

Drug Class: Glucose-elevating agent

PHARMACOLOGY

Action
Elevates blood glucose concentrations (by stimulating production from liver glycogen stores), relaxes smooth muscle of GI tract, decreases gastric and pancreatic secretions in GI tract, and increases myocardial contractility.

Uses
Treatment of severe hypoglycemic reactions in diabetic patients when glucose administration is not possible or during insulin shock therapy in psychiatric patients; diagnostic aid in radiological examination of stomach, duodenum, small bowel, and colon when diminished intestinal motility would be advantageous.

GLUCAGEN: Treatment of severe hypoglycemic reactions that may occur in patients with diabetes treated with insulin; as a diagnostic aid during radiological examinations to temporarily inhibit movement of the GI tract.

Unlabeled Uses
Treatment of propranolol overdose, CV emergencies, and GI disturbances associated with spasms.

Contraindications
Patients with pheochromocytoma or insulinoma; hypersensitivity to any component of the product.

Usual Dosage
Hypoglycemia
ADULTS AND CHILDREN MORE THAN 20 KG: *Subcutaneous/IM/IV:* 1 mg (1 unit). Do not use glucagon at concentrations above 1 mg/mL (1 unit/mL).

CHILDREN LESS THAN 20 KG: *Subcutaneous/IM/IV:* 0.5 mg (0.5 unit) or a dose equivalent to 20 to 30 mcg/kg.

GlucaGen

ADULTS AND CHILDREN WEIGHING 25 KG OR MORE: *Subcutaneous/IM/IV:* 1 mg.

CHILDREN WEIGHING LESS THAN 25 KG OR YOUNGER THAN 8 YR OF AGE: *Subcutaneous/IM/IV:* 0.5 mg. Emergency assistance should be sought if patient fails to respond within 15 min after subcutaneous or IM injection of glucagon. The glucagon injection may be repeated while waiting for emergency assistance. IV glucose must be administered if patient fails to respond to glucagon. When the patient has responded, give oral carbohydrate to restore liver glycogen and prevent recurrence of hypoglycemia.

Pharmacokinetics
ABSORP: Mean C_{max} is 1,686 pg/mL (IM). Median T_{max} is 12.5 min (IM).
METAB: Degraded in liver, kidney, and plasma.
EXCRET: Mean apparent $t_{1/2}$ 45 min (IM).
ONSET: 10 min.
PEAK: 30 min.

➔◀ DRUG INTERACTIONS
No documented drug-drug interactions. The absence of evidence is not evidence of safety.

ADVERSE EFFECTS
CVS: Transient increase in BP and pulse rate; positive inotropic and chronotropic effects (tachycardia).
GI: Nausea; vomiting.
MISC: Generalized allergic reactions, (e.g., urticaria, respiratory distress, hypotension).

CLINICAL IMPLICATIONS
General
- This drug is used to manage hypoglycemia when patient is unconscious and is given parenterally.
- *Children:* TREATMENT OF HYPOGLYCEMIA: Glucagon has been shown to be safe and effective. HYPOGLYCEMIA: Glucagon is effective in treating hypoglycemia only if sufficient liver glycogen is present. Because glucagon is of little or no help in states of starvation, adrenal insufficiency, or chronic hypoglycemia, treat hypoglycemia in these conditions with glucose.
- *Overdosage:* Nausea, vomiting, gastric hypotonicity, diarrhea without consequential toxicity, increased BP and pulse rate.

Pregnancy Risk Category: Category B.

Oral Health Education
When used by DDS:
- Educate patient and family members regarding the risks of prolonged hypoglycemia and the need to arouse the hypoglycemic patient as rapidly as possible.
- Instruct patient or family members to monitor fingerstick blood sugars frequently when treating hypoglycemia until the patient is asymptomatic. Advise family members to call 911 if patient has not responded within 15 min of injection and to administer sec dose of glucagon while awaiting emergency assistance.
- Instruct patient and family members that supplemental carbohydrates must be given as soon as the patient awakens and is able to swallow.
- Advise patient to inform health care provider when hypoglycemic reactions occur so that the treatment regimen may be adjusted if necessary.
- Instruct patient and family members regarding the following measures that may prevent or be used to rapidly treat hypoglycemic reactions caused by insulin: reasonable uniformity from day to day with regard to diet, insulin dose, and exercise; careful adjustment of insulin program; frequent monitoring of fingerstick blood sugars so that a change in insulin requirements can be foreseen; carrying sugar, candy, or other readily absorbable carbohydrate at all times so that it may be taken at the first warning of an oncoming hypoglycemic reaction.

- Caution patient not to take any prescription or OTC drugs, dietary supplements, or herbal preparations unless advised by health care provider.
- Advise patient that follow-up visits and laboratory tests may be necessary to monitor therapy and to keep appointments.

Glucagon Diagnostic Kit — see glucagon

Glucagon Emergency Kit — see glucagon

Glucal — see glyburide

Glucobay — see acarbose

GlucoNorm — see repaglinide

Glucophage — see metformin HCl

Glucophage Forte — see metformin HCl

Glucophage XR — see metformin HCl

Glucotrol — see glipizide

Glucotrol XL — see glipizide

Glucovance — see glyburide/metformin HCl

Glucoven — see glyburide

Glumetza — see metformin HCl

Glupitel — see glipizide

Glyate — see guaifenesin

---

glyburide (glie-BYOO-ride)

DiaBeta, Glynase PresTab, Micronase

■✷■ **Apo-Glyburide, Euglucon, Gen-Glybe, Novo-Glyburide, Nu-Glyburide, PMS-Glyburide, ratio-Glyburide**

■✷■ **Daonil, Euglucon, Gilbenil, Glucal, Glucoven, Nadib, Norboral**

Drug Class: Antidiabetic, sulfonylurea

PHARMACOLOGY

Action
Decreases blood glucose by stimulating insulin release from pancreas. May also decrease hepatic glucose production or increased response to insulin.

Uses
Adjunct to diet to lower blood glucose in patients with type 2 diabetes mellitus (DM) whose hyperglycemia cannot be controlled by diet alone; in combination with metformin when diet and glyburide or diet and metformin alone do not result in adequate glycemic control.

➡◀ DRUG INTERACTIONS RELATED TO DENTAL THERAPEUTICS
No documented drug-drug interactions. The absence of evidence is not evidence of safety.

ADVERSE EFFECTS
⚠ **ORAL:** Thirst; pharyngitis.
CNS: Dizziness; vertigo.
CVS: Arrhythmia; flushing; hypertension; syncope.
GI: Nausea; epigastric fullness; heartburn.

RESP: Dyspnea.

MISC: Disulfiram-like reactions; weakness; paresthesia; fatigue; malaise; hypoglycemia; photosensitivity; leukopenia, thrombocytopenia, agranulocytosis, aplastic and hemolytic anemia.

CLINICAL IMPLICATIONS

General

- Determine degree of disease control and current blood sugar levels. Goals should be <120 mg/dL and A1C <7%. A1C levels ≥8% indicate significant uncontrolled diabetes.
- The routine use of antibiotics in the dental management of diabetic patients is not indicated; however, antibiotic therapy in patients with poorly controlled diabetes has been shown to improve disease control and improve response after periodontal debridement.
- Monitor blood pressure because hypertension and dyslipidemia (CAD) are prevalent in DM.
- *Loss of blood sugar control:* certain medical conditions (e.g., surgery, fever, infection, trauma) and drugs (e.g., corticosteroids) affect glucose control. In these situations, it may be necessary to seek medical consultation before surgical procedures.
- Obtain patient history regarding diabetic ketoacidosis or hypoglycemia with current drug regimen.
- Observe for signs of hypoglycemia (e.g., confusion, argumentativeness, perspiration, altered consciousness). Be prepared to treat hypoglycemic reactions with oral glucose or sucrose.
- Ensure patient has taken medication and eaten meal.
- Monitor vital signs (e.g., BP, pulse pressure, rate and rhythm) at each appointment to assess disease control. Do not provide elective dental treatment when BP is ≥180/110 or in presence of other high-risk CV conditions. Refer to the section entitled "The Patient Taking Cardiovascular Drugs" in Chapter 6: *Clinical Medicine.*
- Determine ability to adapt to stress of dental treatment. Consider short morning appointments.
- Medical consult advised if fasting blood glucose is <70 mg/dL (hypoglycemic risk) or >200 mg/dL (hyperglycemic crisis risk).
- *If insulin is used:* Consider time of peak hypoglycemic effect.
- Blood dyscrasias rarely reported; anticipate increased bleeding, infection, and poor healing.

Oral Health Education

- Explain role of diabetes in periodontal disease and the need to maintain effective plaque control and disease control.
- Advise to bring data on blood sugar values and A1C levels to dental appointments.
- Encourage daily plaque control procedures for effective self-care in patient at risk for cardiovascular disease.

---

glyburide/metformin HCl (glie-BYOO-ride/met-FORE-min HIGH-droe-KLOR-ide)

Synonym: metformin HCl/glyburide

Glucovance

Drug Class: Antidiabetic combination, sulfonylurea and biguanide

PHARMACOLOGY

Action

GLYBURIDE: Decreases blood glucose by stimulating insulin release from pancreas and may decrease hepatic glucose production or increase response to insulin.

METFORMIN: Decreases blood glucose by decreasing hepatic glucose production and may decrease intestinal absorption of glucose and increase response to insulin.

Uses

Adjunct to diet and exercise to improve glycemic control in patients with type 2 diabetes whose hyperglycemia cannot be satisfactorily managed by diet and exercise alone; sec-line therapy when diet, exercise, and initial treatment with a sulfonylurea or metformin do not result in adequate glycemic control in patients with type 2 diabetes.

➜← DRUG INTERACTIONS RELATED TO DENTAL THERAPEUTICS

No documented drug-drug interactions. The absence of evidence is not evidence of safety.

ADVERSE EFFECTS

CNS: Headache, dizziness (>5%).
GI: Diarrhea, nausea, vomiting, abdominal pain (7% to 17%).
RESP: URI (17%); hypoglycemia (6.8%).

CLINICAL IMPLICATIONS

General

- Determine degree of disease control and current blood sugar levels. Goals should be <120 mg/dL and A1C <7%. A1C levels ≥8% indicate significant uncontrolled diabetes.
- The routine use of antibiotics in the dental management of diabetic patients is not indicated; however, antibiotic therapy in patients with poorly controlled diabetes has been shown to improve disease control and improve response after periodontal debridement.
- Monitor blood pressure because hypertension and dyslipidemia (CAD) are prevalent in DM.
- *Loss of blood sugar control:* certain medical conditions (e.g., surgery, fever, infection, trauma) and drugs (e.g., corticosteroids) affect glucose control. In these situations, it may be necessary to seek medical consultation before surgical procedures.
- Obtain patient history regarding diabetic ketoacidosis or hypoglycemia with current drug regimen.
- Observe for signs of hypoglycemia (e.g., confusion, argumentativeness, perspiration, altered consciousness). Be prepared to treat hypoglycemic reactions with oral glucose or sucrose.
- Ensure patient has taken medication and eaten meal.
- Monitor vital signs (e.g., BP, pulse pressure, rate, and rhythm) at each appointment to assess disease control. Do not provide elective dental treatment when BP is ≥180/110 or in presence of other high-risk CV conditions. Refer to the section entitled "The Patient Taking Cardiovascular Drugs" in Chapter 6: *Clinical Medicine.*
- Determine ability to adapt to stress of dental treatment. Consider short morning appointments.
- Medical consult advised if fasting blood glucose is <70 mg/dL (hypoglycemic risk) or >200 mg/dL (hyperglycemic crisis risk).
- *If insulin is used:* Consider time of peak hypoglycemic effect.
- If GI side effects occur, consider semisupine chair position.

Oral Health Education

- Encourage daily plaque control procedures for effective self-care in patient at risk for cardiovascular disease.
- Explain role of diabetes in periodontal disease and the need to maintain effective plaque control and disease control.
- Advise patient to bring data on blood sugar values and A1C levels to dental appointments.

---

glyceryl guaiacolate — see guaifenesin

Glycotuss — see guaifenesin

Glynase PresTab — see glyburide

Glyset — see miglitol

Glytuss — see guaifenesin

gold sodium thiomalate (gold SO-dee-uhm thigh-oh-MAL-ate)
Aurolate

Drug Class: Anti-inflammatory; Antirheumatic; Gold compound

PHARMACOLOGY

Action
Mechanism unknown; suppresses symptoms of rheumatoid arthritis and may slow progression of this disease.

Uses
Symptomatic relief of active adult and juvenile rheumatoid arthritis not adequately controlled by other therapies.

Unlabeled Uses
Treatment of pemphigus and psoriatic arthritis.

➡️◄ DRUG INTERACTIONS RELATED TO DENTAL THERAPEUTICS
Naproxen: Pneumonitis (possible hypersensitivity to gold-naproxen)
- Avoid concurrent use.

ADVERSE EFFECTS
May occur mo after therapy is discontinued.

⚠ **ORAL:** Difficulty swallowing, stomatitis (13%), glossitis; gingivitis; metallic taste.

GI: Diarrhea; nausea; cholestatic jaundice; ulcerative enterocolitis; GI bleeding; abdominal pain and cramping.

RESP: Interstitial pneumonitis; pulmonary fibrosis.

CNS: Confusion; hallucinations.

CVS: "Nitritoid reaction" (e.g., vasomotor reaction with flushing, fainting, weakness, dizziness, sweating, nausea, vomiting, malaise, headache).

MISC: Anaphylactoid reactions within min of injection, arthralgias for several days after injection; thrombocytopenia, anemia, leukopenia, eosinophilia (1% to 3%)

CLINICAL IMPLICATIONS

General
- Determine why drug is being taken. Consider implications of condition on dental treatment.
- Use COX inhibitors with caution; they may exacerbate PUD and GERD.
- *Arthritis:* Consider patient comfort and need for semisupine chair position.
- Blood dyscrasias reported; anticipate increased bleeding, infection, and poor healing.
- If GI side effects occur, consider semisupine chair position.
- Advise products for palliative relief if oral manifestations develop (e.g., stomatitis, mucositis, xerostomia).

Oral Health Education
- Encourage daily plaque control procedures for effective, nontraumatic self-care.
- Evaluate manual dexterity; consider need for power toothbrush.

Gopten — see trandolapril

Graten — see morphine sulfate

Gravol — see dimenhydrinate

Grunicina — see amoxicillin

---

guaifenesin (GWHY-fen-ah-sin)
Synonym: glyceryl guaiacolate

Allfen Jr, Anti-Tuss, Breonesin, Diabetic Tussin EX, Duratuss-G, Fenesin, Gee-Gee, Genatuss, GG-Cen, Glyate, Glycotuss, Glytuss, GuiaCough CF, GuiaCough PE, Guaifenex LA, Guiatuss, Humibid LA, Humibid Sprinkle, Hytuss, Hytuss 2x, Liquibid, Monafed, Mucinex, Muco-Fen-LA, Mytussin, Naldecon Senior EX, Organidin NR, Pneumomist, Robitussin, Scot-tussin Expectorant, Siltussin SA, Sinumist-SR Capsulets, Tusibron, Tussin, Uni-tussin

■✦■ Balminil Expectorant, Benylin E Extra Strength, Robitussin Extra Strength

■◌■ Formula E, Tukol

Drug Class: Expectorant

PHARMACOLOGY

Action

May enhance output of respiratory tract fluid by reducing adhesiveness and surface tension, thus facilitating removal of viscous mucus and making nonproductive coughs more productive and less frequent. Efficacy not well documented.

Uses

Temporary relief of cough associated with respiratory tract infections and related conditions (such as sinusitis, pharyngitis, bronchitis, and asthma) when these conditions are complicated by tenacious mucous or mucous plugs and congestion; effective for productive and nonproductive cough, particularly dry, nonproductive cough that tends to injure mucous membranes of the air passages; helps loosen phlegm and thin bronchial secretions in patients with stable chronic bronchitis.

➡✦ DRUG INTERACTIONS RELATED TO DENTAL THERAPEUTICS

No documented drug-drug interactions. The absence of evidence is not evidence of safety.

ADVERSE EFFECTS

CNS: Dizziness; headache.
GI: Nausea; vomiting.

CLINICAL IMPLICATIONS

General

• Determine why drug is being taken. Take precautions to avoid cross-contamination of microorganisms.
• Monitor respiratory function; uncontrolled respiratory disease is characterized by wheezing, coughing.
• Consider semisupine chair position to assist respiratory function.

Guaifenex LA — see guaifenesin

---

guanabenz acetate (GWAHN-uh-benz ASS-uh-TATE)

Wytensin

Drug Class: Antihypertensive; Antiadrenergic, centrally acting

PHARMACOLOGY

Action

Appears to stimulate central alpha$_2$-adrenergic receptors, inhibiting sympathetic outflow from brain to peripheral circulation.

Uses

Treatment of hypertension alone or with a thiazide diuretic.

➤◆ DRUG INTERACTIONS RELATED TO DENTAL THERAPEUTICS

No documented drug-drug interactions. The absence of evidence is not evidence of safety.

ADVERSE EFFECTS

⚠ **ORAL:** Dry mouth (28% to 38%); taste disorder.

CNS: Drowsiness; sedation; dizziness; anxiety; ataxia; depression; sleep disturbances.

CVS: Chest pain; arrhythmia; palpitations.

GI: Constipation; diarrhea; nausea; vomiting; abdominal discomfort.

RESP: Dyspnea.

MISC: Gynecomastia; muscle or joint pain; weakness.

CLINICAL IMPLICATIONS

General

* Monitor vital signs (e.g., BP, pulse pressure, rate and rhythm) at each appointment to assess disease control. Do not provide elective dental treatment when BP is ≥180/110 or in presence of other high-risk CV conditions. Refer to the section entitled "The Patient Taking Cardiovascular Drugs" in Chapter 6: *Clinical Medicine*.
* Use local anesthetic agents with vasoconstrictor with caution based on functional capacity of the patient and use aspirating technique to prevent intravascular injection.
* Determine ability to adapt to stress of dental treatment. Consider short appointments.
* If GI side effects occur, consider semisupine chair position.
* Chronic dry mouth is possible; anticipate increased caries and candidiasis.

Oral Health Education

* If chronic dry mouth occurs, recommend home fluoride therapy and use of nonalcoholic oral health care products.
* Encourage daily plaque control procedures for effective self-care in patient at risk for cardiovascular disease.

guanadrel (GWAHN-uh-drell)

Hylorel

Drug Class: Antihypertensive; Antiadrenergic, peripherally acting

PHARMACOLOGY

Action

Inhibits vasoconstriction by restraining norepinephrine release from nerve storage sites; depletion of norepinephrine causes relaxation of vascular smooth muscle, decreasing total peripheral resistance and venous return.

Uses

Treatment of hypertension in patients not responding adequately to thiazide-type diuretics.

➤◆ DRUG INTERACTIONS RELATED TO DENTAL THERAPEUTICS

Sympathomimetic amines: Decreased antihypertensive effect (pharmacological antagonism)
* Use local anesthetic agents containing a vasoconstrictor with caution.
* Monitor blood pressure.

ADVERSE EFFECTS

⚠ **ORAL:** Glossitis (8%), dry mouth (2%).

CNS: Fatigue; headache; faintness; drowsiness; paresthesias; confusion; depression; sleep disorders.

CVS: Palpitations, chest pain (28% to 30%), orthostatic hypotension (47%), syncope.

GI: Increased bowel movements; gas pain/indigestion; constipation; anorexia; nausea or vomiting; abdominal distress or pain.

RESP: Shortness of breath; coughing.

MISC: Excessive weight loss or gain; aching limbs; leg cramps; back or neck ache; joint pain or inflammation; gangrene.

CLINICAL IMPLICATIONS

General
- Monitor vital signs (e.g., BP, pulse pressure, rate and rhythm) at each appointment to assess disease control. Do not provide elective dental treatment when BP is ≥180/110 or in presence of other high-risk CV conditions. Refer to the section entitled "The Patient Taking Cardiovascular Drugs" in Chapter 6: *Clinical Medicine*.
- Use local anesthetic agents with vasoconstrictor with caution based on functional capacity of the patient and use aspirating technique to prevent intravascular injection.
- *Postural hypotension:* Monitor BP at the beginning and end of each appointment; anticipate syncope. Have patient sit upright for several min at the end of the dental appointment before dismissing.
- Determine ability to adapt to stress of dental treatment. Consider short appointments.
- Chronic dry mouth is possible; anticipate increased caries activity and candidiasis.
- If GI or musculoskeletal side effects occur, consider semisupine chair position.

Oral Health Education
- Encourage daily plaque control procedures for effective self-care in patient at risk for cardiovascular disease.
- If chronic dry mouth occurs, recommend home fluoride therapy and use of nonalcoholic oral health care products.

---

guanfacine HCl (GWAHN-fay-seen HIGH-droe-KLOR-ide)
Tenex

Drug Class: Antihypertensive; Antiadrenergic, centrally acting

PHARMACOLOGY

Action
Appears to stimulate central alpha$_2$-adrenergic receptors, with decreased sympathetic outflow causing decrease in peripheral vascular resistance and reduction in heart rate.

Uses
Treatment of hypertension.

Unlabeled Uses
Amelioration of heroin withdrawal symptoms.

➡◀ DRUG INTERACTIONS RELATED TO DENTAL THERAPEUTICS
No documented drug-drug interactions. The absence of evidence is not evidence of safety.

ADVERSE EFFECTS
⚠ ORAL: Dry mouth (10% to 54%, dose dependent).
CNS: Somnolence; drowsiness; dizziness; headache; sleep disturbances; insomnia; confusion; depression.
CVS: Postural hypotension; syncope; palpitations.
GI: Constipation; diarrhea; nausea; abdominal discomfort; dyspnea.
MISC: Paresthesia; paresis; leg cramps; hypokinesia.

CLINICAL IMPLICATIONS

General
- Monitor vital signs (e.g., BP, pulse pressure, rate and rhythm) at each appointment to assess disease control. Do not provide elective dental treatment when BP is ≥180/110 or in presence of other high-risk CV conditions. Refer to the section entitled "The Patient Taking Cardiovascular Drugs" in Chapter 6: *Clinical Medicine*.
- Use local anesthetic agents with vasoconstrictor with caution based on functional capacity of the patient and use aspirating technique to prevent intravascular injection.
- Determine ability to adapt to stress of dental treatment. Consider short appointments.
- Chronic dry mouth is possible; anticipate increased caries, candidiasis, and lichenoid mucositis.

- *Postural hypotension:* Monitor BP at the beginning and end of each appointment; antici-pate syncope. Have patient sit upright for several min at the end of the dental appoint-ment before dismissing.
- If GI side effects occur, consider semisupine chair position.

Oral Health Education

- Encourage daily plaque control procedures for effective self-care in patient at risk for car-diovascular disease.
- If chronic dry mouth occurs, recommend home fluoride therapy and use of nonalcoholic oral health care products.

GuiaCough CF — see guaifenesin
GuiaCough PE — see guaifenesin
Guiatuss — see guaifenesin
Gynecort 10 — see hydrocortisone
Gyne-Lotrimin 3 — see clotrimazole
Gyne-Lotrimin 3 Combination Pack — see clotrimazole
Gyne-Lotrimin 7 — see clotrimazole
Gynodiol — see estradiol
Habitrol — see nicotine

---

halcinonide (hal-SIN-oh-nide)

Halog, Halog-E

■■■ **Dermalog**

Drug Class: Corticosteroid, topical

PHARMACOLOGY

Action

Produces anti-inflammatory, antipruritic, and vasoconstrictive effects by an unknown mech-anism.

Uses

Relief of inflammation and pruritus caused by corticosteroid-responsive dermatoses.

➜← DRUG INTERACTIONS RELATED TO DENTAL THERAPEUTICS

No documented drug-drug interactions. The absence of evidence is not evidence of safety.

ADVERSE EFFECTS

⚠ **ORAL:** Dryness; mucosal atrophy; stinging and cracking of skin.
MISC: Numbness of fingers; local skin reactions.

CLINICAL IMPLICATIONS

General

- Determine why drug is being taken. Consider implications of condition on dental treat-ment.
- Due to the anticipated perioperative physiological stress (i.e., minor surgical stress), pa-tients undergoing dental care under local anesthesia should take only their usual daily glucocorticoid dose before dental intervention. No supplementation is justified.
- Anticipate oral candidiasis when steroids are used.

Halcion — see triazolam
Halfprin 81 — see aspirin

halobetasol propionate (hal-oh-BAY-ta-sol PROE-pie-OH-nayt)

Ultravate

Drug Class: Corticosteroid, topical

PHARMACOLOGY

Action
Very high potency topical glucocorticoid with anti-inflammatory, antipruritic, and vasoconstrictive properties. Thought to act by inducing phospholipase A_2 inhibitory proteins, thus controlling biosynthesis of potent mediators of inflammation.

Uses
Relief of inflammatory and pruritic manifestations of corticosteroid-responsive dermatoses.

➡◀ DRUG INTERACTIONS RELATED TO DENTAL THERAPEUTICS
No documented drug-drug interactions. The absence of evidence is not evidence of safety.

ADVERSE EFFECTS
⚠ **ORAL:** Perioral dermatitis; itching; mucosal thinning.
MISC: Burning; stinging; local tissue reactions.

CLINICAL IMPLICATIONS

General
- Determine why drug is being taken. Consider implications of condition on dental treatment.
- Due to the anticipated perioperative physiological stress (i.e., minor surgical stress) in, patients undergoing dental care under local anesthesia should take only their usual daily glucocorticoid dose before dental intervention. No supplementation is justified.
- Anticipate oral candidiasis when steroids are used.

Halofed — see pseudoephedrine

Halog — see halcinonide

Halog-E — see halcinonide

---

haloperidol (HAL-oh-pehr-i-dahl)
(haloperidol decanoate)

■✦■ Apo-Haloperidol, Apo-Haloperidol Decanoate Injection, Haloperidol-LA Omega, Novo-Peridol, PMS-Haloperidol LA, ratio-Haloperidol

Drug Class: Antipsychotic, butyrophenone

PHARMACOLOGY

Action
Has antipsychotic effect, apparently caused by dopamine-receptor blockage in CNS.

Uses
Management of psychotic disorders; control of Tourette disorder in children and adults; management of severe behavioral problems in children; short-term treatment of hyperactive children. Long-term antipsychotic therapy (haloperidol decanoate).

Unlabeled Uses
Treatment of phencyclidine (PCP) psychosis; antiemetic; hiccups.

➡◀ DRUG INTERACTIONS RELATED TO DENTAL THERAPEUTICS
Itraconazole: Possible haloperidol toxicity (decreased metabolism)
- Monitor clinical status.

ADVERSE EFFECTS

⚠ **ORAL:** Dry mouth, tardive dyskinesia; hypersalivation.

CNS: Tardive dystonia; insomnia; restlessness; anxiety; euphoria; agitation; drowsiness; depression; lethargy; headache; confusion; vertigo; seizures; exacerbation of psychotic symptoms; pseudoparkinsonism (e.g., mask-like face, drooling, pill-rolling gestures, shuffling gait, inertia, tremors, cogwheel rigidity); muscle spasms; dyskinesia; akathisia; oculogyric crises; opisthotonos; hyperreflexia.

CVS: Hypertension or hypotension, arrhythmia, tachycardia.

GI: Dyspepsia; anorexia; diarrhea; nausea; vomiting; elevated prolactin levels; adynamic ileus (may lead to death).

RESP: Laryngospasm; bronchospasm; increased depth of respiration; bronchopneumonia.

MISC: Hyperglycemia; hypoglycemia; hyponatremia; photosensitivity; leukocytosis, leukopenia, agranulocytosis.

CLINICAL IMPLICATIONS

General

- Determine why drug is being taken. Consider implications of condition on dental treatment.
- Extrapyramidal behaviors can complicate performance of oral procedures. If present, consult with MD to consider medication changes.
- Chronic dry mouth is possible; anticipate increased caries and candidiasis.
- If GI side effects occur, consider semisupine chair position.
- Monitor vital signs.
- *Geriatric patients:* Use lower dose of opioid.

Oral Health Education

- Evaluate manual dexterity; consider need for power toothbrush.
- If chronic dry mouth occurs, recommend home fluoride therapy and use of nonalcoholic oral health care products.

---

haloperidol decanoate — see haloperidol
Haloperidol-LA Omega — see haloperidol
Haltran — see ibuprofen
Heartline — see aspirin
Hemocyte — see ferrous salts
Hemopad — see microfibrillar collagen hemostat
Hemorrhoidal HC — see hydrocortisone
Hemotene — see microfibrillar collagen hemostat
Hemril-HC Uniserts — see hydrocortisone
Henexal — see furosemide
Hepsera — see adefovir dipivoxil
Heptovir — see lamivudine
Hexadrol — see dexamethasone
Hexadrol Phosphate — see dexamethasone
Hi-Cor 1.0 — see hydrocortisone
Hi-Cor 2.5 — see hydrocortisone
Hidramox — see amoxicillin
Higroton — see chlorthalidone

Hipocol — see niacin
Hivid — see zalcitabine
Hold DM — see dextromethorphan HBr
human insulin injection ([rDNA] origin) NPH — see insulin
human insulin isophane suspension and 30% regular — see insulin
Humibid LA — see guaifenesin
Humibid Sprinkle — see guaifenesin
Humira — see adalimumab
Humulin 70/30 — see insulin
Humulin N — see insulin
Humulin R — see insulin
Hurricaine — see benzocaine
Hydantoina — see phenytoin
Hydeltrasol — see prednisolone
Hyderm — see hydrocortisone

---

hydralazine HCl (high-DRAL-uh-zeen HIGH-droe-KLOR-ide)
Apresoline
■✦■ Nu-Hydral, Novo-Hylazin, Apo-Hydralazine

■✦■ Apresolina

Drug Class: Antihypertensive; Vasodilator

PHARMACOLOGY

Action
Directly relaxes vascular smooth muscle to cause peripheral vasodilation, decreasing arterial BP and peripheral vascular resistance.

Uses
Treatment of essential hypertension (oral form). Treatment of severe essential hypertension (parenteral form).

Unlabeled Uses
Reduction of overload in treatment of CHF, severe aortic insufficiency, and after valve replacement.

➜✦ DRUG INTERACTIONS RELATED TO DENTAL THERAPEUTICS
No documented drug-drug interactions. The absence of evidence is not evidence of safety.

ADVERSE EFFECTS
CNS: Headache; peripheral neuritis with paresthesias, numbness and tingling; dizziness; tremors; depression; disorientation; anxiety.
CVS: Palpitations, tachycardia; hypotension, flushing.
GI: Anorexia; nausea; vomiting; diarrhea; constipation.
RESP: Nasal congestion; dyspnea.
MISC: Hypersensitivity (e.g., rash, urticaria, pruritus, fever, chills, arthralgia, eosinophilia); systemic lupus erythematosus; blood dyscrasias (e.g., reduced hemoglobin, reduced RBC, agranulocytosis, thrombocytopenia, leukopenia).

CLINICAL IMPLICATIONS

General

*   Monitor vital signs (e.g., BP, pulse pressure, rate and rhythm) at each appointment to assess disease control. Do not provide elective dental treatment when BP is ≥180/110 or in the presence of other high-risk CV conditions. Refer to the section entitled "The Patient Taking Cardiovascular Drugs" in Chapter 6: *Clinical Medicine*.
*   Use local anesthetic agents with vasoconstrictor with caution based on functional capacity of the patient and use aspirating technique to prevent intravascular injection.
*   Determine ability to adapt to stress of dental treatment. Consider short appointments.
*   *Postural hypotension:* Monitor BP at the beginning and end of each appointment; anticipate syncope. Have patient sit upright for several min at the end of the dental appointment before dismissing.
*   Blood dyscrasias rarely reported; anticipate increased bleeding, infection, and poor healing.
*   If GI side effects occur, consider semisupine chair position.

Oral Health Education

*   Encourage daily plaque control procedures for effective self-care in patient at risk for cardiovascular disease.

Hydramine Cough — see diphenhydramine HCl

Hydrate — see dimenhydrinate

Hydrocet — see acetaminophen/hydrocodone bitartrate

---

hydrochlorothiazide (HIGH-droe-klor-oh-THIGH-uh-zide)

Esidrix, Ezide, Hydro-DIURIL, Hydro-Par, Microzide, Oretic

■�֍■ Apo-Hydro, Urozide

■֍■ Diclotride

Drug Class: Thiazide diuretic

PHARMACOLOGY

Action

Enhances excretion of sodium, chloride, and water by interfering with transport of sodium ions across renal tubular epithelium.

Uses

Adjunctive therapy for edema associated with CHF, cirrhosis, renal dysfunction, and corticosteroid and estrogen therapy; treatment of hypertension.

Unlabeled Uses

Prevention of formation and recurrence of calcium nephrolithiasis; therapy for nephrogenic diabetes insipidus.

➡◆ DRUG INTERACTIONS RELATED TO DENTAL THERAPEUTICS

COX-1 inhibitors: Decreased antihypertensive effect (reduced prostaglandin synthesis)
*   Monitor blood pressure.

ADVERSE EFFECTS

⚠ **ORAL:** Sialoadenitis.

CNS: Dizziness; lightheadedness; vertigo; headache; paresthesias; weakness; restlessness; insomnia.

CVS: Orthostatic hypotension; arrhythmia.

GI: Anorexia; gastric irritation; nausea; vomiting; abdominal pain or cramping; bloating; diarrhea; constipation; pancreatitis.

RESP: Respiratory distress; pneumonitis; pulmonary edema.

MISC: Muscle cramp or spasm; fever; anaphylactic reactions photosensitivity; electrolyte imbalance; blood dyscrasias (e.g., leukopenia, thrombocytopenia, agranulocytosis, aplastic and hemolytic anemias).

CLINICAL IMPLICATIONS

General

- Monitor vital signs (e.g., BP, pulse pressure, rate and rhythm) at each appointment to assess disease control. Do not provide elective dental treatment when BP is ≥180/110 or in presence of other high-risk CV conditions. Refer to the section entitled "The Patient Taking Cardiovascular Drugs" in Chapter 6: *Clinical Medicine*.
- Use local anesthetic agents with vasoconstrictor with caution based on functional capacity of the patient and use aspirating technique to prevent intravascular injection.
- Determine ability to adapt to stress of dental treatment. Consider short appointments.
- Monitor pulse rhythm to assess for electrolyte imbalance.
- *Postural hypotension:* Monitor BP at the beginning and end of each appointment; anticipate syncope. Have patient sit upright for several min at the end of the dental appointment before dismissing.
- If GI side effects occur, consider semisupine chair position.
- Blood dyscrasias rarely reported; anticipate increased bleeding, infection, and poor healing.

Oral Health Education

- Encourage daily plaque control procedures for effective, nontraumatic self-care.

---

hydrochlorothiazide/losartan potassium — see losartan potassium/ hydrochlorothiazide

hydrochlorothiazide/valsartan — see valsartan/hydrochlorothiazide

hydrocodone bitartrate/acetaminophen — see acetaminophen/ hydrocodone bitartrate

hydrocodone bitartrate/aspirin — see aspirin/hydrocodone bitartrate

hydrocodone bitartrate/ibuprofen — see ibuprofen/hydrocodone bitartrate

---

hydrocortisone (HIGH-droe-CORE-tih-sone)

(hydrocortisone acetate, hydrocortisone buteprate, hydrocortisone butyrate, hydrocortisone cypionate, hydrocortisone phosphate, hydrocortisone sodium succinate, hydrocortisone valerate)

Synonym: cortisol

A-Hydrocort, Ala-Cort, Ala-Scalp, Anucort-HC, Anumed HC, Anusol HC-1 Hydrocortisone Anti-Itch, Anusol-HC, Caldecort Hydrocortisone Anti-Itch, Cetacort, CortaGel Extra Strength, Cortaid Maximum Strength, Cortaid Topical Spray, Cortaid with Aloe, Cort-Dome, Cortef, Cortenema, Cortizone-10 Quickshot Spray, Cortizone for Kids, Cortizone-10, Cortizone-10 Plus Maximum Strength, Cortizone-5, Dermacort, Dermol HC, Dermtex HC Maximum Strength Spray, Gynecort 10 Extra Strength, Hemorrhoidal HC, Hemril-HC Uniserts, Hi-Cor 1.0, Hi-Cor 2.5, Hydrocortisone Phosphate, Hytone, KeriCort-10, LactiCare-HC, Lanacort 10, Lanacort 5, Lanacort Maximum Strength Cool Creme, Locoid, Nutracort, Pandel, Penecort, Proctocort, ProctoCream-HC, Scalpicin, Solu-Cortef, S-T Cort, T/Scalp, U-Cort, Westcort

■✽■ **Aquacort, Claritin Skin Itch Relief, Cortoderm, Emo-Cort, Hyderm, HydroVal, Prevex HC, Sarna HC, Texacort, Uromol HC**

Drug Class: Corticosteroid

PHARMACOLOGY

Action

Short-acting glucocorticoid that depresses formation, release, and activity of endogenous mediators of inflammation including prostaglandins, kinins, histamine, liposomal enzymes, and complement system. Also modifies body's immune response.

Uses

Treatment of primary or secary adrenal cortex insufficiency, rheumatic disorders, collagen diseases, dermatological diseases, allergic states, allergic and inflammatory ophthalmic processes, respiratory diseases, hematological disorders (e.g., idiopathic thrombocytopenic purpura), neoplastic diseases, edematous states (resulting from nephrotic syndrome), GI diseases (e.g., ulcerative colitis and sprue), multiple sclerosis, tuberculous meningitis, trichinosis with neurological or myocardial involvement.

INTRA-ARTICULAR OR SOFT-TISSUE ADMINISTRATION: Treatment of synovitis of osteoarthritis and symptoms of rheumatoid arthritis, bursitis, acute gouty arthritis, epicondylitis, acute nonspecific tenosynovitis, and posttraumatic osteoarthritis.

INTRALESIONAL ADMINISTRATION: Treatment of keloids, lesions of lichen planus, psoriatic plaques, granuloma annulare, lichen simplex chronicus, discoid lupus erythematosus, necrobiosis lipoidica diabeticorum, alopecia areata, and cystic tumors of aponeurosis or tendon.

TOPICAL ADMINISTRATION: Treatment of inflammatory and pruritic manifestations of corticosteroid-responsive dermatoses; management of refractory lesions of psoriasis and other deep-seated dermatoses.

RECTAL ADMINISTRATION: Relief of discomfort associated with hemorrhoids, perianal itching, or irritation.

➜ DRUG INTERACTIONS RELATED TO DENTAL THERAPEUTICS

Midazolam: Possible decreased midazolam effect (increased metabolism)
- Monitor clinical status.

COX-1 inhibitors: Increased risk of peptic ulcers (additive)
- Avoid concurrent use.

ADVERSE EFFECTS

⚠ **ORAL:** Topical: Burning, itching, dryness; topical use may cause same adverse reactions seen with systemic use because of possibility of absorption.

CNS: Convulsions; increased intracranial pressure with papilledema (pseudotumor cerebri); vertigo; headache; neuritis; paresthesias; psychosis.

GI: Pancreatitis; abdominal distension; ulcerative esophagitis; nausea; vomiting; increased appetite and weight gain; peptic ulcer with perforation and hemorrhage; bowel perforation.

MISC: Musculoskeletal effects (e.g., weakness, myopathy, muscle mass loss, osteoporosis, spontaneous fractures); endocrine abnormalities (e.g., menstrual irregularities, cushingoid state, growth suppression in children, sweating, decreased carbohydrate tolerance, hyperglycemia, glycosuria, increased insulin or sulfonylurea requirements in diabetic patients); anaphylactoid or hypersensitivity reactions; aggravation or masking of infections; malaise; fatigue; insomnia.

CLINICAL IMPLICATIONS

General

- Determine why drug is being taken. Consider implications of condition on dental treatment.
- Despite the anticipated perioperative physiological stress (i.e., minor surgical stress), patients undergoing dental care under local anesthesia should take only their usual daily glucocorticoid dose before dental intervention. No supplementation is justified.
- Anticipate oral candidiasis when steroids are used.

hydrocortisone acetate — see hydrocortisone

hydrocortisone buteprate — see hydrocortisone

hydrocortisone butyrate — see hydrocortisone

hydrocortisone cypionate — see hydrocortisone

hydrocortisone phosphate — see hydrocortisone

hydrocortisone sodium succinate — see hydrocortisone

hydrocortisone valerate — see hydrocortisone

Hydro-DIURIL — see hydrochlorothiazide

Hydrogesic — see acetaminophen/hydrocodone bitartrate

Hydromorph Contin — see hydromorphone HCl

---

hydromorphone HCl (HIGH-droe-MORE-phone HIGH-droe-KLOR-ide)

Dilaudid, Dilaudid-HP

■✦■ **Dilaudid-HP Plus, Dilaudid Sterile Powder, Dilaudid-XP, Hydromorph Contin, Hydromorphone HP 10, Hydromorphone HP 20, Hydromorphone HP 50, Hydromorphone HP Forte, PMS-Hydromorphone**

Drug Class: Analgesic, narcotic
DEA Schedule: Schedule II

PHARMACOLOGY

Action
Relieves pain by stimulating opiate receptors in CNS; also causes respiratory depression, inhibition of cough reflex, peripheral vasodilation, inhibition of intestinal peristalsis, sphincter of Oddi spasm, stimulation of chemoreceptors that cause vomiting, and increased bladder tone.

Uses
Relief of moderate to severe pain; control of persistent nonproductive cough.

➜✦ DRUG INTERACTIONS RELATED TO DENTAL THERAPEUTICS

Bupivacaine: Possible respiratory depression (mechanism unknown)
- Avoid concurrent use.

ADVERSE EFFECTS

⚠ **ORAL:** Dry mouth.
CVS: Hypotension; orthostatic hypotension; bradycardia; tachycardia.
CNS: Lightheadedness; dizziness; sedation; disorientation; incoordination; lethargy; anxiety.
GI: Nausea; vomiting; constipation; abdominal pain.
RESP: Respiratory depression; laryngospasm; depression of cough reflex.
MISC: Tolerance; psychological and physical dependence with long-term use.

CLINICAL IMPLICATIONS

General
- *Drug dependence:* Hydromorphone has abuse potential.
- Monitor vital signs (e.g., BP, pulse rate) and respiratory function.
- Chronic dry mouth is possible; anticipate increased caries and candidiasis.
- *Postural hypotension:* Monitor BP at the beginning and end of each appointment; antici-

pate syncope. Have patient sit upright for several min at the end of the dental appointment before dismissing.
• If GI side effects occur, consider semisupine chair position.

Oral Health Education
• If chronic dry mouth occurs, recommend home fluoride therapy and use of nonalcoholic oral health care products.

Hydromorphone HP 10 — see hydromorphone HCl
Hydromorphone HP 20 — see hydromorphone HCl
Hydromorphone HP 50 — see hydromorphone HCl
Hydromorphone HP Forte — see hydromorphone HCl
Hydro-Par — see hydrochlorothiazide
HydroVal — see hydrocortisone

---

hydroxychloroquine sulfate (high-drox-ee-KLOR-oh-kwin SULL-fate)

Plaquenil

Drug Class: Anti-infective; Antimalarial; Antirheumatic

PHARMACOLOGY

Action
May interfere with parasitic nucleoprotein (DNA/RNA) synthesis and parasite growth or cause lysis of parasite or infected erythrocytes. In rheumatoid arthritis, may suppress formation of antigens responsible for symptom-producing hypersensitivity reactions.

Uses
Prophylaxis and treatment of acute attacks of malaria caused by *Plasmodium vivax*, *P. malariae*, *P. ovale*, and susceptible strains of *P. falciparum*. Treatment of chronic discoid and systemic lupus erythematosus (SLE) and acute or chronic rheumatoid arthritis in patients not responding to other therapies.

➡◀ DRUG INTERACTIONS RELATED TO DENTAL THERAPEUTICS
No documented drug-drug interactions. The absence of evidence is not evidence of safety.

ADVERSE EFFECTS
⚠ **ORAL:** Lichen planus–like eruptions.

CVS: Hypotension; ECG changes; cardiomyopathy (rare).

CNS: Headache; irritability; nervousness; emotional changes; nightmares; psychosis; dizziness; vertigo; nystagmus; nerve deafness; convulsions; ataxia.

GI: Anorexia; nausea; vomiting; diarrhea; abdominal cramps.

MISC: Immunoblastic lymphadenopathy; extraocular muscle palsies, photophobia; skeletal muscle weakness; absent or hypoactive deep tendon reflexes; agranulocytosis, blood dyscrasias.

CLINICAL IMPLICATIONS

General
• Determine why drug is being taken. Consider implications of condition on dental treatment.
• *For patients taking this drug on a long term basis:* Monitor vital signs. Blood dyscrasias rarely reported; anticipate increased bleeding, infection, and poor healing.
• If GI side effects occur, consider semisupine chair position.
• *Photophobia:* Direct dental light out of patient's eyes and offer dark glasses for comfort.

hydroxymagnesium aluminate — see magaldrate

hydroxyzine (high-DROX-ih-zeen)
Hydroxyzine Hydrochloride, Vistaril
■✚■ Apo-Hydroxyzine, Novo-Hydroxyzin, Nu-Hydroxyzine, PMS-Hydroxyzine
Drug Class: Antianxiety; Antihistamine; Antiemetic (parenteral)

PHARMACOLOGY
Action
May be caused by suppression of activity in subcortical areas of CNS.

Uses
Symptomatic relief of anxiety and tension associated with psychoneurosis; adjunct therapy in organic disease states with anxiety; management of pruritus caused by allergic conditions; sedative before and after general anesthesia (PO, IM).

➔◆ DRUG INTERACTIONS RELATED TO DENTAL THERAPEUTICS
No documented drug-drug interactions. The absence of evidence is not evidence of safety.

ADVERSE EFFECTS
⚠ ORAL: Dry mouth.
CNS: Transitory drowsiness; involuntary motor activity, including tremor and convulsions.
RESP: Hypersensitivity reactions (e.g., wheezing, shortness of breath).

CLINICAL IMPLICATIONS
General
- Determine why drug is being taken. Consider implications of condition on dental treatment.
- Depressed or anxious patients may neglect self-care. Monitor for plaque control effectiveness.
- Chronic dry mouth is possible; anticipate increased caries and candidiasis.
- *When CNS depressants are used by DDS:* Reduce dose by half.
- *If prescribed by DDS:* Inform patient not to drive, sign important papers, or operate mechanical equipment while taking drug. Short-term use is not likely to cause effects of chronic xerostomia.

Oral Health Education
- Encourage daily plaque control procedures for effective self-care.
- If chronic dry mouth occurs, recommend home fluoride therapy and use of nonalcoholic oral health care products.

Hydroxyzine Hydrochloride — see hydroxyzine
Hygroton — see chlorthalidone
Hylorel — see guanadrel
hyoscine HBr — see scopolamine HBr

hyoscyamine sulfate (hye-oh-SYE-a-mean)
Anaspaz, A-Spas S/L, Cystospaz, Donnamar, Donnatal, ED-SPAZ, Gastrosed, Levbid, Levsin, Levsin Drops, Levsin/SL, Levsinex Timecaps, NuLev
Drug Class: Belladonna alkaloid; Anticholinergic

PHARMACOLOGY

Action

Inhibits the action of acetylcholine on structures innervated by postganglionic cholinergic nerves and on smooth muscles. These receptors are located in the autonomic effector cells of the smooth muscle, cardiac muscle, sinoatrial node, atrioventricular node, and exocrine glands. Inhibits GI propulsive motility and decreases gastric acid secretion. Controls excessive pharyngeal, tracheal, and bronchial secretions.

Uses

To control gastric secretion, visceral spasm, hypermotility in spastic colitis, spastic bladder, cystitis, pylorospasm, and associated abdominal cramps; to reduce symptoms of functional intestinal disorders such as those seen with mild dysentery, diverticulitis, and acute enterocolitis; treatment of infant colic; as a "drying" agent in rhinitis; to reduce rigidity and tremors and to control sialorrhea and hyperhidrosis of Parkinson disease; with morphine or other narcotics, for symptomatic relief of biliary and renal colic; poisoning by anticholinesterase agents; adjunct therapy in treatment of peptic ulcer, irritable bowel syndrome, functional GI disorders, neurogenic bladder, and neurogenic bowel disturbances; preoperative to reduce secretions; block cardiac vagal inhibitory reflexes during anesthesia induction and intubation.

➜← DRUG INTERACTIONS RELATED TO DENTAL THERAPEUTICS

No documented drug-drug interactions. The absence of evidence is not evidence of safety.

ADVERSE EFFECTS

⚠ **ORAL:** Dry mouth; taste disturbance; dysphagia.

CNS: Headache; nervousness; drowsiness; weakness; dizziness; confusion, insomnia; fever; excitability; restlessness; tremor; speech disturbance.

CVS: Palpitations; tachycardia.

GI: Nausea; vomiting; heartburn constipation, bloated feeling; paralytic ileus.

MISC: Suppressed lactation; decreased sweating, photophobia.

CLINICAL IMPLICATIONS

General

- Determine why drug is being taken. Consider implications of condition on dental treatment.
- Anticholinergics have strong xerostomic effects. Anticipate increased caries activity and candidiasis.
- Substernal pain (heartburn) may mimic pain of cardiac origin.
- Use COX inhibitors with caution, they may exacerbate PUD and GERD.
- Monitor vital signs.
- *Photophobia:* Direct dental light out of patient's eyes and offer dark glasses for comfort.

Oral Health Education

- If chronic dry mouth occurs, recommend home fluoride therapy and use of nonalcoholic oral health care products.

Hy-Phen — see acetaminophen/hydrocodone bitartrate

Hyrexin-50 — see diphenhydramine HCl

Hytinic — see ferrous salts

Hytone — see hydrocortisone

Hytrin — see terazosin

Hytuss — see guaifenesin

Hytuss 2x — see guaifenesin

Hyzaar — see losartan potassium/hydrochlorothiazide

ibuprofen (eye-BYOO-pro-fen)

Advil, Advil Liqui-Gels, Children's Advil, Children's Motrin, Genpril, Haltran, Junior Strength Advil, Junior Strength Motrin, Menadol, Midol, Motrin IB, Nuprin, Pedia-Care Fever, Pediatric Advil Drops: Tablets: 100, 200, 400, 600, 800 mg; Caplets: 200 mg; Chewable tablets: 50, 100 mg; Suspension: 100 mg/2.5 mL, 100 mg/5 mL; Oral drops: 40 mg/mL
Advil Migraine, Infant's Motrin, Midol Maximum Strength Cramp Formula, Motrin, Motrin Migraine Pain

■✦■ **Apo-Ibuprofen, Motrin IB Extra Strength, Motrin IB Super Strength, Novo-Profen, Nu-Ibuprofen**

Drug Class: Analgesic; NSAID

PHARMACOLOGY

Action
Decreases inflammation, pain, and fever, probably through inhibition of COX activity and prostaglandin synthesis.

Uses
Relief of symptoms of rheumatoid arthritis, osteoarthritis, mild to moderate pain, primary dysmenorrhea, reduction of fever.

Unlabeled Uses
Symptomatic treatment of juvenile rheumatoid arthritis, sunburn, resistant acne vulgaris.

Contraindications
Hypersensitivity to aspirin, iodides, or any other NSAID.

Usual Dosage
Mild to moderate pain
ADULTS: *PO:* 400 mg q 4 to 6 hr
OTC use (minor aches/pains, dysmenorrhea, fever reduction)
PO: 200 mg q 4 to 6 hr. Do not exceed 1.2 g in 24 hr or take for pain for more than 10 days or for fever for more than 3 days, unless directed by health care provider. Use smallest effective dose.

Pharmacokinetics
ABSORP: T_{max} is 1 to 2 hr. Bioavailability is less than 80%.
DIST: Vd is 0.15 L/kg. 99% protein bound.
EXCRET: Plasma $t_{1/2}$ is 1.8 to 2 hr. 45% to 79% is eliminated through the urine. Cl is 3 to 35 L/hr.

➔✦ DRUG INTERACTIONS

Angiotensin-converting enzyme inhibitors: Decreased antihypertensive effect (decreased prostaglandin
  • Monitor blood pressure.
Anticoagulants, oral: Increased bleeding (platelet inhibition)
  • Avoid concurrent use.
Aspirin: Inhibition of antiplatelet effect of aspirin (blocks access of aspirin to active site)
  • Avoid concurrent use.
Beta-adrenergic blockers: Decreased antihypertensive effect (decreased prostaglandin synthesis)
  • Monitor blood pressure.
Corticosteroids: Increased risk of peptic ulcer disease (additive)
  • Avoid concurrent use.

Furosemide: Decreased antihypertensive effect (decreased prostaglandin synthesis)
- Monitor vital signs.

Lithium: Lithium toxicity (decreased renal excretion)
- Avoid concurrent use.

Methotrexate: Possible methotrexate toxicity (decreased renal excretion)
- Avoid concurrent use.

Naltrexone: Possible increased risk of hepatotoxicity (mechanism unknown)
- Avoid concurrent use.

Thiazide diuretics: Decreased antihypertensive effect (decreased prostaglandin synthesis)
- Monitor blood pressure.

Valproate: Possible increased valproate toxicity (displacement from binding site)
- Monitor clinical status.

ADVERSE EFFECTS

CVS: Peripheral edema; water retention; worsening or precipitation of CHF.

CNS: Dizziness; lightheadedness; drowsiness; vertigo; headaches; aseptic meningitis.

GI: Gastric distress; occult blood loss; diarrhea; vomiting; nausea; heartburn; dyspepsia; anorexia; constipation; abdominal distress/cramps/pain; flatulence; indigestion; GI tract fullness.

MISC: Muscle cramps.

CLINICAL IMPLICATIONS

General
When recommended by DDS:
- *Lactation:* Undetermined.
- *Children:* Safety and efficacy not established.
- *Elderly:* Increased risk of adverse reactions.
- *Renal failure:* Increased risk of dysfunction in patients with preexisting renal disease.
- *GI effects:* Serious GI toxicity (e.g., bleeding, ulceration, perforation) can occur at any time, with or without warning symptoms.
- *Overdosage:* Drowsiness, lethargy, GI irritation/bleeding, nausea, vomiting, tinnitus, sweating, acute renal failure, epigastric pain, metabolic acidosis.

When prescribed by medical facility:
- Determine why drug is being taken. Consider implications of condition on dental treatment.
- If GI side effects occur, consider semisupine chair position.

Pregnancy Risk Category: Undetermined.

Oral Health Education
When recommended by DDS:
- Tell patient to take medication soon after meals or with food, milk, or antacids.
- Advise patient to discontinue drug and notify health care provider if any of the following occur: persistent GI upset or headache, skin rash, itching, visual disturbances, black stools, weight gain or edema, changes in urine pattern, joint pain, fever, blood in urine.
- Instruct patient not to take OTC preparation for more than 3 days for fever and more than 10 days for pain and to notify health care provider if condition does not improve.

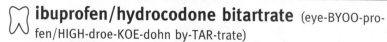 **ibuprofen/hydrocodone bitartrate** (eye-BYOO-pro-fen/HIGH-droe-KOE-dohn by-TAR-trate)

Synonym: hydrocodone bitartrate/ibuprofen

Vicoprofen: Tablets: 7.5 mg hydrocodone bitartrate and 200 mg ibuprofen

Drug Class: Analgesic, Antitussive, NSAID

DEA Schedule: Schedule III

PHARMACOLOGY

Action

HYDROCODONE: Suppresses cough reflex; stimulates opiate receptors in the CNS and peripherally blocks pain impulse generation.

IBUPROFEN: Decreases inflammation, pain, and fever, probably through inhibition of COX activity and prostaglandin synthesis.

Uses

Short-term (generally less than 10 days) management of acute pain. Not indicated for treatment of osteoarthritis or rheumatoid arthritis.

Contraindications

Hypersensitivity to hydrocodone, other opioids, ibuprofen, or other NSAIDs; patients who have experienced asthma, urticaria, or allergic-type reactions after taking aspirin or other NSAIDs.

Usual Dosage

ADULTS AND CHILDREN (16 YR AND OLDER): *PO:* 1 tablet q 4 to 6 hr (max, 5 tablets/24-hr period).

Pharmacokinetics

Ibuprofen

ABSORP: T_{max} is 1 to 2 hr. Bioavailability is less than 80%.

DIST: Vd is 0.15 L/kg. 99% protein bound.

EXCRET: Plasma $t_{1/2}$ is 1.8 to 2 hr. 45% to 79% is eliminated through the urine. Cl is 3 to 35 L/hr.

Hydrocodone

ABSORP: Hydrocodone is rapidly absorbed from the GI tract. T_{max} is acheived at 1.7 hr.

DIST: Distributed throughout the body. Not extensively protein bound.

METAB: Extensively metabolized in the liver to hydromorphone by *O*-demethylation by the CYP2D6 isoenzyme.

EXCRET: Hydrocodone and its metabolites are eliminated primarily in the kidneys.

ONSET: 30 min.

PEAK: 1.7 hr.

DURATION: 4.5 hr.

SPECIAL POP: *Severe renal insufficiency:* The effect of renal insufficiency on the pharmacokinetics of hydrocodone has not been determined.

➨◀ DRUG INTERACTIONS

See also: ibuprofen — Drug Interactions

No specific documented drug-drug interactions with hydrocodone. The absence of evidence is not evidence of safety.

ADVERSE EFFECTS

⚠ **ORAL:** Dry mouth (3% to 9%); mouth ulcer, thirst (<3%).

CVS: Palpitations, vasodilation (<3%); arrhythmia, hypotension, tachycardia (<1%).

CNS: Headache (27%); somnolence (22%); dizziness (14%); anxiety, insomnia, nervousness, paresthesia (3% to 9%); confusion, hypertonia, thinking abnormalities (<3%).

GI: Constipation (22%); nausea (21%); dyspepsia (12%); diarrhea, flatulence, vomiting (3% to 9%); anorexia, gastritis, melena (<3%).

RESP: Dyspnea, hiccups (<3%); pulmonary congestion, pneumonia (<1%).

MISC: Abdominal pain, asthenia, infection (3% to 9%); fever, flu-like symptoms, pain (<3%); allergic reaction (<1%).

CLINICAL IMPLICATIONS

General

When prescribed by DDS:

- Short-term use only; there is no justification for long-term use in the management of dental pain.
- *Lactation:* Undetermined.
- *Children:* Safety and efficacy in children younger than 16 yr not established.
- *Elderly:* Use with caution because of possible increased sensitivity to renal and GI effects of ibuprofen, as well as increased respiratory depression with hydrocodone.
- *Renal failure:* Use with caution and monitor kidney function in patients with advanced kidney disease.
- *Hepatic failure:* As with other NSAIDs, ibuprofen has been reported to cause borderline elevations of one or more liver enzymes; this may occur in up to 15% of patients.
- *Special risk:* Use with caution in elderly or debilitated patients and in those with hepatic or renal dysfunction, hypothyroidism, Addison disease, prostatic hypertrophy, or urethral stricture.
- *Aseptic meningitis:* Aseptic meningitis with fever and coma has been observed on rare occasions in patients on ibuprofen therapy. If signs or symptoms of meningitis develop in a patient on Vicoprofen, the possibility of its being related to ibuprofen should be considered.
- *Cough reflex:* Hydrocodone suppresses the cough reflex; as with opioids, caution should be exercised when Vicoprofen is used postoperatively and in patients with pulmonary disease.
- *Dependence:* Hydrocodone has abuse potential; may be habit forming and cause physical dependence.
- *Fluid retention and edema:* May occur, therefore, use with caution in patients with a history of cardiac decompensation, hypertension, or heart failure.
- *GI effects:* Serious GI toxicity (e.g., bleeding, ulceration, perforation) can occur at any time, with or without warning symptoms.
- *Hematological effects:* Ibuprofen, like other NSAIDs, can inhibit platelet aggregation but the effect is quantitatively less and of shorter duration than that seen with aspirin. Because this prolonged bleeding effect may be exaggerated in patients with underlying hemostatic defects, Vicoprofen should be used with caution in persons with intrinsic coagulation defects and those on anticoagulant therapy.
- *Preexisting asthma:* Patients with asthma may have aspirin-sensitive asthma. The use of aspirin in patients with aspirin-sensitive asthma has been associated with severe bronchospasm, which may be fatal. Because cross-reactivity between aspirin and other NSAIDs has been reported in such aspirin-sensitive patients, Vicoprofen should not be administered to patients with this form of aspirin sensitivity and should be used with caution in patients with preexisting asthma.
- *Overdosage:* HYDROCODONE: Respiratory depression, extreme somnolence progressing to stupor or coma, skeletal muscle flaccidity, cold and clammy skin, bradycardia, hypotension, apnea, circulatory collapse, cardiac arrest, death. IBUPROFEN: GI irritation with erosion; hemorrhage or perforation; kidney, liver, and heart damage; hemolytic anemia; meningitis; headache; dizziness; tinnitus; confusion; blurred vision; mental disturbances; skin rash; stomatitis; edema; reduced retinal sensitivity; corneal deposits; hyperkalemia.

When prescribed by medical facility:

- Determine why drug is being taken. Consider implications of condition on dental treatment.
- If GI side effects occur, consider semisupine chair position.
- Monitor vital signs.
- Chronic dry mouth is possible; anticipate increased caries and candidiasis.

Pregnancy Risk Category: Category C.

Oral Health Education

When prescribed by DDS:

- Explain name, dose, action, and potential side effects of drug.
- Advise patient to take 1 tablet q 4 to 6 hr if needed for pain but to not take more than 5 tablets in 24 hr.

- Advise patient to take without regard to meals but to take with food if GI upset occurs.
- Advise patient that medication is intended to be used for a short period of time (i.e., <10 days) for management of acute pain and is not for long-term use. If pain persists or is not controlled, advise patient to discuss other options for pain management with health care provider.
- Instruct patient to avoid alcoholic beverages and other depressants while taking this medication.
- Advise patient that drug may impair judgment, thinking, or motor skills or cause drowsiness, and to use caution while driving or performing other tasks requiring mental alertness until tolerance is determined.
- Advise patient to stop taking the drug and notify health care provider if any of the following occur: allergic reaction, unusual bleeding or bruising, shortness of breath, black or tarry stools, vomiting of blood or coffee-ground material, blurred vision, edema, excessive sedation.
- Advise women to notify health care provider if pregnant, planning to become pregnant, or breast feeding.
- Warn patient not to take any prescription or OTC drugs or dietary supplements without consulting health care provider.
- Advise patient that follow-up visits may be necessary to monitor therapy and to keep appointments.

When prescribed by medical facility:
- If chronic dry mouth occurs, recommend home fluoride therapy and use of nonalcoholic oral health care products.

 # ibuprofen/oxycodone (eye-BYOO-pro-fen/OX-ee-KOE-dohn)

Synonym: oxycodone/ibuprofen

Combunox: Tablet: 5 mg oxycodone HCl, 400 mg ibuprofen

Drug Class: Opioid/nonopioid analgesic combination

DEA Schedule: Schedule II

PHARMACOLOGY

Action
Oxycodone HCl is a centrally acting semisynthetic opioid analgesic with multiple actions, which involve binding to opiate receptors in the CNS and affects on smooth muscle. Ibuprofen is an NSAID with analgesic and antipyretic properties; action thought to be related to its inhibition of COX activity and prostaglandin synthesis.

Uses
Short-term (no more than 7 days) management of acute, moderate to severe pain.

Contraindications
Hypersensitivity to oxycodone or opioids, ibuprofen; respiratory depression; acute or severe bronchial asthma; hypercarbia; paralytic ileus; allergic-type reactions after taking aspirin or other NSAIDs; head injury; PUD; pregnancy category C (3rd trimester X). Warnings include patient with history of drug abuse or addiction; patients with hypotension or predisposed to circulatory shock; oxycodone affects center that controls respiratory rhythm, may produce irregular and periodic breathing; COPD or cor pulmonale; decreased respiratory reserve, hypoxia, hypercapnia, or preexisting respiratory depression. In these patients, therapeutic doses may decrease respiratory drive to the point of apnea. NSAIDs can promote GI bleeding, ulceration, and perforation of the stomach; be alert for GI symptoms in at-risk patients, as even short-term therapy is not without risk; Combunox not recommended in advanced kidney disease. Precautions include elderly or debilitated patient; severe impairment of hepatic, pulmonary, or renal function; hypothyroidism, Addison disease, acute alcoholism, convulsive disorders, CNS depression or coma, delirium tremens,

kyphoscoliosis associated with respiratory depression; toxic psychosis, prostatic hypertrophy or urethral stricture; biliary tract disease; acute pancreatitis; increased liver enzymes; dehydration; kidney disease; intrinsic coagulation defects; anticoagulant therapy; cardiac decompensation, hypertension, or heart failure; asthma; lactation.

Usual Dosage

Acute moderate to severe pain

ADULTS (AGE 14 AND OLDER): One tablet daily; not to exceed 4 tablets in a 24-hr period and not to exceed 7 days.
CHILDREN: Not studied in patients younger than age 14 yr.

Pharmacokinetics

ABSORP: Rapid absorption of oxycodone after single oral dose within 2 hr; repeated administration q6h does not result in accumulation of ibuprofen; bioavailability of ibuprofen not affected by food.
DIST: Protein binding of oxycodone is ~45%; ibuprofen extensively bound at 99%.
METAB: Liver metabolism of oxycodone to oxymorphone via CYP2D6 isoenzyme; ibuprofen undergoes interconversion in plasma from R-isomer to S-isomer, metabolized to phenyl propionic acids, which circulate in plasma at low levels.
EXCRET: Oxycodone eliminated with $t_{1/2}$ ranging from 1.8 to 2.6 hr after single dose; urinary excretion of unchanged ibuprofen minimal.
ONSET: 2 to 3 hr.
PEAK: 3 hr.
DURATION: 6 hr; no multiple dose efficacy studies have been performed.
SPECIAL POP: *Renal failure:* Precaution in kidney disease.
Elderly: Precaution in elderly.
Hepatic failure: Precaution in liver disease.
Gender: No gender effects on pharmacokinetics.

➥ DRUG INTERACTIONS

See also: ibuprofen — Drug Interactions
Oxycodone is additive with other CNS depressants.
Cimetidine: Oxycodone toxicity (decreased metabolism)
 • Monitor clinical status.

ADVERSE EFFECTS

⚠ ORAL: Dry mouth (<1%).
CNS: Somnolence (7.3%); dizziness (5.1%).
GI: Nausea (8.8%); vomiting (5.3%); flatulence (1%).
MISC: Sweating (1.6%).

CLINICAL IMPLICATIONS

General

 • If oral pain requires additional analgesics, consider nonopioid products.
 • *Geriatric patients:* Use lower dose of opioid.
 • Dry mouth is unlikely in short-term use. No justification for long-term use in the management of dental pain.

Pregnancy Risk Category: Category C (last trimester Category X).

Oral Health Education

 • *If prescribed by DDS:* Warn patient not to drive, sign important papers, or operate mechanical equipment.

Icar — see ferrous salts

Ifa Reduccing S — see phentermine HCl

Ilosone — see erythromycin

Ilotycin — see erythromycin

Ilotycin Gluceptate — see erythromycin
Ilsatec — see lansoprazole
Imdur — see isosorbide mononitrate
Imigran — see sumatriptan

imipramine HCl (im-IPP-ruh-meen HIGH-droe-KLOR-ide)
(imipramine pamoate)
Tofranil, Tofranil-PM
■✦■ Apo-Imipramine, Impril

■▨■ Talpramin

Drug Class: Tricyclic antidepressant

PHARMACOLOGY
Action
Inhibits reuptake of norepinephrine and, to a lesser degree, serotonin in CNS.

Uses
Relief of symptoms of depression; treatment of enuresis in children age 6 yr and older.

Unlabeled Uses
Treatment of chronic pain, panic disorder, eating disorders (bulimia nervosa), and facilitation of cocaine withdrawal.

✦← DRUG INTERACTIONS RELATED TO DENTAL THERAPEUTICS
Tramadol: Increased risk of seizures (additive)
• Avoid concurrent use.
Sympathomimetic amines: Hypertension or hypertensive crisis (additive)
• Monitor vital signs.

ADVERSE EFFECTS
⚠ **ORAL:** Dry mouth; taste disturbance; gingivitis; stomatitis; black tongue; aphthous stomatitis.
CNS: Confusion; hallucinations; delusions; nervousness; restlessness; agitation; panic; insomnia; nightmares; mania; exacerbation of psychosis; drowsiness; dizziness; weakness; numbness; extrapyramidal symptoms; emotional lability; seizures; tremors.
CVS: Arrhythmias; flushing; hypertension or hypotension; palpitations; orthostatic hypotension; tachycardia
GI: Nausea; vomiting; anorexia; GI distress; diarrhea; flatulence; constipation.
RESP: Pharyngitis; rhinitis; sinusitis; laryngitis; coughing.
MISC: Bone marrow depression (e.g., agranulocytosis, leukopenia, aplastic anemia, thrombocytopenia).

CLINICAL IMPLICATIONS
General
• Determine why drug is being taken. Consider implications of condition on dental treatment.
• Chronic dry mouth is possible; anticipate increased caries and candidiasis.
• Determine ability to adapt to stress of dental treatment. Consider short appointments.
• Depressed or anxious patients may neglect self-care. Monitor for plaque control effectiveness.
• *Postural hypotension:* Monitor BP at the beginning and end of each appointment; anticipate syncope. Have patient sit upright for several min at the end of the dental appointment before dismissing.

- Extrapyramidal behaviors can complicate performance of oral procedures. If present, consult with MD to consider medication changes.
- Blood dyscrasias rarely reported; anticipate increased bleeding, infection, and poor healing.
- Monitor vital signs.
- If GI side effects occur, consider semisupine chair position.

Oral Health Education
- Encourage daily plaque control procedures for effective, nontraumatic self-care.
- If chronic dry mouth occurs, recommend home fluoride therapy and use of nonalcoholic oral health care products.

---

imipramine pamoate — see imipramine HCl

Imitrex — see sumatriptan

Imodium — see loperamide HCl

Imodium A-D — see loperamide HCl

Impril — see imipramine HCl

Imuran — see azathioprine

---

indapamide (IN-DAP-uh-mide)
Lozol

■✦■ Apo-Indapamide, Gen-Indapamide, Lozide, Novo-Indapamide, Nu-Indapamide, PMS-Indapamide

Drug Class: Thiazide diuretic

PHARMACOLOGY
Action
Enhances excretion of sodium, chloride, and water by interfering with transport of sodium ions across renal tubular epithelium.

Uses
Treatment of edema associated with CHF, cirrhosis, renal dysfunction, and corticosteroid or estrogen therapy; management of hypertension.

Unlabeled Uses
Treatment of calcium nephrolithiasis, osteoporosis, or diabetes insipidus.

✦✦ DRUG INTERACTIONS RELATED TO DENTAL THERAPEUTICS
COX-1 inhibitors: Decreased antihypertensive effect (decreased prostaglandin synthesis)
- Monitor vital signs.

ADVERSE EFFECTS
⚠ ORAL: Dry mouth (<5%).
CNS: Dizziness; lightheadedness; vertigo; headache; weakness; restlessness; insomnia; drowsiness; fatigue; lethargy; anxiety; depression; nervousness.
CVS: Orthostatic hypotension, palpitations (<5%).
GI: Anorexia; gastric irritation; epigastric distress; nausea; vomiting; abdominal pain/cramping/bloating; diarrhea; constipation.
RESP: Rhinorrhea.
MISC: Muscle cramp or spasm; acute gout.

CLINICAL IMPLICATIONS
General
- Determine why drug is being taken. Consider implications of condition on dental treatment.

- Monitor vital signs (e.g., BP, pulse pressure, rate and rhythm) at each appointment to assess disease control. Do not provide elective dental treatment when BP is ≥180/110 or in presence of other high-risk CV conditions. Refer to the section entitled "The Patient Taking Cardiovascular Drugs" in Chapter 6: *Clinical Medicine*.
- Determine ability to adapt to stress of dental treatment. Consider short appointments.
- Use local anesthetic agents with vasoconstrictor with caution based on functional capacity of the patient and use aspirating technique to prevent intravascular injection.
- Monitor pulse rhythm to assess for electrolyte imbalance.
- Chronic dry mouth is possible; anticipate increased caries, candidiasis, and lichenoid mucositis.
- *Postural hypotension:* Monitor BP at the beginning and end of each appointment; anticipate syncope. Have patient sit upright for several min at the end of the dental appointment before dismissing.

Oral Health Education

- If chronic dry mouth occurs, recommend home fluoride therapy and use of nonalcoholic oral health care products.
- Encourage daily plaque control procedures for effective self-care in patient at risk for cardiovascular disease.

Indarzona — see dexamethasone

Inderal — see propranolol HCl

Inderal LA — see propranolol HCl

Inderalici — see propranolol HCl

---

indinavir sulfate (in-DIN-ah-veer SULL-fate)

Crixivan

Drug Class: Antiretroviral, protease inhibitor

PHARMACOLOGY

Action

Inhibits HIV protease, the enzyme that cleaves viral polyprotein precursors into functional proteins in HIV-infected cells. Inhibition of this enzyme by indinavir results in formation of immature noninfectious viral particles.

Uses

Treatment of HIV infection in adults when antiretroviral therapy is warranted.

➟← DRUG INTERACTIONS RELATED TO DENTAL THERAPEUTICS

No documented drug-drug interactions. The absence of evidence is not evidence of safety.

ADVERSE EFFECTS

⚠ **ORAL:** Dry mouth; altered taste.

CNS: Headache; insomnia; dizziness; somnolence; anxiety.

GI: Nausea; vomiting; diarrhea; anorexia; acid reflux; abdominal pain.

RESP: Cough.

MISC: Asthenia; fatigue; flank pain; back pain; chest pain; malaise; fever; flu-like symptoms.

CLINICAL IMPLICATIONS

General

- Determine why drug is being taken. Consider implications of condition on dental treatment.
- Consider medical consult to determine disease control and influence on dental treatment.

- This drug is frequently prescribed in combination with one or more other antiviral agents. Side effects of all agents must be considered during the drug review process.
- Antibiotic prophylaxis should be considered when <500 PMN/mm³ are reported; elective dental treatment should be delayed until blood values improve.
- Anticipate oral candidiasis when HIV disease is reported.
- Chronic dry mouth is possible; anticipate increased caries and candidiasis.
- If GI side effects occur, consider semisupine chair position.

Oral Health Education

- If chronic dry mouth occurs, recommend home fluoride therapy and use of nonalcoholic oral health care products.
- Encourage daily plaque control procedures for effective self-care.

Indocid — see indomethacin

Indocid P.D.A. — see indomethacin

Indocin — see indomethacin

Indocin IV — see indomethacin

Indocin SR — see indomethacin

---

indomethacin (in-doe-METH-uh-sin)

(indomethacin sodium trihydrate)

Indocin, Indocin IV, Indocin SR

■✦■ **Apo-Indomethacin, Indocid, Indocid P.D.A., Novo-Methacin, Nu-Indo, ratio-Indomethacin, Rhodacine**

■✦■ **Antalgin, Indocid, Malival**

Drug Class: Analgesic; NSAID

PHARMACOLOGY

Action

Decreases inflammation, pain, and fever, probably through inhibition of COX activity and prostaglandin synthesis.

Uses

INDOMETHACIN: Symptomatic treatment of rheumatoid arthritis, osteoarthritis, ankylosing spondylitis, gouty arthritis, acute painful shoulder.
INDOMETHACIN SODIUM TRIHYDRATE (IV): Closure of patent ductus arteriosus.

Unlabeled Uses

Treatment of primary dysmenorrhea; migraine prophylaxis; treatment of cluster headache, polyhydramnios, sunburn; cystoid macular edema.

➜✦ DRUG INTERACTIONS RELATED TO DENTAL THERAPEUTICS

No documented drug-drug interactions. The absence of evidence is not evidence of safety.

ADVERSE EFFECTS

CNS: Dizziness; headache; drowsiness; confusion.
CVS: Edema.
MISC: Ecchymoses, agranulocytosis, leukopenia, hemolytic anemia, aplastic anemia (<1%); fluid retention; hyperkalemia.
GI: Gastric distress; occult blood loss; nausea; diarrhea; vomiting; ulceration; perforation.
RESP: Pulmonary edema; dyspnea.

CLINICAL IMPLICATIONS

General
- Determine why drug is being taken. Consider implications of condition on dental treatment.
- Use COX inhibitors with caution, as they may exacerbate PUD and GERD.
- *Arthritis:* Consider patient comfort and need for semisupine chair position.
- Blood dyscrasias rarely reported; anticipate increased bleeding, infection, and poor healing.
- If GI or respiratory side effects occur, consider semisupine chair position.

Oral Health Education
- Evaluate manual dexterity; consider need for power toothbrush.

---

indomethacin sodium trihydrate — see indomethacin

Infant's Motrin — see ibuprofen

Infants' Pain Reliever — see acetaminophen

Infants' Silapap — see acetaminophen

Inflamase Forte — see prednisolone

Inflamase Mild — see prednisolone

---

infliximab (in-FLICK-sih-mab)

Remicade

Drug Class: Monoclonal antibody

PHARMACOLOGY

Action
Neutralizes the biological activity of TNF-alpha by binding to its soluble and transmembrane forms and inhibits TNF-alpha receptor binding.

Uses
Reduce signs and symptoms and induce and maintain clinical remission of moderate to severe Crohn disease; reduce number of draining enterocutaneous and rectovaginal fistulas and maintain fistula closure in Crohn disease; in combination with methotrexate to reduce signs and symptoms, inhibit progression of structural damage, and improve physical function in patients with moderately to severely active rheumatoid arthritis who have had inadequate response to methotrexate.

Unlabeled Uses
Treatment of plaque psoriasis, ankylosing spondylitis, ulcerative colitis, psoriatic arthritis, psoriasis, Behçet syndrome, uveitis, and juvenile arthritis.

➡◆ DRUG INTERACTIONS RELATED TO DENTAL THERAPEUTICS
No documented drug-drug interactions. The absence of evidence is not evidence of safety.

ADVERSE EFFECTS
CNS: Headache (29%); depression (8%); insomnia (6%); dizziness; confusion; suicide attempt; meningitis; neuritis; peripheral neuropathy.

GI: Nausea (24%); diarrhea (19%); abdominal pain (17%); dyspepsia (10%); vomiting; intestinal obstruction, perforation, and stenosis; pancreatitis; proctalgia; constipation; GI hemorrhage; ileus; peritonitis.

RESP: URI (40%); sinusitis (20%); coughing (18%); pharyngitis (17%); rhinitis (14%); dyspnea (6%); adult respiratory distress syndrome; bronchitis; pleurisy; respiratory insufficiency.

MISC: Infusion reactions (20%); fatigue, fever, back pain, arthralgia (13%); moniliasis (8%);

abscess (6%); lupus-like syndrome; pain; infections; myalgia; tendon disorder; cellulitis; sepsis; cholecystitis; chills; allergic reaction; diaphragmatic hernia; edema; surgical/procedural sequela; intervertebral disc herniation; neoplasms (e.g., blood cell, breast); serum sickness.

POSTMARKETING: Infections have been observed with various pathogens including viral, bacterial, fungal, and protozoal organisms and have been noted in all organ systems in patients receiving infliximab alone or in combination with immunosuppressive agents. Other adverse reactions reported during postmarketing experience include demyelinating disorders (e.g., multiple sclerosis), Guillain-Barré syndrome, interstitial pneumonitis, fibrosis, neuropathies, hemolytic anemia, idiopathic thrombocytic purpura, thrombotic thrombocytopenic purpura, and transverse myelitis. Anaphylactic-like reactions, including laryngeal/pharyngitis edema, severe bronchospasm, and seizure have been associated with infliximab administration.

CLINICAL IMPLICATIONS
General
- Determine why drug is being taken. Consider implications of condition on dental treatment.
- If GI side effects occur, consider semisupine chair position.
- Blood dyscrasias rarely reported; anticipate increased bleeding, infection, and poor healing.
- Most adverse drug reactions were due to infusion reactions. Appoint for dental procedures several days after infusion to avoid adverse effects.

Oral Health Education
- Encourage daily plaque control procedures for effective, nontraumatic self-care.

Infumorph — see morphine sulfate

INH — see isoniazid

Inhibitron — see omeprazole

InnoPran XL — see propranolol HCl

Insogen — see chlorpropamide

Inspiryl — see albuterol

insulin (IN-suh-lin)
(insulin zinc suspension 70% NPH, human insulin isophane suspension and 30% regular, human insulin injection ([rDNA] origin) NPH, isophane insulin suspension regular, insulin injection)

Humulin 70/30, Humulin N, Humulin R, Lente Iletin II, Novolin 70/30, Novolin L, Novolin N, Novolin R, Velosulin BR

■✦■ **Novolin ge 30/70, Novolin ge 40/60, Novolin ge 50/50, Novolin ge Lente, Novolin ge NPH, Novolin ge Toronto, Novolin ge Ultralente**

Drug Class: Antidiabetic, hormone replacement

PHARMACOLOGY
Action
Insulin and its analogs lower blood glucose levels by stimulating peripheral glucose uptake, especially by skeletal muscle and fat, and by inhibiting hepatic glucose production. Insulin inhibits lipolysis, proteolysis, and enhances protein synthesis. Insulin is composed of two amino acid chains (i.e., A [acidic] and B [basic]) joined together by disulfide linkage. Human insulin has minor but important differences from animal insulin with respect to amino acid sequence on the B-chain. It is derived from a biosynthetic process with strains of *Escherichia coli* (recombinant DNA [rDNA]) or yeast. In some patients, human insulin may have a more rapid onset and shorter duration of action than pork insulin. However, the bio-

availability of the insulins is identical when given SC. Human insulin is slightly less anti-genic than pork or beef insulins. Human insulin is also the insulin of choice for patients with insulin allergy, insulin resistance, all pregnant patients with diabetes, and any patient who uses insulin intermittently.

Uses
Management of type 1 diabetes mellitus (insulin-dependent) and type 2 diabetes mellitus (non-insulin-dependent) not properly controlled by diet, exercise, and weight reduction. In hyperkalemia, infusions of glucose and insulin lower serum potassium levels. IV or IM regular insulin may be given for rapid effect in severe ketoacidosis or diabetic coma. Highly purified (single component) and human insulins are used for treatment of local insulin allergy, immunologic insulin resistance, lipodystrophy at injection site, temporary insulin administration, and in newly diagnosed diabetic patients.

➨◀ DRUG INTERACTIONS RELATED TO DENTAL THERAPEUTICS
Aspirin: Possible increased hypoglycemic effect with large doses (mechanism unknown)
• Monitor clinical status.

ADVERSE EFFECTS
CVS: Arrhythmia (associated with hypokalemia).
MISC: Hypersensitivity reaction (e.g., rash, shortness of breath, fast pulse, sweating, hypotension, anaphylaxis, angioedema); local reactions (e.g., redness, swelling, itching at injection site); hypoglycemia; hypokalemia.

CLINICAL IMPLICATIONS
General
• Determine degree of disease control and current blood sugar levels. Goals should be <120 mg/dL and A1C <7%. A1C levels ≥8% indicate significant uncontrolled diabetes.
• The routine use of antibiotics in the dental management of diabetic patients is not indicated; however, antibiotic therapy in patients with poorly controlled diabetes has been shown to improve disease control and improve response after periodontal debridement.
• Monitor blood pressure because hypertension and dyslipidemia (CAD) are prevalent in diabetes mellitus.
• *Loss of blood sugar control:* Certain medical conditions (e.g., surgery, fever, infection, trauma) and drugs (e.g., corticosteroids) affect glucose control. In these situations, it may be necessary to seek medical consultation before surgical dental procedures.
• Obtain patient history regarding diabetic ketoacidosis or hypoglycemia with current drug regimen.
• Observe for signs of hypoglycemia (e.g., confusion, argumentativeness, perspiration, altered consciousness). Be prepared to treat hypoglycemic reactions with oral glucose or sucrose.
• Ensure patient has taken medication and eaten meal.
• Monitor vital signs (e.g., BP, pulse pressure, rate and rhythm) at each appointment to assess disease control. Do not provide elective dental treatment when BP is ≥180/110 or in presence of other high-risk CV conditions. Refer to the section entitled "The Patient Taking Cardiovascular Drugs" in Chapter 6: *Clinical Medicine*.
• Determine ability to adapt to stress of dental treatment. Consider short morning appointments.
• Medical consult advised if fasting blood glucose is <70 mg/dL (hypoglycemic risk) or >200 mg/dL (hyperglycemic crisis risk).
• Consider time of peak hypoglycemic effect of insulin preparation.

Oral Health Education
• Explain role of diabetes in periodontal disease and the need to maintain effective plaque control and disease control.
• Advise patient to bring data on blood sugar values and A1C levels to dental appointments.
• Encourage daily plaque control procedures for effective self-care in patient at risk for cardiovascular disease.

insulin injection — see insulin
insulin zinc suspension 70% NPH — see insulin
Intal — see cromolyn sodium
Invirase — see saquinavir mesylate
Ionamin — see phentermine HCl
Iosopan — see magaldrate

ipratropium bromide (IH-pruh-TROE-pee-uhm BROE-mide)

Atrovent

▮✦▮ **Apo-Ipravent, Combivent Inhalation Solution, Gen-Ipratropium, Novo-Ipramide, Nu-Ipratropium, PMS-Ipratropium, ratio-Ipratropium, ratio-Ipratropium UDV**

Drug Class: Respiratory inhalant; Anticholinergic

PHARMACOLOGY

Action

Antagonizes action of acetylcholine on bronchial smooth muscle in lungs, causing bronchodilation.

Uses

BRONCHOSPASM: Maintenance treatment of bronchospasm associated with COPD, including chronic bronchitis and emphysema, used alone or in combination with other bronchodilators (especially beta-adrenergics).

RHINORRHEA: Symptomatic relief of rhinorrhea associated with allergic and nonallergic rhinitis and symptomatic relief of rhinorrhea associated with the common cold in patients age 12 yr and older for aerosol and solution, 6 yr and older for 0.03% nasal spray, and 5 yr and older for 0.06% nasal spray.

➡◀ DRUG INTERACTIONS RELATED TO DENTAL THERAPEUTICS

No documented drug-drug interactions. The absence of evidence is not evidence of safety.

ADVERSE EFFECTS

⚠ ORAL: Dry mouth.
RESP: Cough; exacerbation of symptoms.
CNS: Nervousness; dizziness; headache.
GI: Nausea; GI distress; constipation.
MISC: Arthritis.

CLINICAL IMPLICATIONS

General

- Monitor vital signs (e.g., BP, pulse rate) and respiratory function. Uncontrolled disease characterized by wheezing, coughing.
- Acute bronchoconstriction can occur during dental treatment; have bronchodilator inhaler available.
- Ensure that bronchodilator inhaler is present at each dental appointment.
- Be aware that sulfites in local anesthetic with vasoconstrictor can precipitate acute asthma attack in susceptible individuals.
- Inhalants can dry oral mucosa; anticipate candidiasis, increased calculus, plaque levels, and caries.
- If GI side effects occur, consider semisupine chair position.

Oral Health Education

- If chronic dry mouth occurs, recommend home fluoride therapy and use of nonalcoholic oral health care products.
- Rinse mouth with water after bronchodilator use to prevent dryness.

---

ipratropium bromide/albuterol sulfate (IH-pruh-TROE-pee-umm BROE-mide al-BYOO-ter-ahl SULL-fate)

Synonym: albuterol sulfate/ipratropium bromide

Combivent, DuoNeb

Drug Class: Bronchodilator

PHARMACOLOGY

Action

ALBUTEROL: Produces bronchodilation by relaxing bronchial smooth muscle through $beta_2$-receptor stimulation.

IPRATROPIUM: Antagonizes action of acetylcholine on bronchial smooth muscle in lungs, causing bronchodilation.

Uses

Treatment of bronchospasm associated with COPD in patients requiring more than one bronchodilator.

➡️⬅ DRUG INTERACTIONS RELATED TO DENTAL THERAPEUTICS

No documented drug-drug interactions. The absence of evidence is not evidence of safety.

ADVERSE EFFECTS

⚠ ORAL: Dry mouth, taste disturbance (<2%).

CNS: Headache (6%); fatigue, dizziness, nervousness, tremor, paresthesia, insomnia (<2%); drowsiness; stimulation; coordination difficulty; weakness.

CVS: Tachycardia, palpitations (<3%).

GI: Nausea (2%); diarrhea, dyspepsia, vomiting (<2%); GI distress; constipation.

RESP: Bronchitis (12%); URI (11%); lung disease (6%); dyspnea (5%); coughing (4%); respiratory disorders (3%); sinusitis (2%); rhinitis, pneumonia (1%); paradoxical bronchospasm; wheezing; exacerbation of COPD symptoms.

MISC: Pain, chest pain (3%); influenza, leg cramps (1%); allergic-type reactions (e.g., skin rash, angioedema of tongue, lips, and face, laryngospasm, anaphylaxis), edema, increased sputum (<2%); heartburn; itching; flushing.

CLINICAL IMPLICATIONS

General

- Acute bronchoconstriction can occur during dental treatment; have bronchodilator inhaler available.
- Monitor vital signs (e.g., BP, pulse rate) and respiratory function. Uncontrolled disease characterized by wheezing, coughing.
- Ensure that bronchodilator inhaler is present at each dental appointment.
- Be aware that sulfites in local anesthetic with vasoconstrictor can precipitate acute asthma attack in susceptible individuals.
- Inhalants can dry oral mucosa; anticipate candidiasis, increased calculus, plaque levels, and caries.
- If GI side effects occur, consider semisupine chair position.

Oral Health Education

- If chronic dry mouth occurs, recommend home fluoride therapy and use of nonalcoholic oral health care products.

• Encourage daily plaque control procedures for effective self-care in patient at risk for cardiovascular disease.

---

irbesartan (ihr-beh-SAHR-tan)

Avapro

■◂▪ Aprovel

Drug Class: Antihypertensive; Angiotensin II antagonist

PHARMACOLOGY

Action

Antagonizes the effect of angiotensin II (vasoconstriction and aldosterone secretion) by blocking the angiotensin II (AT1 receptor) in vascular smooth muscle and the adrenal gland, producing decreased BP.

Uses

Treatment of hypertension; nephropathy in type 2 diabetes.

➡◂ DRUG INTERACTIONS RELATED TO DENTAL THERAPEUTICS

Fluconazole: Possible irbesartan toxicity (decreased metabolism)
• Monitor clinical status.

ADVERSE EFFECTS

CNS: Headache; anxiety/nervousness; dizziness.
CVS: Chest pain, tachycardia.
GI: Diarrhea; dyspepsia/heartburn; abdominal pain; nausea/vomiting.
RESP: Upper respiratory tract infection; influenza; pharyngitis; rhinitis; sinus abnormality.
MISC: Musculoskeletal pain/trauma; fatigue; UTI; rash.

CLINICAL IMPLICATIONS

General

• Monitor vital signs (e.g., BP, pulse pressure, rate and rhythm) at each appointment to assess disease control. Do not provide elective dental treatment when BP is ≥180/110 or in presence of other high-risk CV conditions. Refer to the section entitled "The Patient Taking Cardiovascular Drugs" in Chapter 6: *Clinical Medicine*.
• Use local anesthetic agents with vasoconstrictor with caution based on functional capacity of the patient and use aspirating technique to prevent intravascular injection.
• Determine ability to adapt to stress of dental treatment. Consider short, afternoon appointments.

Oral Health Education

• Encourage daily plaque control procedures for effective self-care in patient at risk for cardiovascular disease.

Ircon — see ferrous salts

Isadol — see zidovudine

Isavir — see acyclovir

ISMO — see isosorbide mononitrate

Isodine — see povidone iodine

Isoket — see isosorbide dinitrate

isoniazid (eye-so-NYE-uh-zid)

Synonym: isonicotinic acid hydrazide; INH

Isoniazid, Nydrazid

■✦■ **Isotamine, PMS-Isoniazid**

Drug Class: Anti-infective; Antitubercular

PHARMACOLOGY

Action
Interferes with lipid and nucleic acid biosynthesis in actively growing tubercle bacilli.

Uses
Treatment of all forms of tuberculosis.

Unlabeled Uses
Improvement of severe tremor in multiple sclerosis.

➡◀ DRUG INTERACTIONS RELATED TO DENTAL THERAPEUTICS

Acetaminophen: Acetaminophen toxicity (increase in toxic metabolites)
• Avoid concurrent use.
Diazepam: Increased IV diazepam toxicity (decreased metabolism)
• Monitor clinical status.
Triazolam: Possible triazolam toxicity (decreased metabolism)
• Monitor clinical status.

ADVERSE EFFECTS

CNS: Peripheral neuropathy; convulsions; toxic encephalopathy; optic neuritis and atrophy; memory impairment; toxic psychosis.
GI: Nausea; vomiting; epigastric distress.
MISC: Gynecomastia; elevated liver enzymes, jaundice; rheumatic syndrome; systemic lupus erythematosus–like syndrome.

CLINICAL IMPLICATIONS

General
• Determine why drug is being taken (prevention or treatment). Consider implications of condition on dental treatment.
• Complete medical consult to ensure noninfectious state exists before providing dental treatment.
• *For dental emergencies:* Follow special precautions to minimize disease transmission (particulate respirators) or refer patient to a hospital-based dental facility.
• This drug causes elevated liver enzymes in 20% of cases and reduced liver function; this may affect drug selection during dental treatment.

---

isonicotinic acid hydrazide — see isoniazid
isophane insulin suspension regular — see insulin
Isoptin — see verapamil HCl
Isoptin I.V. — see verapamil HCl
Isoptin SR — see verapamil HCl
Isopto Atropine — see atropine
Isopto-Carpine — see pilocarpine HCl
Isopto Hyoscine — see scopolamine HBr
Isorbid — see isosorbide dinitrate

Isordil — see isosorbide dinitrate
Isordil Titradose — see isosorbide dinitrate

isosorbide dinitrate (EYE-sos-ORE-bide die-NYE-trate)

Dilatrate-SR, Isordil, Isordil Titradose, Sorbitrate

▌✦▌ APO-ISDN

▌✦▌ Isoket, Isorbid

Drug Class: Antianginal

PHARMACOLOGY

Action
Relaxation of smooth muscle of venous and arterial vasculature.

Uses
Treatment and prevention of angina pectoris.

➧✦ DRUG INTERACTIONS RELATED TO DENTAL THERAPEUTICS
No documented drug-drug interactions. The absence of evidence is not evidence of safety.

ADVERSE EFFECTS
⚠ **ORAL:** Tooth disorder (unspecified).
CNS: Headache; apprehension; weakness; vertigo; dizziness; agitation; insomnia.
CVS: Hypotension, palpitations, arrhythmia, tachycardia, postural hypotension.
GI: Nausea; vomiting; diarrhea; dyspepsia.
RESP: Bronchitis; pneumonia.
MISC: Arthralgia; perspiration; pallor; cold sweat; edema.

CLINICAL IMPLICATIONS

General
- Determine why drug is being taken. Consider implications of condition on dental treatment. Question regarding recent history of angina.
- Monitor vital signs (e.g., BP, pulse pressure, rate; and rhythm) at each appointment to assess disease control. Do not provide elective dental treatment when BP is ≥180/110 or in presence of other high-risk CV conditions. Refer to the section entitled "The Patient Taking Cardiovascular Drugs" in Chapter 6: *Clinical Medicine.*
- Use local anesthetic agents with vasoconstrictor with caution based on functional capacity of the patient and use aspirating technique to prevent intravascular injection.
- Determine ability to adapt to stress of dental treatment. Consider short appointments.
- *Postural hypotension:* Monitor BP at the beginning and end of each appointment; anticipate syncope. Have patient sit upright for several min at the end of the dental appointment before dismissing.

Oral Health Education
- Encourage daily plaque control procedures for effective self-care in patient at risk for cardiovascular disease.

---

isosorbide mononitrate (EYE-sos-ORE-bide MAH-no-NYE-trate)

Imdur, ISMO, Isotrate ER, Monoket

▌✦▌ Elantan, Mono Mack

Drug Class: Antianginal

PHARMACOLOGY

Action
Relaxation of smooth muscle of venous and arterial vasculature.

Uses
Prevention of angina pectoris.

➔← DRUG INTERACTIONS RELATED TO DENTAL THERAPEUTICS

No documented drug-drug interactions. The absence of evidence is not evidence of safety.

ADVERSE EFFECTS

⚠ **ORAL:** Tooth disorder (unspecified).

CNS: Headache; apprehension; weakness; vertigo; dizziness; agitation; insomnia.

CVS: Hypotension; palpitations; arrhythmia; tachycardia; postural hypotension.

GI: Nausea; vomiting; diarrhea; dyspepsia.

MISC: Arthralgia; perspiration; pallor; cold sweat; edema.

CLINICAL IMPLICATIONS

General

- Determine why drug is being taken. Consider implications of condition on dental treatment. Question regarding recent history of angina.
- Monitor vital signs (e.g., BP, pulse pressure, rate and rhythm) at each appointment to assess disease control. Do not provide elective dental treatment when BP is ≥180/110 or in the presence of other high-risk CV conditions. Refer to the section entitled "The Patient Taking Cardiovascular Drugs" in Chapter 6: *Clinical Medicine*.
- Use local anesthetic agents with vasoconstrictor with caution based on functional capacity of the patient and use aspirating technique to prevent intravascular injection.
- Determine ability to adapt to stress of dental treatment. Consider short appointments.
- *Postural hypotension:* Monitor BP at the beginning and end of each appointment; anticipate syncope. Have patient sit upright for several min at the end of the dental appointment before dismissing.

Oral Health Education

- Encourage daily plaque control procedures for effective self-care in patient at risk for cardiovascular disease.

Isotamine — see isoniazid

Isotrate ER — see isosorbide mononitrate

---

isotretinoin (EYE-so-TREH-tih-NO-in)

Synonym: 13-cis-retinoic acid

Accutane, Claravis

■✦■ **Accutane Roche, Isotrex**

■▦■ **Roaccutan**

Drug Class: Acne

PHARMACOLOGY

Action

Reduces sebum secretion and sebaceous gland size, inhibits sebaceous gland differentiation, and alters sebum lipid composition.

Uses

Treatment of severe recalcitrant cystic acne.

Unlabeled Uses

Treatment of keratinization disorders, cutaneous T-cell lymphoma, leukoplakia; prevention of skin cancer in patients with xeroderma pigmentosum.

➔← DRUG INTERACTIONS RELATED TO DENTAL THERAPEUTICS

No documented drug-drug interactions. The absence of evidence is not evidence of safety.

ADVERSE EFFECTS

⚠ **ORAL:** Dry lips, mouth; herpes simplex; gingival bleeding, gingivitis.

CNS: Fatigue; headache; pseudotumor cerebri (e.g., benign intracranial hypertension with headache, visual disturbances, and papilledema); dizziness; drowsiness; insomnia; lethargy; malaise; nervousness; paresthesias; seizures; stroke; weakness; suicidal ideation; suicide attempts; suicide; psychosis; emotional instability; aggression; violent behaviors.
CVS: Palpitations; tachycardia; thrombotic disease; syncope.
GI: Nausea; vomiting; abdominal pain; nonspecific GI symptoms; anorexia; inflammatory bowel disease; esophagitis/esophageal ulceration.
RESP: Bronchospasms, with or without a history of asthma; respiratory infections; voice alterations.
MISC: Flushing; reversibly elevated triglycerides; increased cholesterol level; vasculitis (including Wegener granulomatosis); lymphadenopathy; edema; neutropenia, agranulocytosis; photosensitization.

CLINICAL IMPLICATIONS
General
- Determine why drug is being taken. Consider implications of condition on dental treatment.
- *Dryness and chapping of lips:* Apply protective ointment to lips before oral procedures.
- Chronic dry mouth is possible; anticipate increased caries and candidiasis.
- If GI side effects occur, consider semisupine chair position.

Oral Health Education
- If chronic dry mouth occurs, recommend home fluoride therapy and use of nonalcoholic oral health care products.

Isotrex — see isotretinoin

---

isradipine (iss-RAHD-ih-peen)
DynaCirc, DynaCirc CR
Drug Class: Calcium channel blocker

PHARMACOLOGY
Action
Reduces systemic vascular resistance and BP by inhibiting movement of calcium ions across cell membrane in systemic and coronary vascular smooth muscle and myocardium.
Uses
Treatment of hypertension.

➜← DRUG INTERACTIONS RELATED TO DENTAL THERAPEUTICS
No documented drug-drug interactions. The absence of evidence is not evidence of safety.

ADVERSE EFFECTS
⚠ **ORAL:** Gingival hyperplasia, dry mouth (uncommon).
CNS: Dizziness; lightheadedness; headache; fatigue; lethargy; weakness; shakiness; psychiatric disturbances.
CVS: Tachycardia; palpitations; chest pain.
GI: Nausea; diarrhea; constipation; abdominal discomfort; cramps; dyspepsia; vomiting.
RESP: Shortness of breath; dyspnea; wheezing.
MISC: Transient ischemic attack; stroke; leukopenia (<1%).

CLINICAL IMPLICATIONS
General
- Monitor vital signs (e.g., BP, pulse pressure, rate and rhythm) at each appointment to assess disease control. Do not provide elective dental treatment when BP is ≥180/110 or in presence of other high-risk CV conditions. Refer to the section entitled "The Patient Taking Cardiovascular Drugs" in Chapter 6: *Clinical Medicine*.

- Use local anesthetic agents with vasoconstrictor with caution based on functional capacity of the patient and use aspirating technique to prevent intravascular injection.
- Determine ability to adapt to stress of dental treatment. Consider short appointments.
- Anticipate gingival hyperplasia; consider MD consult to recommend different drug regimen if periodontal health is compromised.
- Blood dyscrasias rarely reported; anticipate increased infection and poor healing.

Oral Health Education
- Encourage daily plaque control procedures for effective self-care in patient at risk for cardiovascular disease.

Istalol — see timolol maleate

Italnik — see ciprofloxacin

---

itraconazole (ih-truh-KAHN-uh-zole)
Sporanox

Drug Class: Anti-infective; Antifungal

PHARMACOLOGY

Action
Inhibits synthesis of ergosterol, which is a vital component of fungal cell membranes. Also inhibits endogenous respiration, causes accumulation of phospholipids and unsaturated fatty acids within fungal cells, and disrupts chitin synthesis.

Uses
INJECTION: Treatment of aspergillosis, blastomycosis, febrile neutropenia, and histoplasmosis.
CAPSULES: Treatment of aspergillosis, blastomycosis, histoplasmosis, and onychomycosis.
ORAL SOLUTION: Treatment of oropharyngeal or esophageal candidiasis and empirical treatment of febrile neutropenia.

Unlabeled Uses
Treatment of other fungal infections (superficial mycoses [e.g., dermatophytoses]; systemic mycoses [e.g., candidiasis, cryptococcus]; and miscellaneous fungal infections [e.g., SC mycoses, cutaneous *Leishmaniasis*]).

➜◆ DRUG INTERACTIONS RELATED TO DENTAL THERAPEUTICS
Midazolam: Midazolam toxicity (decreased metabolism)
- Avoid concurrent use.

ADVERSE EFFECTS
Incidence and type of reactions vary depending on usage and route of administration. In general, the adverse reactions listed occur in at least 1% of the patients treated.
⚠ ORAL: Stomatitis, gingivitis.
CNS: Headache; dizziness; decreased libido; somnolence; vertigo; anxiety; depression; abnormal dreaming.
CVS: Hypertension.
GI: Nausea; vomiting; diarrhea; abdominal pain; anorexia; flatulence; constipation; dyspepsia; gastritis; gastroenteritis; increased appetite; general GI disorders.
RESP: Coughing; dyspnea; pneumonia; sinusitis; sputum increased; rhinitis; URI; pharyngitis.
MISC: Edema; fatigue; fever; malaise; myalgia; bursitis; pain; injury; chest pain; back pain; *Pneumocystis carinii* infection; herpes zoster; application site reaction; vein disorder; asthenia; tremor; hypertriglyceridemia; abnormal liver function, hypokalemia.

CLINICAL IMPLICATIONS

General

- Determine why drug is being taken. Consider implications of condition on dental treatment.
- *If prescribed by the DDS:* Ensure patient knows how to take the drug, how long it should be taken, and to immediately report adverse effects (e.g., rash, difficult breathing, diarrhea, GI upset). See Chapter 4: *Medical Management of Odontogenic Infections*.
- This drug is associated with severe liver failure in patients with no prior history of liver disease; monitor pharmacokinetics of dental drugs used.
- Monitor vital signs (e.g., BP, pulse rate) and respiratory function.
- If GI side effects occur, consider semisupine chair position.

Oral Health Education

- *Oral candidiasis:* Teach patient how to disinfect removable prostheses.
- Recommend new toothbrush be used after resolution of oral infection.

Jaa Prednisone — see prednisone

Junior Strength Advil — see ibuprofen

Junior Strength Motrin — see ibuprofen

K + 8 — see potassium products

K + 10 — see potassium products

Kadian — see morphine sulfate

Kaoch — see potassium products

Kaochlor-20 Concentrate — see potassium products

Kaon — see potassium products

Kaon-Cl — see potassium products

Kaon Cl-10 — see potassium products

Kaon-Cl 20% — see potassium products

Kaopectate II Caplets — see loperamide HCl

Kapanol — see morphine sulfate

Karidium — see sodium fluoride

Karigel — see sodium fluoride

Karigel-N — see sodium fluoride

Kasmal — see ketotifen fumarate

Kay Ciel — see potassium products

Kaylixir — see potassium products

K + Care — see potassium products

K + Care ET — see potassium products

K-Dur 10 — see potassium products

K-Dur 20 — see potassium products

Keduril — see ketoprofen

Keflex — see cephalexin

Keftab — see cephalexin

Kenacort — see triamcinolone

Kenalin — see sulindac

Kenalog-10 — see triamcinolone
Kenalog-40 — see triamcinolone
Kenalog-H — see triamcinolone
Kenalog in Orabase — see triamcinolone
Kenalog — see triamcinolone
Kenamil — see zidovudine
Kenaprol — see metoprolol
Kenoket — see clonazepam
Kenolan — see captopril
Kenopril — see enalapril maleate
Kenzoflex — see ciprofloxacin
Keppra — see levetiracetam
KeriCort-10 — see hydrocortisone
Kerlone — see betaxolol HCl
Ketek — see telithromycin

---

 ketoconazole (KEY-toe-KOE-nuh-zole)

Nizoral: Tablets: 200 mg; Cream: 2% in an aqueous vehicle; Shampoo: 2% in an aqueous suspension

■✦■ **Apo-Ketoconazole, Novo-Ketoconazole**

■■ **Akorazol, Conazol, Cremosan, Fungoral, Konaderm, Mycodib, Onofin-K, Termizol, Tiniazol**

Drug Class: Anti-infective; Antifungal

PHARMACOLOGY

Action
Impairs synthesis of ergosterol, allowing increased permeability in fungal cell membrane and leakage of cellular components.

Uses
Treatment of susceptible systemic and cutaneous fungal infections.
TOPICAL: Seborrheic dermatitis; tinea corporis; tinea cruris; tinea pedis; tinea versicolor.

Contraindications
Fungal meningitis.

Usual Dosage
ADULTS: PO: 200 to 400 mg once a day. *Topical:* Apply to affected and immediate surrounding area once a day for 2 to 4 wk.
CHILDREN OLDER THAN 2 YR: PO: 3.3 to 6.6 mg/kg/day. Treatment may last from 1 wk to 6 mo, depending on infection.

Pharmacokinetics
ABSORP: C_{max} is approximately equal to 3.5 mcg/mL (with a 200-mg dose taken with a meal). T_{max} is 1 to 2 hr. Requires acidity for dissolution and absorption. Absorbed in the GI.
DIST: Approximately 99% protein bound (in vitro), mainly to the albumin fraction. Only a negligible proportion reaches the cerebrospinal fluid.
METAB: Major metabolic pathways are oxidation and degradation of the imidazole and pi-

perazine, oxidative O-dealkylation, and aromatic hydroxylation. It is converted into several inactive metabolites.

EXCRET: Approximately 13% of dose is excreted in urine; 2% to 4% is unchanged drug. The major route of excretion is through the bile into the intestinal tract. Plasma elimination is biphasic with $t_{1/2}$ of 2 hr during the first 10 hr and $t_{1/2}$ of 8 hr after 10 hr.

➜← DRUG INTERACTIONS

Alcohol: Possible disulfiram-like reaction (mechanism unknown)
• Avoid concurrent use.

Amprenavir: Possible toxicity of ketoconazole and amprenavir (decreased metabolism)
• Avoid concurrent use.

Antacids: Decreased ketoconazole effect (decreased absorption)
• Avoid concurrent use or administer 2 hr apart.

Anticoagulants, oral: Increased anticoagulant effect (decreased metabolism)
• Avoid concurrent use or monitor INR.

Benzodiazepines: Benzodiazepine toxicity (decreased metabolism)
• Monitor clinical status.

Bosentan: Possible increased risk of bosentan toxicity (decreased metabolism)
• Monitor clinical status.

Carbamazepine: Possible carbamazepine toxicity (decreased metabolism)
• Monitor clinical status.

Cilostazol: Possible cilostazol toxicity (decreased metabolism)
• Monitor clinical status.

Cimetidine or ranitidine: Decreased ketoconazole effect (decreased absorption)
• Avoid concurrent use.

Corticosteroids: Possible corticosteroid toxicity (decreased metabolism)
• Monitor clinical status.

Cyclosporine: Renal toxicity (decreased metabolism)
• Avoid concurrent use or monitor cyclosporine concentration.

Delavirdine: Possible delavirdine toxicity (decreased metabolism)
• Monitor clinical status.

Desloratadine: Possible desloratadine toxicity (decreased metabolism)
• Monitor clinical status.

Didanosine: Possible decreased didanosine and ketoconazole effect (decreased absorption)
• Administer 2 hr apart.

Dofetilide: Increased risk of cardiac arrhythmias (decreased metabolism)
• Avoid concurrent use.

Ergot alkaloids: Increased risk of serious vasospastic effect (decreased metabolism)
• Avoid concurrent use.

Esomeprazole: Possible decreased ketoconazole effect (decreased absorption)
• Avoid concurrent use.

Galantamine: Possible increased galantamine effect (decreased metabolism)
• Monitor clinical status.

Imatinib: Possible imatinib toxicity (decreased metabolism)
• Monitor clinical status.

Indinavir: Possible indinavir and ketoconazole toxicity (decreased metabolism)
• Avoid concurrent use of monitor concentration of both drugs.

Isoniazid: Decreased ketoconazole concentration (decreased absorption)
• Avoid concurrent use.

Lansoprazole: Possible decreased ketoconazole effect (decreased absorption)
• Avoid concurrent use.

Lopinavir/ritonavir: Possible ketoconazole toxicity (decreased metabolism)
• Avoid ketoconazole dose greater than 200 mg/day.

Loratadine: Possible loratadine toxicity (decreased metabolism)
• Monitor clinical status.

Lovastatin or simvastatin: Rhabdomyolysis (decreased metabolism)
- Avoid concurrent use.

Nisoldipine: Possible increased risk of nisoldipine toxicity (decreased metabolism)
- Monitor clinical status.

Omeprazole: Decreased ketoconazole effect (decreased absorption); possible decreased omeprazole toxicity (decreased metabolism)
- Avoid concurrent use.

Pantoprazole: Possible decreased ketoconazole effect (decreased absorption)
- Avoid concurrent use.

Pimozide: Increased risk of ventricular arrhythmias (decreased metabolism)
- Avoid concurrent use.

Phenytoin: Altered effect of ketoconazole and/or phenytoin (mechanism unknown)
- Avoid concurrent use.

Quinidine: Possible quinidine toxicity (decreased metabolism)
- Avoid concurrent use.

Rabeprazole: Possible decreased ketoconazole effect (decreased absorption)
- Avoid concurrent use.

Rifabutin: Uveitis (decreased metabolism)
- Monitor clinical status.

Rifampin: Decreased ketoconazole effect (increased metabolism)
- Avoid concurrent use.

Ritonavir: Possible ritonavir and ketoconazole toxicity (mutual decreased metabolism)
- Monitor clinical status.

Saquinavir: Possible saquinavir toxicity (decreased metabolism)
- Monitor clinical status.

Sibutramine: Possible sibutramine toxicity (decreased metabolism)
- Monitor clinical status.

Sirolimus: Possible sirolimus toxicity (decreased metabolism)
- Avoid concurrent use.

Sucralfate: Possible decreased ketoconazole effect (decreased metabolism)
- Avoid concurrent use.

Tacrolimus: Possible tacrolimus toxicity (decreased metabolism)
- Avoid concurrent use or monitor tacrolimus concentration.

Theophylline: Possible decreased theophylline effect (increased metabolism)
- Avoid concurrent use or monitor theophylline concentration.

Tolbutamide: Increased risk of hypoglycemia (decreased metabolism)
- Monitor blood glucose.

Triptans: Possible triptan toxicity (decreased metabolism)
- Monitor clinical status.

Verapamil: Possible verapamil toxicity (decreased metabolism)
- Monitor clinical status.

Ziprasidone: Possible increased ziprasidone toxicity (decreased metabolism)
- Monitor clinical status.

Zolpidem: Possible zolpidem toxicity (decreased metabolism)
- Monitor clinical status.

ADVERSE EFFECTS

CNS: Headache; dizziness; somnolence.
GI: Nausea; vomiting; abdominal pain.
MISC: Tablet: Hepatotoxicity; thrombocytopenia, leukopenia, hemolytic anemia.
Cream: Pruritus, stinging (5%); cream contains sulfites.

CLINICAL IMPLICATIONS

General
- Determine why drug is being taken. Blood dyscrasias rarely reported; anticipate increased bleeding, infection, and poor healing.

If prescribed by DDS:
- Ensure patient knows how to take the drug, how long it should be taken and to immediately report adverse effects (e.g., rash, difficult breathing, diarrhea, GI upset). See Chapter 4: *Medical Management of Odontogenic Infections*.
- Be aware that cream contains sulfites; do not prescribe when sulfite sensitivity is reported.
- *Lactation:* Undetermined.
- *Children:* Safety and efficacy in children younger than 2 yr not established (PO). Safety and efficacy not established (topical).
- *Anaphylaxis:* Has occurred after the first dose.
- *Gastric acidity:* Ketoconazole requires acid environment for dissolution and absorption.
- *Hormone levels:* May lower serum testosterone or suppress adrenal corticosteroid secretion.

Pregnancy Risk Category: Category C.

Oral Health Education
- If prescribed by the DDS for oral infection, teach patient to clean and disinfect removable appliances daily and to replace toothbrush following resolution of infection.
- Instruct patient that if a dose is missed, take it as soon as possible. If several hr have passed or if close to the time of next dose, do not double up. Notify health care provider if more than one dose is missed.
- Advise patient not to take medication with antacids. If antacids are required, take ketoconazole 2 hr before antacid.
- Emphasize importance of completing full course of therapy, even if signs and symptoms resolve. Advise patient that maintenance therapy may be required for chronic infections.
- Instruct patient to notify health care provider if severe irritation, itching, or stinging occurs after application.
- Instruct patient to report the following symptoms to the health care provider: fatigue, loss of appetite, nausea, vomiting, yellowing of skin, dark urine, pale stools, abdominal pain, fever, diarrhea.
- Advise patient that drug may cause drowsiness and to use caution while driving or performing other tasks requiring mental alertness.
- Instruct patient not to take OTC medications, including antihistamine, without consulting health care provider.

---

ketoprofen (KEY-toe-PRO-fen)

Orudis, Orudis KT, Oruvail

■✷■ **APO-Keto, APO-Keto SR, APO-Keto-E, Novo-Keto, Novo-Keto-EC, Nu-Ketoprofen, Nu-Ketoprofen-SR, Orudis SR, Rhodis, Rhodis SR, Rhodis-EC, Rhovai**

■✧■ **Keduril, K-Profen, Profenid**

Drug Class: Analgesic; NSAID

PHARMACOLOGY

Action
Decreases inflammation, pain, and fever, probably through inhibition of COX activity and prostaglandin synthesis.

Uses
Treatment of rheumatoid arthritis, osteoarthritis, mild to moderate pain, primary dysmenorrhea.

SUSTAINED-RELEASE FORM ONLY: Treatment of rheumatoid arthritis and osteoarthritis.

OTC USE: Temporary relief of minor aches and pains associated with common cold, headache, toothache, muscular aches, backache, minor arthritis pain, menstrual cramps, and reduction of fever.

Unlabeled Uses

Treatment of juvenile rheumatoid arthritis, sunburn, migraine prophylaxis.

➡️⬅️ DRUG INTERACTIONS RELATED TO DENTAL THERAPEUTICS

No documented drug-drug interactions. The absence of evidence is not evidence of safety.

ADVERSE EFFECTS

⚠️ **ORAL:** Stomatitis (3%), dry mouth, taste disturbance (1%).

CNS: Headache; dizziness; lightheadedness; drowsiness; vertigo.

GI: Peptic ulcer; GI bleeding; dyspepsia (11%); nausea, diarrhea, constipation, abdominal pain (3% to 9%); flatulence; anorexia; vomiting.

RESP: Bronchospasm; laryngeal edema; rhinitis; dyspnea.

MISC: Renal function impairment, increased blood urea nitrogen, edema (3% to 9%); agranulocytosis, thrombocytopenia, anemia (<1%).

CLINICAL IMPLICATIONS

General

- Determine why drug is being taken. Consider implications of condition on dental treatment.
- Use COX inhibitors with caution; they may exacerbate PUD and GERD.
- *Arthritis:* consider patient comfort and need for semisupine chair position.
- If GI side effects occur, consider semisupine chair position.
- Blood dyscrasias rarely reported; anticipate increased bleeding, infection, and poor healing.

Oral Health Education

- If chronic dry mouth occurs, recommend home fluoride therapy and use of nonalcoholic oral health care products.
- Encourage daily plaque control procedures for effective, nontraumatic self-care.
- Evaluate manual dexterity; consider need for power toothbrush.

---

ketorolac tromethamine (KEY-TOR-oh-lak tro-METH-uh-meen)

Acular, Acular LS, Toradol

■✦■ **Apo-Ketorolac, Apo-Ketorolac Injection, Novo-Ketorolac, Toradol I**

■✦■ **Acularen, Alidol, Dola, Dolac, Dolotor, Findol**

Drug Class: Analgesic; NSAID

PHARMACOLOGY

Action

Decreases inflammation, pain, and fever, probably through inhibition of COX activity and prostaglandin synthesis.

Uses

ORAL AND IM FORMS: Short-term management of moderately severe, acute pain.
OPHTHALMIC FORM: Relief of ocular itching caused by seasonal allergic conjunctivitis; treatment of postoperative inflammation in patients who have undergone cataract extraction.

➡️⬅️ DRUG INTERACTIONS RELATED TO DENTAL THERAPEUTICS

No documented drug-drug interactions. The absence of evidence is not evidence of safety.

ADVERSE EFFECTS

⚠️ **ORAL:** Stomatitis (3%); dry mouth.

CNS: Headache (17%); dizziness (7%); drowsiness (6%); sweating (>1%).

CVS: Hypertension (3%).

GI: GI pain (13%); dyspepsia, nausea (12%); diarrhea (7%); constipation, flatulence, GI fullness, vomiting (>1%).

RESP: Bronchospasm.

MISC: Purpura (3%), edema (4%), injection site pain (>1%); muscle cramps; aseptic meningitis; anemia; eosinophilia.

CLINICAL IMPLICATIONS

General
- Determine why drug is being taken and which dose form. Consider implications of condition on dental treatment.
- Side effects least likely to occur with topical dose form.
- Use COX inhibitors with caution; they may exacerbate PUD and GERD.
- *Arthritis:* Consider patient comfort and need for semisupine chair position.
- If GI side effects occur, consider semisupine chair position.
- Monitor vital signs.

Oral Health Education
- Evaluate manual dexterity; consider need for power toothbrush.

---

ketotifen fumarate (KEY-toe-TIF-fen FEW-mah-rate)
Zaditor

■◆■ **Kasmal, Ventisol, Zaditen**

Drug Class: Antihistamine, ophthalmic

PHARMACOLOGY

Action
Inhibits release of mediators from cells involved in hypersensitivity reactions.

Uses
Temporary prevention of itching of eyes caused by allergic conjunctivitis.

➡◀ DRUG INTERACTIONS RELATED TO DENTAL THERAPEUTICS
No documented drug-drug interactions. The absence of evidence is not evidence of safety.

ADVERSE EFFECTS
CNS: Headache (10% to 25%).
MISC: Flu-like syndrome (<5%); photophobia.

CLINICAL IMPLICATIONS

General
- *Photophobia:* Direct dental light out of patient's eyes and offer dark glasses for comfort.

Key-Pred 25 — see prednisolone
Key-Pred 50 — see prednisolone
Key-Pred-SP — see prednisolone
K-G Elixir — see potassium products
Klaricid — see clarithromycin
Klonopin — see clonazepam
Klonopin Wafers — see clonazepam
K-Lor — see potassium products
Klor-Con — see potassium products
Klor-Con 8 — see potassium products

Klor-Con 10 — see potassium products
Klor-Con/25 — see potassium products
Klor-Con/EF — see potassium products
Klor-Con M10 — see potassium products
Klor-Con M15 — see potassium products
Klor-Con M20 — see potassium products
Klorvess — see potassium products
Klotrix — see potassium products
K Lyte — see potassium products
K Lyte DS — see potassium products
K Lyte/Cl — see potassium products
K Lyte/Cl 50 — see potassium products
Koffex DM — see dextromethorphan HBr
Kolyum — see potassium products
Konaderm — see ketoconazole
K-Profen — see ketoprofen
K-10 Solution — see potassium products
K-Tab — see potassium products
K-vescent Potassium Chloride — see potassium products

---

labetalol HCl (la-BET-uh-lahl HIGH-droe-KLOR-ide)

Normodyne, Trandate

■✦■ **Apo-Labetalol**

■✦■ **Midotens**

Drug Class: Alpha-adrenergic blocker; Beta-adrenergic blocker

PHARMACOLOGY

Action
Selectively blocks alpha-1 receptors and nonselectively blocks beta-receptors to decrease BP, heart rate, and myocardial oxygen demand.

Uses
Management of hypertension.

Unlabeled Uses
Treatment of pheochromocytoma; management of clonidine-withdrawal hypertension.

➔← DRUG INTERACTIONS RELATED TO DENTAL THERAPEUTICS

COX-1 inhibitors: Reduced antihypertensive effect (reduced prostaglandin synthesis)
• Monitor blood pressure.
Sympathomimetic amines: Decreased antihypertensive effect (pharmacological antagonism)
• Monitor blood pressure.

ADVERSE EFFECTS
⚠ **ORAL:** Bullous lichen planus.

CNS: Headache; fatigue; dizziness; depression; lethargy; drowsiness; forgetfulness; sleepiness; vertigo; paresthesia; nightmares.

GI: Nausea; vomiting; diarrhea; dyspepsia.

RESP: Bronchospasm; shortness of breath; wheezing.

MISC: Muscle cramps; systemic lupus erythematosus; increased hypoglycemic response to insulin; masking of hypoglycemic signs; asthenia; agranulocytosis; thrombocytopenia; purpura.

CLINICAL IMPLICATIONS

General

- Monitor vital signs (e.g., BP, pulse pressure, rate and rhythm) at each appointment to assess disease control. Do not provide elective dental treatment when BP is ≥180/110 or in the presence of other high-risk CV conditions. Refer to the section entitled "The Patient Taking Cardiovascular Drugs" in Chapter 6: *Clinical Medicine.*
- Use local anesthetic agents with vasoconstrictor with caution based on functional capacity of the patient and use aspirating technique to prevent intravascular injection.
- Determine ability to adapt to stress of dental treatment. Consider short appointments.
- Beta blockers may mask epinephrine-induced signs and symptoms of hypoglycemia in patient with diabetes.
- Blood dyscrasias rarely reported; anticipate increased bleeding, infection, and poor healing.
- If GI side effects occur, consider semisupine chair position.
- Chronic dry mouth is possible; anticipate increased caries candidiasis, and lichenoid mucositis.

Oral Health Education

- Encourage daily plaque control procedures for effective self-care in patient at risk for cardiovascular disease.

Laciken — see acyclovir
LactiCare-HC — see hydrocortisone
Lamictal — see lamotrigine
Lamictal Chewable Dispersible — see lamotrigine
Lamisil — see terbinafine
Lamisil AT — see terbinafine

---

lamivudine (la-MIH-view-deen)

Synonym: 3TCZ

Epivir, Epivir-HBV

■✦■ **Heptovir**

Drug Class: Antiretroviral, nucleoside reverse transcriptase inhibitor

PHARMACOLOGY

Action

Inhibits replication of HIV and hepatitis B virus (HBV).

Uses

HIV Infection

EPIVIR: In combination with other antiretroviral agents for the treatment of HIV infection.

Chronic HBV Infection

EPIVIR-HBV: Treatment of chronic HBV associated with evidence of HBV replication and active liver inflammation.

➡◀ DRUG INTERACTIONS RELATED TO DENTAL THERAPEUTICS

No documented drug-drug interactions. The absence of evidence is not evidence of safety.

ADVERSE EFFECTS

⚠ **ORAL:** Throat infection; stomatitis.

CNS: Headache; neuropathy; dizziness; sleep disturbances; depression; insomnia and other sleep disorders; depressive disorders.

GI: Nausea; vomiting; diarrhea; anorexia; abdominal pain/cramps; dyspepsia.

RESP: Nasal signs and symptoms; cough; paresthesia; abnormal breath sounds/wheezing.

MISC: Malaise; fatigue; fever; chills; myalgia; arthralgia; pancreatitis; elevated liver enzymes; musculoskeletal pain; anaphylaxis; urticaria; rhabdomyolysis; peripheral neuropathy; hepatic steatosis; muscle weakness with creatine phosphokinase elevation; posttreatment exacerbation of hepatitis; redistribution/accumulation of body fat.

CLINICAL IMPLICATIONS

General

- Determine why drug is being taken. Consider implications of condition on dental treatment.
- This drug is frequently prescribed in combination with one or more other antiviral agents. Side effects of all agents must be considered during the drug review process.
- Antibiotic prophylaxis should be considered when <500 PMN/mm^3 are reported; elective dental treatment should be delayed until blood values improve above this level.
- Consider medical consult to determine disease control and influence on dental treatment.
- Anticipate oral candidiasis when HIV disease is reported.

Oral Health Education

- Encourage daily plaque control procedures for effective self care since HIV infection reduces host resistance.

---

lamivudine/zidovudine (la-MIH-view-deen/zie-DOE-view-DEEN)

Synonym: zidovudine/lamivudine

Combivir

Drug Class: Antiviral combination

PHARMACOLOGY

Action

Inhibits replication of HIV by incorporation into HIV DNA and producing an incomplete, nonfunctional DNA.

Uses

Treatment of HIV infection.

➡◀ DRUG INTERACTIONS RELATED TO DENTAL THERAPEUTICS

Fluconazole: Possible zidovudine toxicity (decreased metabolism)
- Avoid concurrent use.

Clarithromycin: Possible decreased zidovudine effect (mechanism unknown)
- Avoid concurrent use.

ADVERSE EFFECTS

CNS: Headache; fatigue; neuropathy; insomnia; dizziness; depression.

GI: Nausea; diarrhea; vomiting; anorexia; abdominal pain; abdominal cramps; dyspepsia.

RESP: Cough.

MISC: Malaise; fever; chills; myalgia; arthralgia; musculoskeletal pain.

CLINICAL IMPLICATIONS
General
- Determine why drug is being taken. Consider implications of condition on dental treatment.
- This drug is frequently prescribed in combination with one or more other antiviral agents. Side effects of all agents must be considered during the drug review process.
- Antibiotic prophylaxis should be considered when <500 PMN/mm³ are reported; elective dental treatment should be delayed until blood values improve above this level.
- Consider medical consult to determine disease control and influence on dental treatment.
- Anticipate oral candidiasis when HIV disease is reported.

Oral Health Education
- Encourage daily plaque control procedures for effective self-care since HIV infection reduces host resistance.

---

lamotrigine (lah-MOE-trih-JEEN)
Lamictal, Lamictal Chewable Dispersible

Drug Class: Anticonvulsant

PHARMACOLOGY
Action
Chemically unrelated to existing antiepileptic drugs (AEDs); precise mechanism(s) unknown. One proposed mechanism suggests inhibition of voltage-sensitive sodium channels, thereby stabilizing neuronal membranes, which modulates presynaptic transmitter release of excitatory amino acids (e.g., glutamate, aspartate).

Uses
BIPOLAR DISORDER: Maintenance treatment of bipolar I disorder to delay the time to occurrence of mood episodes in patients treated for acute mood episodes with standard therapy.

EPILEPSY: Adjunctive therapy in the treatment of partial seizures in adults and as adjunctive therapy in the generalized seizures of Lennox-Gastaut syndrome in pediatric and adult patients. Conversion to monotherapy in adults with partial seizures who are receiving treatment with a single enzyme-inducing AED.

Unlabeled Uses
May be useful in adults with generalized tonic-clonic, absence, atypical absence, and myoclonic seizures.

➡◀ DRUG INTERACTIONS RELATED TO DENTAL THERAPEUTICS
No documented drug-drug interactions. The absence of evidence is not evidence of safety.

ADVERSE EFFECTS
⚠ ORAL: Dry mouth (6%); tooth disorder (3%, unspecified).

CNS: Dizziness (38%); headache (29%); ataxia (22%); somnolence (14%); insomnia (10%); abnormal coordination (7%); incoordination, anxiety (5%); asthenia (≥5%); tremor, depression (4%); convulsions, irritability, speech disorder (3%); concentration disturbance, seizure exacerbation (2%).

GI: Nausea (19%); vomiting (9%); dyspepsia (7%); abdominal pain, diarrhea (6%); constipation (5%); anorexia (2%).

RESP: Rhinitis (14%); pharyngitis (10%); increased cough (8%); sinusitis (≥5%).

MISC: Back pain, fatigue (8%); flu-like syndrome (7%); fever (6%); lymphadenopathy, infection, pain, weight decrease (≥5%); neck pain, arthralgia (2%); photosensitivity (2%).

CLINICAL IMPLICATIONS

General

- Determine why drug is being taken. Consider implications of condition on dental treatment.
- Determine ability to adapt to stress of dental treatment. Consider short appointments.
- Determine level of disease control, type and frequency of seizure, and compliance with medication regimen.
- Monitor for respiratory side effects; consider semisupine chair position.
- Chronic dry mouth is possible; anticipate increased caries and candidiasis.

Oral Health Education

- Evaluate manual dexterity; consider need for power toothbrush.
- If chronic dry mouth occurs, recommend home fluoride therapy and use of nonalcoholic oral health care products.

Lampicin — see ampicillin

Lanacort 5 — see hydrocortisone

Lanacort 10 — see hydrocortisone

Lanacort Maximum Strength Cool Creme — see hydrocortisone

Lanexat — see flumazenil

Lanophyllin — see theophylline

Lanoxicaps — see digoxin

Lanoxin — see digoxin

---

lansoprazole (lan-SO-pruh-zole)

Prevacid, Prevacid I.V.

■■■ **Ilsatec, Ogastro, Ulpax**

Drug Class: GI

PHARMACOLOGY

Action

Suppresses gastric acid secretion by blocking "acid (proton) pump" within gastric parietal cells.

Uses

ORAL: Short-term treatment of active duodenal ulcer; to maintain healing of duodenal ulcers; short-term treatment of all grades of erosive esophagitis; maintenance of healing of erosive esophagitis; long-term treatment of pathological hypersecretory conditions, including Zollinger-Ellison syndrome; in combination with amoxicillin plus clarithromycin or amoxicillin alone (in patients intolerant of or resistant to clarithromycin) for the eradication of *Helicobacter pylori* in patients with active or recurrent duodenal ulcers; short-term treatment and symptomatic relief of active benign gastric ulcer (including NSAID-associated gastric ulcer in patients who continue NSAID use and for reducing risk of NSAID-associated gastric ulcer in patients with a history of NSAID-associated gastric ulcer); treatment of heartburn and other symptoms of GERD.

IV: Short-term treatment (up to 7 days) of all grades of erosive esophagitis.

➔ DRUG INTERACTIONS RELATED TO DENTAL THERAPEUTICS

Ketoconazole and itraconazole: Possible decreased ketoconazole and itraconazole effect (decreased absorption)

- Monitor clinical status.

Clarithromycin: Possible stomatitis, glossitis, and black tongue (mechanism unknown)
- Avoid concurrent use.

ADVERSE EFFECTS
CNS: Headache (>1%).
GI: Diarrhea (4%); abdominal pain (2%); constipation, nausea (1%); pancreatitis; vomiting.
MISC: Injection site pain/reaction (IV, 1%); anaphylactoid reactions.

CLINICAL IMPLICATIONS
General
- If patient has GI disease, consider semisupine chair position.
- Drugs that lower acidity in intestinal tract may interfere with absorption of some antibiotics (e.g., penicillin, tetracyclines).
- Use COX inhibitors with caution, they may exacerbate PUD and GERD.
- Anticipate chemical erosion of teeth.
- Substernal pain (heartburn) may mimic pain of cardiac origin.

Oral Health Education
- Inform patient that toothbrushing should not be done after reflux, but to only rinse mouth with water, then use home fluoride product to minimize chemical-erosion caries.

Largactil — see chlorpromazine HCl
Lasix — see furosemide
Lasix Special — see furosemide

---

latanoprost (lah-TAN-oh-prahst)
Xalatan

Drug Class: Ophthalmic prostaglandin agonist

PHARMACOLOGY
Action
Prostaglandin F_{2a} analog that reduces intraocular pressure (IOP) by increasing the output of aqueous humor.

Uses
For reduction of elevated IOP in patients with open-angle glaucoma or ocular hypertension.

➡️⬅ DRUG INTERACTIONS RELATED TO DENTAL THERAPEUTICS
No documented drug-drug interactions. The absence of evidence is not evidence of safety.

ADVERSE EFFECTS
RESP: URI, cold, flu (4%).
MISC: Muscle/joint/back pain; photophobia.

CLINICAL IMPLICATIONS
General
- *Photophobia:* Direct dental light out of patient's eyes and offer dark glasses for comfort.

Latotryd — see erythromycin
Lauricin — see erythromycin
Lauritran — see erythromycin
L-deprenyl — see selegiline HCl
Ledercort — see triamcinolone

Lederpax — see erythromycin
Ledertrexate — see methotrexate

leflunomide (leh-FLEW-nah-mide)
Arava
Drug Class: Antirheumatic agent

PHARMACOLOGY
Action
An isoxazole immunomodulatory agent that inhibits dihydro-orotate dehydrogenase and has antiproliferative and anti-inflammatory activity.

Uses
Treatment of active rheumatoid arthritis to reduce signs and symptoms and to retard structural damage.

➶➕ DRUG INTERACTIONS RELATED TO DENTAL THERAPEUTICS
No documented drug-drug interactions. The absence of evidence is not evidence of safety.

ADVERSE EFFECTS
⚠ **ORAL:** Dry mouth, mouth ulcers (3%); gingivitis; aphthous stomatitis; tooth disorder; taste disturbance; candidiasis.
CNS: Dizziness; headache; paresthesia; anxiety; depression; insomnia; neuralgia; neuritis; sleep disorder; vertigo; migraine.
CVS: Hypertension (10%), chest pain (2%), palpitations; tachycardia.
GI: Abdominal pain; anorexia; diarrhea; dyspepsia; gastroenteritis; nausea; vomiting.
RESP: Bronchitis; increased cough; respiratory infection; pharyngitis; pneumonia; rhinitis; sinusitis; asthma; dyspnea; epistaxis; lung disorder.
MISC: Peripheral edema; weight loss; UTI; asthenia; flu-like syndrome; infection; injury, accident; pain; back pain; fever; hernia; malaise; neck pain; pelvic pain; increased sweating; anemia; ecchymoses.

CLINICAL IMPLICATIONS
General
• Determine why drug is being taken. Consider implications of condition on dental treatment.
• *Arthritis:* Consider patient comfort and need for semisupine chair position.
• Monitor vital signs.
• Chronic dry mouth is possible; anticipate increased caries and candidiasis.
• If GI side effects occur, consider semisupine chair position.
• Place on frequent maintenance schedule to avoid periodontal inflammation.

Oral Health Education
• If hands are affected, consider recommendation of powered devices for plaque control.
• If chronic dry mouth occurs, recommend home fluoride therapy and use of nonalcoholic oral health care products.

Lenpryl — see captopril
Lente Iletin II — see insulin
Leponex — see clozapine
Leptilan — see valproic acid and derivatives
Leptopsique — see perphenazine
Lertamine — see loratadine

Lertamine-D — see pseudoephedrine
Lescol — see fluvastatin
Lescol XL — see fluvastatin

---

levalbuterol HCl (lev-al-BYOO-ter-ol HIGH-droe-KLOR-ide)
Xopenex, Xopenex HFA
Drug Class: Bronchodilator; Sympathomimetic

PHARMACOLOGY
Action
Produces bronchodilation by relaxing bronchial smooth muscles via beta$_2$-adrenergic receptor stimulation.

Uses
Treatment or prevention of bronchospasm in patients with reversible obstructive airway disease.

➡️ DRUG INTERACTIONS RELATED TO DENTAL THERAPEUTICS
Pilocarpine: Increased myopia (mechanism unknown)
• Monitor clinical status.

ADVERSE EFFECTS
⚠ **ORAL:** Dry mouth.

CNS: Dizziness, nervousness, tremor, anxiety, hypesthesia of the hand, insomnia, paresthesia; headache (children 6 to 11 yr of age).

GI: Dyspepsia; diarrhea; gastroenteritis; nausea.

RESP: Increased cough; viral infection.

MISC: Flu-like symptoms, accidental injury, pain, leg cramps, lymphadenopathy, myalgia; abdominal pain, asthma, fever (children 6 to 11 yr of age).

CLINICAL IMPLICATIONS
General
• Monitor vital signs (e.g., BP, pulse rate) and respiratory function. Uncontrolled disease characterized by wheezing, coughing.
• Acute bronchoconstriction can occur during dental treatment; have bronchodilator inhaler available.
• Ensure that bronchodilator inhaler is present at each dental appointment.
• Be aware that sulfites in local anesthetic with vasoconstrictor can precipitate acute asthma attack in susceptible individuals.
• Inhalants can dry oral mucosa; anticipate candidiasis, increased calculus, plaque levels, and caries.

Oral Health Education
• Rinse mouth with water after bronchodilator use to prevent dryness.
• If chronic dry mouth occurs, recommend home fluoride therapy and use of nonalcoholic oral health care products.

Levaquin — see levofloxacin
Levatol — see penbutolol sulfate
Levbid — see hyoscyamine sulfate

---

levetiracetam (lev-eh-TEER-ah-see-tam)
Keppra
Drug Class: Anticonvulsant

PHARMACOLOGY

Action

Mechanism unknown; may selectively prevent hypersynchronization of epileptiform burst firing and propagation of seizure activity.

Uses

Adjunctive therapy in partial onset seizures in adults with epilepsy.

➜← DRUG INTERACTIONS RELATED TO DENTAL THERAPEUTICS

No documented drug-drug interactions. The absence of evidence is not evidence of safety.

ADVERSE EFFECTS

The following adverse reaction figures were obtained when levetiracetam was added to concomitant antiepileptic drug therapy. The reported frequencies provide one basis to estimate the relative contribution to adverse event incidences.

⚠ **ORAL:** Gingivitis.

CNS: Somnolence (15%); headache (14%); dizziness (9%); depression, nervousness (4%); ataxia, vertigo (3%); amnesia, anxiety, emotional lability, hostility, paresthesia (2%); confusion, convulsion, grand mal convulsion, insomnia, abnormal thinking, tremor ($\geq$1%).

GI: Anorexia (3%); constipation, diarrhea, dyspepsia, gastroenteritis, nausea, vomiting ($\geq$1%).

RESP: Increased cough (2%); bronchitis ($\geq$1%).

MISC: Asthenia (15%); infection (13%, unspecified); pain (7%); abdominal pain, accidental injury, back pain, fever, flu-like syndrome, fungal infection, chest pain, weight gain ($\geq$1%); leukopenia; thrombocytopenia; neutropenia; pancytopenia.

CLINICAL IMPLICATIONS

General

- Determine why drug is being taken. Consider implications of condition on dental treatment.
- Determine ability to adapt to stress of dental treatment. Consider short appointments.
- Determine level of disease control, type and frequency of seizure, and compliance with medication regimen.
- Blood dyscrasias rarely reported; anticipate increased bleeding, infection, and poor healing.
- This drug is often used in combination with other anticonvulsants that have their own side effect profile to consider.

Oral Health Education

- Evaluate manual dexterity; consider need for power toothbrush.

Levitra — see vardenafil HCl

---

levodopa/carbidopa (LEE-voe-DOE-puh/CAR-bih-doe-puh)

Synonym: carbidopa/levodopa

Sinemet 10/100, Sinemet 25/100, Sinemet 25/250, Sinemet CR

■✦■ **Apo-Levocarb, Novo-Levocarbidopa, Nu-Levocarb**

■✦■ **Racovel**

Drug Class: Antiparkinson

PHARMACOLOGY

Action

Levodopa is precursor of dopamine, which is deficient in parkinsonism patients. Carbidopa has no activity of its own but inhibits decarboxylation of levodopa, making it more available to brain.

Uses

Treatment of symptoms of idiopathic Parkinson disease (paralysis agitans), postencephalitic parkinsonism, and symptomatic parkinsonism associated with carbon monoxide and manganese poisoning.

➜← DRUG INTERACTIONS RELATED TO DENTAL THERAPEUTICS

Benzodiazepines: Decreased levodopa effect (mechanism unknown)
- Use benzodiazepines with caution.

ADVERSE EFFECTS

⚠ **ORAL:** Dry mouth; burning tongue; bitter taste.

CNS: Paranoid delusions; psychotic episodes; depression; suicidal ideation; dementia; convulsions; hallucinations; dizziness; choreiform; dystonic and other involuntary movements.

CVS: Postural hypotension (5%).

GI: Nausea; anorexia; vomiting; GI distress; epigastric pain; GI bleeding; duodenal ulcer.

MISC: Positive Coombs test result; flushing; malaise.

CLINICAL IMPLICATIONS

General

- Determine why drug is being taken. Consider implications of condition on dental treatment.
- Extrapyramidal behaviors associated with Parkinson disease can complicate access to oral cavity and complicate oral procedures.
- Chronic dry mouth is possible; anticipate increased caries and candidiasis.
- *Postural hypotension:* Monitor BP at the beginning and end of each appointment; anticipate syncope. Have patient sit upright for several min at the end of the dental appointment before dismissing.
- If GI side effects occur, consider semisupine chair position.

Oral Health Education

- Evaluate manual dexterity; consider need for power toothbrush.
- If chronic dry mouth occurs, recommend home fluoride therapy and use of nonalcoholic oral health care products.

---

levofloxacin (lee-voe-FLOX-ah-sin)

Levaquin, Quixin

▉◆▉ **Elequine, Tavanic**

Drug Class: Antibiotic, fluoroquinolone

PHARMACOLOGY

Action

Interferes with microbial DNA synthesis.

Uses

Treatment of acute maxillary sinusitis, acute bacterial exacerbation of chronic bronchitis, nosocomial pneumonia, community-acquired pneumonia, skin and skin structure infections, chronic bacterial prostatitis, UTI, and acute pyelonephritis caused by susceptible strains of specific microorganisms.

OPHTHALMIC USE: Treatment of conjunctivitis caused by susceptible strains of aerobic gram-positive and aerobic gram-negative microorganisms.

➜← DRUG INTERACTIONS RELATED TO DENTAL THERAPEUTICS

Corticosteroids: Possible increased risk of Achilles tendon disorder (mechanism unknown)
- Consider risk/benefit.

ADVERSE EFFECTS

⚠ **ORAL:** Dry, painful mouth (>1%).

CNS: Headache (6%); insomnia (5%); dizziness (3%); anxiety, fatigue (1%); abnormal EEG; encephalopathy.

GI: Nausea (7%); diarrhea (6%); constipation, abdominal pain (3%); dyspepsia, vomiting (2%); flatulence (1%).

RESP: Dyspnea (1%); allergic pneumonitis.

MISC: Pain, chest pain, back pain (1%); anaphylactic shock; anaphylactoid reactions; dysphonia; multisystem organ failure; leukopenia; tendon rupture.

CLINICAL IMPLICATIONS

General

- Determine why drug is being taken. Take precautions to avoid cross-contamination of microorganisms.
- If oral infection occurs that requires antibiotic therapy, select an appropriate product from a different class of anti-infectives.
- Prolonged use of antibiotics may result in bacterial or fungal overgrowth of nonsusceptible microorganisms; anticipate candidiasis.

Levothroid — see levothyroxine sodium

---

levothyroxine sodium (lee-voe-thigh-ROX-een SO-dee-uhm)

Synonym: L-thyroxine; T4

Levothroid, Levoxyl, Synthroid

◼◗◼ **Eutirox, Tiroidine**

Drug Class: Thyroid hormone

PHARMACOLOGY

Action

Increases metabolic rate of body tissues; is needed for normal growth and maturation.

Uses

Replacement or supplemental therapy in hypothyroidism; TSH suppression (in thyroid cancer, nodules, goiters, and enlargement in chronic thyroiditis).

➡◀ DRUG INTERACTIONS RELATED TO DENTAL THERAPEUTICS

No documented drug-drug interactions. The absence of evidence is not evidence of safety.

ADVERSE EFFECTS

CNS: Tremors; headache; nervousness; insomnia.

CVS: Palpitations, tachycardia, hypertension, increased pulse pressure, arrhythmia (high doses).

GI: Diarrhea; vomiting.

MISC: Hypersensitivity; weight loss; menstrual irregularities; sweating; heat tolerance; fever; decreased bone density (in women using levothyroxine long term).

CLINICAL IMPLICATIONS

General

- Be aware that uncontrolled thyroid disease poses a risk for CV events during dental treatment; elevated doses of thyroid hormone mimic signs of hyperthyroid disease.
- Monitor blood pressure and pulse rate to determine degree of thyroid disease control.
- Use local anesthetic agents with a vasoconstrictor with caution. Thyroid hormones and epinephrine are synergistic; use aspiration technique.

Levoxyl — see levothyroxine sodium
Levsin — see hyoscyamine sulfate
Levsin Drops — see hyoscyamine sulfate
Levsinex Timecaps — see hyoscyamine sulfate
Levsin/SL — see hyoscyamine sulfate
Lexapro — see escitalopram oxalate
Librium — see chlordiazepoxide
Lidex — see fluocinonide
Lidex-E — see fluocinonide

 lidocaine HCl (LIE-doe-cane HIGH-droe-KLOR-ide)

DentiPatch: Patch: 23/2 cm² patch, 46.1/2 cm² patch
Octocaine: Injection: 2% with 1:50,000 epinephrine, 2% with 1:100,000 epinephrine
Xylocaine: Solution: 4%; Jelly: 2%
Xylocaine Viscous: Solution: 2%
Xylocaine HCl: Injection: 0.5% with 1:200,000 epinephrine, 1% with 1:100,000 epinephrine, 1% with 1:200,000 epinephrine, 2% with 1:50,000 epinephrine, 2% with 1:100,000 epinephrine, 2% with 1:200,000 epinephrine, 1.5% with 7.5% dextrose
Xylocaine MPF: Injection: 1% with 1:200,000 epinephrine, 1.5% with 1:200,000 epinephrine, 2% with 1:200,000 epinephrine
Zilactin-L: Liquid: 2.5%
Anestacon, Burn-o-Jel, DermaFlex, Dilocaine, Duo-Trach Kit, ELA-Max, Lidocaine HCl for Cardiac Arrhythmias, Lidocaine HCl in 5% Dextrose, Lidoject-1, Lidoject-2, Lidopen Auto-Injector, Nervocaine, Numby Stuff, Solarcaine Aloe Extra Burn Relief, Xylocaine HCl IV for Cardiac Arrhythmias, Xylocaine MPF

■✦■ **Lidodan Endotracheal, Lidodan Ointment, Lidodan Viscous, Xylocaine CO2, Xylocaine Endotracheal, Xylocaine 4% Sterile Solution, Xylocaine Spinal 5%, Xylocard**

■✦■ **Pisacaina, Uvega, Xylocaina**

Drug Class: Antiarrhythmic; Local anesthetic

PHARMACOLOGY

Action
Attenuates phase 4 diastolic depolarization, decreases automaticity, decreases action potential duration, and raises ventricular fibrillation threshold; inhibits conduction of nerve impulses from sensory nerves.

Uses
Acute management of ventricular arrhythmias; topical anesthesia in local skin disorders; local anesthesia of accessible mucous membranes.

Unlabeled Uses
Intraosseous or endotracheal administration to pediatric patients with cardiac arrest.

Contraindications
Hypersensitivity to amide local anesthetics; Stokes-Adams syndrome; Wolff-Parkinson-White syndrome; severe degrees of sinuatrial, AV, or intraventricular block in absence of pacemaker; ophthalmic use.

Usual Dosage

4.5 mg/kg (not to exceed 300 mg).
ADULTS: *IM:* 300 mg. May be repeated after 60 to 90 min. *Patch:* Apply patch and allow to remain in place until the desired anesthetic effect is produced for up to 15 min. Use the lowest dosage for effectiveness. *Topical:* Apply as needed to affected area; use lowest dose possible when applying to mucous membranes.

Pharmacokinetics

ABSORP: Completely absorbed after parenteral administration. Its rate of absorption depends on the site of administration and the presence or absence of a vasoconstrictor.
DIST: Permeates all tissues and crosses the blood-brain and placental barriers.
METAB: Metabolized rapidly by oxidative *N*-dealkylation in the liver.
EXCRET: Metabolites and unchanged drug are excreted in the kidneys. Elimination half-life after an intravenous bolus injection is typically 1.5 to 2 hr.

➔✚ DRUG INTERACTIONS

Amprenavir: Possible serious toxicity (decreased metabolism)
  • Avoid concurrent use.
Arbutamine: Possible increased risk of cardiac arrhythmias (mechanism unknown)
  • Avoid concurrent use.
Bupivacaine: Possible lidocaine toxicity (displacement from binding)
  • Avoid concurrent use.
Propranolol or metoprolol: Lidocaine toxicity (decreased metabolism)
  • Use lidocaine judiciously.

ADVERSE EFFECTS

⚠ **ORAL:** Stinging at injection site; burning, stinging, sloughing, tenderness (with topical application); numbness of lips or tongue and other paresthesias, including heat and cold.
CVS: Hypotension; bradycardia; cardiovascular collapse; cardiac arrest.
CNS: Dizziness; lightheadedness; nervousness; drowsiness; apprehension; confusion; mood changes; hallucinations; tremors.
GI: Nausea; vomiting.
RESP: Respiratory depression or arrest.
MISC: Hypersensitivity reactions. Local reactions, including soreness at IM injection site; venous thrombosis or phlebitis; extravasation; difficulty in speaking, breathing, and swallowing.

CLINICAL IMPLICATIONS

General

When used by dental professional:
  • *Lactation:* Excreted in breast milk.
  • *Hypersensitivity:* May occur.
  • *Renal failure:* Use caution with repeated doses or prolonged use in patients with renal impairment.
  • *Hepatic failure:* Use caution with repeated doses or prolonged use in patients with hepatic impairment.
  • *Cardiac effects:* Use with caution and in lower doses in patients with CHF, reduced cardiac output, digitalis toxicity, and in the elderly.
  • *Malignant hyperthermia:* Has been reported with administration of amide local anesthetics.
  • *Methemoglobinemia:* Do not use in patients with congenital or idiopathic methemoglobinemia or in infants younger than 12 mo who are receiving methemoglobin-inducing drugs.
  • *Topical use:* May impair swallowing and enhance danger of aspiration; avoid food for 1 hr if used in mouth or throat. Systemic effects can occur following topical use; use lowest possible dose to avoid serious toxicity, shock, or heart block. Monitor blood pressure and pulse.
  • *Overdosage:* Confusion, drowsiness, unconsciousness, tremors, convulsions, hypotension, bradycardia, cardiovascular collapse, cardiac arrest, tinnitus, diplopia.

Pregnancy Risk Category: Category B.

Oral Health Education

When used by dental professional:

- Explain that adverse reactions related to the CNS (e.g., drowsiness, confusion, paresthesias, convulsions, respiratory arrest) can occur and are related to CNS toxicity.
- Emphasize importance of not allowing topical solution to come in contact with eyes or broken skin.
- Advise patient not to chew gum or eat food until 60 min after oral anesthetic has been administered.
- Advise patient that drug may cause dizziness or drowsiness and to avoid getting out of bed or walking without assistance.

Lidocaine HCl for Cardiac Arrhythmias — see lidocaine HCl

Lidocaine HCl in 5% Dextrose — see lidocaine HCl

---

lidocaine HCl/prilocaine (LIE-doe-cane HIGH-droe-KLOR-ide/PRILL-oh-cane)

Synonym: prilocaine/lidocaine HCl

EMLA: Cream: 2.5% lidocaine and 2.5% prilocaine; Anesthetic Disc: 1 g EMLA emulsion (2.5% lidocaine, 2.5% prilocaine); contact surface approximately 10 cm²

Oraqix: Gel: 2.5% lidocaine and 2.5% prilocaine; Locally applied by injector device (1.7 g per cartridge)

■✦■ EMLA Patch

Drug Class: Local anesthetic

PHARMACOLOGY

Action

Stabilizes neuronal membranes by inhibiting the ionic fluxes required for the initiation and conduction of impulses, thereby effecting local anesthetic action.

Uses

As a topical anesthetic for use on normal intact skin for local analgesia or genital mucous membranes for superficial minor surgery and as pretreatment for infiltration anesthesia.

Contraindications

Sensitivity to local anesthetics of the amide type or any component of the product. Precaution in individuals at risk for methemoglobinemia.

Usual Dosage

Periodontal anesthesia

ADULTS AND CHILDREN: *Topical:* Apply thick layer of cream or anesthetic disc to designated site on mucosa. When using an injector devise, insert blunt tip applicator into pocket and inject small amount to fill pocket. Maximum dose is 5 cartridges over a 3-hr period.

Pediatrics (intact skin)

CHILDREN 0 TO 3 MO OR LESS THAN 5 KG: *Topical:* Apply 1 g per 10 cm² for a max of 1 hr.

CHILDREN 3 TO 12 MO AND MORE THAN 5 KG: *Topical:* Apply 2 g per 20 cm² for a max of 4 hr.

CHILDREN 1 TO 6 YR AND MORE THAN 10 KG: *Topical:* Apply 10 g per 100 cm² for a max of 4 hr.

CHILDREN 7 TO 12 YR AND MORE THAN 20 KG: *Topical:* Apply 20 g per 200 cm² for a max of 4 hr.

Note: If a patient is older than 3 mo and does not meet the min weight requirement, the max total dose should be restricted to that which corresponds to the patient's weight.

Pharmacokinetics

Lidocaine
ABSORP: Completely absorbed after parenteral administration. Its rate of absorption depends on the site of administration and the presence or absence of a vasoconstrictor.

DIST: Permeates all tissues and crosses the blood-brain and placental barriers.

METAB: Metabolized rapidly by oxidative N-dealkylation in the liver.

EXCRET: Metabolites and unchanged drug are excreted in the kidneys. Elimination half-life after an intravenous bolus injection is typically 1.5 to 2 hr.

➡️⬅️ DRUG INTERACTIONS

See: lidocaine — Drug Interactions

See: prilocaine — Drug Interactions

ADVERSE EFFECTS

⚠️ **ORAL:** Application site reactions (e.g., stinging, ulceration, edema, abscess, erythema); taste disturbance.

CVS: Bradycardia; hypotension; cardiovascular collapse leading to arrest.

CNS: CNS excitement or depression; lightheadedness; nervousness; apprehension; euphoria; confusion; dizziness; drowsiness; sensations of hot, cold, or numbness; twitching; tremors; convulsions, unconsciousness; respiratory depression and arrest.

MISC: Allergic and anaphylactoid reactions characterized by urticaria, angioedema, bronchospasm, and shock.

CLINICAL IMPLICATIONS

General
When used by dental professional:
- *Lactation:* Lidocaine and probably prilocaine are excreted in human milk.
- *Children:* Children younger than 7 yr have shown less overall benefit than older children or adults. Do not use in neonates with a gestational age of 37 wk or less.
- *Application:* Application to larger areas or for longer than recommended could result in sufficient absorption causing serious adverse reactions.
- *Methemoglobinemia:* Do not use in patients with congenital or idiopathic methemoglobinemia or in infants younger than 12 mo of age who are receiving treatment with methemoglobin-inducing agents (e.g., acetaminophen, nitrates, phenytoin, sulfonamides).
- *Overdosage:* Confusion, drowsiness, unconsciousness, tremors, convulsions, hypotension, bradycardia, cardiovascular collapse, cardiac arrest, tinnitus, diplopia. (**Caution:** If injectable local anesthetics are used, additive systemic toxicity can occur.)

Pregnancy Risk Category: Category B.

Oral Health Education
When used by dental professional:
- Explain name, dose, action, and potential side effects of medication.
- Caution patient, parent, or guardian that medication may block all skin sensations and to avoid trauma to the treated area by scratching, rubbing, or exposure to extremely hot or cold temperatures until complete sensation has returned.
- Avoid contact of agent with eyes; use protective lenses.

Lidodan Endotracheal — see lidocaine HCl

Lidodan Ointment — see lidocaine HCl

Lidodan Viscous — see lidocaine HCl

Lidoject-1 — see lidocaine HCl

Lidoject-2 — see lidocaine HCl

Lidopen Auto-Injector — see lidocaine HCl
Lifenac — see diclofenac
Lifenal — see diclofenac
Lin-Amox — see amoxicillin
Lin-Buspirone — see buspirone HCl

linezolid (lin-EH-zoe-lid)

Zyvox

|✦| Zyvoxam, Zyvoxam IV

Drug Class: Antibiotic; Anti-infective

PHARMACOLOGY

Action

Prevents the formation of a functional 70S initiation complex, which is essential to the bacterial translation process.

Uses

Treatment of vancomycin-resistant *Enterococcus faecium* infections; treatment of nosocomial pneumonia, complicated and uncomplicated skin and skin structure infections, and community-acquired pneumonia caused by susceptible strains of specific organisms.

➡◀ DRUG INTERACTIONS RELATED TO DENTAL THERAPEUTICS

Sympathomimetic amines: Hypertension (mechanism unknown)
• Monitor blood pressure.

ADVERSE EFFECTS

⚠ **ORAL:** Altered taste (2%); tongue discoloration, candidiasis (1%).
CNS: Headache (7%); insomnia, convulsions (3%); dizziness (2%); vertigo (1%); neuropathy.
GI: Diarrhea (11%); vomiting (9%); nausea (6%); generalized and localized abdominal pain; GI bleeding; loose stools; constipation.
RESP: URI (4%); pneumonia, dyspnea (3%); cough, apnea (2%).
MISC: Fever (14%); sepsis (8%); trauma, injection site reactions (3%); fungal infections, localized pain (2%); blood dyscrasias (anemia [5.6%], thrombocytopenia [4.7%], eosinophilia [1%], thrombocythemia [2.8%]).

CLINICAL IMPLICATIONS

General

• Determine why drug is being taken. Take precautions to avoid cross-contamination of microorganisms.
• Monitor respiratory function; consider semisupine chair position.
• Prolonged use of antibiotics may result in bacterial or fungal overgrowth of nonsusceptible microorganisms; anticipate candidiasis.
• If GI side effects occur, consider semisupine chair position.
• Blood dyscrasias reported; anticipate increased bleeding, infection, and poor healing.
• If oral infection occurs that requires antibiotic therapy, select an appropriate product from a different class of anti-infectives.

Oral Health Education

• Encourage daily plaque control procedures for effective, nontraumatic self-care.

Lin-Nefazodone — see nefazodone HCl

liothyronine sodium (lie-oh-THIGH-row-neen SO-dee-uhm)

Synonyms: T3; triiodothyronine

Cytomel, Triostat

■◆■ **Triyotex**

Drug Class: Thyroid hormone

PHARMACOLOGY

Action

Increases metabolic rate of body tissues; needed for normal growth and maturation.

Uses

Replacement or supplemental therapy in hypothyroidism; thyroid-stimulating hormone suppression for treatment or prevention of euthyroid goiters (e.g., thyroid nodules, multinodular goiters, enlargement in chronic thyroiditis); diagnostic agent in suppression tests to differentiate suspected hyperthyroidism from euthyroidism; treatment of myxedema coma/precoma (IV).

➤◆ DRUG INTERACTIONS RELATED TO DENTAL THERAPEUTICS

No documented drug-drug interactions. The absence of evidence is not evidence of safety.

ADVERSE EFFECTS

CNS: Tremors; headache; nervousness; insomnia.
CVS: Palpitations; tachycardia; hypertension; increased pulse pressure; arrhythmia (high doses).
GI: Diarrhea; vomiting.
MISC: Hypersensitivity; weight loss; menstrual irregularities; sweating; heat intolerance; fever; decreased bone density (in women using drug long term).

CLINICAL IMPLICATIONS

General

- Determine why drug is being taken. Consider implications of condition on dental treatment.
- Be aware that uncontrolled thyroid disease poses a risk for cardiovascular events during dental treatment; elevated doses of thyroid hormone mimic signs of hyperthyroid disease.
- Monitor blood pressure and pulse rate to determine degree of thyroid disease control.
- Use local anesthetic agents with a vasoconstrictor with caution. Thyroid hormones and epinephrine are synergistic; use aspiration technique.

liotrix (LIE-oh-trix)

Thyrolar 1, Thyrolar 1/2, Thyrolar 1/4, Thyrolar 2, Thyrolar 3

Drug Class: Thyroid hormone

PHARMACOLOGY

Action

Increases metabolic rate of body tissues; is needed for normal growth and maturation.

Uses

Replacement or supplemental therapy in hypothyroidism; pituitary thyroid-stimulating hormone suppression in treatment or prevention of various types of euthyroid goiters, including thyroid nodules, subacute or chronic lymphocytic thyroiditis (Hashimoto), multinodular goiter, and management of thyroid cancer; diagnostic agent in suppression tests to differentiate suspected and hyperthyroidism or thyroid gland autonomy.

➜← DRUG INTERACTIONS RELATED TO DENTAL THERAPEUTICS
No documented drug-drug interactions. The absence of evidence is not evidence of safety.

ADVERSE EFFECTS
No adverse drug effects reported.

CLINICAL IMPLICATIONS
General
- Be aware that uncontrolled thyroid disease poses a risk for cardiovascular events during dental treatment; elevated doses of thyroid hormone mimic signs of hyperthyroid disease.
- Use local anesthetic agents with a vasoconstrictor with caution. Thyroid hormones and epinephrine are synergistic; use aspiration technique.
- Monitor blood pressure and pulse rate to determine degree of thyroid disease control.

Lipidil — see fenofibrate

Lipidil Micro — see fenofibrate

Lipidil Supra — see fenofibrate

Lipitor — see atorvastatin calcium

Liquibid — see guaifenesin

Liquid Pred — see prednisone

Liquiprin Drops for Children — see acetaminophen

Liroken — see diclofenac

---

lisinopril (lie-SIN-oh-prill)
Prinivil, Zestril

■✦■ Apo-Lisinopril

Drug Class: Antihypertensive; ACE inhibitor

PHARMACOLOGY
Action
Competitively inhibits angiotensin I-converting enzyme (ACE), prevention of angiotensin I conversion to angiotensin II, a potent vasoconstrictor that also stimulates aldosterone secretion. Results in decrease in sodium and fluid retention, decrease in BP, and increase in diuresis.

Uses
Treatment of hypertension; treatment of heart failure not responding to diuretics and digitalis; treatment of acute MI within 24 hr in hemodynamically stable patients.

➜← DRUG INTERACTIONS RELATED TO DENTAL THERAPEUTICS
COX-1 inhibitors: Decreased antihypertensive effect (decreased prostaglandin synthesis)
- Monitor blood pressure.

ADVERSE EFFECTS
⚠ **ORAL:** Dry mouth, taste disturbance (1%).
CNS: Dizziness (12%); headache (6%); fatigue (3%).
CVS: Chest pain (3.4%), hypotension (9%), postural hypotension (>1%).
GI: Diarrhea (4%); nausea (2%); vomiting (1%).
RESP: Cough (4%); URI (2%); common cold (1%).
MISC: Chest pain (3%); abdominal pain (2%); asthenia (1%); anaphylactoid reactions; neutropenia, agranulocytosis, leukopenia, thrombocytopenia (rare).

CLINICAL IMPLICATIONS

General

- Monitor vital signs (e.g., BP, pulse pressure, rate and rhythm) at each appointment to assess disease control. Do not provide elective dental treatment when BP is ≥180/110 or in the presence of other high-risk CV conditions. Refer to the section entitled "The Patient Taking Cardiovascular Drugs" in Chapter 6: *Clinical Medicine.*
- Use local anesthetic agents with vasoconstrictor with caution based on functional capacity of the patient and use aspirating technique to prevent intravascular injection.
- Determine ability to adapt to stress of dental treatment. Consider short appointments.
- If coughing is problematic, consider semisupine chair position for treatment.
- *Postural hypotension:* Monitor BP at the beginning and end of each appointment; anticipate syncope. Have patient sit upright for several min at the end of the dental appointment before dismissing.
- Blood dyscrasias rarely reported; anticipate increased bleeding, infection, and poor healing.
- Susceptible patient with DM may experience severe recurrent hypoglycemia.
- Chronic dry mouth is possible; anticipate increased caries, candidiasis, and lichenoid mucositis.

Oral Health Education

- Encourage daily plaque control procedures for effective self care in patient at risk for cardiovascular disease.
- If chronic dry mouth occurs, recommend home fluoride therapy and use of nonalcoholic oral health care products.

Lithane — see lithium
Litheum — see lithium

---

lithium (LITH-ee-uhm)

Eskalith, Eskalith CR, Lithobid, Lithonate, Lithotabs
■✦■ Carbolith, Duralith, Lithane, PMS-Lithium Carbonate, PMS-Lithium Citrate
■◑■ Carbolit, Litheum

Drug Class: Antipsychotic; Antimanic

PHARMACOLOGY

Action

Specific mechanism unknown; alters sodium transport in nerve and muscle cells and effects shift toward intraneuronal metabolism of catecholamines.

Uses

Management of bipolar disorder and manic episodes of manic-depressive illness.

Unlabeled Uses

Treatment of neutropenia; unipolar depression; schizoaffective disorder; prophylaxis of cluster headaches; premenstrual tension; tardive dyskinesia; hyperthyroidism; syndrome of inappropriate diuretic hormone (SIADH) secretion; postpartum affective psychosis; corticosteroid-induced psychosis.

✦← DRUG INTERACTIONS RELATED TO DENTAL THERAPEUTICS

COX-1 inhibitors: Lithium toxicity (decreased renal excretion)
- Avoid concurrent use.

Metronidazole: Lithium toxicity (mechanism unknown)
- Avoid concurrent use.

Tetracyclines: Lithium toxicity (decreased renal excretion)
- Avoid concurrent use.

ADVERSE EFFECTS

⚠ **ORAL:** Dry mouth; parotitis; dental caries; taste disturbance; thirst; tongue movements.
CNS: Fine hand tremor; muscle hyperirritability; headache; fatigue; ataxia; dizziness; psychomotor retardation; confusion; dystonia; hallucinations; blackouts; seizures; pseudotumor cerebri; drowsiness; poor memory and intellectual function; muscular weakness; slurred speech.
CVS: Arrhythmia; hypotension; bradycardia.
GI: Anorexia; nausea; vomiting; diarrhea.
MISC: Fever; swollen joints.

CLINICAL IMPLICATIONS

General
- Determine why drug is being taken. Consider implications of condition on dental treatment.
- Depressed or anxious patients may neglect self-care. Monitor for plaque control effectiveness.
- Extrapyramidal behaviors can complicate performance of oral procedures. If present, consult with MD to consider medication changes.
- *Geriatric patients:* Use lower dose of opioid.
- Chronic dry mouth is possible; anticipate increased caries activity and candidiasis.
- Monitor vital signs.

Oral Health Education
- Determine need for power toothbrush for self-care.
- If chronic dry mouth occurs, recommend home fluoride therapy and use of nonalcoholic oral health care products.

Lithobid — see lithium
Lithonate — see lithium
Lithotabs — see lithium
LoCHOLEST — see cholestyramine
LoCHOLEST Light — see cholestyramine
Locoid — see hydrocortisone
Lodimol — see dipyridamole
Lodine — see etodolac
Lodine XL — see etodolac
Lodrane 24 — see brompheniramine
Lodrane XR — see brompheniramine
Lofibra — see fenofibrate
Logesic — see diclofenac
Logimax — see felodipine
LoHist 12 — see brompheniramine
Lomacin — see lomefloxacin HCl

---

lomefloxacin HCl (low-MUH-FLOX-uh-sin HIGH-droe-KLOR-ide)

Maxaquin

 Lomacin

Drug Class: Antibiotic, fluoroquinolone

PHARMACOLOGY

Action
Interferes with microbial DNA synthesis.

Uses
Treatment of infections of the lower respiratory tract and urinary tract caused by suscepti-ble organisms; prevention of UTI in patients undergoing transurethral or transrectal proce-dures.

➡◀ DRUG INTERACTIONS RELATED TO DENTAL THERAPEUTICS
Corticosteroids: Possible increased risk of Achilles tendon disorders (mechanism unknown)
  • Consider risk/benefit.

ADVERSE EFFECTS
⚠ ORAL: Stomatitis, tongue discoloration, taste perversion, dry mouth, candidiasis (<1%).
CNS: Headache (4%); dizziness (2%).
MISC: Photosensitivity (2.3%).
GI: Nausea (4%); diarrhea, abdominal pain (1%).

CLINICAL IMPLICATIONS

General
  • Determine why drug is being taken. Take precautions to avoid cross-contamination of mi-croorganisms.
  • If GI side effects occur, consider semisupine chair position.
  • If oral infection occurs that requires antibiotic therapy, select an appropriate product from a different class of anti-infectives.
  • Prolonged use of antibiotics may result in bacterial or fungal overgrowth of nonsuscepti-ble microorganisms; anticipate candidiasis.

Lomine — see dicyclomine HCl
Loniten — see minoxidil

---

loperamide HCl (low-PEHR-uh-mide HIGH-droe-KLOR-ide)
Diar-aid, Imodium, Imodium A-D, Kaopectate II Caplets, Neo-Diaral, Pepto Diarrhea Control
■✦■ **Apo-Loperamide, PMS-Loperamide Hydrochloride, Rhoxal-loperamide**
■✦■ **Acanol, Cryoperacid, Pramidal, Raxedin, Top-Dal**
Drug Class: Antidiarrheal

PHARMACOLOGY

Action
Slows intestinal motility, affects water and electrolyte movement through intestine, inhibits peristalsis, reduces daily fecal volume, increases viscosity and bulk density of stool, dimin-ishes loss of fluid and electrolytes.

Uses
Control and symptomatic relief of acute nonspecific or chronic diarrhea; reduction in vol-ume of ileostomy output.

➡◀ DRUG INTERACTIONS RELATED TO DENTAL THERAPEUTICS
No documented drug-drug interactions. The absence of evidence is not evidence of safety.

ADVERSE EFFECTS
⚠ ORAL: Dry mouth.

CNS: Fatigue; drowsiness; dizziness.
GI: Abdominal pain; distention or discomfort; constipation; nausea; vomiting.

CLINICAL IMPLICATIONS

General

- Determine why drug is being taken. Consider implications of condition on dental treatment.
- Chronic dry mouth is possible; anticipate increased caries activity and candidiasis.
- If GI side effects occur, consider semisupine chair position.

Oral Health Education

- If chronic dry mouth occurs, recommend home fluoride therapy and use of nonalcoholic oral health care products.

Lopid — see gemfibrozil
Lopresor — see metoprolol
Lopressor — see metoprolol
Lorabid — see loracarbef

---

loracarbef (lor-a-KAR-bef)

Lorabid

■◉■ **Carbac**

Drug Class: Antibiotic, cephalosporin

PHARMACOLOGY

Action

Binds to proteins in bacterial cell wall, which inhibits cell wall synthesis.

Uses

Treatment of otitis media, acute maxillary sinusitis, pharyngitis, tonsillitis, infections of lower respiratory tract, skin and skin structures, and urinary tract caused by susceptible strains of specific microorganisms.

➡️⬅️ DRUG INTERACTIONS RELATED TO DENTAL THERAPEUTICS

No documented drug-drug interactions. The absence of evidence is not evidence of safety.

ADVERSE EFFECTS

⚠️ **ORAL:** Candidiasis; glossitis; thirst.
CNS: Headache; somnolence.
CVS: Hypotension; syncope; chest pain; palpitations.
GI: Diarrhea; abdominal pain; nausea; vomiting; anorexia.
RESP: Rhinitis.
MISC: Hypersensitivity; hypoprothrombinemia, platelet dysfunction; pseudomembranous colitis; multiple blood dyscrasias (e.g., thrombocytopenia, leukopenia).

CLINICAL IMPLICATIONS

General

- Determine why drug is being taken. Take precautions to avoid cross-contamination of microorganisms.
- Blood dyscrasias rarely reported; anticipate increased bleeding, infection, and poor healing.
- If GI side effects occur, consider semisupine chair position.
- Prolonged use of antibiotics may result in bacterial or fungal overgrowth of nonsusceptible microorganisms; anticipate candidiasis.

- If oral infection occurs that requires antibiotic therapy, select an appropriate product from a different class of anti-infectives.

Oral Health Education

- Encourage daily plaque control procedures for effective, nontraumatic self-care.

loratadine (lore-AT-uh-DEEN)

Alavert, Claritin, Claritin Hives Relief, Claritin Non-Drowsy Allergy, Claritin RediTabs, Tavist ND

■✦■ Apo-Loratadine, Claritin Kids

■◆■ Clarityne, Lertamine, Lowadina, Sensibit

Drug Class: Antihistamine

PHARMACOLOGY

Action

Competitively antagonizes histamine at the H_1 receptor site.

Uses

Temporarily relieves symptoms caused by hay fever or other upper respiratory allergies (e.g., runny nose, sneezing, itchy/watery eyes, itching of the nose or throat); treatment of chronic idiopathic urticaria.

➡✦ DRUG INTERACTIONS RELATED TO DENTAL THERAPEUTICS

No documented drug-drug interactions. The absence of evidence is not evidence of safety.

ADVERSE EFFECTS

⚠ **ORAL:** Dry mouth (3%), thirst; stomatitis.

CNS: Headache (12%); somnolence (8%); fatigue, nervousness (4%); hyperkinesia (3%); paresthesia; dizziness; migraine; tremor; vertigo; impaired concentration; depression; agitation; anxiety; confusion; insomnia; seizures.

CVS: Palpitations; postural hypotension; bradycardia or tachycardia; hypertension or hypotension.

GI: Abdominal pain (2%); anorexia; increased appetite and weight gain; nausea; vomiting; diarrhea; constipation; flatulence; gastritis; dyspepsia; hiccup.

RESP: Wheezing (4%); URI (2%); nasal dryness; pharyngitis; epistaxis; nasal congestion; dyspnea; coughing; rhinitis; hemoptysis; sinusitis; sneezing; bronchospasm; bronchitis; laryngitis.

MISC: Breast pain; arthralgia; myalgia; malaise; chest pain; leg cramps; asthenia; back pain; fever; peripheral edema; blood dyscrasias (e.g., anemia, thrombocytopenia, leukopenia, agranulocytosis).

CLINICAL IMPLICATIONS

General

- Determine why drug is being taken. Consider implications of condition on dental treatment.
- Consider semisupine chair position to control effects of postnasal drainage.
- Be aware that patients with multiple allergies are at increased risk for allergy to dental drugs.
- Chronic dry mouth is possible; anticipate increased caries activity and candidiasis.
- Monitor vital signs (e.g., BP, pulse rate) and respiratory function. Uncontrolled disease characterized by postnasal drainage, coughing.
- *Postural hypotension:* Monitor BP at the beginning and end of each appointment; anticipate syncope. Have patient sit upright for several min at the end of the dental appointment before dismissing.
- If GI side effects occur, consider semisupine chair position.
- Blood dyscrasias rarely reported; anticipate increased bleeding, infection, and poor healing.

Oral Health Education
- If chronic dry mouth occurs, recommend home fluoride therapy and use of nonalcoholic oral health care products.
- Determine need for power toothbrush for self-care.

---

 lorazepam (lore-AZE-uh-pam)

Ativan: Injection: 2, 4 mg/mL
Lorazepam: Tablets: 0.5, 1, 2 mg
Lorazepam Intensol: Oral Solution, concentrated: 2 mg/mL

■✦■ **Apo-Lorazepam, Novo-Lorazem, Nu-Loraz**

■✦■ **Sinestron**

Drug Class: Antianxiety; Benzodiazepine

PHARMACOLOGY
Action
Potentiates action of GABA, resulting in increased neuronal inhibition and CNS depression, especially in limbic system and reticular formation.

Uses
Treatment of anxiety, anxiety associated with depression (oral); preanesthetic medication for sedation/anxiety and decreased recall, status epilepticus (IV).

Unlabeled Uses
Relief of chemotherapy-induced nausea and vomiting; acute alcohol withdrawal; psychogenic catatonia.

Usual Dosage
Antianxiety
Adults: *PO:* Usual dose: 2 to 6 mg/day (range, 1 to 10 mg/day) in divided doses; largest dose at bedtime.
Elderly/Debilitated patients: *Initial dose:* 1 to 2 mg/day in divided doses; increase gradually.

Status epilepticus
Adults: *IV:* Recommended dose 4 mg given at rate of 2 mg/min. If seizures continue or recur after a 10- to 15-min observation period, an additional 4 mg IV may be administered slowly.

Pharmacokinetics
ABSORP: Absolute bioavailability is 90%. T_{max} is about 2 hr. C_{max} is 20 ng/mL after 2 mg dose (dose-dependent).
DIST: 85% protein bound.
METAB: Rapidly conjugated at its 3-hydroxy group into lorazepam glucuronide.
EXCRET: The $t_{1/2}$ is approximately 12 hr for unconjugated lorazepam and approximately 18 hr for lorazepam glucuronide.

➜← DRUG INTERACTIONS
No documented drug-drug interactions. The absence of evidence is not evidence of safety.

ADVERSE EFFECTS
⚠ **ORAL:** Dry mouth; coated tongue; difficulty swallowing; gingival pain; salivation.
CNS: Drowsiness; confusion; ataxia; dizziness; lethargy; fatigue; apathy; memory impairment; disorientation; anterograde amnesia, restlessness; headache; slurred speech; aphonia; stupor; coma; euphoria; irritability; vivid dreams; psychomotor retardation; paradoxical reactions (e.g., anger, hostility, mania, insomnia).

CVS: Bradycardia or tachycardia; hypertension or hypotension; palpitations.

GI: Constipation; diarrhea; nausea; anorexia; vomiting.

RESP: Partial airway obstruction (injection); respiratory depression.

MISC: Dependence/withdrawal syndrome (e.g., confusion, abnormal perception of movement, depersonalization, muscle twitching, psychosis, paranoid delusions, seizures); pain, burning, redness at IM injection site; blood dyscrasias (e.g., leukopenia, agranulocytosis, thrombocytopenia, others).

CLINICAL IMPLICATIONS

General

- Determine why drug is being taken. Consider implications of condition on dental treatment.
- Depressed or anxious patients may neglect self-care. Monitor for plaque control effectiveness.
- Extrapyramidal behaviors can complicate performance of oral procedures. If present consult with MD to consider medication changes.
- Chronic dry mouth is possible; anticipate increased caries and candidiasis.
- Monitor vital signs.
- Blood dyscrasias rarely reported; anticipate increased bleeding, infection and poor healing.
- *When prescribed by DDS:* May produce sedation, interfere with eye-hand coordination, and the ability to operate mechanical equipment. Inform patient not to drive, sign important papers, or operate mechanical equipment.

Pregnancy Risk Category: Category D. Avoid use, especially during first trimester because of possible increased risk of congenital malformations. Advise women of childbearing age to use effective contraceptive method. Not recommended during labor and delivery.

Oral Health Education

- *When prescribed by DDS:* Warn patient not to drink alcoholic products while taking the drug.
- Evaluate manual dexterity; consider need for power toothbrush.
- If chronic dry mouth occurs, recommend home fluoride therapy and use of nonalcoholic oral health care products.
- Encourage daily plaque control procedures for effective, nontraumatic self-care.

Lorazepam Intensol — see lorazepam

Lorcet 10/650 — see acetaminophen/hydrocodone bitartrate

Lorcet-HD — see acetaminophen/hydrocodone bitartrate

Lorcet Plus — see acetaminophen/hydrocodone bitartrate

Lortab 5/500 — see acetaminophen/hydrocodone bitartrate

Lortab 7.5/500 — see acetaminophen/hydrocodone bitartrate

Lortab 10/500 — see acetaminophen/hydrocodone bitartrate

Lortab ASA — see aspirin/hydrocodone bitartrate

Lortab ASA Tablets — see narcotic analgesic combinations

Lortab Elixir — see narcotic analgesic combinations

---

losartan potassium (low-SAHR-tan poe-TASS-ee-uhm)

Cozaar

Drug Class: Antihypertensive; Angiotensin II antagonist

PHARMACOLOGY

Action

Antagonizes the effect of angiotensin II (vasoconstriction and aldosterone secretion) by blocking the angiotensin II receptor (AT_1 receptor) in vascular smooth muscle and the adrenal gland, producing decreased BP.

Uses

Treatment of hypertension; nephropathy in type 2 diabetic patients; reduce risk of stroke in patients with hypertension and left ventricular hypertrophy.

➡◀ DRUG INTERACTIONS RELATED TO DENTAL THERAPEUTICS

Fluconazole: Possible losartan toxicity (decreased metabolism)
• Monitor blood pressure.

ADVERSE EFFECTS

⚠ **ORAL:** Dental pain, dry mouth (1%).
CNS: Dizziness; insomnia; headache.
GI: Diarrhea; dyspepsia; abdominal pain; nausea.
RESP: Cough; sinusitis; upper respiratory infection; pharyngitis.
MISC: Muscle cramps; myalgia; back pain; leg pain; chest pain; edema/swelling; photosensitivity (1%).

CLINICAL IMPLICATIONS

General

• Monitor vital signs (e.g., BP, pulse pressure, rate and rhythm) at each appointment to assess disease control. Do not provide elective dental treatment when BP is ≥180/110 or in the presence of other high-risk CV conditions. Refer to the section entitled "The Patient Taking Cardiovascular Drugs" in Chapter 6: *Clinical Medicine*.
• Use local anesthetic agents with vasoconstrictor with caution based on functional capacity of the patient and use aspirating technique to prevent intravascular injection.
• Determine ability to adapt to stress of dental treatment. Consider short appointments.
• If coughing is problematic, consider semisupine chair position for treatment.
• Susceptible patient with DM may experience severe recurrent hypoglycemia.
• Chronic dry mouth is possible; anticipate increased caries, candidiasis, and lichenoid mucositis.

Oral Health Education

• Encourage daily plaque control procedures for effective self-care in patient at risk for cardiovascular disease.

losartan potassium/hydrochlorothiazide (low-SAHR-tan poe-TASS-ee-uhm/high-droe-klor-oh-THIGH-uh-zide)

Synonym: hydrochlorothiazide/losartan potassium

Hyzaar

Drug Class: Antihypertensive, Angiotensin Receptor Blocker

PHARMACOLOGY

Action

Losartan antagonizes the effect of angiotensin II (i.e., vasoconstriction and aldosterone secretion) by blocking the angiotensin II receptor (AT1 receptor) in vascular smooth muscle and the adrenal gland, producing decreased BP; hydrochlorothiazide inhibits reabsorption of sodium and chloride in ascending loop of Henle and early distal tubules.

Uses

Hypertension.

➡️← DRUG INTERACTIONS RELATED TO DENTAL THERAPEUTICS

COX-1 inhibitors: Decreased antihypertensive effect (decreased prostaglandin synthesis)
- Monitor blood pressure.

ADVERSE EFFECTS

⚠️ **ORAL:** Dental pain, dry mouth (losartan); sialadenitis (hydrochlorothiazide).

CNS: Dizziness; syncope, anxiety, ataxia, confusion, depression, dream abnormality, hyperesthesia, insomnia, decreased libido, memory impairment, migraine, nervousness, panic disorder, paresthesia, peripheral neuropathy, sleep disorder, somnolence, tremor, vertigo (losartan); restlessness (hydrochlorothiazide).

CVS: Chest pain, edema (>1%).

GI: Abdominal pain; anorexia, constipation, dyspepsia, flatulence, gastritis, vomiting (losartan); pancreatitis, cramping, gastric irritation (hydrochlorothiazide).

RESP: URI; dyspnea, epistaxis, respiratory congestion (losartan); respiratory distress (e.g., pneumonitis, pulmonary edema) (hydrochlorothiazide).

MISC: Back pain; chest pain, facial edema, arm pain, arthralgia, arthritis, fibromyalgia, hip pain, joint swelling, knee pain, leg pain, muscle cramps, muscle weakness, musculoskeletal pain, myalgia, shoulder pain, stiffness (losartan); weakness, fever, muscle spasm (hydrochlorothiazide).

CLINICAL IMPLICATIONS

General

- Monitor vital signs (e.g., BP, pulse pressure, rate and rhythm) at each appointment to assess disease control. Do not provide elective dental treatment when BP is ≥180/110 or in the presence of other high-risk CV conditions. Refer to the section entitled "The Patient Taking Cardiovascular Drugs" in Chapter 6: *Clinical Medicine.*
- Use local anesthetic agents with vasoconstrictor with caution based on functional capacity of the patient and use aspirating technique to prevent intravascular injection.
- Determine ability to adapt to stress of dental treatment. Consider short appointments.
- Susceptible patient with DM may experience severe recurrent hypoglycemia.
- Chronic dry mouth is possible; anticipate increased caries candidiasis, and lichenoid mucositis.
- If GI or musculoskeletal side effects occur, consider semisupine chair position.

Oral Health Education

- Determine need for power toothbrush for self-care.
- If chronic dry mouth occurs, recommend home fluoride therapy and use of nonalcoholic oral health care products.

Losec — see omeprazole

Lotensin — see benazepril HCl

Lotrel — see amlodipine/benazepril HCl

Lotrimin — see clotrimazole

Lotrimin AF — see clotrimazole

Lotronex — see alosetron

---

lovastatin (LOW-vuh-STAT-in)

Altoprev, Mevacor
■✦■ Apo-Lovastatin, Gen-Lovastatin, ratio-Lovastatin
Drug Class: Antihyperlipidemic, HMG-CoA reductase inhibitor

PHARMACOLOGY

Action

Increases rate at which body removes cholesterol from blood and reduces production of cholesterol in body by inhibiting enzyme that catalyzes early rate-limiting step in cholesterol synthesis; increases HDL; reduces LDL, VLDL, and triglycerides.

Uses

To reduce elevated cholesterol and LDL cholesterol levels in patients with primary hyper-cholesterolemia (types IIa and IIb [immediate-release only]); to slow progression of coronary atherosclerosis in patients with coronary heart disease; to reduce risk of MI, unstable angina, and coronary revascularization procedures; as an adjunct to diet to reduce total and LDL cholesterol and apolipoprotein B levels in adolescent boys and girls (who are at least 1 yr postmenarche) age 10 to 17 yr with heterozygous familial hypercholesterolemia (immediate-release only). As an adjunct to diet for reduction of elevated total and LDL cholesterol, apolipoprotein B, and triglycerides and to increase HDL cholesterol in patients with primary hypercholesterolemia (heterozygous familial and nonfamilial) and mixed dyslipidemia (Fredrickson types IIa and IIb) when response to diet restricted in saturated fat and cholesterol and to nonpharmacological measures alone has been inadequate (extended-release only).

➥➡ DRUG INTERACTIONS RELATED TO DENTAL THERAPEUTICS

Fluconazole, ketoconazole, or itraconazole: Rhabdomyolysis (decreased metabolism)
• Avoid concurrent use.
Clarithromycin: Rhabdomyolysis (decreased metabolism)
• Avoid concurrent use.

ADVERSE EFFECTS

⚠ **ORAL:** Dry mouth; taste disturbance.
CNS: Headache; dizziness; paresthesia; insomnia.
CVS: Arrhythmia; palpitations; postural hypotension.
GI: Nausea; vomiting; diarrhea; abdominal pain; constipation; flatulence; heartburn; dyspepsia; pancreatitis.
RESP: Sinusitis (6%).
MISC: Myalgia; muscle cramps; myopathy; rhabdomyolysis with increased CPK; arthralgias; infection (11% to 15%, unspecified); hypersensitivity syndrome (e.g., anaphylaxis, angioedema, lupus erythematosus–like syndrome, polymyalgia rheumatica, vasculitis, purpura, thrombocytopenia, leukopenia, hemolytic anemia, arthritis, arthralgia, urticaria, fever, chills, dyspnea, toxic epidermal necrolysis, erythema multiforme).

CLINICAL IMPLICATIONS

General

• High LDL cholesterol concentration is the major cause of atherosclerosis, which leads to CAD (angina, MI); determine degree of CV health and ability to withstand stress of dental treatment.
• Monitor vital signs (e.g., BP, pulse pressure, rate and rhythm) at each appointment to assess disease control. Do not provide elective dental treatment when BP is ≥180/110 or in the presence of other high-risk CV conditions. Refer to the section entitled "The Patient Taking Cardiovascular Drugs" in Chapter 6: *Clinical Medicine.*
• *Postural hypotension:* Monitor BP at the beginning and end of each appointment; anticipate syncope. Have patient sit upright for several min at the end of the dental appointment before dismissing.
• If GI side effects occur, consider semisupine chair position.
• Chronic dry mouth is possible; anticipate increased caries and candidiasis.
• Blood dyscrasias rarely reported; anticipate increased bleeding, infection and poor healing.

Oral Health Education

• If chronic dry mouth occurs, recommend home fluoride therapy and use of nonalcoholic oral health care products.
• Encourage daily plaque control procedures for effective self-care in patient at risk for cardiovascular disease.

lovastatin/niacin — see niacin/lovastatin

Lovenox — see enoxaparin sodium

Lovenox HP — see enoxaparin sodium

Lowadina — see loratadine

Lozide — see indapamide

Lozol — see indapamide

L-thyroxine — see levothyroxine sodium

Luminal Sodium — see phenobarbital

Lunelle — see estradiol cypionate/medroxyprogesterone acetate

Lunesta — see eszopiclone

Luride — see sodium fluoride

Luride Lozi-Tabs — see sodium fluoride

Luride-SF Lozi-Tabs — see sodium fluoride

Luritran — see erythromycin

Luvox — see fluvoxamine maleate

Luxiq — see betamethasone

Lyphocin — see vancomycin

Mabicrol — see clarithromycin

Macrobid — see nitrofurantoin

Macrodantin — see nitrofurantoin

Macrodantina — see nitrofurantoin

---

magaldrate (MAG-al-drate)

Synonym: Hydroxymagnesium aluminate

Iosopan, Riopan

Drug Class: Antacid

PHARMACOLOGY

Action

Neutralizes gastric acid, thereby increasing pH of stomach and duodenal bulb. Increases lower esophageal sphincter tone and inhibits smooth muscle contraction and gastric emptying.

Uses

Symptomatic relief of upset stomach associated with hyperacidity, including heartburn, gastroesophageal reflux, acid indigestion and sour stomach; relief of hyperacidity associated with peptic ulcer, gastritis, peptic esophagitis, gastric hyperacidity, and hiatal hernia.

➡◀ DRUG INTERACTIONS RELATED TO DENTAL THERAPEUTICS

Ketoconazole or itraconazole: Decreased ketoconazole or itraconazole effect (decreased absorption)
- Administer as far apart as possible.

Clorazepate: Decreased oral clorazepate effect (decreased absorption)
- Administer as far apart as possible.

Corticosteroids: Decreased oral corticosteroid effect (decreased metabolism)
- Administer as far apart as possible.

Metronidazole: Decreased metronidazole effect (decreased metabolism)
- Avoid concurrent use.

Tetracyclines: Decreased tetracycline effect (decreased metabolism)
- Avoid concurrent use.

ADVERSE EFFECTS

CNS: Neurotoxicity; encephalopathy.

GI: Diarrhea; constipation; intestinal obstruction; rebound hyperacidity.

MISC: Osteomalacia; bone pain; muscular weakness; malaise; decreased fluoride absorption; aluminum accumulation in serum, bone and CNS; milk-alkali syndrome.

CLINICAL IMPLICATIONS

General
- If patient has GI disease, consider semisupine chair position.

Magnidol — see acetaminophen

Malival — see indomethacin

Mapap Extra Strength — see acetaminophen

Mapap Infant Drops — see acetaminophen

Mapap Regular Strength — see acetaminophen

Mapluxin — see digoxin

Maranox — see acetaminophen

Marcaine — see bupivacaine

Margesic H — see acetaminophen/hydrocodone bitartrate

Marovilina — see ampicillin

Masflex — see meloxicam

Mavik — see trandolapril

Maxair Autohaler — see pirbuterol acetate

Maxalt — see rizatriptan

Maxalt-MLT — see rizatriptan

Maxalt RPD — see rizatriptan

Maxaquin — see lomefloxacin HCl

Maxeran — see metoclopramide

Maxidex — see dexamethasone

Maximum Bayer — see aspirin

Maximum Strength Nytol — see diphenhydramine HCl

Maximum Strength Sleepinal Capsules and Soft Gels — see diphenhydramine HCl

Maximum Strength Unisom SleepGels — see diphenhydramine HCl

Maxivate — see betamethasone

Maxolon — see metoclopramide

Mebaral — see mephobarbital

meclizine (MEK-lih-zeen)

Antivert, Antrizine, Dramamine Less Drowsy, Meni-D, Vergon

▌✦▌ Bonamine

Drug Class: Antiemetic; Antivertigo; Anticholinergic

PHARMACOLOGY

Action

Acts on CNS to decrease vestibular stimulation and depress labyrinthine activity.

Uses

Prevention and treatment of nausea, vomiting, and dizziness of motion sickness; possibly effective treatment for vertigo of vestibular dysfunction origin.

➡✦ DRUG INTERACTIONS RELATED TO DENTAL THERAPEUTICS

No documented drug-drug interactions. The absence of evidence is not evidence of safety.

ADVERSE EFFECTS

⚠ **ORAL:** Dry mouth, nose, throat.

CNS: Drowsiness; excitation; nervousness; restlessness; insomnia; euphoria; vertigo; hallucinations.

CVS: Hypotension; palpitations; tachycardia.

GI: Nausea; vomiting; diarrhea; constipation; anorexia.

CLINICAL IMPLICATIONS

General

- Determine why drug is being taken. Consider implications of condition on dental treatment.
- Anticholinergics have strong xerostomic effects. Anticipate increased caries and candidiasis.
- Monitor vital signs.
- If GI side effects occur, consider semisupine chair position.

Oral Health Education

- If chronic dry mouth occurs, recommend home fluoride therapy and use of nonalcoholic oral health care products.

---

meclofenamate sodium (mek-loe-FEN-uh-mate SO-dee-uhm)

Meclofenamate sodium

Drug Class: Analgesic; NSAID

PHARMACOLOGY

Action

Decreases inflammation, pain and fever, probably through inhibition of COX activity and prostaglandin synthesis.

Uses

Treatment of rheumatoid and osteoarthritis; treatment of primary dysmenorrhea; relief of mild to moderate pain; idiopathic heavy menstrual blood loss.

Unlabeled Uses

Relief of sunburn; pain; migraine (aborts acute attacks).

➡◄ DRUG INTERACTIONS RELATED TO DENTAL THERAPEUTICS
No documented drug-drug interactions. The absence of evidence is not evidence of safety.

ADVERSE EFFECTS
⚠ **ORAL:** Stomatitis.

CNS: Headache; vertigo; drowsiness; dizziness; tinnitus.

MISC: Blood dyscrasias (<1%) (e.g., agranulocytosis, hemolytic anemia, leukopenia, neutropenia).

GI: Diarrhea; vomiting; nausea; abdominal pain; dyspepsia; peptic ulcer; GI bleeding; constipation; flatulence; anorexia; heartburn.

RESP: Breathing difficulties in aspirin-sensitive individuals.

CLINICAL IMPLICATIONS
General
- Determine why drug is being taken. Consider implications of condition on dental treatment.
- Use COX inhibitors with caution, they may exacerbate PUD and GERD.
- *Arthritis:* consider patient comfort and need for semisupine chair position.
- If GI side effects occur, consider semisupine chair position.
- Blood dyscrasias rarely reported; anticipate increased bleeding, infection, and poor healing.

Oral Health Education
- Evaluate manual dexterity; consider need for power toothbrush.

Meclomid — see metoclopramide
Meda Cap — see acetaminophen
Meda Tab — see acetaminophen
Med-Atenolol — see atenolol
Medralone 40 — see methylprednisolone
Medralone 80 — see methylprednisolone
Medrol — see methylprednisolone

---

medroxyprogesterone acetate (meh-DROX-ee-pro-JESS-tuh-rone ASS-uh-TATE)

Amen, Curretab, Cycrin, Depo-Provera, Provera
■✦■ **Gen-Medroxy, Novo-Medrone, ratio-MPA**

Drug Class: Progestin

PHARMACOLOGY
Action
Inhibits secretion of pituitary gonadotropins, thereby preventing follicular maturation and ovulation (contraceptive effect); inhibits spontaneous uterine contraction; transforms proliferative endometrium into secretory endometrium; produces antineoplastic effect in advanced endometrial or renal carcinoma.

Uses
PO: Treatment of secondary amenorrhea and abnormal uterine bleeding caused by hormonal imbalance; reduction of incidence of endometrial hyperplasia in nonhysterectomized postmenopausal women receiving 0.625 mg conjugated estrogen.

PARENTERAL: Prevention of pregnancy; adjunctive and palliative treatment of inoperable, recurrent, and metastatic endometrial or renal carcinoma.

➡✚ DRUG INTERACTIONS RELATED TO DENTAL THERAPEUTICS

No documented drug-drug interactions. The absence of evidence is not evidence of safety.

ADVERSE EFFECTS

CNS: Depression; headache; nervousness; dizziness; insomnia; fatigue; somnolence.

GI: Abdominal pain or discomfort; nausea.

RESP: Pulmonary embolism.

MISC: Breast tenderness; masculinization of female fetus; edema; weight changes, especially weight gain; anaphylactoid reactions; bone mineral density changes, increasing risk of osteoporosis; hyperglycemia; pyrexia; galactorrhea.

CLINICAL IMPLICATIONS

General

- Determine why drug is being taken. Consider implications of condition on dental treatment.

---

medroxyprogesterone acetate/conjugated estrogens — see estrogens, conjugated/medroxyprogesterone acetate

medroxyprogesterone acetate/estradiol cypionate — see estradiol cypionate/medroxyprogesterone acetate

---

mefenamic acid (MEH-fen-AM-ik ASS-id)

Ponstel

■✚■ Apo-Mefenamic, Nu-Mefenamic, PMS-Mefenamic Acid, Ponstan

■▬■ Ponstan

Drug Class: Analgesic; NSAID

PHARMACOLOGY

Action

Decreases inflammation, pain, and fever, probably through inhibition of COX activity and prostaglandin synthesis.

Uses

Relief of moderate pain lasting less than 1 wk; treatment of primary dysmenorrhea.

Unlabeled Uses

Treatment of sunburn, migraine (acute attack), premenstrual syndrome.

➡✚ DRUG INTERACTIONS RELATED TO DENTAL THERAPEUTICS

No documented drug-drug interactions. The absence of evidence is not evidence of safety.

ADVERSE EFFECTS

⚠ **ORAL:** Dry mouth; pharyngitis.

CNS: Headache; vertigo; drowsiness; dizziness; insomnia.

GI: Diarrhea; vomiting; abdominal pain; dyspepsia; GI bleeding; nausea; constipation; flatulence.

RESP: Bronchospasm; laryngeal edema; rhinitis; dyspnea; hemoptysis; shortness of breath.

MISC: Autoimmune hemolytic anemia may occur if used long term.

CLINICAL IMPLICATIONS
General
- Determine why drug is being taken. Consider implications of condition on dental treatment.
- If GI side effects occur, consider semisupine chair position.
- Chronic dry mouth is possible with long-term use; anticipate increased caries and candidiasis.

Oral Health Education
- If chronic dry mouth occurs, recommend home fluoride therapy and use of nonalcoholic oral health care products.

Mellaril — see thioridazine HCl
Melleril — see thioridazine HCl

---

meloxicam (mell-OX-ih-kam)
Mobic

■✴■ **Mobicox**

■◆■ **Masflex**

Drug Class: Analgesic; NSAID

PHARMACOLOGY
Action
Decreases inflammation, pain, and fever, probably through inhibition of COX activity and prostaglandin synthesis.

Uses
Relief of signs and symptoms of osteoarthritis and rheumatoid arthritis.

✦← DRUG INTERACTIONS RELATED TO DENTAL THERAPEUTICS
No documented drug-drug interactions. The absence of evidence is not evidence of safety.

ADVERSE EFFECTS
⚠ **ORAL:** Dry mouth; ulcerative stomatitis.

CNS: Dizziness, headache, insomnia (4%); fatigue, convulsions, paresthesia, tremor, vertigo, abnormal dreaming, anxiety, increased appetite, confusion, depression, nervousness, somnolence (<2%).

CVS: Palpitations, arrhythmia, hypertension or hypotension, syncope (<2%); hot flushes.

GI: Diarrhea (8%); nausea (7%); dyspeptic signs and symptoms (6%); abdominal pain (5%); constipation, flatulence, vomiting (3%); colitis, duodenal ulcer, eructation, esophagitis, gastric ulcer, gastritis, gastroesophageal reflux, GI hemorrhage, hematemesis, hemorrhagic duodenal ulcer, hemorrhagic gastric ulcer, intestinal perforation, melena, pancreatitis, perforated duodenal ulcer, perforated gastric ulcer (<2%).

RESP: URI (8%); coughing (2%); asthma, bronchospasm, dyspnea (<2%).

MISC: Influenza-like symptoms (6%); household accidents, edema, pain (5%); falls (3%); allergic reaction, face edema, fever, malaise, photosensitivity (<2%); anaphylactic reactions including shock; blood dyscrasias (anemia [4%], leukopenia, thrombocytopenia, purpura [<2%]).

CLINICAL IMPLICATIONS
General
- Determine why drug is being taken. Consider implications of condition on dental treatment.
- Use COX inhibitors with caution; they may exacerbate PUD and GERD.

- *Arthritis:* consider patient comfort and need for semisupine chair position.
- Chronic dry mouth is possible; anticipate increased caries activity and candidiasis.
- Monitor vital signs.
- If GI side effects occur, consider semisupine chair position.
- Blood dyscrasias rarely reported; anticipate increased bleeding, infection, and poor healing.

Oral Health Education
- Evaluate manual dexterity; consider need for power toothbrush.
- If chronic dry mouth occurs, recommend home fluoride therapy and use of nonalcoholic oral health care products.

memantine HCl (meh-MAN-teen HIGH-droe-KLOR-ide)

Namenda

Drug Class: NMDA receptor antagonist

PHARMACOLOGY

Action
It is postulated that memantine exerts its therapeutic effect as a low to moderate affinity, uncompetitive nervous system *N*-methyl-D-aspartate (NMDA) receptor antagonist by binding preferentially to the NMDA receptor-operated cation channels.

Uses
Treatment of moderate to severe dementia of the Alzheimer type.

Unlabeled Uses
Treatment of vascular dementia.

➡◄ DRUG INTERACTIONS RELATED TO DENTAL THERAPEUTICS
No documented drug-drug interactions. The absence of evidence is not evidence of safety.

ADVERSE EFFECTS
CNS: Dizziness (7%); headache, confusion (6%); somnolence, hallucination (3%); transient ischemic attack, cerebrovascular accident, vertigo, ataxia, hypokinesia, aggressive reaction (≥1%).
CVS: Hypertension (4%), syncope (1%).
GI: Constipation (5%); vomiting (3%).
RESP: Coughing (4%); dyspnea (2%); pneumonia (≥1%).
MISC: Pain (3%); fatigue (2%).

CLINICAL IMPLICATIONS

General
- Patient may experience hypotension or hypertension. Monitor vital signs at each appointment; anticipate syncope.
- Ensure that caregiver is present at every dental appointment and understands informed consent.
- If coughing is problematic, consider semisupine chair position for treatment.

Oral Health Education
- Evaluate manual dexterity; consider need for power toothbrush.
- Teach caregiver to assist patient with oral self-care practices.

Menadol — see ibuprofen

Menest — see estrogens, conjugated or esterified

Meni-D — see meclizine

meperidine HCl (meh-PEHR-ih-deen HIGH-droe-KLOR-ide)
Demerol

Drug Class: Narcotic analgesic

PHARMACOLOGY
Action
Relieves pain by stimulating opiate receptors in CNS; also causes respiratory depression, peripheral vasodilation, inhibition of intestinal peristalsis, sphincter of Oddi spasm, stimulation of chemoreceptors that cause vomiting and increased bladder tone.

Uses
ORAL AND PARENTERAL: Relief of moderate to severe pain.
PARENTERAL: Preoperative sedation; support of anesthesia; obstetrical analgesia.

➦◀ DRUG INTERACTIONS RELATED TO DENTAL THERAPEUTICS
No documented drug-drug interactions. The absence of evidence is not evidence of safety.

ADVERSE EFFECTS
⚠ ORAL: Dry mouth; taste disturbance.
CNS: Lightheadedness; dizziness; sedation; disorientation; incoordination; seizures.
CVS: Bradycardia (frequent); orthostatic hypotension, arrhythmia.
GI: Nausea; vomiting; constipation; abdominal pain.
RESP: Respiratory depression; laryngospasm; depression of cough reflex.

CLINICAL IMPLICATIONS
General
- Determine why drug is being taken. Consider implications of condition on dental treatment.
- If oral pain requires additional analgesics, consider nonopioid products.
- *Geriatric patients:* Use lower dose of opioid.
- Monitor vital signs (e.g., BP, pulse rate) and respiratory function.
- *Postural hypotension:* Monitor BP at the beginning and end of each appointment; anticipate syncope. Have patient sit upright for several min at the end of the dental appointment before dismissing.
- If GI side effects occur, consider semisupine chair position.
- Chronic dry mouth is unlikely because this drug is used on a short-term basis for pain management or during surgery.
- *When prescribed by DDS:* Short-term use only; there is no justification for long-term use in the management of dental pain.

Oral Health Education
- If chronic dry mouth occurs, recommend home fluoride therapy and use of nonalcoholic oral health care products.

mephobarbital (meh-foe-BAR-bih-tahl)
Mebaral

Drug Class: Sedative and hypnotic; Barbiturate; Anticonvulsant

PHARMACOLOGY
Action
Depresses sensory cortex, decreases motor activity, alters cerebellar function, and produces drowsiness, sedation, and hypnosis.

Uses

As a sedative for relief of anxiety, tension, and apprehension; as an anticonvulsant for the treatment of grand mal and petit mal epilepsy.

➕ DRUG INTERACTIONS RELATED TO DENTAL THERAPEUTICS

Doxycycline: Decreased doxycycline effect (increased metabolism)
- Avoid concurrent use.

ADVERSE EFFECTS

CNS: Agitation; confusion; hyperkinesia; ataxia; CNS depression; nightmares; nervousness; psychiatric disturbance; hallucinations; insomnia; anxiety; dizziness; thinking abnormality; headache.

CVS: Bradycardia, hypotension, syncope (1%).

GI: Nausea; vomiting; constipation.

RESP: Hypoventilation; apnea.

MISC: Hypersensitivity reactions including angioedema, skin rashes, exfoliative dermatitis, fever.

CLINICAL IMPLICATIONS

General

- Determine why drug is being taken. Consider implications of condition on dental treatment.
- Determine ability to adapt to stress of dental treatment. Consider short appointments.
- Determine level of disease control, type and frequency of seizure and compliance with medication regimen.
- Depressed or anxious patients may neglect self care. Monitor for plaque control effectiveness.
- Monitor vital signs.

Oral Health Education

- Determine need for power toothbrush for self-care.

🔲 mepivacaine HCl (meh-PIHV-ah-cane HIGH-droe-KLOR-ide)

Carbocaine: Injection: Mepivacaine HCl 1%, 1.5%, 2%, 3%
Carbocaine with Neo-Cobefrin: Injection: Mepivacaine HCl 2% with 1:20,000 levonordefrin
Mepivacaine HCl: Injection: Mepivacaine HCl 3%
Mepivacaine HCl and Levonordefrin: Injection: Mepivacaine HCl 2% with 1:20,000 levonordefrin
Polocaine: Injection: Mepivacaine HCl 1%, 2%, 3%
Polocaine MPF: Injection: Mepivacaine HCl 1.5%, 2%
Polocaine with Levonordefrin: Injection: Mepivacaine HCl 2% with 1:20,000 levonordefrin

Drug Class: Injectable local anesthetic, amide

PHARMACOLOGY

Action

Inhibits ion fluxes across membranes to block nerve action potential.

Uses

Peripheral nerve block (e.g., cervical, brachial, intercostal, pudendal): 1% or 2% solution.
Transvaginal block (paracervical plus pudendal): 1% solution.

Paracervical block in obstetrics: 1% solution.
Caudal and epidural block: 1%, 1.5%, or 2% solution.
Infiltration: 0.5% (via dilution) or 1% solution.
Therapeutic block (pain management): 1% or 2% solution.
Dental procedures (infiltration or nerve block): 3% solution or 2% solution with levonordefrin.

Usual Dosage
Regional anesthesia in the oral health care setting
3% PLAIN OR 2% WITH LEVONORDEFRIN 1:20,000
ADULTS AND CHILDREN: 6.6 mg/kg of body weight, not to exceed 400 mg (3% formulation) or 550 mg (2% with levonordefrin 1:20,000 formulation).

Pharmacokinetics
METAB: Liver.
EXCRET: Kidney (metabolites).
ONSET: 3 to 5 min.
DURATION: 0.75 to 1.50 hr; 2 to 6 hr with epinephrine.
SPECIAL POP: *Renal failure:* Use with caution in patients with renal disease.
Elderly: Repeated doses may cause accumulation of the drug or its metabolites or slow metabolic degradation; give reduced doses.

➡⬅ DRUG INTERACTIONS
Intercurrent use: Mixtures of local anesthetics are sometimes employed to compensate for the slower onset of one drug and the shorter duration of action of the sec drug. Toxicity is probably additive with mixtures of local anesthetics, but some experiments suggest synergisms. Exercise caution regarding toxic equivalence when mixtures of local anesthetics are employed. Some preparations contain vasoconstrictors. Keep this in mind when using concurrently with other drugs that may interact with vasoconstrictors.
Sedatives: If employed to reduce patient apprehension during dental procedures, use reduced doses, since local anesthetics used in combination with CNS depressants may have additive effects. Give young children minimal doses of each agent.
Bupivacaine: Mepivacaine toxicity (displacement from binding site)
  • Avoid concurrent use.

ADVERSE EFFECTS
⚠ **ORAL:** Trismus; tingling.
CNS: Convulsions, loss of consciousness (overdose).
CVS: Myocardial depression; cardiac arrest; dysrhythmias; bradycardia.
RESP: Status asthmaticus, respiratory arrest, anaphylaxis (allergy).
MISC: Discoloration at injection site; tissue necrosis.

CLINICAL IMPLICATIONS
General
  • *Lactation:* Safety for use during lactation has not been established.
  • Use the lowest dosage that results in effective anesthesia to avoid high plasma levels and serious adverse effects. Inject slowly, with frequent aspirations before and during the injection, to avoid intravascular injection. Perform syringe aspirations before and during each supplemental injection in continuous (intermittent) catheter techniques. During the administration of epidural anesthesia, it is recommended that a test dose be administered initially and that the patient be monitored for CNS toxicity and cardiovascular toxicity, as well as for signs of unintended intrathecal administration, before proceeding.
  • *Inflammation or sepsis:* Use local anesthetic procedures with caution when there is inflammation or sepsis in the region of proposed injection.
  • *CNS toxicity:* Monitor cardiovascular and respiratory vital signs and state of consciousness after each injection. Restlessness, anxiety, incoherent speech, lightheadedness, numbness, and tingling of the mouth and lips, metallic taste, tinnitus, dizziness, blurred vision, tremors, twitching, depression, or drowsiness may be early signs of CNS toxicity.

- *Malignant hyperthermia:* Many drugs used during anesthesia are considered potential triggering agents for familial malignant hyperthermia. It is not known whether local anesthetics may trigger this reaction and the need for supplemental general anesthesia cannot be predicted in advance; therefore, have a standard protocol for management available.
- *Vasoconstrictors:* Use solutions containing a vasoconstrictor with caution and in carefully circumscribed quantities in areas of the body supplied by end arteries or having otherwise compromised blood supply (e.g., digits, nose, external ear, penis). Use with extreme caution in patients whose medical history and physical evaluation suggest the existence of hypertension, peripheral vascular disease, arteriosclerotic heart disease, cerebral vascular insufficiency, or heart block; these individuals may exhibit exaggerated vasoconstrictor response. Serious dose-related cardiac arrhythmias may occur if preparations containing a vasoconstrictor such as epinephrine are employed in patients during or following the administration of potent inhalation agents.

Pregnancy Risk Category: Category C.

Oral Health Education

- Advise the patient to exert caution to avoid inadvertent trauma to the lips, tongue, cheek, mucosae, or soft palate when these structures are anesthetized. The ingestion of food should therefore be postponed until normal function returns.
- Advise the patient to consult the dentist if anesthesia persists or a rash develops.

Mepivacaine HCl and Levonordefrin — see mepivacaine HCl

Mepron — see atovaquone

Meridia — see sibutramine HCl

Merxil — see diclofenac

Mesacal — see mesalamine

---

mesalamine (me-SAL-uh-MEEN)

Synonym: 5-aminosalicylic acid; 5-ASA

Asacol, Pentasa, Rowasa

█✦█ Mesacal, Novo-5 ASA, Salofalk

Drug Class: Intestinal anti-inflammatory, Aminosalicylic acid derivative

PHARMACOLOGY

Action

Reduces inflammation of colon topically by preventing production of substances involved in inflammatory processes (e.g., arachidnoic acid).

Uses

Treatment of active, mild to moderate, distal ulcerative colitis, proctosigmoiditis, or proctitis.

Unlabeled Uses

Treatment of Crohn disease.

✦← DRUG INTERACTIONS RELATED TO DENTAL THERAPEUTICS

No documented drug-drug interactions. The absence of evidence is not evidence of safety.

ADVERSE EFFECTS

⚠ **ORAL:** Pharyngitis (11%); oral ulceration; dry mouth; candidiasis; lichen planus; taste perversion.

CNS: Headache; asthenia; chills; dizziness; fever; sweating; malaise.

GI: Abdominal pain; cramps; discomfort; colitis exacerbation; constipation; diarrhea; dyspepsia; vomiting; flatulence; nausea; eructation; rectal pain; soreness; burning.

RESP: Cough.

MISC: Arthralgia; back pain; hypertonia; myalgia; dysmenorrhea; edema; flu-like syndrome; pain; photosensitivity; blood dyscrasias (e.g., agranulocytosis, leukopenia, thrombocytopenia, others).

CLINICAL IMPLICATIONS

General
- If patient has GI disease, consider semisupine chair position.
- Use COX inhibitors with caution; they may exacerbate PUD and GERD.
- Chronic dry mouth is possible; anticipate increased caries and candidiasis.
- Blood dyscrasias rarely reported; anticipate increased bleeding, infection, and poor healing.

Oral Health Education
- If chronic dry mouth occurs, recommend home fluoride therapy and use of nonalcoholic oral health care products.

M-Eslon — see morphine sulfate
Metadate CD — see methylphenidate HCl
Metadate ER — see methylphenidate HCl
Metadol — see methadone HCl
Metaglip — see glipizide/metformin HCl

---

metaprotereno sulfate (MEH-tuh-pro-TEHR-uh-nahl SULL-fate)
Alupent

Drug Class: Bronchodilator; Sympathomimetic

PHARMACOLOGY

Action
Relaxes bronchial smooth muscle through beta-2 receptor stimulation.

Uses
Treatment of bronchial asthma and reversible bronchospasm associated with bronchitis and emphysema; control of acute asthma attacks in children at least 6 yr of age (inhalation solution only).

➤◀ DRUG INTERACTIONS RELATED TO DENTAL THERAPEUTICS
No documented drug-drug interactions. The absence of evidence is not evidence of safety.

ADVERSE EFFECTS
⚠ **ORAL:** Dry mouth, throat; pharyngitis; taste disturbance.
CNS: Tremor; dizziness; nervousness; weakness; headache; shakiness/nervousness/tension; drowsiness; insomnia.
CVS: Tachycardia (<17%); palpitations (4%).
GI: GI distress; nausea; vomiting.
RESP: Cough; asthma exacerbation; asthma exacerbation; hoarseness; nasal congestion.
MISC: Fatigue; skin reaction.

CLINICAL IMPLICATIONS

General
- Monitor vital signs (e.g., BP, pulse rate) and respiratory function. Uncontrolled disease characterized by wheezing, coughing.
- Acute bronchoconstriction can occur during dental treatment; have bronchodilator inhaler available.

- Ensure that bronchodilator inhaler is present at each dental appointment.
- Be aware that sulfites in local anesthetic with vasoconstrictor can precipitate acute asthma attack in susceptible individuals.
- Inhalants can dry oral mucosa; anticipate candidiasis and increased calculus, plaque levels, and caries activity.

Oral Health Education

- If chronic dry mouth occurs, recommend home fluoride therapy and use of nonalcoholic oral health care products.

---

metaxalone (me-TAX-a-lone)

Skelaxin

Drug Class: Skeletal muscle relaxant

PHARMACOLOGY

Action

Mechanism of action not established but may be caused by general CNS depression. No direct action on the contractile mechanism of striated muscle, the motor endplate, or the nerve fiber. Does not directly relax tense skeletal muscles.

Uses

As an adjunct to rest, physical therapy, and other measures for the relief of discomfort associated with acute, painful, musculoskeletal conditions.

➔⬅ DRUG INTERACTIONS RELATED TO DENTAL THERAPEUTICS

No documented drug-drug interactions. The absence of evidence is not evidence of safety.

ADVERSE EFFECTS

CNS: Drowsiness; dizziness; headache; nervousness; irritability.

GI: Nausea; vomiting; GI upset.

MISC: Hypersensitivity reaction (i.e., light rash with or without pruritus); leukopenia; hemolytic anemia; jaundice; anaphylactoid reactions (rare).

CLINICAL IMPLICATIONS

General

- Determine why drug is being taken. Consider implications of condition on dental treatment.
- If GI side effects occur, consider semisupine chair position.
- Blood dyscrasias rarely reported; anticipate increased infection and poor healing.

Oral Health Education

- Encourage daily plaque control procedures for effective, nontraumatic self-care.

---

metformin HCl (met-FORE-min HIGH-droe-KLOR-ide)

Fortamet, Glucophage, Glucophage XR, Glumetza, Riomet

🇨🇦 Apo-Metformin, Gen-Metformin, Novo-Metformin, Nu-Metformin, PMS-Metformin, ratio-Metformin, Rhoxal-metformin, Rhoxal-metformin FC

🇲🇽 Dabex, Dimefor, Glucophage Forte

Drug Class: Antidiabetic, biguanide

PHARMACOLOGY

Action

Decreases blood glucose by decreasing hepatic glucose production. May also decrease intestinal absorption of glucose and increase response to insulin.

Uses

Adjunct to diet and exercise to lower blood glucose in patients with type 2 diabetes mellitus. Metformin immediate-release (IR) tablets and oral solution are indicated in patients 10 yr of age and older. The extended-release (ER) tablets are indicated in patients 17 yr of age and older. In combination with a sulfonylurea or insulin to improve glycemic control, metformin is indicated in patients 17 yr of age and older.

➪◆ DRUG INTERACTIONS RELATED TO DENTAL THERAPEUTICS

No documented drug-drug interactions. The absence of evidence is not evidence of safety.

ADVERSE EFFECTS

⚠ **ORAL:** Taste disorder (1% to 5%).

CNS: METFORMIN IR: Asthenia, headache (≥5%); lightheadedness (1% to 5%). METFORMIN ER: Dizziness, headache (1% to 5%).

CVS: Palpitation (1% to 5%).

GI: METFORMIN IR: Abdominal discomfort, diarrhea, flatulence, indigestion, nausea/vomiting (≥5%); abnormal stools (1% to 5%). METFORMIN ER: Diarrhea, nausea/vomiting (≥5%); abdominal distention, abdominal pain, constipation, dyspepsia/heartburn, flatulence (1% to 5%).

RESP: METFORMIN IR: Dyspnea (1% to 5%). METFORMIN ER: URI (1% to 5%).

MISC: METFORMIN IR: Chest discomfort, chills, flu-like syndrome (1% to 5%).

CLINICAL IMPLICATIONS

General

- Determine degree of disease control and current blood sugar levels. Goals should be <120 mg/dL and A1C <7%. A1C levels ≥8% indicate significant uncontrolled diabetes.
- The routine use of antibiotics in the dental management of diabetic patients is not indicated; however, antibiotic therapy in patients with poorly controlled diabetes has been shown to improve disease control and improve response after periodontal debridement.
- Monitor BP because hypertension and dyslipidemia (CAD) are prevalent in DM.
- Monitor vital signs (e.g., BP, pulse pressure, rate and rhythm) at each appointment to assess disease control. Do not provide elective dental treatment when BP is ≥180/110 or in the presence of other high-risk CV conditions. Refer to the section entitled "The Patient Taking Cardiovascular Drugs" in Chapter 6: *Clinical Medicine.*
- *Loss of blood sugar control:* Certain medical conditions (e.g., surgery, fever, infection, trauma) and drugs (e.g., corticosteroids) affect glucose control. In these situations, it may be necessary to seek medical consultation before surgical procedures.
- Obtain patient history regarding diabetic ketoacidosis or hypoglycemia with current drug regimen.
- Observe for signs of hypoglycemia (e.g., confusion, argumentativeness, perspiration, altered consciousness). Be prepared to treat hypoglycemic reactions with oral glucose or sucrose.
- Ensure patient has taken medication and eaten meal.
- Determine ability to adapt to stress of dental treatment. Consider short, morning appointments.
- Medical consult advised if fasting blood glucose is <70 mg/dL (hypoglycemic risk) or >200 mg/dL (hyperglycemic crisis risk).
- *If insulin is used:* Consider time of peak hypoglycemic effect.
- If GI side effects occur, consider semisupine chair position.

Oral Health Education

- Explain role of diabetes in periodontal disease and the need to maintain effective plaque control and disease control.
- Advise to bring data on blood sugar values and A1C levels to dental appointments.

metformin HCl/glipizide — see glipizide/metformin HCl
metformin HCl/glyburide — see glyburide/metformin HCl
metformin HCl/rosiglitazone maleate — see rosiglitazone maleate/ metformin HCl

methadone HCl (METH-uh-dohn HIGH-droe-KLOR-ide)

Dolophine HCl, Methadose

■✦■ **Metadol**

Drug Class: Narcotic analgesic

PHARMACOLOGY

Action
Relieves pain by stimulating opiate receptors in CNS; also causes respiratory depression, peripheral vasodilation, inhibition of intestinal peristalsis, sphincter of Oddi spasm, stimulation of chemoreceptors that cause vomiting and increased bladder tone.

Uses
Management of severe pain; detoxification and temporary maintenance treatment of narcotic addiction.

➧✦ DRUG INTERACTIONS RELATED TO DENTAL THERAPEUTICS

Fluconazole: Possible methadone toxicity (decreased metabolism)
- Monitor clinical status.

ADVERSE EFFECTS

⚠ **ORAL:** Dry mouth.
CNS: Lightheadedness; euphoria; dysphoria; headache; insomnia; dizziness; sedation; disorientation; incoordination.
CVS: Circulatory depression, bradycardia (frequent).
GI: Nausea; vomiting; constipation; abdominal pain.
RESP: Laryngospasm; respiratory depression; depression of cough reflex.
MISC: Tolerance; psychological and physical dependence with long-term use.

CLINICAL IMPLICATIONS

General
- Determine why drug is being taken. Consider implications of condition on dental treatment.
- If oral pain requires additional analgesics, consider nonopioid products.
- Chronic dry mouth is possible; anticipate increased caries activity and candidiasis.
- Monitor vital signs.
- Be aware that patient may be taking opioid antagonists and other CNS depressant drugs.

Oral Health Education
- Most patients who abuse substances have poor oral health because of neglect. Encourage daily self-care to prevent periodontal disease.
- If chronic dry mouth occurs, recommend home fluoride therapy and use of nonalcoholic oral health care products.

Methadose — see methadone HCl

methimazole (meth-IMM-uh-zole)

Tapazole

Drug Class: Antithyroid

PHARMACOLOGY

Action

Inhibits synthesis of thyroid hormones.

Uses

Long-term therapy of hyperthyroidism; amelioration of hyperthyroidism in preparation for subtotal thyroidectomy or radioactive iodine therapy.

➜◀ DRUG INTERACTIONS RELATED TO DENTAL THERAPEUTICS

No documented drug-drug interactions. The absence of evidence is not evidence of safety.

ADVERSE EFFECTS

⚠ **ORAL:** Taste loss.

CNS: Paresthesias; neuritis; headache; vertigo; drowsiness; neuropathies; CNS stimulation; depression.

GI: Nausea; vomiting; epigastric distress.

MISC: Abnormal hair loss; arthralgia; myalgia; edema; lymphadenopathy; drug fever; interstitial pneumonitis; insulin autoimmune syndrome; agranulocytosis; thrombocytopenia; hypoprothrombinemia; bleeding.

CLINICAL IMPLICATIONS

General

- Be aware that uncontrolled hyperthyroid disease poses a risk for cardiovascular events during dental treatment.
- Monitor blood pressure and pulse rate to determine degree of thyroid disease control.
- Use local anesthetic agents with a vasoconstrictor with caution. Thyroid hormones and epinephrine are synergistic; use aspiration technique.
- Blood dyscrasias rarely reported; anticipate increased bleeding, infection, and poor healing.

Oral Health Education

- Encourage daily plaque control procedures for effective, nontraumatic self-care.

methocarbamol (meth-oh-CAR-buh-mahl)

Robaxin, Robaxin-750

Drug Class: Skeletal muscle relaxant, centrally acting

PHARMACOLOGY

Action

May cause relaxation of skeletal muscle via general CNS depression. Does not directly relax tense skeletal muscles.

Uses

Adjunctive therapy for relief of painful, acute musculoskeletal conditions; control of neuromuscular manifestations of tetanus.

➜◀ DRUG INTERACTIONS RELATED TO DENTAL THERAPEUTICS

No documented drug-drug interactions. The absence of evidence is not evidence of safety.

ADVERSE EFFECTS

⚠ **ORAL:** Metallic taste.

CNS: Headache; amnesia; confusion; dizziness/lightheadedness; drowsiness; insomnia; mild muscular incoordination; sedation; seizures (including grand mal); vertigo.

GI: Dyspepsia; nausea; vomiting.
MISC: Hypersensitivity reactions, anaphylactic reactions; angioneurotic edema; fever.

CLINICAL IMPLICATIONS

General
- Determine why drug is being taken. Consider implications of condition on dental treatment.
- *For back pain:* Consider semisupine chair position for patient comfort.

---

methotrexate (meth-oh-TREK-sate)

Synonym: amethopterin; MTX

Methotrexate LPF Sodium, Methotrexate Sodium, Methotrexate Sodium, Rheumatrex Dose Pack, Trexall,

■✦■ **ratio-Methotrexate**

■✦■ **Ledertrexate, Texate, Trixilem**

Drug Class: Antineoplastic; Antimetabolite; Antipsoriatic; Antiarthritic

PHARMACOLOGY

Action
Competitively inhibits dihydrofolic acid reductase and thereby inhibits DNA synthesis and cellular replication. In rheumatoid arthritis, believed to reduce immune function.

Uses
Antineoplastic chemotherapy for treatment of gestational choriocarcinoma, chorioadenoma destruens, hydatidiform mole; treatment and prophylaxis of acute (meningeal) lymphocytic leukemia; treatment of breast cancer, epidermoid cancers of head and neck, advanced mycosis fungoides, and lung cancer; in combination therapy in advanced-stage non-Hodgkin lymphoma; as adjunct in high doses followed by leucovorin rescue in nonmetastatic osteosarcoma (postsurgically); symptomatic control of severe psoriasis and severe rheumatoid arthritis; polyarticular-course juvenile rheumatoid arthritis.

➠✦ DRUG INTERACTIONS RELATED TO DENTAL THERAPEUTICS

COX-1 inhibitors: Possible methotrexate toxicity (decreased renal clearance)
- Avoid concurrent use.

Tetracyclines: Possible methotrexate toxicity (mechanism unknown)
- Avoid concurrent use.

ADVERSE EFFECTS

⚠ **ORAL:** Stomatitis (3% to 10%).
CNS: Dizziness (1% to 3%); fatigue; headache; aphasia; hemiparesis; paresis; convulsions; leukoencephalopathy (IV after craniospinal irradiation); chemical arachnoiditis; transient paresis; neurotoxicity.
GI: Nausea, vomiting (10%); enteritis (3% to 10%); diarrhea (1% to 3%); abdominal distress (common); anorexia; hematemesis; melena; GI ulceration and bleeding.
RESP: Deaths from interstitial pneumonitis; chronic interstitial obstructive pulmonary disease.
MISC: Malaise; chills; fever; lower resistance to infections; arthralgia; myalgia; diabetes; osteoporosis; anaphylactoid reaction; sudden death; thrombocytopenia, leukopenia; elevated liver function tests (15%); decreased hematocrit.

CLINICAL IMPLICATIONS

General
- Determine why drug is being taken. Consider implications of condition on dental treatment.

- Consider medical consult to determine disease control and influence on dental treatment.
- Liver and kidney function tests should be completed every 1 to 2 mo; discuss risks associated with using or prescribing drugs.
- Blood dyscrasias reported; anticipate increased bleeding, infection, and poor healing.
- *Arthritis:* Consider patient comfort and need for semisupine chair position.
- Advise products for palliative relief of oral manifestations (e.g., stomatitis, mucositis, xerostomia).

Oral Health Education
- Evaluate manual dexterity; consider need for power toothbrush.

Methotrexate LPF Sodium — see methotrexate
Methotrexate Sodium — see methotrexate

---

methyldopa and methyldopate HCl (meth-ill-DOE-puh and meth-ill-DOE-pate HIGH-droe-KLOR-ide)

Synonym: methyldopate HCl and methyldopa

Aldomet

■✦■ Apo-Methyldopa, Nu-Medopa,

Drug Class: Antihypertensive; Antiadrenergic, centrally acting

PHARMACOLOGY
Action
Causes central alpha-adrenergic stimulation, which inhibits sympathetic cardioaccelerator and vasoconstrictor centers; reduces plasma renin activity; reduces standing and supine BP.

Uses
Treatment of hypertension.

✦← DRUG INTERACTIONS RELATED TO DENTAL THERAPEUTICS
Sympathomimetic amines: Reduced antihypertensive effect (physiological antagonism)
- Monitor blood pressure.

ADVERSE EFFECTS
⚠ **ORAL:** Dry mouth; sialoadenitis; discolored tongue; sore tongue.
CNS: Dizziness; sedation; nightmares; headache; asthenia or weakness; paresthesias; lightheadedness; symptoms of cerebrovascular insufficiency; parkinsonism; Bell palsy; decreased mental acuity; involuntary choreoathetotic movements.
CVS: Postural hypotension; bradycardia; edema leading to CHF.
GI: Constipation; nausea; vomiting; distention; flatus; diarrhea.
MISC: Fever; lupus-like syndrome; mild arthralgia or myalgia; bone marrow depression; blood dyscrasias (e.g., leukopenia, granulocytopenia, thrombocytopenia, hemolytic anemia).

CLINICAL IMPLICATIONS
General
- Monitor vital signs (e.g., BP, pulse pressure, rate and rhythm) at each appointment to assess disease control. Do not provide elective dental treatment when BP is ≥180/110 or in the presence of other high-risk CV conditions. Refer to the section entitled "The Patient Taking Cardiovascular Drugs" in Chapter 6: *Clinical Medicine.*
- Use local anesthetic agents with vasoconstrictor with caution based on functional capacity of the patient and use aspirating technique to prevent intravascular injection.

- Determine ability to adapt to stress of dental treatment. Consider short appointments.
- *Postural hypotension:* Monitor BP at the beginning and end of each appointment; anticipate syncope. Have patient sit upright for several min at the end of the dental appointment before dismissing.
- Extrapyramidal behaviors can complicate performance of oral procedures. If symptoms present, consult with MD to consider medication changes.
- Blood dyscrasias rarely reported; anticipate increased bleeding, infection, and poor healing.
- Chronic dry mouth is possible; anticipate increased caries and candidiasis.

Oral Health Education
- Encourage daily plaque control procedures for effective self-care in patient at risk for cardiovascular disease.
- If chronic dry mouth occurs, recommend home fluoride therapy and use of nonalcoholic oral health care products.

---

methyldopate HCl and methyldopa — see methyldopa and methyldopate HCl

Methylin — see methylphenidate HCl

Methylin ER — see methylphenidate HCl

---

methylphenidate HCl (meth-ill-FEN-ih-date HIGH-droe-KLOR-ide)
Concerta, Metadate CD, Metadate ER, Methylin, Methylin ER, Ritalin, Ritalin LA, Ritalin-SR

▮✦▮ **PMS-Methylphenidate, ratio-Methylphenidate**

Drug Class: Psychotherapeutic; CNS stimulant

PHARMACOLOGY

Action
Acts as mild cortical stimulant with CNS action; exact mechanism of action unknown.

Uses
Treatment of ADHD; treatment of narcolepsy (Ritalin, Ritalin SR, Metadate ER, Methylin).

➡◀ DRUG INTERACTIONS RELATED TO DENTAL THERAPEUTICS

Pilocarpine: Increased myopia (mechanism unknown)
- Monitor clinical status.

ADVERSE EFFECTS

CNS: Nervousness; insomnia; dizziness; headache; dyskinesias; drowsiness; convulsions; toxic psychosis; motor tics.

CVS: Arrhythmia, palpitations, blood pressure changes (both increased and decreased).

GI: Anorexia; nausea; abdominal pain; weight loss during prolonged therapy.

RESP: URI; cough; pharyngitis; sinusitis.

MISC: Tourette syndrome; hypersensitivity reactions (e.g., rash, itching, fever, joint pain, exfoliative dermatitis, erythema multiforme, thrombocytopenia, purpura).

CLINICAL IMPLICATIONS

General
- Determine why drug is being taken. Consider implications of condition on dental treatment.
- Patients with ADHD may have short attention spans; consider short appointment.
- Monitor vital signs.
- If GI side effects occur, consider semisupine chair position.

Oral Health Education
- Evaluate manual dexterity; consider need for power toothbrush.

---

methylprednisolone (METH-ill-pred-NIH-suh-lone)
(methylprednisolone acetate, methylprednisolone sodium succinate)

A-Methapred, depMedalone 40, depMedalone 80, Depo-Medrol, Depopred-40, Depopred-80, Duralone-40, Duralone-80, Medralone 40, Medralone 80, Medrol, Solu-Medrol,

▌✦▌ Depo-Medrol

▌✦▌ Cryosolona

Drug Class: Corcticosteroid

PHARMACOLOGY

Action
Depresses formation, release, and activity of endogenous mediators of inflammation including prostaglandins, kinins, histamine, liposomal enzymes, and complement system. Modifies body's immune response.

Uses
Replacement therapy in primary or secary adrenal cortex insufficiency; adjunctive therapy for short-term administration in rheumatic disorders; exacerbation or maintenance therapy in collagen diseases; treatment of dermatological diseases; control of allergic states or allergic and inflammatory ophthalmic processes; management of respiratory diseases; treatment of hematological disorders; palliative management of neoplastic diseases; management of cerebral edema associated with primary or metastatic brain tumor, craniotomy, or head injury; induction of diuresis in edematous states (due to nephrotic syndrome); management of critical exacerbations of GI diseases; management of acute exacerbations of multiple sclerosis; treatment of tuberculous meningitis; management of trichinosis with neurological or myocardial involvement.

INTRA-ARTICULAR OR SOFT-TISSUE ADMINISTRATION: Adjunctive therapy for short-term administration in synovitis of osteoarthritis, rheumatoid arthritis, bursitis, acute gouty arthritis, epicondylitis, acute nonspecific tenosynovitis, and posttraumatic osteoarthritis.

INTRALESIONAL ADMINISTRATION: Management of keloids; treatment of localized hypertrophic, infiltrated, inflammatory lesions of lichen planus, psoriatic plaques, granuloma annulare, lichen simplex chronicus; treatment of discoid lupus erythematosus, necrobiosis lipoidica diabeticorum, alopecia areata, and cystic tumors of aponeurosis or tendon.

TOPICAL ADMINISTRATION: Treatment of inflammatory and pruritic manifestations of corticosteroid-responsive dermatoses.

Unlabeled Uses
Reduction of mortality in severe alcoholic hepatitis; prevention of respiratory distress syndrome; treatment of septic shock; improvement of neurological function in acute spinal cord injury.

➜◆ DRUG INTERACTIONS RELATED TO DENTAL THERAPEUTICS

Ketoconazole, itraconazole, or clarithromycin: Possible toxicity of methylprednisolone (decreased metabolism)
- Monitor clinical status.

Metronidazole: Decreased metronidazole effect (increased metabolism)
- Avoid concurrent use.

COX-1 inhibitors: Increased risk of peptic ulcers (decreased prostaglandin synthesis)
- Avoid concurrent use.

ADVERSE EFFECTS

⚠ **ORAL:** Ulcerative esophagitis; poor wound healing; masking of infections.

CNS: Convulsions; pseudotumor cerebri (increased intracranial pressure with papilledema); vertigo; headache; neuritis; paresthesias; psychosis.

CVS: Cardiovascular collapse (IV administration).

GI: Pancreatitis; abdominal distention; nausea; vomiting; increased appetite and weight gain; peptic ulcer with perforation and hemorrhage; bowel perforation.

MISC: Musculoskeletal effects (e.g., weakness, myopathy, muscle mass loss, osteoporosis, spontaneous fractures); endocrine abnormalities (e.g., menstrual irregularities, cushingoid state, growth suppression in children, sweating, decreased carbohydrate tolerance, hyperglycemia, glycosuria, increased insulin or sulfonylurea requirements in diabetic patients, hirsutism); anaphylactoid or hypersensitivity reactions; aggravation of infections; fatigue; insomnia; osteonecrosis, tendon rupture, infection, skin atrophy, postinjection flare, hypersensitivity, facial flushing (intra-articular administration). Topical application may produce adverse reactions seen with systemic use because of absorption.

CLINICAL IMPLICATIONS

General

- Determine why drug is being taken. Consider implications of condition on dental treatment.
- Parenterally administered steroids have greater and more severe side effects than oral dose forms.
- Despite the anticipated perioperative physiological stress (i.e., minor surgical stress), patients undergoing dental care under local anesthesia should take only their usual daily glucocorticoid dose before dental intervention. No supplementation is justified.
- Be aware that signs of bacterial oral infection may be masked and anticipate oral candidiasis.
- If GI side effects occur, consider semisupine chair position.
- *Arthritis:* Consider patient comfort and need for semisupine chair position.
- Place on frequent maintenance schedule to avoid periodontal inflammation.

Oral Health Education

- Evaluate manual dexterity; consider need for power toothbrush.

---

methylprednisolone acetate — see methylprednisolone
methylprednisolone sodium succinate — see methylprednisolone
Meticorten — see prednisone

---

metoclopramide (MET-oh-kloe-PRA-mide)

Maxolon, Octamide, Octamide PFS, Reglan

■✦■ APO-Metoclop, Maxeran, Metoclopramide Omega, Nu-Metoclopramide,

■✦■ Carnotprim, Clorimet, Meclomid, Plasil, Pramotil

Drug Class: Dopamine antagonist; Antiemetic agent

PHARMACOLOGY

Action

Stimulates upper GI tract motility, resulting in accelerated gastric emptying and intestinal transit and increased resting tone of lower esophageal sphincter. Exerts antiemetic properties through antagonism of central and peripheral dopamine receptors.

Uses

PO: Relief of symptoms associated with acute and recurrent diabetic gastroparesis; short-term therapy of symptomatic, documented gastroesophageal reflux disease in adults who fail to respond to conventional therapy.

PARENTERAL: Prevention of nausea and vomiting associated with emetogenic cancer chemotherapy; prophylaxis of postoperative nausea and vomiting when nasogastric suction is undesirable; facilitation of small bowel intubation when tube does not pass pylorus with conventional maneuvers.

Unlabeled Uses

Treatment of hiccups, migraines, postoperative gastric bezoars, improvement in lactation, radiation-induced emesis.

➡️⬅️ DRUG INTERACTIONS RELATED TO DENTAL THERAPEUTICS

No documented drug-drug interactions. The absence of evidence is not evidence of safety.

ADVERSE EFFECTS

⚠️ **ORAL:** Tardive dyskinesia.

CNS: Dizziness; drowsiness; depression; hallucinations; extrapyramidal symptoms that respond rapidly to treatment with anticholinergic agents (e.g., diphenhydramine IV); exacerbation of Parkinson disease; akathisia.

CVS: Hypertension or hypotension; tachycardia or bradycardia.

GI: Diarrhea.

CLINICAL IMPLICATIONS

General

- Determine why drug is being taken. Consider implications of condition on dental treatment.
- If patient has GI disease, consider semisupine chair position.
- Use COX inhibitors with caution; they may exacerbate PUD and GERD.
- Extrapyramidal behaviors can complicate performance of oral procedures. If symptoms present, consult with MD to consider medication change.
- Monitor vital signs.

Oral Health Education

- Inform patient that toothbrushing should not be done after reflux, but to only rinse mouth with water, then use home fluoride product to minimize chemical erosion caries.
- Determine need for power toothbrush for self-care.

Metoclopramide Omega — see metoclopramide

---

metolazone (meh-TOLE-uh-ZONE)

Mykrox, Zaroxolyn

Drug Class: Thiazide-like diuretic

PHARMACOLOGY

Action

Increases urinary excretion of sodium and chloride by inhibiting reabsorption in ascending limb of loop of Henle and early distal tubules.

Uses

Treatment of edema and hypertension.

Unlabeled Uses

Prevention of calcium nephrolithiasis; reduction of postmenopausal osteoporosis; reduction of urine volume in diabetes insipidus.

➡️⬅️ DRUG INTERACTIONS RELATED TO DENTAL THERAPEUTICS

COX-1 inhibitors: Decreased antihypertensive effect (decreased prostaglandin synthesis)
- Monitor blood pressure.

ADVERSE EFFECTS
⚠ **ORAL:** RAPID-ACTING FORMULATION: Dry mouth (<2%).

CNS: RAPID-ACTING FORMULATION: Dizziness; headache; weakness; "weird" feeling; neuropathy; fatigue; lethargy; lassitude; depression. SLOW-ACTING FORMULATION: Dizziness; syncope; neuropathy; vertigo; headache; weakness; fatigue; lethargy; lassitude; anxiety; depression; nervousness.

CVS: RAPID-ACTING FORMULATION: Orthostatic hypotension, palpitations (<2%); chest pain.

GI: RAPID-ACTING FORMULATION: Nausea. SLOW-ACTING FORMULATION: Nausea; anorexia; pancreatitis.

RESP: RAPID-ACTING FORMULATION: Cough; epistaxis; sinus congestion; sore throat.

MISC: RAPID-ACTING FORMULATION: Impotence; joint pain; back pain; itching eyes; tinnitus; muscle cramps and spasms. SLOW-ACTING FORMULATION: Swelling; chills; acute gouty attack; hyperglycemia; glucosuria; muscle cramps and spasms; leukopenia, agranulocytosis, aplastic anemia.

CLINICAL IMPLICATIONS
General
- Determine why drug is being taken. Consider implications of condition on dental treatment.
- Monitor vital signs (e.g., BP, pulse pressure, rate and rhythm) at each appointment to assess disease control. Do not provide elective dental treatment when BP is ≥180/110 or in the presence of other high-risk CV conditions. Refer to the section entitled "The Patient Taking Cardiovascular Drugs" in Chapter 6: *Clinical Medicine*.
- Use local anesthetic agents with vasoconstrictor with caution based on functional capacity of the patient and use aspirating technique to prevent intravascular injection.
- Determine ability to adapt to stress of dental treatment. Consider short appointments.
- Monitor pulse rhythm to assess for electrolyte imbalance.
- Chronic dry mouth is possible; anticipate increased caries, candidiasis, and lichenoid mucositis.
- *Postural hypotension:* Monitor BP at the beginning and end of each appointment; anticipate syncope. Have patient sit upright for several min at the end of the dental appointment before dismissing.
- If GI side effects occur, consider semisupine chair position.
- Blood dyscrasias rarely reported; anticipate increased bleeding, infection, and poor healing.

Oral Health Education
- Encourage daily plaque control procedures for effective self-care in patient at risk for cardiovascular disease.
- If chronic dry mouth occurs, recommend home fluoride therapy and use of nonalcoholic oral health care products.

---

metoprolol (meh-TOE-pro-lahl)
Lopressor, Toprol XL

■✦■ **Apo-Metoprolol, Apo-Metoprolol (Type L), Betaloc, Betaloc Durules, Gen-Metoprolol, Novo-Metoprol, Nu-Metop, PMS-Metoprolol-B, PMS-Metoprolol-B**

■▸■ **Kenaprol, Lopresor, Proken M, Prolaken, Ritmolol, Selectadril, Seloken, Selopres**

Drug Class: Beta-adrenergic blocker

PHARMACOLOGY
Action
Blocks beta receptors, primarily affecting CV system (e.g., decreases heart rate, decreases contractility, decreases BP) and lungs (e.g., promotes bronchospasm).

Uses

Used alone or in combination with other antihypertensive agents, for management of hypertension, long-term management of angina pectoris, MI (immediate-release tablets and injection), treatment of stable, symptomatic (New York Heart Association class II or III) heart failure of ischemic, hypertensive, or cardiomyopathic origin (Toprol-XL 25 mg only).

➡⬅ DRUG INTERACTIONS RELATED TO DENTAL THERAPEUTICS

Diazepam or clonazepam: Possible diazepam or clonazepam toxicity (decreased metabolism)
- Monitor clinical status.

Lidocaine: Lidocaine toxicity (decreased metabolism)
- Minimize lidocaine dosage.

COX-1 inhibitors: Decreased antihypertensive effect (decreased prostaglandin synthesis)
- Monitor vital signs.

Sympathomimetic amines: Decreased antihypertensive effect (pharmacological antagonism)
- Monitor vital signs.

ADVERSE EFFECTS

⚠ **ORAL:** Dry mouth; taste disturbances.

CNS: Headache; fatigue; dizziness (10%); depression (5%); lethargy; drowsiness; forgetfulness; sleepiness (10%); vertigo; paresthesias.

CVS: Bradycardia; hypotension; arrhythmia.

GI: Nausea; vomiting; diarrhea (5%); gastric pain; constipation; heartburn; flatulence.

RESP: Shortness of breath (3%); bronchospasm; dyspnea; wheezing.

MISC: Increased hypoglycemic response to insulin; may mask hypoglycemic signs; muscle cramps; asthenia; systemic lupus erythematosus; cold extremities; photosensitivity; blood dyscrasias (e.g., leukopenia, agranulocytosis, thrombocytopenia).

CLINICAL IMPLICATIONS

General
- Determine why drug is being taken. Consider implications of condition on dental treatment.
- Monitor vital signs (e.g., BP, pulse pressure, rate and rhythm) at each appointment to assess disease control. Do not provide elective dental treatment when BP is ≥180/110 or in the presence of other high-risk CV conditions. Refer to the section entitled "The Patient Taking Cardiovascular Drugs" in Chapter 6: *Clinical Medicine*.
- Determine ability to adapt to stress of dental treatment. Consider short appointments.
- Use local anesthetic agents with vasoconstrictor with caution based on functional capacity of the patient and use aspirating technique to prevent intravascular injection.
- Beta blockers may mask epinephrine-induced signs and symptoms of hypoglycemia in patient with diabetes.
- Chronic dry mouth is possible; anticipate increased caries activity and candidiasis.
- *Postural hypotension:* Monitor BP at the beginning and end of each appointment; anticipate syncope. Have patient sit upright for several min at the end of the dental appointment before dismissing.
- Blood dyscrasias rarely reported; anticipate increased bleeding, infection, and poor healing.

Oral Health Education
- Encourage daily plaque control procedures for effective self-care in patient at risk for cardiovascular disease.
- If chronic dry mouth occurs, recommend home fluoride therapy and use of nonalcoholic oral health care products.

Metric 21 — see metronidazole

MetroCream — see metronidazole

MetroGel MetroGel-Vaginal — see metronidazole
MetroLotion — see metronidazole

---

 metronidazole (meh-troe-NID-uh-zole)

Flagyl, Protostat : Tablets: 250, 500 mg
Flagyl ER: Tablets, extended-release: 750 mg
Flagyl 375: Capsules: 375 mg
Flagyl I.V.: Powder for Injection, lyophilized: 500 mg
Flagyl I.V. RTU: Injection: 5 mg/mL
Metric 21: Tablets: 250 mg
MetroCream: Cream: 0.75%
MetroGel MetroGel-Vaginal, : Gel: 0.75%
MetroLotion: Lotion: 0.75%
Noritate: Cream: 1%

■✦■ **Apo-Metronidazole, Florazole ER, Nida Gel, Novo-Nidazol**

■▶■ **Ameblin, Flagenase, Fresenizol, Milezzol, Nidrozol, Otrozol, Selegil, Servizol, Vatrix-S, Vertisal**

Drug Class: Anti-infective

PHARMACOLOGY

Action
Enters bacterial or protozoal cell and impairs synthesis of DNA, resulting in cell death.

Uses
Treatment of serious infections caused by susceptible anaerobic bacteria; prophylaxis of postoperative infection in patients undergoing colorectal surgery; treatment of amebiasis; treatment of trichomoniasis and asymptomatic partners of infected patients; bacterial vaginosis (Flagyl ER only).
TOPICAL: Treatment of inflammatory papules, pustules, and erythema of acne rosacea.
VAGINAL: Treatment of bacterial vaginosis.

Unlabeled Uses
Treatment of hepatic encephalopathy, Crohn disease, antibiotic-associated pseudomembranous colitis, *Helicobacter pylori* infection.

Contraindications
Hypersensitivity to nitroimidazole derivatives or any component of the products; first trimester of pregnancy in patients with trichomoniasis.

Usual Dosage
Anaerobic bacterial infections
ADULTS: *PO:* (Flagyl 375, Flagyl 250-mg tablets) Usual dosage is 7.5 mg/kg (approximately 500 mg for a 70-kg adult) q 6 hr (max, 4 g per 24 hr) for 7 to 10 days.

Pharmacokinetics
ABSORP: Oral metronidazole is well absorbed; topical application is less complete and more prolonged. Following administration, T_{max} is 1 to 2 hr, and C_{max} is 25 mg/mL. Oral bioavailability is not affected by food, but peak serum levels will be delayed to 2 hr.

DIST: Metronidazole appears in cerebrospinal fluid, saliva, and breast milk in concentrations similar to those found in plasma. Less than 20% is protein bound.

METAB: Metabolites are 2-hydroxymethyl and acidic metabolite.

EXCRET: Routes of elimination are via urine (60% to 80%) and feces (6% to 15%). Renal Cl is approximately 10 mL/min per 1.73 m². The $t_{1/2}$ is 8 hr in healthy adults, and the hydroxy-metabolite $t_{1/2}$ is 15 hr.

SPECIAL POP: *Hepatic failure:* Patients with hepatic dysfunction metabolized metronidazole more slowly: accumulation of drug may occur. Cautiously administer doses below the usual recommended dose.

Elderly: Because the pharmacokinetics of metronidazole may be altered in the elderly, monitoring of serum levels may be necessary to adjust the dosage accordingly.

➡️⬅️ DRUG INTERACTIONS

Alcohol: Mild disulfiram-like syndrome (inhibition of intermediary metabolism of alcohol)
- Avoid concurrent use.

Cyclophosphamide: Possible increased risk of cyclophosphamide toxicity (mechanism unknown)
- Avoid concurrent use.

Antacids: Possible decreased metronidazole effect (decreased metabolism)
- Avoid clinical use.

Anticoagulants, oral: Increased anticoagulant effect (decreased metabolism)
- Avoid concurrent use.

Phenobarbital: Decreased metronidazole effect (increased metabolism)
- Avoid concurrent use.

Carbamazepine: Possible carbamazepine toxicity
- Avoid concurrent use.

Corticosteroids: Decreased metronidazole effect (increased metabolism)
- Avoid concurrent use.

Cyclosporine: Possible cyclosporine toxicity (decreased metabolism)
- Avoid concurrent use.

Disulfiram: Organic brain syndrome (mechanism unknown)
- Avoid concurrent use.

Fluorouracil: Metronidazole toxicity (decreased metabolism)
- Avoid concurrent use.

Lithium: Lithium toxicity (mechanism unknown)
- Avoid concurrent use.

Phenytoin: Possible phenytoin toxicity (decreased metabolism)
- Avoid concurrent use.

Tacrolimus: Possible tacrolimus toxicity (decreased metabolism)
- Avoid concurrent use.

ADVERSE EFFECTS

When known, dose form and percentage are stated.

⚠ **ORAL:** Furry tongue; glossitis; stomatitis.
Flagyl ER: Metallic taste (9%), dry mouth (2%).
MetroGel Vaginal: Unusual taste (2%).

CVS: Flattening of T-wave.

CNS: Seizures; peripheral neuropathy; dizziness; vertigo; incoordination; ataxia; confusion; depression; insomnia; syncope; irritability; weakness.
Flagyl ER: Headache (18%); dizziness (4%).
MetroGel Vaginal: Headache (5%); dizziness (2%).

GI: Nausea; anorexia; vomiting; diarrhea; constipation; epigastric distress; cramps; pseudomembranous colitis.
Flagyl ER: Nausea (10%); abdominal pain, diarrhea (4%).

RESP: Flagyl ER: URI (4%).

MISC: Hypersensitivity reactions including dermatological reactions, nasal congestion, dry vagina, and fever; fleeting joint pain; pancreatitis. Topical or vaginal use may cause similar adverse effects. After prolonged IV use, thrombophlebitis may occur.

Flagyl ER: Bacterial infection (7%); influenza-like symptoms (6%); moniliasis (3%).

CLINICAL IMPLICATIONS
General
When prescribed by DDS:
- Antibiotic-associated diarrhea can occur. Have patient contact DDS immediately if signs develop.
- *Lactation:* Excreted in breast milk.
- *Children:* Safety and efficacy not established, except for amebiasis.
- *Elderly:* Monitoring serum levels may be necessary for proper dosing.
- *Hepatic failure:* Patients with severe hepatic disease metabolize drug slowly; use caution and lower dose.
- *Candidiasis:* Known or previously unrecognized candidiasis may present more prominent symptoms during therapy.
- *Hematologic effects:* Use with caution in patients with a history of blood dyscrasia.
- *Neurologic effects:* Seizures and peripheral neuropathy have occurred. Use extra caution with prolonged use, high doses, or history of CNS disease.
- *Overdosage:* Nausea, vomiting, ataxia, seizures, peripheral neuropathy.

When prescribed by medical facility:
- Determine why drug is being taken. If oral infection occurs that requires antibiotic therapy, select an appropriate product from a different class of anti-infectives.
- If GI side effects occur, consider semisupine chair position.

Pregnancy Risk Category: Category B.

Oral Health Education
When prescribed by DDS:
- Explain name, dose, action, and potential side effects of drug.
- Ensure patient knows how to take the drug, how long it should be taken, and to immediately report adverse effects (e.g., rash, difficult breathing, diarrhea, GI upset). See Chapter 4: *Medical Management of Odontogenic Infections*.
- Instruct patient to notify health care provider if infection does not appear to be improving or appears to be getting worse.
- Caution patient to avoid alcoholic beverages while taking metronidazole and for at least 3 days following completion of therapy.
- Advise patient that metallic taste is a common side effect of therapy but that this will resolve when therapy has been discontinued.
- Advise patient to report any other bothersome side effects to health care provider and to immediately report any abnormal neurological signs or symptoms (e.g., seizures, extremity numbness, abnormal skin sensations).
- Advise women to notify health care provider if pregnant, planning to become pregnant, or breastfeeding.
- Instruct patient not to take any prescription or OTC medications, dietary supplements, or herbal preparations unless advised by health care provider.
- Advise patient that follow-up examinations and laboratory tests may be required to monitor therapy and to keep appointments.

Tablets and capsules:
- Advise patient to take prescribed dose without regard to meals but to take with food if GI upset occurs.

Extended-release tablets:
- Advise patient to take prescribed dose daily, 1 hr before or 2 hr after a meal.
- Caution patient to swallow extended-release tablet whole and not crush, chew, or divide.

Mevacor — see lovastatin

mexiletine HCl (MEX-ih-leh-teen HIGH-droe-KLOR-ide)

Mexitil

■✦■ Novo-Mexiletine

Drug Class: Antiarrhythmic

PHARMACOLOGY

Action

Reduces rate of rise of action potential; decreases effective refractory period in Purkinje fibers; has local anesthetic actions.

Uses

Treatment of documented life-threatening ventricular arrhythmias (e.g., sustained ventricular tachycardia).

➡◆ DRUG INTERACTIONS RELATED TO DENTAL THERAPEUTICS

No documented drug-drug interactions. The absence of evidence is not evidence of safety.

ADVERSE EFFECTS

⚠ **ORAL:** Dry mouth (3%), taste disturbance; mucous membrane changes (unspecified).

CNS: Dizziness, lightheadedness (26%); tremor (13%); nervousness (11%); coordination difficulties (10%); headache (8%); changes in sleep habits (7%); weakness (5%); paresthesias, numbness, fatigue (4%); speech difficulties, confusion, clouded sensorium (3%); depression (2%); drowsiness; ataxia.

CVS: Palpitations, chest pain (7.5%); ventricular arrhythmia (2%).

GI: Nausea, vomiting, heartburn (40%); diarrhea (5%); constipation (4%); changes in appetite (3%); abdominal pain, cramps or discomfort (1%); dyspepsia.

RESP: Dyspnea (6%).

MISC: Nonspecific edema (4%); fever (1%); hypersensitivity; blood dyscrasias (e.g., thrombocytopenia, leukopenia, agranulocytosis, neutropenia).

CLINICAL IMPLICATIONS

General

- Monitor vital signs (e.g., BP, pulse pressure, rate and rhythm) at each appointment to assess disease control. Do not provide elective dental treatment when BP is ≥180/110 or in the presence of other high-risk CV conditions. Refer to the section entitled "The Patient Taking Cardiovascular Drugs" in Chapter 6: *Clinical Medicine*.
- Use local anesthetic agents with vasoconstrictor with caution based on functional capacity of the patient and use aspirating technique to prevent intravascular injection.
- Determine ability to adapt to stress of dental treatment. Consider short appointments.
- Chronic dry mouth is possible; anticipate increased caries, candidiasis, and lichenoid mucositis.
- Blood dyscrasias rarely reported; anticipate increased bleeding, infection, and poor healing.
- If GI side effects occur, consider semisupine chair position.

Oral Health Education

- Encourage daily plaque control procedures for effective self-care in patient at risk for cardiovascular disease.
- If chronic dry mouth occurs, recommend home fluoride therapy and use of nonalcoholic oral health care products.

Mexitil — see mexiletine HCl

Miacalcic — see calcitonin-salmon

Miacalcin — see calcitonin-salmon

Miacalcin NS — see calcitonin-salmon

Micardis — see telmisartan
Miccil — see bumetanide
Micostatin — see nystatin

---

 microfibrillar collagen hemostat

Synonym: collagen: MCH

Avitene: Fibrous form: 1 g, 5 g; Web form: 70 mm × 70 mm, 70 mm × 35 mm, 35 mm × 35 mm
Hemopad: Fibrous form: 2.5 cm × 5 cm, 5 cm × 8 cm, 8 cm × 10 cm
Hemotene: Fibrous form: 1 g

Drug Class: Hemostat, topical

PHARMACOLOGY
Action
An absorbable topical hemostatic agent that attracts platelets that adhere to the fibrils, triggering aggregation of platelets into thrombi in the collagen mass.

Uses
Adjunct to hemostasis.

Contraindications
Hypersensitivity to any component of the product; contaminated wounds.

Usual Dosage
Bleeding when other means of control are ineffective or impractical
Apply directly to source of bleeding as needed.

Pharmacokinetics
SPECIAL POP: No well-controlled studies for use in pregnant women. Safety for use during pregnancy has not been established.

➡️⬅️ DRUG INTERACTIONS
No documented drug-drug interactions. The absence of evidence is not evidence of safety.

ADVERSE EFFECTS
MISC: Allergic reaction; foreign body reaction; potentiation of infection/abscess formation; hematoma; wound dehiscence; and mediastinitis.

CLINICAL IMPLICATIONS
General
- Several min after placement, remove excess material.
- The use of a MCH in dental extraction sockets increases the incidence of alveolalgia.
- Compress with dry sponges immediately prior to application of the dry product, then apply pressure over the hemostat with dry sponge; length of time varies with force and severity of bleeding.
- Adheres to wet gloves, instruments, or tissue surfaces. To facilitate handling, use dry smooth forceps. Do not use gloved fingers to apply pressure.
- Moistening or wetting with saline or thrombin impairs the hemostatic efficacy; use dry and discard any unused portion.

Pregnancy Risk Category: Category C.

Micro-K Extencaps — see potassium products
Micro-K LS — see potassium products
Micronase — see glyburide

microNefrin — see epinephrine
Microrgan — see ciprofloxacin
Microzide — see hydrochlorothiazide
Midamor — see amiloride HCl

---

 midazolam HCl (meh-DAZE-oh-lam HIGH-droe-KLOR-ide)

Versed: Syrup: 2 mg/mL; Injection: 1, 5 mg (as hydrochloride)/mL

■✦■ **Apo-Midazolam**

■✦■ **Dormicum**

Drug Class: General anesthetic; Benzodiazepine
DEA Schedule: Schedule IV

PHARMACOLOGY

Action
Depresses all levels of CNS, including limbic and reticular formation, probably through increased action of GABA, which is major inhibitory neurotransmitter in brain.

Uses
Preoperative sedative; conscious sedation prior to diagnostic, therapeutic, or endoscopic procedures; induction of general anesthesia; supplement to nitrous oxide and oxygen for short surgical procedures; infusion for sedation of intubated and mechanically ventilated patients as a component of anesthesia or during treatment in critical care setting.

Unlabeled Uses
Treatment of epileptic seizures; alternative for the termination of refractory status epilepticus.

Contraindications
Hypersensitivity to benzodiazepines; uncontrolled pain; existing CNS depression; shock; acute narrow-angle glaucoma; acute alcohol intoxication; coma.

Usual Dosage
Preoperative sedative
ADULTS: *IM:* 0.07 to 0.08 mg/kg approximately 1 hr before surgery.
Conscious sedation
ADULTS: *IV:* 1 to 2.5 mg as 1 mg/mL dilution over 2 min. Increase by small increments to total dose of no more than 5 mg in at least 2-min intervals; use less if patient is premedicated with other CNS depressants.
CHILDREN: *IM:* 0.1 to 0.15 mg/kg. Doses up to 0.5 mg/kg have been used for more anxious patients. Total dose usually does not exceed 10 mg.
CHILDREN (YOUNGER THAN 6 MO): *IV:* Titrate in small increments to clinical effect and monitor carefully.
CHILDREN (6 MO TO 5 YR): *IV:* 0.05 to 0.1 mg/kg. Total dose up to 0.6 mg/kg may be necessary. Do not exceed 6 mg.
CHILDREN (6 TO 12 YR): *IV:* 0.025 to 0.05 mg/kg. Total dose up to 0.4 mg/kg. Do not exceed 10 mg.
CHILDREN (12 TO 16 YR): *IV:* Dose as adults.

Pharmacokinetics
ABSORP: Midazolam is rapidly absorbed. The oral AUC ratio of metabolite to midazolam is higher than IV. Mean T_{max} is 0.17 to 2.65 hr and the absolute bioavailability is 36%.

DIST: Midazolam exhibits linear pharmacokinetics (dose 0.25 to 1 mg/kg). Approximately 97% is protein bound (mainly to albumin). The mean steady-state Vd is 1.24 to 2.02 L/kg in children 6 mo to less than 16 yr old receiving 0.15 mg/kg IV.

METAB: Midazolam is subject to substantial intestinal and hepatic first-pass metabolism by cytochrome P450 3A4. Active metabolite is alpha-hydroxymidazolam.

EXCRET: Metabolites excreted in urine.

ONSET: Onset is 10 to 20 min.

SPECIAL POP: *Hepatic failure:* Following oral administration (15 mg), C_{max} and bioavailability were 43% and 100% higher, respectively. The clearance was reduced 40% and $t_{1/2}$ increased 90%. Doses should be titrated.

CHF: Following oral administration (7.5 mg), $t_{1/2}$ increased 43%.

➜← DRUG INTERACTIONS

Alfentanil: Hypotension (decreased sympathetic tone)
- Avoid concurrent use.

Amprenavir: Possible serious life-threatening midazolam toxicity (decreased metabolism)
- Avoid concurrent use.

Corticosteroids: Possible decreased midazolam effect (increased metabolism)
- Monitor clinical status.

Erythromycin, clarithromycin, or roxithromycin: Possible midazolam toxicity (decreased metabolism)
- Avoid concurrent use.

Fluconazole, itraconazole, or ketoconazole: Midazolam toxicity (decreased metabolism)
- Avoid concurrent use.

Lopinavir/ritonavir: Increased midazolam effect (decreased metabolism)
- Avoid concurrent use.

Nelfinavir: Possible midazolam toxicity (decreased metabolism)
- Monitor clinical status.

Propofol: Possible increased midazolam effect (decreased metabolism)
- Monitor clinical status.

Ranitidine: Altered midazolam effect (mechanism unknown)
- Monitor clinical status.

Saquinavir: Prolonged midazolam effect (decreased metabolism)
- Monitor clinical status.

St. John's wort: Decreased midazolam effect (increased metabolism)
- Monitor clinical status.

Theophylline: Decreased midazolam effect (receptor blockade)
- Avoid concurrent use.

Valproate: Possible midazolam toxicity (displacement from binding site)
- Monitor clinical status.

ADVERSE EFFECTS

⚠ **ORAL:** Excessive salivation; taste disturbance; toothache (unspecified).

CVS: Hypotension (2.3%), vasovagal episode, variations in blood pressure and pulse rate.

CNS: Headache; oversedation; retrograde amnesia; euphoria or dysphoria; confusion; argumentative; anxiety; emergence delirium and dreaming; nightmares; tonic/clonic movements; tremor; athetoid movements; ataxia; dizziness; slurred speech; paresthesia; weakness; loss of balance; drowsiness; nervousness; agitation; restlessness; prolonged emergence from anesthesia; insomnia; dysphonia.

GI: Nausea; vomiting; retching.

RESP: Respiratory depression or arrest; decreased tidal volume, decreased respiratory rate; apnea, coughing; laryngospasm; bronchospasm; dyspnea; hyperventilation; wheezing; shallow respirations; airway obstruction; tachypnea.

MISC: Pain, tenderness, and induration at injection site; yawning; chills; lethargy; weakness; toothache; faint feeling; hematoma; desaturation, apnea, hypotension, paradoxical reactions, hiccups, seizure-like activity, nystagmus (children).

CLINICAL IMPLICATIONS

General

When used or prescribed by DDS:

- Monitor vital signs.
- Geriatric, debilitated, and pediatric patients are more sensitive to the CNS effects of benzodiazepines.
- Warn patient not to drink alcoholic products while taking the drug.
- May produce sedation and interfere with eye-hand coordination and the ability to operate mechanical equipment. Inform patient not to drive, sign important papers, or operate mechanical equipment.
- *Lactation:* Midazolam is excreted in breast milk. Exercise caution when administering to a nursing mother.
- *Children:* As a group, pediatric patients generally require higher dosages of midazolam (mg/kg) than do adults. Pediatric patients (younger than 6 yr) may require higher dosages (mg/kg) than older pediatric patients and may require closer monitoring. In obese pediatric patients, calculate the dose based on ideal body weight.
- *Elderly:* May need to decrease dosage. Titration should be more gradual.
- *Renal failure:* Patients with renal impairment may have longer $t_{1/2}$ for midazolam, which may result in slower recovery.
- *Special risk:* High-risk surgical patients require lower doses. Patients with COPD are unusually sensitive to respiratory depressant effects. In renal or heart failure patients, give less frequently. Exercise care when administering to patients with uncompensated acute illness (e.g., severe fluid or electrolyte disturbances).
- *Hazardous tasks:* No patient should operate hazardous machinery or motor vehicle until the side effects of the drug have subsided or until the day after anesthesia and surgery, whichever is longer.
- *Benzyl alcohol:* The midazolam injection contains benzyl alcohol, which has been associated with a fatal "gasping syndrome" in premature infants.
- *Debilitated patients:* May need to decrease dosage. Titration should be more gradual.
- Serious cardiorespiratory events have occurred, including respiratory depression, airway obstruction, desaturation, permanent neurologic injury, apnea, respiratory arrest or cardiac arrest, sometimes resulting in death.
- *Improper dosing:* Reactions such as agitation, involuntary movements, hyperactivity, and combativeness have been reported.
- *Ophthalmic:* Moderate lowering of intraocular pressure following induction with midazolam.
- *Intracranial pressure/circulatory side effects:* Does not protect against the increase in intracranial pressure or circulatory effects associated with endotracheal intubation under light general anesthesia.
- *Overdosage:* Sedation, impaired coordination and reflexes, hypotension, hypoventilation, somnolence, coma, confusion.
- Continuously monitor patient for hypoventilation or apnea.
- Assist with ambulation after procedure until drowsiness resolves.
- Because serious life-threatening cardiorespiratory events have been reported, make provision for monitoring, detection, and correction of these reactions for every patient regardless of health status.

Pregnancy Risk Category: Category D.

Oral Health Education

When used or prescribed by DDS:

- Inform patient and family preoperatively about possibility of temporary postoperative amnesia.
- Advise patient that drug may cause drowsiness and to use caution while driving or performing other tasks requiring mental alertness until drowsiness has subsided or until day after administration, whichever is longer.
- Advise patient to avoid alcohol and other CNS depressants for 24 hr following administration.
- The patient should inform her health care provider if she is pregnant, planning to become pregnant, or is breast feeding.

- Patients receiving continuous infusion in critical care settings over an extended period of time may experience symptoms of withdrawal following abrupt discontinuation.

Midol — see ibuprofen
Midol Maximum Strength Cramp Formula — see ibuprofen
Midol PM — see diphenhydramine HCl
Midotens — see labetalol HCl

miglitol (mig-LIH-tall)

Glyset

Drug Class: Antidiabetic, alpha-glucosidase inhibitor

PHARMACOLOGY

Action

Inhibits intestinal enzymes that digest carbohydrates, thereby reducing carbohydrate digestion after meals, which lowers postprandial glucose elevation in diabetic patients.

Uses

Patients with type 2 diabetes mellitus who have been failed by dietary therapy. May be used alone or in combination with sulfonylureas.

➡◀ DRUG INTERACTIONS RELATED TO DENTAL THERAPEUTICS

No documented drug-drug interactions. The absence of evidence is not evidence of safety.

ADVERSE EFFECTS

GI: Abdominal pain; diarrhea; flatulence.

CLINICAL IMPLICATIONS

General

- Determine degree of disease control and current blood sugar levels. Goals should be <120 mg/dL and A1C <7%. A1C levels ≥8% indicate significant uncontrolled diabetes.
- The routine use of antibiotics in the dental management of diabetic patients is not indicated; however, antibiotic therapy in patients with poorly controlled diabetes has been shown to improve disease control and improve response following periodontal debridement.
- Monitor blood pressure because hypertension and dyslipidemia (CAD) are prevalent in diabetes mellitus.
- Monitor vital signs (e.g., BP, pulse pressure, rate and rhythm) at each appointment to assess disease control. Do not provide elective dental treatment when BP is ≥180/110 or in presence of other high-risk CV conditions. Refer to the section entitled "The Patient Taking Cardiovascular Drugs" in Chapter 6: *Clinical Medicine*.
- *Loss of blood sugar control:* Certain medical conditions (e.g., surgery, fever, infection, trauma) and drugs (e.g., corticosteroids) affect glucose control. In these situations, it may be necessary to seek medical consultation before surgical procedures.
- Obtain patient history regarding diabetic ketoacidosis or hypoglycemia with current drug regimen.
- Combination therapy with insulin or sulfonylurea: Observe for signs of hypoglycemia (e.g., confusion, argumentative, perspiration, altered consciousness). Be prepared to treat hypoglycemic reactions with oral glucose.
- Determine ability to adapt to stress of dental treatment. Consider short, morning appointments.
- Medical consult advised if fasting blood glucose is <70 mg/dL (hypoglycemic risk) or >200 mg/dL (hyperglycemic crisis risk).
- *If insulin is used:* Consider time of peak hypoglycemic effect.
- If GI side effects occur, consider semisupine chair position.

Oral Health Education
- Explain role of diabetes in periodontal disease and the need to maintain effective plaque control and disease control.
- Advise to bring data on blood sugar values and A1C levels to dental appointments.
- Encourage daily plaque control procedures for effective self-care in patient at risk for CV disease.

Miles Nervine — see diphenhydramine HCl

Milezzol — see metronidazole

Minidyne — see povidone iodine

Minims Atropine — see atropine

Minims-Pilocarpine — see pilocarpine HCl

Minims Prednisolone — see prednisolone

Minipres — see prazosin HCl

Minipress — see prazosin HCl

Mini Thin Pseudo — see pseudoephedrine

Minitran — see nitroglycerin

Minocin — see minocycline HCl

---

 minocycline HCl (min-oh-SIGH-kleen HIGH-droe-KLOR-ide)

Arestin: Microspheres, sustained-release: 1 mg (as hydrochloride)
Dynacin: Tablets: 50 mg (as hydrochloride); Tablets: 75 mg (as hydrochloride); Tablets: 100 mg (as hydrochloride); Capsules: 50 mg (as hydrochloride); Capsules: 100 mg (as hydrochloride)
Minocin: Capsules, pellet-filled: 50 mg (as hydrochloride); Capsules, pellet-filled: 100 mg (as hydrochloride); Powder for injection, cryodesiccated: 100 mg

Apo-Minocycline, Gen-Minocycline, Novo-Minocycline, PMS-Minocycline, ratio-Minocycline, Rhoxal-minocycline

Drug Class: Antibiotic, tetracycline

PHARMACOLOGY

Action
Inhibits bacterial protein synthesis.

Uses
Treatment of periodontitis as an adjunct to scaling and root planing. Treatment of infections caused by susceptible strains of gram-positive and gram-negative bacteria, *Rickettsia* and *Mycoplasma* pneumonia, and trachoma; treatment for susceptible infections when penicillins are contraindicated; adjunctive treatment of acute intestinal amebiasis; treatment of asymptomatic carriers of *Neisseria meningitidis* to eliminate meningococci from nasopharynx, chlamydia, inflammatory acne, syphilis, gonorrhea.

Contraindications
Standard considerations.

Usual Dosage
Periodontitis
ADULTS: Subgingival 1-mg microspheres are to be inserted by an oral health care professional.

Susceptible infections

ADULTS: *PO/IV:* 200 mg initially, *then PO/IV:* 100 mg q 12 hr *or PO:* 50 mg qid (max, parenteral 400 mg per 24 hr). Renal impairment: do not exceed 200 mg/24 hr.

CHILDREN OLDER THAN 8 YR OF AGE: *PO/IV:* 4 mg/kg initially, then 2 mg/kg q 12 hr (max, usual adult dose).

Pharmacokinetics

ABSORP: T_{max} is 1 to 4 hr after a single dose. Food does not affect extent of absorption, but C_{max} is slightly decreased and delayed by 1 hr.

DIST: Minocycline has very high lipid solubility, readily penetrates cerebrospinal fluid, and displays a good penetration of saliva, brain, eye, and prostate. 70% to 80% is protein bound.

METAB: Metabolism is concentrated by the liver in the bile.

EXCRET: 1% to 12% is excreted unchanged in urine. Serum $t_{1/2}$ is approximately 11 to 23 hr in healthy volunteers. Hemodialysis and peritoneal dialysis have little effect.

SPECIAL POP: *Renal failure:* Serum $t_{1/2}$ is 18 to 69 hr.
Hepatic failure: Serum $t_{1/2}$ is 11 to 16 hr.

➡◀ DRUG INTERACTIONS

Amitriptyline: Localized hemosiderosis (possible synergism)
• Avoid concurrent use.

ADVERSE EFFECTS

⚠ ORAL: Stomatitis; glossitis; dysphagia; enamel hypoplasia (e.g., in utero, lactation); candidiasis; esophageal ulceration; tooth discoloration; oral cavity discoloration (e.g., tongue, lips, gingivae); Microspheres: taste disturbance

CNS: Convulsions; dizziness; hypoesthesia; paresthesia; sedation; vertigo; bulging fontanelles in infants; benign intracranial hypertension (i.e., pseudotumor cerebri) in adults; headache.

GI: Anorexia; nausea; vomiting; diarrhea; dyspepsia; enterocolitis; pseudomembranous colitis; pancreatitis; inflammatory lesions (with monilial overgrowth) in oral and anogenital regions.

RESP: Cough; dyspnea; bronchospasm; exacerbation of asthma; pneumonitis.

MISC: Fever, discoloration of secretions; brown-black microscopic discoloration of the thyroid gland; photosensitivity; blood dyscrasias (e.g., thrombocytopenia, hemolytic anemia, leukopenia).

CLINICAL IMPLICATIONS

General

When prescribed by DDS:
• *Lactation:* Excreted in breast milk. Advise patient against nursing.
• *Children:* Avoid in children younger than 8 yr of age unless other appropriate drugs are ineffective or contraindicated because abnormal bone formation and discoloration of teeth may occur.
• *Renal failure:* May increase BUN; may lead to azotemia, hyperphosphatemia, and acidosis.
• *Superinfection:* Prolonged use may result in bacterial or fungal overgrowth.
• *Photosensitivity:* May cause exaggerated sunburn reactions.
• *Hepatotoxicity:* Has been reported. Use with caution in patients with hepatic dysfunction and in conjunction with hepatotoxic drugs.
• *Pseudotumor cerebri (benign intracranial hypertension):* Has been reported in adults. Usual manifestations are headache and blurred vision.
• *Tooth discoloration:* May cause permanent discoloration of the teeth.
• *Overdosage:* Dizziness, nausea, vomiting.
• Ensure patient knows how to take the drug, how long it should be taken, and to immedi-

ately report adverse effects (e.g., rash, difficult breathing, diarrhea, GI upset). See Chapter 4: *Medical Management of Odontogenic Infections*.

When prescribed by medical facility:
- Determine why drug is being taken. If GI side effects occur, consider semisupine chair position.
- Blood dyscrasias rarely reported; anticipate increased bleeding, infection, and poor healing.
- If oral infection occurs that requires antibiotic therapy, select an appropriate product from a different class of anti-infectives.
- Prolonged use of antibiotics may result in bacterial or fungal overgrowth of nonsusceptible microorganisms; anticipate candidiasis.

Pregnancy Risk Category: Category D.

Oral Health Education

When prescribed by DDS:
- Explain name, dose, action, and potential side effects of drug.
- Review dosing schedule and prescribed length of therapy with patient. Advise patient that dose and duration of therapy are dependent on site and cause of infection.
- Instruct patient using capsules to take prescribed dose with a full glass of water.
- Instruct patient or caregiver using oral suspension to measure and administer prescribed dose using dosing spoon, dosing syringe, or medicine cup.
- Advise patient to take without regard to meals, but to take with food if GI upset occurs.
- Advise patient to take 1 hr before or 2 hr after antacids containing aluminum, calcium, or magnesium, or preparations containing iron or zinc.
- Instruct patient to complete entire course of therapy, even if symptoms of infection have disappeared.
- Advise patient to discontinue therapy and contact health care provider immediately if skin rash, hives, itching, shortness of breath, headache, or blurred vision occurs.
- Advise patient that medication may cause photosensitivity and to avoid unnecessary exposure to sunlight or tanning lamps and to use sunscreens and wear protective clothing to avoid photosensitivity reactions.
- Caution women taking oral contraceptives that minocycline may make birth control pills less effective and to use nonhormonal forms of contraception during treatment.
- Advise women to notify health care provider if pregnant, planning to become pregnant, or breast feeding.
- Caution patient that drug may cause dizziness, light-headedness, or blurred vision and to use caution while driving or performing other hazardous tasks until tolerance is determined.
- Advise patient to report signs of superinfection to health care provider: black furry tongue, white patches in mouth, foul-smelling stools, or vaginal itching or discharge.
- Warn patient that diarrhea containing blood or pus may be a sign of a serious disorder and to seek medical care if noted and not treat at home.
- Caution patient not to take any prescription or OTC medications, dietary supplements, or herbal preparations unless advised by health care provider.
- Advise patient to discard any unused minocycline by the expiration date noted on the label.
- Advise patient that follow-up examinations and laboratory tests may be required to monitor therapy and to keep appointments.

Subgingival Microspheres
- Caution patient to avoid touching treated areas and to avoid brushing for 12 hr following treatment. Advise patient to avoid eating hard, crunchy, or sticky foods for 1 wk following treatment and postpone use of interproximal cleaning devices for 10 days.
- Advise patient that mild to moderate sensitivity is expected after treatment, but to notify dental professional immediately if pain, swelling, or other problems occur.

When prescribed by medical facility:
- Encourage daily plaque control procedures for effective, nontraumatic self-care.

Minodiab — see glipizide
Minofen — see acetaminophen

minoxidil (min-OX-ih-dill)
Loniten, Minoxidil for Men, Monoxidil, Rogaine
█✦█ **APO-Gain Topical Solution**
█▄█ **Regaine**
Drug Class: Antihypertensive; Topical hair growth

PHARMACOLOGY
Action
Directly dilates vascular smooth muscle by mechanism possibly related to blockade of calcium uptake or stimulation of catecholamine release; reduces elevated systolic and diastolic BP by decreasing peripheral arteriolar resistance; triggers sympathetic, vagal inhibitory, and renal homeostatic mechanisms including increased renin release, which results in increased cardiac rate and output and fluid retention; stimulates hair growth by unknown mechanism, but likely is related to its arterial vasodilating action.

Uses
ORAL FORM: Management of severe hypertension associated with target organ damage in patients who have failed to respond to maximal doses of a diuretic plus two other antihypertensive drugs.
TOPICAL FORM: Treatment of androgenic alopecia.

Unlabeled Uses
Treatment of alopecia areata (topical).

➜◆ DRUG INTERACTIONS RELATED TO DENTAL THERAPEUTICS
No documented drug-drug interactions. The absence of evidence is not evidence of safety.

ADVERSE EFFECTS
CNS: Headache; dizziness, faintness (topical); fatigue (systemic).
CVS: Tachycardia.
GI: Diarrhea; nausea; vomiting.
MISC: Temporary edema (7%); breast tenderness (<1%); darkening of skin; thrombocytopenia, leukopenia (rare) (systemic).

CLINICAL IMPLICATIONS
General
- Determine why drug is being taken. Consider implications of condition on dental treatment.
- Monitor vital signs (e.g., BP, pulse pressure, rate and rhythm) at each appointment to assess disease control. Do not provide elective dental treatment when BP is ≥180/110 or in the presence of other high-risk CV conditions. Refer to the section entitled "The Patient Taking Cardiovascular Drugs" in Chapter 6: *Clinical Medicine*.
- Use local anesthetic agents with vasoconstrictor with caution based on functional capacity of the patient and use aspirating technique to prevent intravascular injection.
- Determine ability to adapt to stress of dental treatment. Consider short appointments.
- Blood dyscrasias rarely reported; anticipate increased bleeding, infection, and poor healing.

Oral Health Education
- Encourage daily plaque control procedures for effective self-care in patient at risk for cardiovascular disease.

Minoxidil for Men — see minoxidil
MiraLax — see polyethylene glycol (peg)
Mirapex — see pramipexole dihydrochloride

mirtazapine (mer-TAZ-ah-peen)

Remeron
Drug Class: Tetracyclic antidepressant

PHARMACOLOGY

Action
Unknown. May enhance central nonadrenergic and serotonergic activity.

Uses
Treatment of depression.

➡️⬅️ DRUG INTERACTIONS RELATED TO DENTAL THERAPEUTICS
No documented drug-drug interactions. The absence of evidence is not evidence of safety.

ADVERSE EFFECTS
⚠️ **ORAL:** Dry mouth (25%), thirst; glossitis; candidiasis; aphthous ulceration.
CNS: Somnolence; asthenia; dizziness; abnormal dreams; abnormal thinking; tremor; confusion; hypesthesia; apathy; depression; hypokinesis; twitching; agitation; anxiety; amnesia; hyperkinesia; paresthesia.
CVS: Hypertension, vasodilatation (>1%).
GI: Nausea; constipation; vomiting; appetite changes; abdominal pain.
RESP: Cough; dyspnea.
MISC: Flu-like syndrome; back pain; myasthenia; myalgia; arthralgia; peripheral edema.

CLINICAL IMPLICATIONS

General
- Determine why drug is being taken. Consider implications of condition on dental treatment.
- Determine ability to adapt to stress of dental treatment. Consider short appointments.
- Depressed or anxious patients may neglect self-care. Monitor for plaque control effectiveness.
- Extrapyramidal behaviors can complicate performance of oral procedures. If symptoms present, consult with MD to consider medication changes.
- Chronic dry mouth is possible; anticipate increased caries and candidiasis.
- Monitor vital signs.

Oral Health Education
- Encourage daily plaque control procedures for effective self-care.
- *Tremor, extrapyramidal signs:* Determine need for power toothbrush for self-care.
- If chronic dry mouth occurs, recommend home fluoride therapy and use of nonalcoholic oral health care products.

misoprostol (MY-so-PRAHST-ole)

Cytotec
█✚█ **Apo-Misoprostol, Novo-Misoprostol**
Drug Class: Prostaglandin

PHARMACOLOGY

Action
Synthetic prostaglandin E_1 analog that inhibits gastric acid secretion and exerts mucosal-protective properties.

Uses
Prevention of gastric ulcers in high-risk patients who are taking NSAIDs.

➡← DRUG INTERACTIONS RELATED TO DENTAL THERAPEUTICS
No documented drug-drug interactions. The absence of evidence is not evidence of safety.

ADVERSE EFFECTS
CNS: Headache (2%).
GI: Diarrhea (14% to 40% [dose-related]); abdominal pain (13% to 20%); nausea, flatulence (3%); dyspepsia (2%); vomiting, constipation (1%).

CLINICAL IMPLICATIONS
General
• Determine why drug is being taken. Consider implications of condition on dental treatment.
• Avoid prescribing opioids for dental pain. Acetaminophen is appropriate if GI bleeding is present.
• If GI side effects occur, consider semisupine chair position.
• Consider acetaminophen for oral pain control.

Mitroken — see ciprofloxacin
Mobic — see meloxicam
Mobicox — see meloxicam

---

modafinil (moe-DAFF-ih-nill)
Provigil
■✦■ **Alertec**

Drug Class: CNS stimulant; Analeptic

PHARMACOLOGY
Action
Wakefulness-promoting agent; however, precise mechanism(s) unknown.

Uses
Improve wakefulness in patients with excessive daytime sleepiness associated with narcolepsy, obstructive sleep apnea/hypopnea syndrome, and shift work sleep disorder.

Unlabeled Uses
Treatment of fatigue associated with multiple sclerosis.

➡← DRUG INTERACTIONS RELATED TO DENTAL THERAPEUTICS
Triazolam: Reduced triazolam effect (increased metabolism)
• Monitor clinical status.

ADVERSE EFFECTS
⚠ **ORAL:** Dry mouth (4%), mouth ulceration, thirst, taste disturbance (1%).
CNS: Headache (34%); nervousness (7%); anxiety, dizziness, insomnia (5%); depression, emotional lability, paresthesia, somnolence (2%); anxiety, confusion, dyskinesia, hyperkinesias, hypertonia, tremor, vertigo (1%); symptoms of mania or psychosis.
CVS: Hypertension (3%); tachycardia, vasodilation, palpitation (2%).
GI: Nausea (11%); diarrhea (6%); dyspepsia (5%); anorexia, constipation (2%); flatulence.
RESP: Lung disorder (2%); asthma (1%).
MISC: Flu-like syndrome (4%); chest pain (3%); chills (1%); agranulocytosis.

CLINICAL IMPLICATIONS

General

- Determine why drug is being taken. Consider implications of condition on dental treatment. Anticipate short attention span.
- Extrapyramidal behaviors can complicate performance of oral procedures. If symptoms present, consult with MD to consider medication changes.
- Chronic dry mouth is possible; anticipate increased caries and candidiasis.
- Monitor vital signs.
- If GI side effects occur, consider semisupine chair position.

Oral Health Education

- Determine need for power toothbrush for self-care.
- If chronic dry mouth occurs, recommend home fluoride therapy and use of nonalcoholic oral health care products.

Modecate — see fluphenazine
Modecate Concentrate — see fluphenazine
Moditen hydrochloride — see fluphenazine

---

moexipril HCl (moe-EX-ah-pril HIGH-droe-KLOR-ide)

Univasc

Drug Class: Antihypertensive; ACE inhibitor

PHARMACOLOGY

Action

Competitively inhibits angiotensin I-converting enzyme, preventing conversion of angiotensin I to angiotensin II, which is a potent vasoconstrictor and also stimulates aldosterone secretion from the adrenal cortex. This results in decrease in sodium and fluid retention, decrease in BP, and increase in diuresis.

Uses

Treatment of hypertension.

➡️⬅ DRUG INTERACTIONS RELATED TO DENTAL THERAPEUTICS

COX-1 inhibitors: Reduced antihypertensive effect (decreased prostaglandin synthesis)
- Monitor blood pressure.

ADVERSE EFFECTS

CNS: Dizziness (4%); fatigue (2%).
GI: Diarrhea (3%).
RESP: Cough (6%).
MISC: Flu syndrome (3%); flushing (2%); anaphylactoid reactions.

CLINICAL IMPLICATIONS

General

- Monitor vital signs (e.g., BP, pulse pressure, rate and rhythm) at each appointment to assess disease control. Do not provide elective dental treatment when BP is ≥180/110 or in presence of other high-risk CV conditions. Refer to the section entitled "The Patient Taking Cardiovascular Drugs" in Chapter 6: *Clinical Medicine*.
- Use local anesthetic agents with vasoconstrictor with caution based on functional capacity of the patient and use aspirating technique to prevent intravascular injection.
- Determine ability to adapt to stress of dental treatment. Consider short appointments.
- If coughing is problematic, consider semisupine chair position for treatment.
- Susceptible patient with DM may experience severe recurrent hypoglycemia.

Oral Health Education

- Encourage daily plaque control procedures for effective self-care in patient at risk for CV disease.

---

mometasone furoate (moe-MET-uh-SONE FYU-roh-ate)

Asmanex Twisthaler, Elocon, Nasonex

∎✦∎ **Elocom**

Drug Class: Corticosteroid

PHARMACOLOGY

Action

Medium-potency topical corticosteroid that depresses formation, release, and activity of endogenous mediators of inflammation including prostaglandins, kinins, histamine, liposomal enzymes, and complement system; modifies body's immune response.

Uses

TOPICAL: Relief of inflammatory and pruritic manifestations of corticosteroid-responsive dermatoses.

INTRANASAL: Treatment of nasal symptoms of seasonal allergic and perennial allergic rhinitis; prophylaxis of nasal symptoms of seasonal allergic rhinitis; treatment of nasal polyps.

ORAL INHALATION: Maintenance treatment of asthma as prophylactic therapy; in asthma patients requiring oral corticosteroid therapy, adding Asmanex Twisthaler may reduce or eliminate the need for oral corticosteroids.

➜◆ DRUG INTERACTIONS RELATED TO DENTAL THERAPEUTICS

No documented drug-drug interactions. The absence of evidence is not evidence of safety.

ADVERSE EFFECTS

CNS: INTRANASAL: Headache ($\geq$5%).
ORAL INHALATION: Headache ($\geq$3%); insomnia (1% to 3%).

Oral: INTRANASAL: Taste disturbance, dysphagia.
ORAL INHALATION: Oral candidiasis ($\geq$3%).

GI: INTRANASAL: Vomiting ($\geq$5%); diarrhea, nausea (2% to 5%).
ORAL INHALATION: Abdominal pain, dyspepsia, nausea ($\geq$3%); anorexia, flatulence, gastroenteritis, vomiting (1% to 3%).

RESP: INTRANASAL: Coughing, epistaxis, sinusitis, upper respiratory tract infection ($\geq$5%); asthma, bronchitis, wheezing (2% to 5%).
ORAL INHALATION: Sinusitis, upper respiratory infection ($\geq$3%); dysphonia, epistaxis, respiratory disorder (1% to 3%).

MISC: Systemic absorption may produce reversible hypothalamic pituitary adrenal axis suppression, manifestations of Cushing syndrome, hyperglycemia, and glycosuria.
INTRANASAL: Viral infection ($\geq$5%); chest pain, flu-like symptoms (2% to 5%); anaphylaxis (postmarketing).
ORAL INHALATION: Allergic rhinitis ($\geq$3%); fatigue, flu-like symptoms, accidental injury, infection, pain, postprocedure pain (1% to 3%).

CLINICAL IMPLICATIONS

General

- Determine why drug is being taken. Consider implications of condition on dental treatment.
- Consider semisupine chair position to control effects of postnasal drainage.
- Anticipate oral candidiasis when steroids are used.

Oral Health Education
- Teach patient to rinse mouth and gargle vigorously with water after inhaled steroid use to minimize the potential for candidiasis.

Monafed — see guaifenesin
Monitan — see acebutolol HCl
Monodox — see doxycycline hyclate
Monoket — see isosorbide mononitrate
Mono Mack — see isosorbide mononitrate
Monopril — see fosinopril sodium
Monoxidil — see minoxidil

---

montelukast sodium (mahn-teh-LOO-kast SO-dee-uhm)
Singulair

Drug Class: Leukotriene receptor antagonist

PHARMACOLOGY

Action
Blocks the effects of specific leukotrienes in the respiratory airways, thereby reducing bronchoconstriction, edema, and inflammation.

Uses
Prophylaxis and chronic treatment of asthma in patients 12 mo and older; relief of symptoms of seasonal allergic rhinitis in patients 2 yr and older.

➡◀ DRUG INTERACTIONS RELATED TO DENTAL THERAPEUTICS
No documented drug-drug interactions. The absence of evidence is not evidence of safety.

ADVERSE EFFECTS
⚠ **ORAL:** Thirst; dental pain (unspecified).
CNS: Dizziness; headache.
GI: Dyspepsia; gastroenteritis; nausea; diarrhea; abdominal pain.
RESP: Bronchitis.
MISC: Asthenia; fatigue; viral infection; influenza; pyuria; fever; leg pain.

CLINICAL IMPLICATIONS

General
- Determine why drug is being taken. Consider implications of condition on dental treatment.
- Monitor vital signs (e.g., BP, pulse rate, respiratory rate and function); uncontrolled disease characterized by wheezing and coughing.
- Acute bronchoconstriction can occur during dental treatment; have bronchodilator inhaler available.
- Ensure that bronchodilator inhaler is present at each dental appointment.
- Be aware that sulfites in local anesthetic with vasoconstrictor can precipitate acute asthma attack in susceptible individuals.

Monurol — see fosfomycin tromethamine
Morphine HP — see morphine sulfate

morphine sulfate (moRE-feen SULL-fate)

Astramorph PF, Duramorph, Infumorph, Kadian, MS Contin, MSIR, OMS Concentrate, Oramorph SR, RMS, Roxanol, Roxanol 100, Roxanol Rescudose, Roxanol T, Roxanol UD

■✦■ M.O.S.-Sulfate, M-Eslon, Morphine HP, ratio-Morphine SR, Statex

■▩■ Analfin, Duralmor LP, Graten, Kapanol, MST Continus

Drug Class: Narcotic analgesic

PHARMACOLOGY

Action

Relieves pain by stimulating opiate receptors in CNS; also causes respiratory depression, peripheral vasodilation, inhibition of intestinal peristalsis, sphincter of Oddi spasm, stimulation of chemoreceptors that cause vomiting, and increased bladder tone.

Uses

Relief of moderate to severe acute and chronic pain; relief of pain in patients who require opioid analgesics for more than a few days (sustained-release only); management of pain not responsive to nonnarcotic analgesics; dyspnea associated with acute left ventricular failure and pulmonary edema; preoperative sedation; adjunct to anesthesia; analgesia during labor.

➡✦ DRUG INTERACTIONS RELATED TO DENTAL THERAPEUTICS

Bupivacaine: Possible respiratory depression (mechanism unknown)
  • Avoid concurrent use.
Lidocaine: Possible increased CNS and respiratory depression (additive)
  • Minimize lidocaine dosage and monitor clinical status.

ADVERSE EFFECTS

⚠ **ORAL:** Dry mouth; taste alteration.
CNS: Lightheadedness; dizziness; drowsiness; sedation; euphoria; dysphoria; delirium; disorientation; incoordination.
CVS: Circulatory depression; shock; hypotension; bradycardia.
GI: Nausea; vomiting; constipation; abdominal pain.
RESP: Respiratory depression; apnea; respiratory arrest; laryngospasm; depression of cough reflex.
MISC: Tolerance; psychological and physical dependence with chronic use; pain at injection site; local irritation and induration after SC use.

CLINICAL IMPLICATIONS

General

• Determine why drug is being taken. Consider implications of condition on dental treatment.
• Avoid prescribing opioids for dental pain. Acetaminophen is appropriate if GI bleeding is present.
• Chronic dry mouth is possible; anticipate increased caries activity and candidiasis.
• Monitor vital signs.

Oral Health Education

• Determine need for power toothbrush for self-care.
• If chronic dry mouth occurs, recommend home fluoride therapy and use of nonalcoholic oral health care products.

M.O.S.-Sulfate — see morphine sulfate
Motrin — see ibuprofen

Motrin IB — see ibuprofen
Motrin IB Extra Strength — see ibuprofen
Motrin IB Super Strength — see ibuprofen
Motrin Migraine Pain — see ibuprofen
MouthKote F/R — see sodium fluoride

---

moxifloxacin HCl (mox-ih-FLOX-ah-sin HIGH-droe-KLOR-ide)

Avelox, Avelox IV, Vigamox

Drug Class: Antibiotic, fluoroquinolone

PHARMACOLOGY

Action

Interferes with microbial DNA synthesis.

Uses

Treatment of acute bacterial sinusitis, acute bacterial exacerbation of chronic bronchitis, community-acquired pneumonia, uncomplicated skin and skin structure infections, and conjunctivitis caused by susceptible organisms.

➡◀ DRUG INTERACTIONS RELATED TO DENTAL THERAPEUTICS

Corticosteroids: Possible increased risk of Achilles tendon disorder (mechanism unknown)
• Consider risk/benefit.

ADVERSE EFFECTS

⚠ **ORAL:** Dry mouth, candidiasis, stomatitis, glossitis, taste disorder (<3%).
CNS: Dizziness (3%); headache, insomnia, nervousness, anxiety, confusion, somnolence, tremor, vertigo, paresthesia (<3%); psychotic reaction.
CVS: Syncope.
GI: Nausea (7%); diarrhea (6%); vomiting, abnormal LFT, dyspepsia, constipation, anorexia, flatulence, GI disorder (<3%); pseudomembranous colitis.
RESP: Dyspnea (<3%).
MISC: Abdominal pain, asthenia, moniliasis, pain, malaise, allergic reaction, leg pain, back pain, chest pain (<3%); angioedema (including laryngeal edema), anaphylactic reaction, anaphylactic shock; decreased hemoglobin/hematocrit (>2%).

CLINICAL IMPLICATIONS

General

• Determine why drug is being taken. Take precautions to avoid cross-contamination of microorganisms.
• If oral infection occurs that requires antibiotic therapy, select an appropriate product from a different class of anti-infectives.
• Chronic dry mouth is possible; anticipate increased caries and candidiasis.
• If GI side effects occur, consider semisupine chair position.

Moxlin — see amoxicillin
M-oxy — see oxycodone HCl
MS Contin — see morphine sulfate
MSD Enteric Coated ASA — see aspirin

MSIR — see morphine sulfate
MST Continus — see morphine sulfate
MTX — see methotrexate
Mucinex — see guaifenesin
Muco-Fen-LA — see guaifenesin
Munobal — see felodipine
Mupiban — see mupirocin

---

mupirocin (myoo-PIHR-oh-sin)
Synonym: pseudomonic acid A

Bactroban, Bactroban Nasal

■▪■ **Mupiban**

Drug Class: Anti-infective, topical

PHARMACOLOGY

Action
Inhibits bacterial protein synthesis.

Uses
Treatment of impetigo caused by *Staphylococcus aureus* and *Streptococcus pyogenes* (topical ointment); treatment of secarily infected traumatic skin lesions (up to 10 cm in length or 100 cm² in area) caused by susceptible strains of *Staphylococcus aureus* and *Streptococcus pyogenes* (topical cream); eradication of nasal colonization with methicillin-resistant *Staphylococcus aureus* in adult patients and healthcare workers (nasal).

➤◆ DRUG INTERACTIONS RELATED TO DENTAL THERAPEUTICS
No documented drug-drug interactions. The absence of evidence is not evidence of safety.

ADVERSE EFFECTS
CNS: TOPICAL: Headache (2%).
NASAL: Headache (9%).
GI: TOPICAL: Nausea (5%) (secary infected eczema).
RESP: NASAL: Respiratory disorder (5%); cough (2%).

CLINICAL IMPLICATIONS

General
• Determine why drug is being taken. Take precautions to avoid cross-contamination of microorganisms.

Myambutol — see ethambutol HCl
Mycelex — see clotrimazole
Mycelex-7 — see clotrimazole
Mycelex-7 Combination Pack — see clotrimazole
Mycobutin — see rifabutin
Mycodib — see ketoconazole

mycophenolate mofetil/mycophenolic acid (my-koe-
FEN-oh-late moE-feh-till/MY-koe-fen-AHL-ik ASS-id)

Synonym: mycophenolic acid/mycophenolate mofetil

CellCept, Myfortic

■✦■ **CellCept I.V.**

Drug Class: Immunosuppressive

PHARMACOLOGY

Action

Inhibits immune-mediated inflammatory responses but exact mechanism not known.

Uses

CELLCEPT: In combination with cyclosporine and corticosteroids for prophylaxis of organ rejection in patients receiving allogeneic renal, cardiac, or hepatic transplants.

MYFORTIC: In combination with cyclosporine and corticosteroids for prophylaxis of organ rejection in patients receiving allogeneic renal transplants.

➡◀ DRUG INTERACTIONS RELATED TO DENTAL THERAPEUTICS

No documented drug-drug interactions. The absence of evidence is not evidence of safety.

ADVERSE EFFECTS

⚠ **ORAL:** Candidiasis (11%); gingivitis, gingival hyperplasia, stomatitis, thirst, dry mouth (3% to 10%).

CNS: Headache (54%); insomnia (52%); asthenia (43%); tremor (34%); dizziness (29%); anxiety (28%); paresthesia (21%); depression, convulsion (17%); hypertonia (16%); agitation (13%); somnolence, nervousness (11%); emotional lability, neuropathy, hallucinations, abnormal thinking, vertigo, delirium, hypesthesia, psychosis (3% to <10%).

CVS: Chest pain (26%); hypertension (77%); hypotension (32%); tachycardia or bradycardia, arrhythmia (17% to 20%)

GI: Abdominal pain (63%); nausea (55%); diarrhea (51%); constipation (41%); vomiting (34%); anorexia (25%); dyspepsia (22%); enlarged abdomen (19%); flatulence, cholangitis (14%); hepatitis (13%); cholestatic jaundice (12%); esophagitis, flatulence, gastritis, gastroenteritis, GI hemorrhage, ileus, infection, rectal disorder, GI disorder, dysphagia, GI moniliasis, melena, stomach ulcer (3% to <10%); colitis, pancreatitis.

RESP: Infection, dyspnea (37%); pleural effusion (34%); increased cough (31%); lung disorder (30%); sinusitis (26%); rhinitis (19%); pneumonia (14%); atelectasis (13%); asthma (11%); lung edema, hiccups, pneumothorax, increased sputum, epistaxis, apnea, voice alteration, pain, hemoptysis, neoplasm, respiratory acidosis, bronchitis, respiratory disorder, hyperventilation, respiratory moniliasis (3% to <10%); interstitial lung disorder including fatal pulmonary fibrosis.

MISC: Pain (75%); fever (52%); sepsis, infection (27%); chest pain (26%); ascites (24%); accidental injury (19%); hernia (12%); chills (11%); peritonitis (10%); face edema, cyst, flu-like syndrome, malaise, pelvic pain, neck pain, cellulitis (with IV), phlebitis, abnormal healing, abscess, gout (3% to <10%); life-threatening infections (e.g., meningitis, infectious endocarditis), increased frequency of tuberculosis and atypical mycobacterial infection; blood dyscrasias (16% to 42%) (e.g., leukopenia, leukocytosis, thrombocytopenia, anemia).

CLINICAL IMPLICATIONS

General

- Determine why drug is being taken. Consider implications of condition on dental treatment.
- Consider medical consult to determine disease control and influence on dental treatment.

- Blood dyscrasias reported; anticipate increased bleeding, infection, and poor healing.
- Chronic dry mouth is possible; anticipate increased caries activity and candidiasis.
- Place on frequent maintenance schedule to avoid periodontal inflammation.

Oral Health Education

- Encourage daily plaque control procedures for effective, nontraumatic self-care.

---

mycophenolic acid/mycophenolate mofetil — see mycophenolate mofetil/mycophenolic acid

Mycostatin — see nystatin

Mycostatin Pastilles — see nystatin

Myfortic — see mycophenolate mofetil/mycophenolic acid

Mykrox — see metolazone

Myotonachol — see bethanechol chloride

Mysoline — see primidone

Mytelase — see ambenonium Cl

Mytussin — see guaifenesin

---

nabumetone (nab-YOU-meh-TONE)

Relafen

■✦■ **Apo-Nabumetone, Gen-Nabumetone, Rhoxal-nabumetone**

■◈■ **Relifex**

Drug Class: Analgesic; NSAID

PHARMACOLOGY

Action
Decreases inflammation, pain, and fever, probably through inhibition of COX activity and prostaglandin synthesis.

Uses
Relief of symptoms of chronic and acute rheumatoid arthritis and osteoarthritis.

➦◀ DRUG INTERACTIONS RELATED TO DENTAL THERAPEUTICS
No documented drug-drug interactions. The absence of evidence is not evidence of safety.

ADVERSE EFFECTS
⚠ **ORAL:** Dry mouth (3%); stomatitis.

CNS: Dizziness; lightheadedness; drowsiness; confusion; increased sweating; vertigo; headaches; nervousness; migraine; anxiety; aggravated Parkinson disease or epilepsy; paresthesia; peripheral neuropathy; myalgia; tremors; fatigue.

GI: Diarrhea; ulceration; heartburn; dyspepsia; nausea; vomiting; anorexia; diarrhea; constipation; flatulence; indigestion; appetite changes; abdominal cramps; epigastric pain; hematemesis; peptic ulcer.

RESP: Bronchospasm; laryngeal edema; dyspnea; hemoptysis; shortness of breath.

MISC: Photosensitivity; leukopenia, thrombocytopenia (<1%).

CLINICAL IMPLICATIONS

General
- Determine why drug is being taken. Consider implications of condition on dental treatment.
- *Arthritis:* Consider patient comfort and need for semisupine chair position.
- Chronic dry mouth is possible; anticipate increased caries and candidiasis.

- If GI side effects occur, consider semisupine chair position.
- Blood dyscrasias rarely reported; anticipate increased bleeding, infection, and poor healing.

Oral Health Education
- Evaluate manual dexterity; consider need for power toothbrush.

---

n-acetyl-p-aminophenol — see acetaminophen
Nadib — see glyburide

---

nadolol (nay-DOE-lahl)

Corgard

■✦■ **Apo-Nadol, Novo-Nadolol, ratio-Nadolol**

Drug Class: Beta-adrenergic blocker

PHARMACOLOGY

Action
Blocks beta-receptors, which primarily affect cardiovascular system (decreases heart rate, contractility, and BP) and lungs (promotes bronchospasm).

Uses
Management of hypertension and angina pectoris.

➦← DRUG INTERACTIONS RELATED TO DENTAL THERAPEUTICS

COX-1 inhibitors: Decreased antihypertensive effect (decreased prostaglandin synthesis)
- Monitor blood pressure.

Sympathomimetic amines: Decreased antihypertensive effect (pharmacological antagonism)
- Monitor blood pressure.

ADVERSE EFFECTS

⚠ **ORAL:** Dry mouth; taste disturbance; stomatitis.

CNS: Depression; fatigue; lethargy; drowsiness; short-term memory loss; headache; dizziness.

CVS: Bradycardia; arrhythmia; chest pain; hypotension or hypertension; orthostatic hypotension.

GI: Nausea; vomiting; diarrhea.

RESP: Wheezing; bronchospasm; difficulty breathing.

MISC: Increased sensitivity to cold; blood dyscrasias (e.g., thrombocytopenia, leukopenia, agranulocytosis, anemia).

CLINICAL IMPLICATIONS

General
- Monitor vital signs (e.g., BP, pulse pressure, rate and rhythm) at each appointment to assess disease control. Do not provide elective dental treatment when BP is ≥180/110 or in presence of other high-risk CV conditions. Refer to the section entitled "The Patient Taking Cardiovascular Drugs" in Chapter 6: *Clinical Medicine*.
- Use local anesthetic agents with vasoconstrictor with caution based on functional capacity of the patient and use aspirating technique to prevent intravascular injection.
- Determine ability to adapt to stress of dental treatment. Consider short appointments.
- *Postural hypotension:* Monitor BP at the beginning and end of each appointment; anticipate syncope. Have patient sit upright for several min at the end of the dental appointment before dismissing.
- Beta blockers may mask epinephrine-induced signs and symptoms of hypoglycemia in patient with diabetes.
- Chronic dry mouth is possible; anticipate increased caries and candidiasis.
- If GI side effects occur, consider semisupine chair position.

- Blood dyscrasias rarely reported; anticipate increased bleeding, infection, and poor healing.

Oral Health Education

- Encourage daily plaque control procedures for effective self-care in patient at risk for cardiovascular disease.
- If chronic dry mouth occurs, recommend home fluoride therapy and use of nonalcoholic oral health care products.

Nadopen-V — see penicillin V

Nalcrom — see cromolyn sodium

Naldecon Senior EX — see guaifenesin

Nalfon Pulvules — see fenoprofen calcium

---

 naloxone HCl (NAL-ox-ohn HIGH-droe-KLOR-ide)

Naloxone HCl: Neonatal injection: 0.02 mg/mL
Narcan: Injection: 0.4 mg/mL, 1 mg/mL

■◄■ **Narcanti**

Drug Class: Narcotic antagonist

PHARMACOLOGY

Action

Evidence suggests that naloxone antagonizes opioid effects by competing for opiate receptor sites in the CNS.

Uses

Complete or partial reversal of opioid depression, including respiratory depression, induced by natural and synthetic opioids, including propoxyphene; diagnosis of suspected or known opioid overdosage; adjunctive agent to increase BP in management of septic shock.

Contraindications

Standard considerations.

Usual Dosage

Opioid overdosage

ADULTS: *IV:* (*IM/SC* if IV route is not available) 0.4 to 2 mg; dose may be repeated at 2- to 3-min intervals if desired degree of counteraction and improvement in respiratory function are not obtained. If no response is observed after administration of 10 mg of naloxone, question the diagnosis.

CHILDREN: *IV:* (*IM/SC* if IV route is not available) Initial dose is 0.01 mg/kg; may give a subsequent dose of 0.1 mg/kg.

Postoperative opioid depression

ADULTS: *IV:* Small doses are usually sufficient. Titrate dose in increments of 0.1 to 0.2 mg IV at 2- to 3-min intervals to the desired degree of reversal (e.g., adequate ventilation without significant pain). Repeat doses may be required at 1- or 2-hr intervals, depending on amount, type, and time interval since last administration of an opiate.

CHILDREN: *IV:* Inject in increments of 0.005 to 0.01 mg at 2- to 3-min intervals to the desired degree of reversal of respiratory depression. Follow recommendation and cautions for adults.

Pharmacokinetics

DIST: Rapidly distributed in the body and readily crosses the placenta. Plasma protein binding is relatively weak.

METAB: Metabolized in the liver primarily by glucuronidation (major metabolite naloxone-3-glucuronide).

EXCRET: In adults the $t_{1/2}$ ranges from 30 to 81 min, while in neonates the $t_{1/2}$ is about 3 hr. Approximately 25% to 40% is excreted as metabolites in the urine within 6 hr, about 50% in 24 hr, and 60% to 70% in 72 hr.

ONSET: Following IV administration, the onset of action is usually apparent within 2 min.

DURATION: Duration of effect is more prolonged after IM injection compared with IV administration.

➡️⬅️ DRUG INTERACTIONS

Clonidine: Decreased clonidine effect (blockade of clonidine effect)
- Monitor blood pressure and clinical status.

ADVERSE EFFECTS

CVS: Hypotension; hypertension; ventricular tachycardia and fibrillation; pulmonary edema; cardiac arrest; death.

CNS: Agitation; seizures; convulsions; paresthesia; hallucinations; tremulousness.

GI: Nausea; vomiting.

RESP: Dyspnea; respiratory depression; hypoxia.

MISC: Coma; encephalopathy; withdrawal.

CLINICAL IMPLICATIONS

General
When used by DDS:
- *Lactation:* Undetermined.
- *Children:* May be given IV in children to reverse the effects of opiates. IM/SC route for opiate intoxication is not endorsed by the American Academy of Pediatrics because absorption may be erratic or delayed.
- *Elderly:* Use with caution because of the greater frequency of decreased hepatic, renal, or cardiac function, and of concomitant diseases or other drug therapy.
- *Renal failure:* Use with caution.
- *Hepatic failure:* Use with caution.
- *Opiate duration:* Because duration of action of some opiates may exceed that of naloxone, keep patients under continuous surveillance.
- *Postoperative:* Abrupt postoperative reversal of opioid depression may result in nausea, vomiting, sweating, tremulousness, tachycardia, increased BP, seizures, ventricular tachycardia and fibrillation, pulmonary edema, and cardiac arrest, which may result in death.
- *Withdrawal:* Use with caution in patients, including neonates of mothers suspected to be physically dependent on opioids, because an acute withdrawal syndrome may be precipitated.
- *Overdosage:* Seizures, severe hypertension, bradycardia, cognitive impairment, behavioral symptoms (including irritability, anxiety, tension, suspiciousness, sadness, difficulty concentrating, lack of appetite), somatic symptoms (including dizziness, heaviness, sweating, nausea, stomachaches).

Pregnancy Risk Category: Category B.

Oral Health Education
When used by DDS:
- Explain name, action, and potential side effects of drug.
- Advise patient or caregiver that medication will be prepared and administered by a health care professional in a medical setting.

---

naloxone HCl/buprenorphine HCl — see buprenorphine HCl/naloxone HCl

---

naltrexone HCl (nal-TREX-ohn HIGH-droe-KLOR-ide)
ReVia

Drug Class: Narcotic antagonist

PHARMACOLOGY

Action
Opioid receptor antagonist, markedly attenuating or completely blocking, reversibly, the subjective effects of IV administered opioids.

Uses
Treatment of alcohol dependence; blockade of exogenously administered opioids.

Unlabeled Uses
Eating disorders; postconcussional syndrome unresponsive to other treatments.

➡◀ DRUG INTERACTIONS RELATED TO DENTAL THERAPEUTICS
No documented drug-drug interactions. The absence of evidence is not evidence of safety.

ADVERSE EFFECTS
⚠ ORAL: Increased thirst (<10%); dry mouth (<1%).

CNS: Headache (7%); dizziness, fatigue (4%); insomnia (3%); anxiety, somnolence (2%); nervousness, low energy (>10%); increased energy, feeling down, irritability, loss of appetite (>10%); depression (0% to 15%); suicidal attempt/ideation (0% to 1%).

GI: Abdominal cramps (>10%); nausea (10%); diarrhea, constipation, vomiting (3%).

CLINICAL IMPLICATIONS

General
- Determine why drug is being taken. Consider implications of condition on dental treatment.
- Avoid prescribing opioids for dental pain. Acetaminophen is appropriate if GI bleeding is present. GI bleeding is associated with alcoholism.
- Determine if patient is in a professional treatment program.
- Alcohol and tobacco use and abuse predisposes to oral squamous cell carcinoma; perform oral cancer examination routinely.
- Do not recommend or prescribe alcohol-containing mouth rinses.

Oral Health Education
- Most substance abusers have poor oral health because of neglect. Encourage daily self-care to prevent periodontal disease.

Namenda — see memantine HCl
Naprelan — see naproxen
Naprodil — see naproxen
Naprosyn — see naproxen

---

 naproxen (nay-PROX-ehn)
(naproxen sodium)

Aleve: Tablets: 200 mg (220 mg naproxen sodium)
Anaprox: Tablets: 250 mg (275 mg naproxen sodium)
Anaprox DS: Tablets: 500 mg (550 mg naproxen sodium)
EC Naprosyn: Tablets, delayed-release: 375, 500 mg
Naprelan: Tablets, controlled-release: 375 mg (412.5 mg naproxen sodium), 500 mg (550 mg naproxen sodium)
Naprosyn: Tablets: 250, 375, 500 mg; Suspension: 125 mg/5 mL

◼✦◼ Apo-Naproxen, Apo-Naproxen SR, Gen-Naproxen EC, Naxen, Novo-Naprox, Novo-Naprox EC, Nu-Naprox, ratio-Naproxen, Apo-Napro-Na, Apo-Napro-Na DS, Novo-Naprox Sodium, Novo-Naprox SR, Novo-Naprox Sodium DS

■■■ **Artron, Atiflan, Atiquim, Dafloxen, Faraxen, Flanax, Flexen, Flogen, Fuxen, Naprodil, Naxen, Naxil, Neonaxil, Nixal, Novaxen, Pactens, Pronaxil, Supradol, Tandax, Velsay**

Drug Class: Analgesic; NSAID

PHARMACOLOGY

Action

Decreases inflammation, pain, and fever, probably through inhibition of COX activity and prostaglandin synthesis.

Uses

Rx: Management of mild to moderate pain, symptoms of rheumatoid or osteoarthritis, bursitis, tendinitis, ankylosing spondylitis, primary dysmenorrhea, acute gout. Naproxen (not naproxen sodium) also indicated for treatment of juvenile rheumatoid arthritis. Delayed-release naproxen is not recommended for initial treatment of acute pain because absorption is delayed compared with other naproxen formulations.

OTC: Temporary relief of minor aches and pains associated with the common cold, headache, toothache, muscular aches, backache, minor arthritis pain, pain of menstrual cramps, and reduction of fever.

Unlabeled Uses

Sunburn, migraine, premenstrual syndrome.

Contraindications

Allergy to aspirin, iodides or any NSAID; patients in whom aspirin or other NSAIDs induce symptoms of asthma, rhinitis, or nasal polyps.

Usual Dosage

Pain, dysmenorrhea, bursitis, tendinitis

NAPROXEN

ADULTS: *PO:* 500 mg initially, then 250 mg q 6 to 8 hr. Do not exceed 1,250 mg/day.

NAPROXEN SODIUM

ADULTS: *PO:* 550 mg initially, then 275 mg q 6 to 8 hr. Do not exceed 1,375 mg/day.

CONTROLLED RELEASE

PO: 750 to 1,000 mg once daily. Individualize dosage. Do not exceed 1,500 mg/day.

Pharmacokinetics

ABSORP: Naproxen is completely absorbed from the GI tract. Tablet T_{max} is 2 to 4 hr (immediate-release); suspension T_{max} is 1 to 4 hr; fasted patients' T_{max} is 4 to 6 hr (delayed-release); bioavailability is 95%; steady state is reached in 4 to 5 days.

DIST: Vd is 0.16 L/kg and protein binding is 99% albumin-bound.

METAB: Liver.

EXCRET: Naproxen is eliminated in urine (95%), primarily as naproxen less than 1%, 6-o-desmethylnaproxen less than 1%, or their conjugates (66% to 92%). Naproxen $t_{1/2}$ is 12 to 17 hr; clearance is 0.13 mL/min/kg; $t_{1/2}$ of metabolites and conjugates is less than 12 hr.

SPECIAL POP: *Renal failure:* Metabolites and conjugates may accumulate.

➡◀ DRUG INTERACTIONS

Alendronate: Increased risk of gastric ulcers (additive)
• Avoid concurrent use.

Angiotensin-converting enzyme inhibitors: Decreased antihypertensive effect (decreased prostaglandin synthesis)
• Monitor blood pressure.

Famotidine or ranitidine: Possible decreased naproxen effect (mechanism unknown)
• Monitor clinical status.

Diazepam: Possible decreased onset of action of naproxen (delayed absorption)
• Monitor clinical status.

Cholestyramine: Possible decreased naproxen effect (delayed absorption)
- Monitor clinical status.

Clopidogrel: Increased gastrointestinal bleeding (additive)
- Avoid concurrent use.

Corticosteroids: Increased risk of peptic ulcer disease (additive)
- Avoid concurrent use.

Furosemide: Decreased antihypertensive effect (decreased prostaglandin synthesis)
- Monitor blood pressure.

Misoprostol: Ataxia (mechanism unknown)
- Monitor clinical status.

Naltrexone: Possible increased risk of hepatotoxicity (mechanism unknown)
- Avoid concurrent use.

Probenecid: Possible naproxen toxicity (decreased renal excretion)
- Avoid concurrent use.

Thiazide diuretics: Hypertensive crisis (decreased diuretic effect)
- Monitor blood pressure.

ADVERSE EFFECTS

CVS: Edema; weight gain; CHF; alterations in BP; vasodilation; palpitations; tachycardia; chest pain; bradycardia.

CNS: Headache; dizziness; drowsiness; vertigo; lightheadedness; mental depression; nervousness; irritability; fatigue; malaise; insomnia; sleep disorders; dream abnormalities; aseptic meningitis.

GI: Constipation; heartburn; abdominal pain; peptic ulceration and bleeding; nausea; dyspepsia; diarrhea; vomiting; anorexia; colitis; flatulence.

RESP: Bronchospasm; laryngeal edema; dyspnea; shortness of breath.

CLINICAL IMPLICATIONS

General

When recommended by DDS:
- *Lactation:* Excreted in breast milk.
- *Children:* Safety and efficacy in children younger than 2 yr not established (Rx); do not give to children younger than 12 yr except under the advice and supervision of an M.D. (OTC).
- *Elderly:* Increased risk of adverse reactions.
- *Renal failure:* Assess function before and during therapy in patients with renal impairment because NSAID metabolites are eliminated renally.
- *Hepatic failure:* May need to reduce dosage in patients with hepatic failure.
- *Cardiovascular disease:* Drug may worsen CHF and may decrease hypertension control.
- *GI effects:* Serious GI toxicity (e.g., bleeding, ulceration, perforation) can occur at any time, with or without warning symptoms.
- *Overdosage:* Drowsiness, nausea, heartburn, vomiting, indigestion, seizures.

When recommended by medical facility:
- Determine why drug is being taken. Consider implications of condition on dental treatment.
- Monitor vital signs.
- If GI side effects occur, consider semisupine chair position.
- *Arthritis:* Consider patient comfort and need for semisupine chair position.

Pregnancy Risk Category: Category B.

Oral Health Education

When recommended by DDS:
- Tell patient to take with milk, meals, or antacids; follow with 1/2 to 1 glass of water to reduce GI upset.
- Advise patient to shake oral suspension before measuring.
- Explain that it may take 2 to 4 wk with naproxen and 1 to 2 days with naproxen sodium for anti-inflammatory effects to occur. Peak analgesic effect may occur in 1 to 2 hr.
- Caution patient that use with aspirin, alcohol, steroids, and other GI irritants may cause increased GI upset.

- Instruct patient to report the following symptoms to health care provider: visual problems, abdominal pain, symptoms of gastric bleeding.
- Caution patient to avoid consumption of alcoholic beverages and smoking.
- Advise patient to use caution while driving or performing other activities that require coordinated motor movements and mental alertness.

When recommended for arthritis:

- Evaluate manual dexterity; consider need for power toothbrush.

---

naproxen sodium — see naproxen

Naramig — see naratriptan

---

naratriptan (NAHR-ah-trip-tan)

Amerge

Naramig

Drug Class: Analgesic, migraine

PHARMACOLOGY

Action

Binds to serotonin (5-HT) 1_B and 1_D receptors in intracranial arteries leading to vasoconstriction and subsequent relief of migraine headache.

Uses

Treatment of acute migraine attacks with or without aura.

DRUG INTERACTIONS RELATED TO DENTAL THERAPEUTICS

No documented drug-drug interactions. The absence of evidence is not evidence of safety.

ADVERSE EFFECTS

⚠ **ORAL:** Dry mouth (1%).

CNS: Dizziness, drowsiness, malaise/fatigue, paresthesia (2%); vertigo (≥1%); cerebral vascular accident, including transient ischemic attack, subarachnoid hemorrhage, and cerebral infarction.

GI: Nausea (5%); vomiting (≥1%); colonic ischemia (postmarketing).

RESP: Dyspnea.

MISC: Atypical sensation (4%); pain and pressure in neck and throat (2%); warm/cold temperature sensation, sensations of pressure, tightness, and heaviness (≥1%); photosensitivity.

CLINICAL IMPLICATIONS

General

- Monitor vital signs (e.g., BP and pulse). Drugs for prevention are sympatholytic; drugs for treatment of acute attack are sympathomimetic.
- If GI side effects occur, consider semisupine chair position.
- This drug is for acute use during migraine attack. Patient is unlikely to present for oral health care appointment.

Narcan — see naloxone HCl

Narcanti — see naloxone HCl

---

narcotic analgesic combinations

Narcotic analgesics

Codeine, hydrocodone bitartrate, dihydrocodeine bitartrate, opium, oxycodone HCl, oxycodone terephthalate, meperidine HCl, propoxyphene HCl, propoxyphene napsylate, tramadol.

Barbiturates, acetylcarbromal, carbromal, and bromisovalum

Barbiturates, acetylcarbromal, carbromal, and bromisovalum are used for their sedative effects.

Alor 5/500, Lortab ASA Tablets: 1 or 2 tablets q 4 to 6 hr up to 8 tablets daily: 5 mg hydrocodone bitartrate, 500 mg aspirin
Lortab Elixir: 15 mL q 4 to 6 hr: 2.5 hydrocodone bitartrate, 167 mg acetaminophen per 5 mL. 7% alcohol, saccharin, sorbitol, sucrose, parabens
Synalgos-DC: 2 capsules q 4 hr: 16 mg dihydrocodeine bitartrate, 356.4 mg aspirin, 30 mg caffeine
Percodan-Demi Tablets: 1 or 2 tablets q 6 hr: 2.25 mg oxycodone HCl and 0.19 mg oxycodone terephthalate, 325 mg aspirin
Percodan Tablets, Roxiprin Tablets: 1 tablets q 6 hr: 4.5 mg oxycodone HCl and 0.38 mg oxycodone terephthalate, 325 mg aspirin
Darvon Compound-32 Pulvules: 1 tablet q 4 hr: 32 mg propoxyphene, 389 mg aspirin, 32.4 caffeine
Darvon Compound-65 Pulvules: 1 tablet q 4 hr: 65 mg propoxyphene, 389 mg aspirin, 32.4 mg caffeine
B & O Supprettes No. 15A Suppositories: 1 or 2 suppositories daily: 30 mg powdered opium, 16.2 mg powdered belladonna extract, polyethylene glycol base
B & O Supprettes No. 16A Suppositories: 1 or 2 suppositories daily: 60 mg powdered opium, 16.2 mg powdered belladonna extract, polyethylene glycol base

ADVERSE EFFECTS

Refer to monographs for each component included in combination for complete adverse effect profile. High-dose combination products are more likely to experience adverse drug effects.
⚠ **ORAL:** Dry mouth.
GI: Nausea; vomiting.
RESP: Depression of respiration.
CNS: Sedation; dizziness.
CVS: Hypotension.

Nardil — see phenelzine sulfate
Nasacort AQ — see triamcinolone
Nasacort HFA — see triamcinolone
NasalCrom — see cromolyn sodium
Nasarel — see flunisolide
Nasonex — see mometasone furoate

---

nateglinide (nah-TEG-lih-nide)
Starlix
Drug Class: Antidiabetic, Meglitinide

PHARMACOLOGY

Action
Lowers blood glucose levels by stimulating insulin secretion from the pancreas.

Uses
As monotherapy to lower blood glucose in patients with type 2 diabetes mellitus whose hyperglycemia cannot be adequately controlled by diet and exercise and who have not been treated long-term with other antidiabetic agents; in combination with metformin or a thiazolidinedione, in patients whose hyperglycemia is inadequately controlled with metformin, or after a therapeutic response to a thiazolidinedione. Do not use as a substitute for those drugs.

➤← DRUG INTERACTIONS RELATED TO DENTAL THERAPEUTICS

No documented drug-drug interactions. The absence of evidence is not evidence of safety.

ADVERSE EFFECTS

CNS: Dizziness (4%).
GI: Diarrhea (3%).
RESP: URI (11%); bronchitis (3%); coughing (2%).
MISC: Back pain, flu-like symptoms (4%); arthropathy, accidental trauma (3%); hypoglycemia (2.4%).

CLINICAL IMPLICATIONS

General

- Determine degree of disease control and current blood sugar levels. Goals should be <120 mg/dL and A1C <7%. A1C levels ≥8% indicate significant uncontrolled diabetes.
- The routine use of antibiotics in the dental management of diabetic patients is not indicated; however, antibiotic therapy in patients with poorly controlled diabetes has been shown to improve disease control and improve response after periodontal debridement.
- Monitor blood pressure because hypertension and dyslipidemia (CAD) are prevalent in diabetes mellitus.
- Monitor vital signs (e.g., BP, pulse pressure, rate and rhythm) at each appointment to assess disease control. Do not provide elective dental treatment when BP is ≥180/110 or in presence of other high-risk CV conditions. Refer to the section entitled "The Patient Taking Cardiovascular Drugs" in Chapter 6: *Clinical Medicine*.
- *Loss of blood sugar control:* Certain medical conditions (e.g., surgery, fever, infection, trauma) and drugs (e.g., corticosteroids) affect glucose control. In these situations, it may be necessary to seek medical consultation before surgical dental procedures.
- Obtain patient history regarding diabetic ketoacidosis or hypoglycemia with current drug regimen.
- Observe for signs of hypoglycemia (e.g., confusion, argumentativeness, perspiration, altered consciousness). Be prepared to treat hypoglycemic reactions with oral glucose or sucrose.
- Ensure patient has taken medication and eaten meal.
- Determine ability to adapt to stress of dental treatment. Consider short, morning appointments.
- Medical consult advised if fasting blood glucose is <70 mg/dL (hypoglycemic risk) or >200 mg/dL (hyperglycemic crisis risk).
- *If insulin is used:* Consider time of peak hypoglycemic effect.
- If GI side effects occur, consider semisupine chair position.

Oral Health Education

- Explain role of diabetes in periodontal disease and the need to maintain effective plaque control and disease control.
- Advise to bring data on blood sugar values and A1C levels to dental appointments.

Navane — see thiothixene

Naxen — see naproxen

Naxifelar — see cephalexin

Naxil — see naproxen

---

nedocromil sodium (NEH-doe-KROE-mill SO-dee-uhm)

Alocril, Tilade

Drug Class: Respiratory inhalant

PHARMACOLOGY

Action

Inhibits release of mediators from inflammatory cell types associated with asthma, including histamine from mast cells and beta glucuronidase from macrophages. May also suppress local production of leukotrienes and prostaglandins. Inhibits development of broncho-constriction responses to inhaled antigen and other challenges such as cold air.

Uses

Maintenance of mild to moderate bronchial asthma; treatment of itching caused by allergic conjunctivitis.

➡️⬅ DRUG INTERACTIONS RELATED TO DENTAL THERAPEUTICS

No documented drug-drug interactions. The absence of evidence is not evidence of safety.

ADVERSE EFFECTS

⚠️ ORAL: Taste disturbance.
CNS: Headache.
GI: Nausea; vomiting; dyspepsia; abdominal pain.
RESP: Rhinitis; URI; asthma.
MISC: Infection (8%); flu-like syndrome (3%); chills, fever (2%); neck rigidity (1%); anaphylactic reactions, angioedema, serotonin syndrome, photophobia, photosensitization (1%); leukopenia, ecchymosis, anemia (0.1% to 1%).

CLINICAL IMPLICATIONS

General
- Determine why drug is being taken. Consider implications of condition on dental treatment.
- Monitor vital signs (e.g., BP, pulse rate, respiratory rate and function); uncontrolled disease characterized by wheezing and coughing.
- Acute bronchoconstriction can occur during dental treatment; have bronchodilator inhaler available.
- Be aware that sulfites in local anesthetic with vasoconstrictor can precipitate acute asthma attack in susceptible individuals.
- Inhalants can dry oral mucosa; anticipate candidiasis, increased calculus, plaque levels, and caries.

Oral Health Education
- If chronic dry mouth occurs, recommend home fluoride therapy and use of nonalcoholic oral health care products.
- Ensure that bronchodilator inhaler is present at each dental appointment.

---

nefazodone HCl (neff-AZE-oh-dohn HIGH-droe-KLOR-ide)

Serzone

▌✚▌ Apo-Nefazodone, Lin-Nefazodone, Serzone-5HT2

Drug Class: Antidepressant

PHARMACOLOGY

Action
Undetermined; inhibits neuronal uptake of serotonin and norepinephrine; antagonizes alpha$_1$-adrenergic receptors.

Uses
Treatment of depression.

➡️⬅ DRUG INTERACTIONS RELATED TO DENTAL THERAPEUTICS

Alprazolam or triazolam: Possible alprazolam or triazolam toxicity (decreased metabolism)
- Monitor clinical status.

ADVERSE EFFECTS

⚠️ ORAL: Dry mouth (25%); taste disturbance; thirst.
CNS: Headache (36%); somnolence (28%); dizziness (22%); asthenia, insomnia (11%); lightheadedness (10%); confusion (8%); memory impairment, paresthesia (4%); abnormal dreams, decreased concentration (3%); ataxia, incoordination, psychomotor retardation, tremor (2%); hypertonia, decreased libido (1%); convulsions.

CVS: Postural hypotension (4%), hypotension (2%).

GI: Nausea (23%); constipation (17%); dyspepsia (9%); diarrhea (8%); increased appetite (5%); nausea and vomiting (2%); gastroenteritis (≥1%).

RESP: Increased cough (3%); dyspnea, bronchitis (≥1%).

MISC: Infection (8%); flu-like syndrome (3%); chills, fever (2%); neck rigidity (1%); anaphylactic reactions, angioedema, serotonin syndrome; photophobia, photosensitization (1%); leukopenia, ecchymosis, anemia (0.1% to 1%).

CLINICAL IMPLICATIONS
General
- Determine why drug is being taken. Consider implications of condition on dental treatment.
- Depressed or anxious patients may neglect self-care. Monitor for plaque control effectiveness.
- Determine ability to adapt to stress of dental treatment. Consider short appointments.
- Chronic dry mouth is possible; anticipate increased caries and candidiasis.
- *Postural hypotension:* Monitor BP at the beginning and end of each appointment; anticipate syncope. Have patient sit upright for several min at the end of the dental appointment before dismissing.
- If GI side effects occur, consider semisupine chair position.
- *Photophobia:* Direct dental light out of patient's eyes and offer dark glasses for comfort.

Oral Health Education
- Encourage daily plaque control procedures for effective self-care.
- Evaluate manual dexterity; consider need for power toothbrush.
- If chronic dry mouth occurs, recommend home fluoride therapy and use of nonalcoholic oral health care products.

---

nelfinavir mesylate (nell-FIN-ah-veer MES-il-ayt)
Viracept

Drug Class: Antiretroviral, protease inhibitor

PHARMACOLOGY
Action
Inhibits HIV protease, the enzyme required to form functional proteins in HIV-infected cells.

Uses
Treatment of HIV infection in combination with other antiretroviral agents.

➡◆ DRUG INTERACTIONS RELATED TO DENTAL THERAPEUTICS
Midazolam or triazolam: Possible midazolam or triazolam toxicity (decreased metabolism)
- Monitor clinical status.

ADVERSE EFFECTS
⚠ **ORAL:** Mouth ulcerations (unspecified).

CNS: Headache; paresthesia; dizziness; insomnia; somnolence; anxiety; depression; seizures; emotional lability; hyperkinesia; migraine; sleep disorder.

CVS: Torsades de pointes, prolonged QT interval.

GI: Anorexia; diarrhea (20%); dyspepsia; flatulence; nausea (3%); vomiting; abdominal pain; pancreatitis; bleeding.

RESP: Dyspnea.

MISC: Asthenia; fever; myalgia; back pain; malaise; arthralgia; myasthenia; myopathy; accidental injury; allergic reaction; arthralgia; cramps; anemia, leukopenia, thrombocytopenia (<2%).

CLINICAL IMPLICATIONS
General
- Determine why drug is being taken. Consider implications of condition on dental treatment.

- Consider medical consult to determine disease control and influence on dental treatment.
- This drug is frequently prescribed in combination with one or more other antiviral agents. Side effects of all agents must be considered during the drug review process.
- Antibiotic prophylaxis should be considered when <500 PMN/mm^3 are reported; elective dental treatment should be delayed until blood values improve.
- Anticipate oral candidiasis when HIV disease is reported.
- Monitor vital signs.
- Blood dyscrasias rarely reported; anticipate increased bleeding, infection, and poor healing.

Oral Health Education
- Encourage daily plaque control procedures for effective, nontraumatic self-care.

Nembutal Sodium — see pentobarbital sodium

Neo-Diaral — see loperamide HCl

Neodol — see acetaminophen

Neodolito — see acetaminophen

Neofomiral — see fluconazole

Neonaxil — see naproxen

Neopap — see acetaminophen

Neopulmonier — see dextromethorphan HBr

Neoral — see cyclosporine

Nephro-Fer — see ferrous salts

Nervocaine — see lidocaine HCl

Neugeron — see carbamazepine

Neurontin — see gabapentin

Neurosine — see buspirone HCl

NeutraGard Advanced — see sodium fluoride

---

nevirapine (nuh-VEER-uh-peen)

Viramune

Drug Class: Antiretroviral, non-nucleoside reverse transcriptase inhibitor

PHARMACOLOGY

Action
Inhibits replication of retroviruses, including HIV.

Uses
In combination with other antiretroviral agents for treatment of HIV-1 infection.

➡️⬅️ DRUG INTERACTIONS RELATED TO DENTAL THERAPEUTICS
No documented drug-drug interactions. The absence of evidence is not evidence of safety.

ADVERSE EFFECTS
⚠️ **ORAL:** Ulcerative stomatitis; oral lesions (unspecified).
CNS: Fatigue (5%); headache (4%); somnolence; paresthesia; malaise.
GI: Nausea (9%); abdominal pain, diarrhea (2%); vomiting.
MISC: Fever; eosinophilia; granulocytopenia; thrombocytopenia.

CLINICAL IMPLICATIONS

General
- Determine why drug is being taken. Consider implications of condition on dental treatment.

- Consider medical consult to determine disease control and influence on dental treatment.
- Anticipate oral candidiasis when HIV disease is reported.
- Advise products for palliative relief of oral manifestations (e.g., stomatitis, mucositis, xerostomia).
- If GI side effects occur, consider semisupine chair position.
- Blood dyscrasias rarely reported; anticipate increased bleeding, infection, and poor healing.

Oral Health Education

- Encourage daily plaque control procedures for effective, nontraumatic self-care.

Nexium — see esomeprazole magnesium

---

niacin (NYE-uh-sin)

Synonyms: B3; nicotinic acid

Niaspan, Slo-Niacin

■■■ Hipocol, Pepevit

Drug Class: Vitamin; Antihyperlipidemic

PHARMACOLOGY

Action

Necessary for lipid metabolism, tissue respiration, and glycogenolysis. At pharmacological doses, it reduces total cholesterol, LDL cholesterol, and triglycerides while increasing HDL cholesterol. Also causes peripheral vasodilation, especially cutaneous vessels.

Uses

Prevention and treatment of niacin deficiency or pellagra; treatment of hyperlipidemia (types IV and V); adjunct to diet for the reduction of elevated total and LDL levels in patients with primary hypercholesterolemia when the response to diet and other nonpharmacologic measures alone has been inadequate.

➥◀ DRUG INTERACTIONS RELATED TO DENTAL THERAPEUTICS

No documented drug-drug interactions. The absence of evidence is not evidence of safety.

ADVERSE EFFECTS

CNS: Dizziness; syncope; headache.
CVS: Postural hypotension; atrial fibrillation and other cardiac arrhythmias.
GI: Nausea; bloating; flatulence; hunger; vomiting; heartburn; diarrhea; activation of peptic ulcer; abdominal pain; dyspepsia.
MISC: Hyperuricemia; hyperglycemia; decreased glucose tolerance test results; toxic amblyopia; sensation of warmth; cystoid macular edema.

CLINICAL IMPLICATIONS

General

- Determine why drug is being taken. Consider implications of condition on dental treatment.
- High LDL cholesterol concentration is the major cause of atherosclerosis, which leads to CAD (angina, MI); determine degree of CV health and ability to withstand stress of dental treatment.
- Determine ability to adapt to stress of dental treatment. Consider short appointments.
- Monitor vital signs (e.g., BP, pulse pressure, rate and rhythm) at each appointment to assess disease control. Do not provide elective dental treatment when BP is ≥180/110 or in the presence of other high-risk CV conditions. Refer to the section entitled "The Patient Taking Cardiovascular Drugs" in Chapter 6: *Clinical Medicine*.

- *Postural hypotension:* Monitor BP at the beginning and end of each appointment; antici-pate syncope. Have patient sit upright for several min at the end of the dental appoint-ment before dismissing.
- If GI side effects occur, consider semisupine chair position.

Oral Health Education
- Encourage daily plaque control procedures for effective self-care in patient at risk for car-diovascular disease.

---

niacin/lovastatin (NYE-uh-sin/LOW-vuh-STAT-in)

Synonym: lovastatin/niacin

Advicor

Drug Class: Antihyperlipidemic combination

PHARMACOLOGY

Action

NIACIN: Necessary for lipid metabolism, tissue respiration, and glycogenolysis; reduces total cholesterol, LDL cholesterol, and triglycerides (TG) while increasing HDL cholesterol. LOVASTATIN: Increases rate at which body removes cholesterol from blood and reduces pro-duction of cholesterol in the body by inhibiting enzyme that catalyses early rate-limiting step in cholesterol synthesis; increases HDL; reduces LDL, VLDL, and TG.

Uses

Treatment of primary hypercholesterolemia (heterozygous familial and nonfamilial) and mixed dyslipidemia (Frederickson Types IIa and IIb) in patients treated with lovastatin who require further TG-lowering or HDL-raising who may benefit from having niacin added to their regimen; patients treated with niacin who require further LDL-lowering who may bene-fit from having lovastatin added to their regimen.

➡️⬅️ DRUG INTERACTIONS RELATED TO DENTAL THERAPEUTICS

Fluconazole, ketoconazole, or itraconazole: Rhabdomyolysis (decreased lovastatin metabo-lism)
- Avoid concurrent use.

Clarithromycin: Rhabdomyolysis (decreased lovastatin metabolism)
- Avoid concurrent use.

ADVERSE EFFECTS

The incidence stated for the following adverse reactions were reported with Advicor (nia-cin/lovastatin) administration. Adverse reactions occurring with administration of either nia-cin or lovastatin listed in their respective monographs.

⚠️ **ORAL:** Dry mouth, taste disturbance.
CNS: Headache (9%); asthenia (5%).
CVS: Flushing, postural hypotension.
GI: Nausea (7%); diarrhea (6%); abdominal pain (4%); dyspepsia, vomiting (3%).
MISC: Infection (20%); pain (8%); flu-like syndrome (6%); blood dyscrasias, including thrombocytopenia, leukopenia, others.

CLINICAL IMPLICATIONS

General
- High LDL cholesterol concentration is the major cause of atherosclerosis, which leads to CAD (e.g., angina, MI); determine degree of CV health and ability to withstand stress of dental treatment.
- Monitor vital signs (e.g., BP, pulse pressure, rate and rhythm) at each appointment to as-sess disease control. Do not provide elective dental treatment when BP is ≥180/110 or

in the presence of other high-risk CV conditions. Refer to the section entitled "The Patient Taking Cardiovascular Drugs" in Chapter 6: *Clinical Medicine.*
- Determine ability to adapt to stress of dental treatment. Consider short appointments.
- *Postural hypotension:* Monitor BP at the beginning and end of each appointment; anticipate syncope. Have patient sit upright for several min at the end of the dental appointment before dismissing.
- If GI side effects occur, consider semisupine chair position.
- Chronic dry mouth is possible; anticipate increased caries and candidiasis.
- Blood dyscrasias rarely reported; anticipate increased bleeding, infection, and poor healing.

Oral Health Education
- Encourage daily plaque control procedures for effective self-care in patient at risk for cardiovascular disease.
- If chronic dry mouth occurs, recommend home fluoride therapy and use of nonalcoholic oral health care products.

Niar — see selegiline HCl

Niaspan — see niacin

---

nicardipine HCl (NYE-CAR-dih-peen HIGH-droe-KLOR-ide)
Cardene, Cardene I.V., Cardene SR

■◆■ **Ridene**

Drug Class: Calcium channel blocker

PHARMACOLOGY
Action
Inhibits movement of calcium ions across cell membrane in systemic and coronary vascular smooth muscle and myocardium.

Uses
Treatment of chronic stable (effort-associated) angina (immediate-release capsules); management of hypertension (immediate- and sustained-release capsules; IV when oral therapy not feasible or desirable).

➜◆ DRUG INTERACTIONS RELATED TO DENTAL THERAPEUTICS
No documented drug-drug interactions. The absence of evidence is not evidence of safety.

ADVERSE EFFECTS
⚠ **ORAL:** Dry mouth; gingival hyperplasia.
CNS: Dizziness; lightheadedness; asthenia; psychiatric disturbances; headache; paresthesia; somnolence; weakness.
CVS: Flushing (9.7%); palpitations (4%), postural hypotension (1%), tachycardia (3%).
GI: Nausea; abdominal discomfort; cramps; dyspepsia.
MISC: Flushing; allergic reaction; myalgia; hypokalemia.

CLINICAL IMPLICATIONS
General
- Determine why drug is being taken. Consider implications of condition on dental treatment.
- Monitor vital signs (e.g., BP, pulse pressure, rate and rhythm) at each appointment to assess disease control. Do not provide elective dental treatment when BP is ≥180/110 or in the presence of other high-risk CV conditions. Refer to the section entitled "The Patient Taking Cardiovascular Drugs" in Chapter 6: *Clinical Medicine.*
- Use local anesthetic agents with vasoconstrictor with caution based on functional capacity of the patient and use aspirating technique to prevent intravascular injection.

- Determine ability to adapt to stress of dental treatment. Consider short appointments.
- *Angina:* Ensure patient brings personal acute-use nitroglycerin prescription to all dental appointments; verify expiration date to ensure drug activity.
- Anticipate gingival hyperplasia; consider MD consult to recommend different drug regimen if periodontal health is compromised.
- Chronic dry mouth is possible; anticipate increased caries activity and candidiasis.

Oral Health Education
- Encourage daily plaque control procedures for effective self-care in patient at risk for CV disease.

NicoDerm — see nicotine

Nicolan — see nicotine

Nicorette — see nicotine

Nicorette DS — see nicotine

Nicorette Plus — see nicotine

---

nicotine (NIK-oh-TEEN)

Commit, Habitrol, NicoDerm, Nicorette, Nicorette DS, Nicotrol, Nicotrol Inhaler, Nicotrol NS, ProStep

■✦■ **Nicorette Plus**

■✦■ **Nicolan, Nicotinell TTS**

Drug Class: Smoking deterrent

PHARMACOLOGY

Action
Reduces nicotine withdrawal symptoms by providing nicotine levels lower than those associated with smoking.

Uses
Aid to smoking cessation. Part of comprehensive behavioral smoking-cessation program.

➡◀ DRUG INTERACTIONS RELATED TO DENTAL THERAPEUTICS

No documented drug-drug interactions. The absence of evidence is not evidence of safety.

ADVERSE EFFECTS

⚠ **ORAL:** Local irritation (mouth, throat); taste disturbance, pain in jaw; gum disorder, tooth disorder (unspecified) (≥3%); excess salivation.

CNS: Insomnia; dizziness; lightheadedness; irritability; headache; impaired concentration; confusion; convulsions; depression; paresthesia; abnormal dreams.

CVS: Hypertension (≥3%).

GI: GI distress; belching; indigestion; nausea; vomiting; hiccups; anorexia; constipation; diarrhea.

RESP: Increased cough; pharyngitis; sinusitis; difficulty breathing; hoarseness; sneezing.

MISC: Pain; myalgia; arthralgia; dysmenorrhea.

CLINICAL IMPLICATIONS

General
- Determine why drug is being taken. Consider implications of condition on dental treatment.
- Monitor vital signs (e.g., BP, pulse pressure, rate, and rhythm) at each appointment to assess disease control. Do not provide elective dental treatment when BP is ≥180/110 or in the presence of other high-risk CV conditions. Refer to the section entitled "The Patient Taking Cardiovascular Drugs" in Chapter 6: *Clinical Medicine*.

- Perform oral cancer examination because of increased risk with tobacco use.
- If GI side effects occur, consider semisupine chair position.

Oral Health Education
- Inform patient about the risks of using tobacco products and the relationship between tobacco use and oral cancer.
- Explain role of tobacco use in periodontal disease and the need to consider a smoking cessation program.
- Encourage daily plaque control procedures for effective self-care.

Nicotinell TTS — see nicotine

nicotinic acid — see niacin

Nicotrol — see nicotine

Nicotrol Inhaler — see nicotine

Nicotrol NS — see nicotine

Nida Gel — see metronidazole

Nidrozol — see metronidazole

Nifedical XL — see nifedipine

---

nifedipine (nye-FED-ih-peen)
Adalat, Adalat CC, Afeditab CR, Nifedical XL, Procardia, Procardia XL

■✦■ **Adalat XL, Apo-Nifed, Apo-Nifed PA, Novo-Nifedin, Nu-Nifed, Nu-Nifedipine**

■✦■ **Corogal, Corotrend, Nifedipres, Noviken-N**

Drug Class: Calcium channel blocker

PHARMACOLOGY
Action
Inhibits movement of calcium ions across cell membrane in systemic and coronary vascular smooth muscle and myocardium. Increases carbon monoxide and decreases peripheral vascular resistance. Minimal effect on sinuatrial and AV nodal conduction. Reduces myocardial oxygen demand; relaxes and prevents coronary artery spasm.

Uses
Treatment of vasospastic (Prinzmetal or variant) angina; chronic stable angina; hypertension (sustained-release tablets only).

➡◀ DRUG INTERACTIONS RELATED TO DENTAL THERAPEUTICS
No documented drug-drug interactions. The absence of evidence is not evidence of safety

ADVERSE EFFECTS
⚠ **ORAL:** Gingival hyperplasia; dry mouth; thirst.

CNS: Dizziness; lightheadedness; giddiness; nervousness; headache; sleep disturbances; insomnia; abnormal dreams; blurred vision; equilibrium disturbances; weakness; jitteriness; paresthesia; somnolence; malaise; anxiety.

CVS: Flushing (25%); edema (30%); palpitations (7%).

GI: Nausea (11%); diarrhea; constipation; abdominal discomfort; cramps; dyspepsia; flatulence.

RESP: Nasal or chest congestion; shortness of breath; wheezing; cough; respiratory infection.

MISC: Flushing; sweating; muscle cramps, pain and inflammation; joint stiffness, pain, or arthritis; chills; fever.

CLINICAL IMPLICATIONS

General
- Determine why drug is being taken. Consider implications of condition on dental treatment.
- Monitor vital signs (e.g., BP, pulse pressure, rate, and rhythm) at each appointment to assess disease control. Do not provide elective dental treatment when BP is ≥180/110 or in the presence of other high-risk CV conditions. Refer to the section entitled "The Patient Taking Cardiovascular Drugs" in Chapter 6: *Clinical Medicine*.
- Use local anesthetic agents with vasoconstrictor with caution based on functional capacity of the patient and use aspirating technique to prevent intravascular injection.
- Determine ability to adapt to stress of dental treatment. Consider short appointments.
- *Angina:* Ensure patient brings personal acute-use nitroglycerin prescription to all dental appointments; verify expiration date to ensure drug activity.
- Anticipate gingival hyperplasia; consider MD consult to recommend different drug regimen if periodontal health is compromised.
- Chronic dry mouth is possible; anticipate increased caries and candidiasis.
- If GI side effects occur, consider semisupine chair position.

Oral Health Education
- Encourage daily plaque control procedures for effective self care in patient at risk for CV disease.

Nifedipres — see nifedipine

Niferex — see ferrous salts

Niferex-150 — see ferrous salts

Nilstat — see nystatin

Niravam — see alprazolam

---

nisoldipine (nye-SOLD-ih-peen)

Sular

 Syscor

Drug Class: Calcium channel blocker

PHARMACOLOGY

Action
Inhibits movement of calcium ions across cell membrane in systemic and coronary vascular smooth muscle and myocardium.

Uses
Treatment of hypertension, alone or in combination with other antihypertensive agents.

➡◀ DRUG INTERACTIONS RELATED TO DENTAL THERAPEUTICS

Ketoconazole: Possible increased nisoldipine toxicity (decreased metabolism)
- Avoid concurrent use.

ADVERSE EFFECTS

⚠ **ORAL:** Gingival hyperplasia
CNS: Headache; dizziness.
CVS: Chest pains, peripheral edema (7% to 29%); palpitations; vasodilation.
GI: Nausea.
RESP: Pharyngitis, rhinitis.

CLINICAL IMPLICATIONS

General
- Monitor vital signs (e.g., BP, pulse pressure, rate, and rhythm) at each appointment to assess disease control. Do not provide elective dental treatment when BP is ≥180/110 or

in the presence of other high-risk CV conditions. Refer to the section entitled "The Patient Taking Cardiovascular Drugs" in Chapter 6: *Clinical Medicine*.
- Use local anesthetic agents with vasoconstrictor with caution based on functional capacity of the patient and use aspirating technique to prevent intravascular injection.
- Determine ability to adapt to stress of dental treatment. Consider short appointments.
- Anticipate gingival hyperplasia; consider MD consult to recommend different drug regimen if periodontal health is compromised.
- Chronic dry mouth is possible; anticipate increased caries and candidiasis.
- If GI side effects occur, consider semisupine chair position.

Oral Health Education
- Encourage daily plaque control procedures for effective self-care in patient at risk for CV disease.

Nistaken — see propafenone
Nistaquim — see nystatin
Nitradisc — see nitroglycerin
Nitrek — see nitroglycerin
Nitro-Bid — see nitroglycerin
Nitro-Bid IV — see nitroglycerin
Nitroderm TTS — see nitroglycerin
Nitrodisc — see nitroglycerin
Nitro-Dur — see nitroglycerin

---

nitrofurantoin (nye-troe-FYOOR-an-toyn)
Furadantin, Macrobid, Macrodantin

■✦■ Apo-Nitrofurantoin, Novo-Furantoin

■✦■ Furadantina, Macrodantina

Drug Class: Anti-infective, urinary

PHARMACOLOGY
Action
May interfere with bacterial cell wall formation and bacterial duplication. Inhibits bacterial carbohydrate metabolism. Bacteriostatic in low concentrations; bactericidal at higher concentrations.

Uses
Treatment of urinary tract infections caused by susceptible strains of *Escherichia coli*, enterococci, *Staphylococcus aureus*, certain strains of *Klebsiella*, *Enterobacter*, and *Proteus* species.

➤✦ DRUG INTERACTIONS RELATED TO DENTAL THERAPEUTICS
No documented drug-drug interactions. The absence of evidence is not evidence of safety.

ADVERSE EFFECTS
⚠ **ORAL:** Sialadenitis.
CNS: Peripheral neuropathy; headache; dizziness; nystagmus; drowsiness.
GI: Anorexia; nausea; emesis; abdominal pain; diarrhea; parotiditis; pancreatitis.
RESP: Acute, subacute or chronic pulmonary reaction (e.g., shortness of breath, chest pain, cough, fever, chills); permanent pulmonary impairment.
MISC: Anaphylaxis; asthmatic attack in patient with history of asthma; drug fever; arthralgia; photosensitivity; muscular aches; blood dyscrasias (e.g., agranulocytosis, anemia, leukopenia, thrombocytopenia).

CLINICAL IMPLICATIONS

General
- Determine why drug is being taken. Consider implications of condition on dental treatment.
- Blood dyscrasias rarely reported; anticipate increased bleeding, infection, and poor healing.

Oral Health Education
- Encourage daily plaque control procedures for effective, nontraumatic self-care.

Nitrogard — see nitroglycerin

---

 nitroglycerin (nye-troe-GLIH-suh-rin)

Deponit: Transdermal systems: 16, 32 mg
Minitran: Transdermal systems: 9, 18, 36, 54 mg
Nitrek: Transdermal systems: 22.4, 44.8, 67.2 mg
Nitro-Bid: Ointment, topical: 2% in a lanolin-petrolatum base
Nitro-Bid IV: Injection, IV: 5 mg/mL
Nitro-Dur: Transdermal systems: 20, 40, 60, 80, 100, 120, 160 mg
Nitro-Time: Capsules, sustained-release: 2.5, 6.5, 9 mg
Nitrodisc: Transdermal systems: 16, 24, 32 mg
Nitrogard: Tablets, buccal, controlled-release (transmucosal): 2, 3 mg
Nitrol: Ointment, topical: 2% in a lanolin-petrolatum base
Nitrolingual: Aerosol spray, translingual: 0.4 mg/metered dose
NitroQuick, Nitrostat: Tablets, sublingual: 0.3, 0.4, 0.6 mg
Transderm-Nitro: Transdermal systems: 12.5, 25, 50, 75 mg

▌✦▌ Gen-Nitro, Nitrolingual Pumpspray

▌✦▌ Anglix, Cardinit, Nitradisc, Nitroderm TTS

Drug Class: Antianginal

PHARMACOLOGY

Action
Relaxation of smooth muscle of venous and arterial vasculature.

Uses
Treatment of acute angina (SL, translingual, IV, transmucosal); prophylaxis of angina (SL, transmucosal, translingual, sustained release, transdermal, topical); control of BP in perioperative or intraoperative hypertension (IV); CHF associated with MI (IV).

Unlabeled Uses
Reduce cardiac workload in patients with MI and in refractory CHF (SL, topical, oral, IV); adjunctive treatment of Raynaud disease (topical); treatment of hypertensive crisis (IV).

Contraindications
Hypersensitivity to nitrates; severe anemia; closed-angle glaucoma; orthostatic hypotension; early MI; pericarditis or pericardial tamponade; head trauma or cerebral hemorrhage; allergy to adhesives (transdermal); hypotension or uncorrected hypovolemia (IV); increased intracranial pressure or decreased cerebral perfusion (IV).

Usual Dosage
Angina
ADULTS: *SL:* 0.15 to 0.6 mg dissolved under tongue or in buccal pouch at first sign of acute angina attack; repeat q 5 min (do not exceed 3 tablets in 15 min).

Translingual: 1 to 2 sprays onto or under tongue at first onset of attack.

Transmucosal: 1 mg q 3 to 5 hr during waking hours; tablet placed between lip or cheek and gum.

Pharmacokinetics

ABSORP: Rapid.

DIST: Vd: 3 L/kg. Plasma protein binding is approximately 60% (parent); 1,2 dinitroglycerin 60%; 1,3 dinitroglycerin 30%.

METAB: Extensive in liver by nitrate reductase; known sites of extrahepatic metabolism include red blood cells and vascular walls. Metabolized to inorganic nitrate and the active 1,2 and 1,3 dinitroglycerols, which are less effective vasodilators but have longer plasma half-lives than parent compound.

EXCRET: Eliminated by urine as inactive metabolites. Serum $t_{1/2}$ is 3 min (IV) and 1 to 4 min (SL). Clearance is 1 L/kg/min.

ONSET: 1 to 2 min (IV) and 1 to 3 min (SL).

DURATION: 3 to 5 min (IV), 30 to 60 min (SL), and 3 to 5 hr (buccal).

➡◀ DRUG INTERACTIONS

Diazoxide: Severe hypotension (additive)
- Monitor clinical status.

Diltiazem: Hypotension (additive)
- Monitor clinical status.

ADVERSE EFFECTS

⚠ **ORAL:** SL TABLETS: Burning, tingling sensation; tooth disorder (unspecified).

CVS: Tachycardia; palpitations; hypotension; syncope; arrhythmias.

CNS: Headache; apprehension; weakness; vertigo; dizziness; agitation; insomnia.

GI: Nausea; vomiting; diarrhea; dyspepsia.

RESP: Bronchitis; pneumonia.

MISC: Arthralgia; perspiration; pallor; cold sweat; edema.

CLINICAL IMPLICATIONS

General

- Determine why drug is being taken. Consider implications of condition on dental treatment.
- Monitor vital signs (e.g., BP, pulse pressure, rate, and rhythm) at each appointment to assess disease control. Do not provide elective dental treatment when BP is ≥180/110 or in presence of other high-risk CV conditions. Refer to the section entitled "The Patient Taking Cardiovascular Drugs" in Chapter 6: *Clinical Medicine*.
- Use local anesthetic agents with vasoconstrictor with caution based on functional capacity of the patient and use aspirating technique to prevent intravascular injection.
- Determine ability to adapt to stress of dental treatment. Consider short appointments.
- *Angina:* Ensure patient brings personal acute-use nitroglycerin prescription to all dental appointments; verify expiration date to ensure drug activity.
- *Postural hypotension:* Monitor BP at the beginning and end of each appointment; anticipate syncope. Have patient sit upright for several min at the end of the dental appointment before dismissing.
- If used to relieve acute anginal attack, ensure patient is sitting down.

When used by DDS:

- *Angina:* May aggravate angina caused by hypertrophic cardiomyopathy.
- *Defibrillation:* Do not discharge cardioverter/defibrillator through paddle electrode.
- *MI:* Safety of oral or sublingual products in acute MI not established; use only with close observation and monitoring. However, IV nitroglycerin is drug of choice in acute MI.
- *Orthostatic hypotension:* May occur even with small doses; alcohol accentuates this reaction.
- *Sublingual administration:* Absorption is dependent on salivary secretion; dry mouth decreases absorption.
- *Overdosage:* Hypotension, tachycardia, flushing, excessive sweating, headache, vertigo,

palpitations, visual disturbances, nausea, vomiting, confusion, and dyspnea may occur as a result of vasodilation and methemoglobinemia.

Pregnancy Risk Category: Category C.

Oral Health Education

- Encourage daily plaque control procedures for effective self-care in patients at risk for cardiovascular disease.

When used by DDS:

- Review with patient and family the following signs of angina: pressure-like chest pain of acute onset, often associated with physical activity, which may radiate down to left arm or up to neck and jaw.

Sublingual

- Advise patient to dissolve tablet under tongue and not to swallow. If pain remains, the dose may be repeated q 5 min until 3 tablets are taken. If pain still persists or becomes more intense, patient should be taught to call 911 or appropriate local number to obtain emergency services.
- Tell patient to place tablet between gum and cheek if stinging sensation occurs.
- Caution patient to sit or lie down while taking and for 20 min after initial dose. If dizziness occurs, instruct patient to lie down.
- Teach patient storage instructions (per Administration/Storage information).
- Advise patient to discard 6 mo after opening package.
- Instruct patient to report these symptoms to health care provider: severe headache, blurred vision, dry mouth, dizziness, or flushing.

Nitrol — see nitroglycerin

Nitrolingual — see nitroglycerin

Nitrolingual Pumpspray — see nitroglycerin

NitroQuick — see nitroglycerin

Nitrostat — see nitroglycerin

Nitro-Time — see nitroglycerin

Nivoflox — see ciprofloxacin

Nixal — see naproxen

---

nizatidine (nye-ZAT-ih-deen)

Axid AR, Axid Pulvules

⬛✦⬛ **Apo-Nizatidine, Novo-Nizatidine, PMS-Nizatidine**

Drug Class: Histamine H_2 antagonist

PHARMACOLOGY

Action

Reversibly and competitively blocks histamine at H_2-receptors, particularly those in gastric parietal cells, leading to inhibition of gastric acid secretion.

Uses

Treatment and maintenance of duodenal ulcer, GERD (including erosive or ulcerative disease), and benign gastric ulcer. Prevention of heartburn, acid indigestion, and sour stomach brought on by consuming irritating food and beverages.

➡◆ DRUG INTERACTIONS RELATED TO DENTAL THERAPEUTICS

No documented drug-drug interactions. The absence of evidence is not evidence of safety.

ADVERSE EFFECTS

CNS: Headache; somnolence; fatigue; dizziness.

GI: Diarrhea; constipation; nausea; vomiting; abdominal discomfort; anorexia; cholestatic or hepatocellular effects.

MISC: Gynecomastia; sweating; fever; eosinophilia, thrombocytopenia.

CLINICAL IMPLICATIONS

General

- Determine why drug is being taken. Consider implications of condition on dental treatment.
- If patient has GI disease, consider semisupine chair position.
- Use COX inhibitors with caution; they may exacerbate PUD and GERD.
- If GI side effects occur, consider semisupine chair position.
- Blood dyscrasias rarely reported; anticipate increased bleeding.
- Anticipate chemical erosion of teeth.
- Substernal pain (heartburn) may mimic pain of cardiac origin.
- Drugs that lower acidity in intestinal tract may interfere with absorption of some antibiotics (penicillin, tetracyclines).

Oral Health Education

- *GERD:* Inform patient that toothbrushing should not be done after reflux, but to only rinse mouth with water, then use home fluoride product to minimize chemical erosion caries.

Nizoral — see ketoconazole

No Pain-HP — see capsaicin

Nobligan — see tramadol HCl

Nolvadex — see tamoxifen citrate

Nolvadex-D — see tamoxifen citrate

Norboral — see glyburide

Norco — see acetaminophen/hydrocodone bitartrate

---

norethindrone acetate (nor-eth-IN-drone ASS-uh-TATE)

Aygestin

■✦■ **Norlutate**

■◐■ **Syngestal**

Drug Class: Progestin

PHARMACOLOGY

Action

Inhibits secretion of pituitary gonadotropins, thereby preventing follicular maturation and ovulation.

Uses

Treatment of secary amenorrhea; endometriosis; abnormal uterine bleeding caused by hormonal imbalance in the absence of organic pathology (e.g., uterine cancer).

➡◀ DRUG INTERACTIONS RELATED TO DENTAL THERAPEUTICS

No documented drug-drug interactions. The absence of evidence is not evidence of safety.

ADVERSE EFFECTS

CVS: Thrombophlebitis; cerebral thrombosis and embolism; hypertension; edema.

CNS: Depression; changes in libido; changes in appetite; headache; nervousness; dizziness; fatigue.

RESP: Pulmonary embolism.

MISC: Premenstrual syndrome; backache.

CLINICAL IMPLICATIONS

General
• Monitor vital signs.

Oral Health Education
• Caution patient who reports cigarette smoking of increased risk of blood clot formation.

Norfenon — see propafenone

---

norfloxacin (nor-FLOX-uh-SIN)
Chibroxin, Noroxin

▮✦▮ **Apo-Norflox, Novo-Norfloxacin**

▮✦▮ **Difoxacil, Floxacin, Oranor**

Drug Class: Antibiotic, fluoroquinolone

PHARMACOLOGY

Action
Interferes with microbial DNA synthesis.

Uses
Oral treatment of urinary tract infections caused by susceptible organisms; treatment of sexually transmitted diseases caused by *Neisseria gonorrhoeae*; ocular solution for treatment of superficial ocular infections from strains of susceptible organisms; prostatitis caused by *Escherichia coli*.

➡◀ DRUG INTERACTIONS RELATED TO DENTAL THERAPEUTICS

Corticosteroids: Possible increased risk of Achilles tendon disorder (mechanism unknown)
• Consider risk/benefit.

ADVERSE EFFECTS

⚠ **ORAL:** Dry, painful mouth (1%).
CNS: Headache; dizziness; fatigue; drowsiness.
MISC: Eosinophilia, leukopenia, neutropenia, increase or decrease in platelets (1% to 1.5%).
GI: Diarrhea; nausea; vomiting; abdominal pain/discomfort.

CLINICAL IMPLICATIONS

General
• Determine why drug is being taken. Consider implications of condition on dental treatment.
• If GI side effects occur, consider semisupine chair position.
• If oral infection occurs that requires antibiotic therapy, select an appropriate product from a different class of anti-infectives.
• Prolonged use of antibiotics may result in bacterial or fungal overgrowth of nonsusceptible microorganisms; anticipate candidiasis.
• Blood dyscrasias rarely reported; anticipate increased bleeding, infection, and poor healing.

Oral Health Education
• Encourage daily plaque control procedures for effective, nontraumatic self-care.

Noritate — see metronidazole
Norlutate — see norethindrone acetate
Normodyne — see labetalol HCl

Noroxin — see norfloxacin

Norpace — see disopyramide phosphate

Norpace CR — see disopyramide phosphate

Norpramin — see desipramine HCl

Norpril — see enalapril maleate

---

nortriptyline HCl (nor-TRIP-tih-leen HIGH-droe-KLOR-ide)

Aventyl HCl, Aventyl HCl Pulvules, Pamelor

■✦■ Apo-Nortriptyline, Gen-Nortriptyline, Novo-Nortriptyline, Nu-Nortriptyline, PMS-Nortriptyline, ratio-Nortriptyline

Drug Class: Tricyclic antidepressant

PHARMACOLOGY

Action
Inhibits reuptake of norepinephrine and serotonin in CNS.

Uses
Relief of symptoms of depression.

Unlabeled Uses
Treatment of panic disorder; premenstrual depression; dermatologic disorders (e.g., chronic urticaria, angioedema, nocturnal pruritus in atopic eczema).

➡◆ DRUG INTERACTIONS RELATED TO DENTAL THERAPEUTICS

Fluconazole: Possible nortriptyline toxicity (decreased metabolism)
 • Monitor clinical status.

Tramadol: Increased risk of seizure (additive)
 • Avoid concurrent use.

Sympathomimetic amines: Hypertension and hypertensive crisis (additive)
 • Monitor blood pressure.

ADVERSE EFFECTS

⚠ **ORAL:** Dry mouth; gingivitis; ulcerative stomatitis; taste disturbance.

CNS: Confusion; hallucinations; delusions; nervousness; restlessness; agitation; panic; insomnia; nightmares; mania; exacerbation of psychosis; drowsiness; dizziness; weakness; fatigue; emotional lability; seizures; tremors; extrapyramidal symptoms (e.g., pseudoparkinsonism, movement disorders, akathisia).

CVS: Arrhythmias; hypertension or hypotension; orthostatic hypotension; palpitations; tachycardia.

GI: Nausea; vomiting; anorexia; GI distress; diarrhea; flatulence; constipation.

RESP: Pharyngitis; rhinitis; sinusitis; laryngitis; coughing.

MISC: Numbness; breast enlargement; bone marrow depression, including agranulocytosis, aplastic anemia, eosinophilia, leukopenia, thrombocytopenia.

CLINICAL IMPLICATIONS

General
 • Determine why drug is being taken. Consider implications of condition on dental treatment.
 • Chronic dry mouth is possible; anticipate increased caries and candidiasis.
 • Determine ability to adapt to stress of dental treatment. Consider short appointments.
 • Depressed or anxious patients may neglect self-care. Monitor for plaque control effectiveness.
 • *Postural hypotension:* Monitor BP at the beginning and end of each appointment; anticipate syncope. Have patient sit upright for several min at the end of the dental appointment before dismissing.

- Extrapyramidal behaviors can complicate performance of oral procedures. If present, consult with MD to consider medication changes.
- Blood dyscrasias rarely reported; anticipate increased bleeding, infection, and poor healing.
- Monitor vital signs.
- If GI side effects occur, consider semisupine chair position.

Oral Health Education

- Encourage daily plaque control procedures for effective, nontraumatic self-care.
- Determine need for power toothbrush for self-care.
- If chronic dry mouth occurs, recommend home fluoride therapy and use of nonalcoholic oral health care products.

Norvas — see amlodipine

Norvasc — see amlodipine

Norvir — see ritonavir

Norwich Extra-Strength — see aspirin

Novacef — see cefixime

Novamoxin — see amoxicillin

Novasen — see aspirin

Novaxen — see naproxen

Noviken-N — see nifedipine

Novo Ampicillin — see ampicillin

Novo-5 ASA — see mesalamine

Novo-Acebutolol — see acebutolol HCl

Novo-Alprazol — see alprazolam

Novo-Amiodarone — see amiodarone

Novo-Atenol — see atenolol

Novo-AZT — see zidovudine

Novo-Buspirone — see buspirone HCl

Novo-Butamide — see tolbutamide

Novo-Captoril — see captopril

Novo-Carbamaz — see carbamazepine

Novo-Cefaclor — see cefaclor

Novo-Cefadroxil — see cefadroxil

Novo-Cholamine — see cholestyramine

Novo-Cholamine Light — see cholestyramine

Novo-Cimetine — see cimetidine

Novo-Clobetasol — see clobetasol propionate

Novo-Clonazepam — see clonazepam

Novo-Clonidine — see clonidine HCl

Novo-Clopamine — see clomipramine HCl

Novo-Clopate — see clorazepate dipotassium

Novo-Cycloprine — see cyclobenzaprine HCl

Novo-Desipramine — see desipramine HCl

Novo-Difenac — see diclofenac
Novo-Difenac K — see diclofenac
Novo-Difenac SR — see diclofenac
Novo-Diflunisal — see diflunisal
Novo-Diltiazem — see diltiazem HCl
Novo-Diltiazem SR — see diltiazem HCl
Novo-Divalproex — see valproic acid and derivatives
Novo-Doxazosin — see doxazosin mesylate
Novo-Doxepin — see doxepin HCl
Novo-Doxylin — see doxycycline hyclate
Novo-Famotidine — see famotidine
Novo-Fluoxetine — see fluoxetine HCl
Novo-Flupam — see flurazepam HCl
Novo-Flurbiprofen — see flurbiprofen
Novo-Flurprofen — see flurbiprofen
Novo-Fluvoxamine — see fluvoxamine maleate
Novo-Furantoin — see nitrofurantoin
Novo-Gabapentin — see gabapentin
Novo-Gemfibrozil — see gemfibrozil
Novo-Glyburide — see glyburide
Novo-Hydroxyzin — see hydroxyzine
Novo-Hylazin — see hydralazine HCl
Novo-Indapamide — see indapamide
Novo-Ipramide — see ipratropium bromide
Novo-Keto — see ketoprofen
Novo-Ketoconazole — see ketoconazole
Novo-Keto-EC — see ketoprofen
Novo-Ketorolac — see ketorolac tromethamine
Novo-Levocarbidopa — see levodopa/carbidopa
Novo-Lexin — see cephalexin
Novolin 70/30 — see insulin
Novolin ge 30/70 — see insulin
Novolin ge 40/60 — see insulin
Novolin ge 50/50 — see insulin
Novolin ge Lente — see insulin
Novolin ge NPH — see insulin
Novolin ge Toronto — see insulin
Novolin ge Ultralente — see insulin
Novolin L — see insulin
Novolin N — see insulin

Novolin R — see insulin
Novo-Lorazem — see lorazepam
Novo-Medrone — see medroxyprogesterone acetate
Novo-Metformin — see metformin HCl
Novo-Methacin — see indomethacin
Novo-Metoprol — see metoprolol
Novo-Mexiletine — see mexiletine HCl
Novo-Minocycline — see minocycline HCl
Novo-Misoprostol — see misoprostol
Novo-Nadolol — see nadolol
Novo-Naprox — see naproxen
Novo-Naprox EC — see naproxen
Novo-Naprox Sodium — see naproxen
Novo-Naprox Sodium DS — see naproxen
Novo-Naprox SR — see naproxen
Novo-Nidazol — see metronidazole
Novo-Nifedin — see nifedipine
Novo-Nizatidine — see nizatidine
Novo-Norfloxacin — see norfloxacin
Novo-Nortriptyline — see nortriptyline HCl
Novo-Oxybutynin — see oxybutynin Cl
Novo-Pen-VK — see penicillin V
Novo-Peridol — see haloperidol
Novo-Pindol — see pindolol
Novo-Pirocam — see piroxicam
Novo-Prazin — see prazosin HCl
Novo-Prednisolone — see prednisolone
Novo-Profen — see ibuprofen
Novo-Purol — see allopurinol
Novoquin — see ciprofloxacin
Novo-Ranitidine — see ranitidine HCl
Novorythro Encap — see erythromycin
Novo-Salmol — see albuterol
Novo-Selegiline — see selegiline HCl
Novo-Sertraline — see sertraline HCl
Novo-Sotalol — see sotalol HCl
Novo-Spiroton — see spironolactone
Novo-Spirozine — see spironolactone
Novo-Sucralfate — see sucralfate
Novo-Sundac — see sulindac

Novo-Tamoxifen — see tamoxifen citrate
Novo-Temazepam — see temazepam
Novo-Terazosin — see terazosin
Novo-Terbinafine — see terbinafine
Novo-Tetra — see tetracycline HCl
Novo-Theophyl SR — see theophylline
Novo-Timol Tablets — see timolol maleate
Novo-Trazodone — see trazodone HCl
Novo-Trimel — see trimethoprim/sulfamethoxazole
Novo-Trimel D.S. — see trimethoprim/sulfamethoxazole
Novo-Valproic — see valproic acid and derivatives
Novo-Veramil — see verapamil HCl
Novo-Veramil SR — see verapamil HCl
Nu-Acebutolol — see acebutolol HCl
Nu-Acyclovir — see acyclovir
Nu-Alpraz — see alprazolam
Nu-Amoxi — see amoxicillin
Nu-Ampi — see ampicillin
Nu-Atenol — see atenolol
Nu-Beclomethasone — see beclomethasone dipropionate
Nu-Buspirone — see buspirone HCl
Nu-Capto — see captopril
Nu-Carbamazepine — see carbamazepine
Nu-Cefaclor — see cefaclor
Nu-Cephalex — see cephalexin
Nu-Cimet — see cimetidine
Nu-Clonazepam — see clonazepam
Nu-Clonidine — see clonidine HCl
Nu-Cotrimox — see trimethoprim/sulfamethoxazole
Nu-Cromolyn — see cromolyn sodium
Nu-Cyclobenzaprine — see cyclobenzaprine HCl
Nu-Desipramine — see desipramine HCl
Nu-Diclo — see diclofenac
Nu-Diclo-SR — see diclofenac
Nu-Diflunisal — see diflunisal
Nu-Diltiaz — see diltiazem HCl
Nu-Diltiaz-CD — see diltiazem HCl
Nu-Divalproex — see valproic acid and derivatives
Nu-Doxycycline — see doxycycline hyclate
Nu-Erythromycin-S — see erythromycin

Nu-Famotidine — see famotidine
Nu-Fenofibrate — see fenofibrate
Nu-Fluoxetine — see fluoxetine HCl
Nu-Flurbiprofen — see flurbiprofen
Nu-Fluvoxamine — see fluvoxamine maleate
Nu-Gemfibrozil — see gemfibrozil
Nu-Glyburide — see glyburide
Nu-Hydral — see hydralazine HCl
Nu-Hydroxyzine — see hydroxyzine
Nu-Ibuprofen — see ibuprofen
Nu-Indapamide — see indapamide
Nu-Indo — see indomethacin
Nu-Ipratropium — see ipratropium bromide
Nu-Iron — see ferrous salts
Nu-Iron 150 — see ferrous salts
Nu-Ketoprofen — see ketoprofen
Nu-Ketoprofen-SR — see ketoprofen
NuLev — see hyoscyamine sulfate
Nu-Levocarb — see levodopa/carbidopa
Nu-Loraz — see lorazepam
Numby Stuff — see lidocaine HCl
Nu-Medopa — see methyldopa and methyldopate HCl
Nu-Mefenamic — see mefenamic acid
Nu-Metformin — see metformin HCl
Nu-Metoclopramide — see metoclopramide
Nu-Metop — see metoprolol
Nu-Naprox — see naproxen
Nu-Nifed — see nifedipine
Nu-Nifedipine — see nifedipine
Nu-Nortriptyline — see nortriptyline HCl
Nu-Oxybutynin — see oxybutynin Cl
Nu-Pen-VK — see penicillin V
Nu-Pindol — see pindolol
Nu-Pirox — see piroxicam
Nu-Pravastatin — see pravastatin sodium
Nu-Prazo — see prazosin HCl
Nuprin — see ibuprofen
Nu-Propranolol — see propranolol HCl
Nu-Ranit — see ranitidine HCl
Nu-Salbutamol Solution — see albuterol

Nu-Selegiline — see selegiline HCl
Nu-Sotalol — see sotalol HCl
Nu-Sucralfate — see sucralfate
Nu-Sulindac — see sulindac
Nu-Temazepam — see temazepam
Nu-Terazosin — see terazosin
Nu-Tetra — see tetracycline HCl
Nu-Ticlopidine — see ticlopidine HCl
Nu-Timolol — see timolol maleate
Nutracort — see hydrocortisone
Nu-Trazodone — see trazodone HCl
Nu-Trazodone-D — see trazodone HCl
Nu-Valproic — see valproic acid and derivatives
Nu-Verap — see verapamil HCl
Nyaderm — see nystatin
Nydrazid — see isoniazid

---

 nystatin (nye-STAT-in)

Mycostatin: Vaginal tablets: 100,000 units; Ointment: 100,000 units/g; Powder: 100,000 units/g
Mycostatin Pastilles: Troches/pastilles: 200,000 units
Nilstat: Oral suspension: 100,000 units; Bulk powder: 150 million units, 1 billion units, 2 billion units; Cream: 100,000 units; Ointment: 100,000 units
Pedi-Dri: Powder: 100,000 units/g

■✦■ **Candistatin, Nyaderm, PMS-Nystatin, ratio-Nystatin**

■✦■ **Micostatin, Nistaquim**

Drug Class: Anti-infective; Antifungal

PHARMACOLOGY

Action
Binds to fungal cell membrane, changing membrane permeability and allowing leakage of intracellular components.

Uses
Treatment of intestinal, oral, vulvovaginal, cutaneous, or mucocutaneous candidiasis.

Contraindications
Standard considerations.

Usual Dosage
Oral or mucocutaneous candidiasis
ADULTS AND CHILDREN: *PO:* (suspension) 200,000 to 600,000 units qid; swish and swallow, or (oral pastilles) 1 to 2 pastilles (200,000 to 400,000 units) dissolved in mouth 4 to 5 times/day.
INFANTS *PO:* 200,000 units qid.

➔◆ DRUG INTERACTIONS

No documented drug-drug interactions. The absence of evidence is not evidence of safety.

ADVERSE EFFECTS

GI: Diarrhea; GI distress; nausea; vomiting (with large oral doses).

CLINICAL IMPLICATIONS

General

When prescribed by DDS:
- *Lactation:* Undetermined.
- *Effectiveness:* Has no activity against bacteria or trichomonads. Not indicated for systemic mycoses.
- *Overdosage:* Nausea, diarrhea, vomiting.

When prescribed by medical facilities:
- Determine why drug is being taken. Take precautions to avoid cross-contamination of microorganisms.
- If GI side effects occur, consider semisupine chair position.

Pregnancy Risk Category: Category C (oral).

Oral Health Education

If prescribed by DDS:
- Instruct patient that long-term therapy may be needed to clear infection and that patient should complete entire course of medication. Take drug for 2 days after symptoms have disappeared or as directed.
- Advise patient to notify health care provider if irritation occurs.
- Assure patient that relief from itching may occur after 24 to 72 hr.
- Instruct patient to carefully wash hands before and after each application of topical medication.
- Advise patient with oral candidiasis not to use mouthwash, which may alter normal flora and promote infections.

Nytol — see diphenhydramine HCl

Nytol Extra Strength — see diphenhydramine HCl

Obe-Nix 30 — see phentermine HCl

Octamide — see metoclopramide

Octamide PFS — see metoclopramide

Octocaine — see lidocaine HCl

Ocufen — see flurbiprofen

Ocuflox — see ofloxacin

Ocupress — see cargteolol HCl

Ocusert Pilo-20 — see pilocarpine HCl

Ocusert Pilo-40 — see pilocarpine HCl

Oestrogel — see estradiol

---

ofloxacin (oh-FLOX-uh-SIN)

Floxin, Ocuflox

◼◈◼ **Apo-Oflox**

Drug Class: Antibiotic, fluoroquinolone

PHARMACOLOGY

Action

Interferes with microbial DNA synthesis.

Uses

Treatment of acute bacterial exacerbations of chronic bronchitis, community acquired pneumonia, uncomplicated skin and skin structure infections, acute uncomplicated urethral and cervical gonorrhea, nongonococcal urethritis, cervicitis, acute pelvic inflammatory disease, uncomplicated cystitis, complicated UTI, prostatitis caused by *Escherichia coli*.

OPHTHALMIC: Treatment of conjunctivitis and corneal ulcer infections caused by susceptible organisms.

OTIC: Treatment of otitis externa and chronic suppurative otitis media in patients with perforated tympanic membranes; treatment of acute otitis media in pediatric patients with tympanostomy tubes.

➡◀ DRUG INTERACTIONS RELATED TO DENTAL THERAPEUTICS

Corticosteroids: Possible increased risk of Achilles tendon disorder (mechanism unknown)
  • Consider risk-benefit.

ADVERSE EFFECTS

⚠ ORAL: Painful or dry mouth, dysgeusia; taste disturbance (7%, otic).

CNS: Dizziness, vertigo (1%, otic); headache; dizziness; fatigue; lethargy; drowsiness; insomnia; nervousness.

CVS: Chest pain (3%).

GI: Diarrhea; nausea; vomiting; abdominal pain or discomfort; flatulence.

MISC: Application site reaction (3%), paresthesia (otic); vaginitis; fever; decreased appetite; photosensitivity; blood dyscrasias (leukopenia, eosinophilia, neutropenia, anemia). Ophthalmic use may possibly cause same adverse reactions seen with systemic use because of absorption.

CLINICAL IMPLICATIONS

General

• Determine why drug is being taken. Take precautions to avoid cross-contamination of microorganisms.
• If GI side effects occur, consider semisupine chair position.
• If an oral infection requires antibiotic therapy, select an appropriate product from a different class of anti-infectives.
• Prolonged use of antibiotics may result in bacterial or fungal overgrowth of nonsusceptible microorganisms; anticipate candidiasis.
• Blood dyscrasias are rarely reported; anticipate increased bleeding, infection, and poor healing.

Oral Health Education

• Encourage daily plaque control procedures for effective, nontraumatic self-care.

Ogastro — see lansoprazole

Ogen — see estropipate

---

olanzapine (oh-LAN-zah-peen)

Zyprexa, Zyprexa Intramuscular, Zyprexa Zydis

Drug Class: Atypical antipsychotic

PHARMACOLOGY

Action

Unknown. May control psychotic symptoms through antagonism of selected dopamine and serotonin receptors in the CNS.

Uses

Treatment of schizophrenia (oral); short-term treatment of acute mixed or manic episodes with bipolar I disorder (oral); in combination with lithium or valproate for short-term treatment of acute episodes associated with bipolar I disorder (oral); agitation associated with schizophrenia and bipolar I mania (IM).

➡️⬅️ DRUG INTERACTIONS RELATED TO DENTAL THERAPEUTICS

Diazepam: Increased orthostatic hypotension (mechanism unknown)
• Avoid concurrent use.
Tramadol: Possible increased risk of serotonin syndrome (mechanism unknown)
• Monitor clinical status.

ADVERSE EFFECTS

⚠️ **ORAL:** Dry mouth (22%); increased salivation and thirst, dental caries (1%).

CNS: Somnolence (35%); dizziness (18%); parkinsonism (14%); insomnia (12%); personality disorder (8%); tremor, abnormal gait, increased appetite (6%); akathisia (5%); hypertonia, dystonia (3%); articulation impairment (2%); abnormal dreams, emotional lability, euphoria, decreased libido, paresthesia, schizophrenic reaction (≥1%).

CVS: Hypotension (3% to 5%); tachycardia, chest pain (3%); hypertension (2%).

GI: Constipation, dyspepsia (11%); nausea (9%); increased appetite (6%); vomiting (4%).

RESP: Increased cough, rhinitis (6%); pharyngitis (4%); dyspnea (≥1%).

MISC: Asthenia (15%); accidental injury (12%); fever (6%); back pain, extremity pain, joint pain (5%); flu-like syndrome, suicide attempt, intentional injury, joint stiffness and twitching (≥1%); allergic reactions (e.g., anaphylactoid reaction, angioedema, pruritus, urticaria), pancreatitis, rhabdomyolysis; ecchymosis; leukopenia (>1%); thrombocytopenia.

CLINICAL IMPLICATIONS

General

• Determine why drug is being taken. Consider implications of condition on dental treatment.
• Determine ability to adapt to stress of dental treatment. Consider short appointments.
• Monitor vital signs (e.g., BP, pulse, respiration).
• *Postural hypotension*: Monitor BP at the beginning and end of each appointment; anticipate syncope. Have patient sit upright for several min at the end of the dental appointment before dismissing.
• Depressed or anxious patients may neglect self-care. Monitor for plaque control effectiveness.
• Chronic dry mouth is possible; anticipate increased caries and candidiasis.
• Extrapyramidal behaviors can complicate performance of oral procedures. If present consult with MD to consider medication changes.
• If GI side effects occur consider semisupine chair position.
• Blood dyscrasias are rarely reported; anticipate increased bleeding, infection, and poor healing.

Oral Health Education

• Encourage daily plaque control procedures for effective, nontraumatic self-care.
• If chronic dry mouth occurs, recommend home fluoride therapy and use of nonalcoholic oral health care products.

Olexin — see omeprazole

---

olmesartan medoxomil (ole-mih-SAR-tan meh-DOX-oh-mill)

Benicar

Drug Class: Antihypertensive; Angiotensin II antagonist

PHARMACOLOGY

Action

Blocks vasoconstrictor effects of angiotensin II by selectively blocking the binding of angiotensin II to the AT_1 receptor in vascular smooth muscle.

Uses

Treatment of hypertension.

➡◀ DRUG INTERACTIONS RELATED TO DENTAL THERAPEUTICS

No documented drug-drug interactions. The absence of evidence is not evidence of safety.

ADVERSE EFFECTS

CNS: Dizziness; fatigue; vertigo; insomnia.
GI: Abdominal pain; dyspepsia; gastroenteritis; nausea.
MISC: Chest pain; peripheral edema; arthritis; myalgia; skeletal pain.

CLINICAL IMPLICATIONS

General

- Monitor vital signs (e.g., BP, pulse pressure, rate and rhythm) at each appointment to assess disease control. Do not provide elective dental treatment when BP is ≥180/110 or in the presence of other high-risk CV conditions. Refer to the section entitled "The Patient Taking Cardiovascular Drugs" in Chapter 6: *Clinical Medicine*.
- Use local anesthetic agents with vasoconstrictor with caution based on functional capacity of the patient and use aspirating technique to prevent intravascular injection.
- Determine ability to adapt to stress of dental treatment. Consider short afternoon appointments.

Oral Health Education

- Encourage daily plaque control procedures for effective self-care in patient at risk for cardiovascular disease.

---

olopatadine HCl (oh-low-pat-AD-een HIGH-droe-KLOR-ide)

Patanol

Drug Class: Ophthalmic antihistaminic agent

PHARMACOLOGY

Action

Inhibits release of histamine from mast cells and relatively selective histamine H_1 antagonist. Inhibits type 1 immediate hypersensitivity reactions.

Uses

Temporary relief of itching caused by allergic conjunctivitis.

➡◀ DRUG INTERACTIONS RELATED TO DENTAL THERAPEUTICS

No documented drug-drug interactions. The absence of evidence is not evidence of safety.

ADVERSE EFFECTS

⚠ **ORAL:** Taste disturbance.
RESP: Pharyngitis, rhinitis, sinusitis; cold syndrome.
MISC: Asthenia; headache.

CLINICAL IMPLICATIONS

General

- Determine why drug is being taken. Consider implications of condition on dental treatment.
- *Photophobia*: Direct dental light out of patient's eyes and offer dark glasses for comfort.

Olux — see clobetasol propionate

omalizumab (oh-mah-lie-ZOO-mab)

Xolair

Drug Class: Monoclonal antibody

PHARMACOLOGY

Action

Selectively binds to human IgE, inhibiting the binding of IgE to the high-affinity IgE receptor on the surface of mast cells and basophils and limiting the degree of release of mediators of the allergic response.

Uses

Treatment of moderate to severe persistent asthma in patients who have a positive skin test result or in vitro reactivity to a perennial aeroallergen and whose symptoms are inadequately controlled with inhaled corticosteroids.

Unlabeled Uses

Seasonal allergic rhinitis.

➡◆ DRUG INTERACTIONS RELATED TO DENTAL THERAPEUTICS

No documented drug-drug interactions. The absence of evidence is not evidence of safety.

ADVERSE EFFECTS

CNS: Headache (15%); fatigue, dizziness (3%).

RESP: URI (20%); viral infections (23%); sinusitis, pharyngitis.

MISC: Injection site reactions (e.g., bruising, redness, warmth, burning, stinging, itching, hive formation, pain, indurations, mass, inflammation [45%]); viral infections (23%); arthralgia (8%); pain (7%); leg pain (4%); fracture, arm pain (2%); malignancy (0.5%); hypersensitivity (e.g., urticaria, dermatitis, pruritus, anaphylaxis).

CLINICAL IMPLICATIONS

General

- This is a single-dose, SC administration product.
- Determine why drug is being taken. Consider implications of condition on dental treatment.
- Acute bronchoconstriction can occur during dental treatment; have bronchodilator inhaler available.
- Be aware that sulfites in local anesthetic with vasoconstrictor can precipitate acute asthma attack in susceptible individuals.
- Consider semisupine chair position to assist respiratory function.

Oral Health Education

- Instruct patient to bring bronchodilator inhaler to each dental appointment.

omeprazole (oh-MEH-pray-ZAHL)

Prilosec, Prilosec OTC, Zegerid

■✦■ **Losec**

■✦■ **Inhibitron, Olexin, Osiren, Ozoken, Prazidec, Prazolit, Ulsen**

Drug Class: GI; Proton pump inhibitor

PHARMACOLOGY

Action

Suppresses gastric acid secretion by blocking acid (proton) pump within gastric parietal cell.

Uses

Short-term treatment of active duodenal ulcer, gastroesophageal reflux disease (GERD), including erosive esophagitis and symptomatic GERD; long-term treatment of pathological hypersecretory conditions (e.g., Zollinger-Ellison syndrome, multiple endocrine adenomas, systemic mastocytosis); to maintain healing of erosive esophagitis; in combination with clarithromycin to eradicate *Helicobacter pylori*, use clarithromycin and amoxicillin in combination with omeprazole in patients with a 1-yr history of duodenal ulcers or active duodenal ulcers to eradicate *H. pylori*; short-term treatment of active benign gastric ulcer; heartburn.

Unlabeled Uses

Posterior laryngitis; enhanced efficacy of pancreatin for treatment of steatorrhea in patients with cystic fibrosis.

➡️⬅️ DRUG INTERACTIONS RELATED TO DENTAL THERAPEUTICS

Ketoconazole or itraconazole: Decreased ketoconazole or itraconazole effect (decreased absorption)
- Avoid concurrent use.

Ketoconazole: Possible omeprazole toxicity (decreased metabolism)
- Avoid concurrent use.

Benzodiazepams: Possible increased benzodiazepam toxicity (decreased metabolism)
- Monitor clinical status.

ADVERSE EFFECTS

CNS: Headache (7%); dizziness (2%); asthenia.
MISC: Back pain.
GI: Diarrhea, nausea (4%); flatulence, vomiting (3%); abdominal pain; acid regurgitation; constipation.
RESP: Cough, URI ($\geq$1%).

CLINICAL IMPLICATIONS

General
- Determine why drug is being taken. Consider implications of condition on dental treatment.
- If patient has GI disease, consider semisupine chair position.
- Anticipate chemical erosion of teeth.
- Substernal pain (heartburn) may mimic pain of cardiac origin.

Oral Health Education
- Inform patient that toothbrushing should not be done following reflux, but to only rinse mouth with water, then use home fluoride product to minimize chemical erosion caries.

Omnicef — see cefdinir

Omnipen — see ampicillin

OMS Concentrate — see morphine sulfate

---

ondansetron HCl (ahn-DAN-SEH-trahn HIGH-droe-KLOR-ide)
Zofran, Zofran ODT

Drug Class: Antiemetic; Antivertigo

PHARMACOLOGY

Action
Selective serotonin (5-HT$_3$) receptor antagonist that inhibits serotonin receptors in GI tract or chemoreceptor trigger zone.

Uses

PARENTERAL AND ORAL: Prevention of nausea and vomiting with initial and repeat courses of emetogenic cancer chemotherapy, including high-dose cisplatin; prevention of postoperative nausea or vomiting.

ORAL: Prevention of nausea and vomiting associated with radiation therapy in patients receiving either total body irradiation, single high-dose fraction to the abdomen, or daily fractions to the abdomen; prevention of nausea and vomiting associated with highly emetogenic cancer chemotherapy, including cisplatin (50 mg/m^2).

Unlabeled Uses

Treatment of nausea and vomiting associated with acetaminophen poisoning or prostacyclin therapy; treatment of acute levodopa-induced psychosis (e.g., visual hallucinations); reduction in bulimic episodes due to bulimia nervosa; treatment of spinal or epidural morphine-induced pruritus; management of social anxiety disorder.

➡← DRUG INTERACTIONS RELATED TO DENTAL THERAPEUTICS

Tramadol: Possible decreased analgesic effect (pharmacologic antagonism)
• Avoid concurrent use.

ADVERSE EFFECTS

⚠ ORAL: Dry mouth (2%).
CNS: Headache; seizures.
CVS: Arrhythmias (6%); hypotension (3% to 5%); chest pain (2%); hypertension (2.5%).
GI: Constipation (9%); abdominal pain.
RESP: Bronchospasm.
MISC: Fever; anaphylaxis; weakness.

CLINICAL IMPLICATIONS

General

• Determine why drug is being taken. Consider implications of condition on dental treatment.
• Consider medical consult to determine disease control and influence on dental treatment.
• This drug is used for short-course therapy to prevent nausea. If dental care is needed, consider semisupine chair position.
• Monitor vital signs.

Oral Health Education

• Encourage daily plaque control procedures to increase oral health.

Onofin-K — see ketoconazole
Opthavir — see acyclovir
Optivar — see azelastine HCl
Optomicin — see erythromycin
Oracort — see triamcinolone
Orajel Mouth-Aid — see benzocaine
Oramorph SR — see morphine sulfate
Oranor — see norfloxacin
Oraphen-PD — see acetaminophen
Oraqix — see lidocaine HCl/prilocaine
Orasone — see prednisone
Orelox — see cefpodoxime proxetil

Oretic — see hydrochlorothiazide
Organidin NR — see guaifenesin
Orinase — see tolbutamide
Orinase Diagnostic — see tolbutamide

orlistat (ORE-lih-stat)
Xenical

Drug Class: Gastrointestinal lipase inhibitor

PHARMACOLOGY
Action
Reversible lipase inhibitor for obesity management that acts by inhibiting absorption of dietary fats.

Uses
Obesity management including weight loss and weight maintenance when used in combination with a reduced-calorie diet; reduction of risk for weight regain after prior weight loss.

➤◀ DRUG INTERACTIONS RELATED TO DENTAL THERAPEUTICS
No documented drug-drug interactions. The absence of evidence is not evidence of safety.

ADVERSE EFFECTS
⚠ **ORAL:** Gingival disorder (4%); unspecified tooth disorder (4%).

CNS: Anxiety; depression; dizziness; headache.

GI: Abdominal pain/discomfort (25.5%); oily spotting, fatty/oily stool, oily evacuation; flatus with discharge; fecal urgency, increased defecation, fecal incontinence; infectious diarrhea; nausea; rectal pain/discomfort; vomiting.

RESP: Ear, nose, and throat symptoms; influenza (40%); lower respiratory tract infection; URI (38%).

MISC: Fatigue; pedal edema; sleep disorder; urinary tract infection.

CLINICAL IMPLICATIONS
General
- Determine why drug is being taken. Consider implications of condition on dental treatment.
- If GI side effects occur, consider semisupine chair position.

Ortho-Est — see estropipate
Ortopsique — see diazepam
Or-Tyl — see dicyclomine HCl
Orudis — see ketoprofen
Orudis KT — see ketoprofen
Orudis SR — see ketoprofen
Oruvail — see ketoprofen

oseltamivir phosphate (oh-sell-TAM-ih-veer FOSS-fate)
Tamiflu

Drug Class: Anti-infective; Antiviral

PHARMACOLOGY

Action
Inhibition of influenza virus neuraminidase with possible alteration of virus particle aggregation and release.

Uses
Treatment of uncomplicated acute illness caused by influenza infection in patients >1 yr who have been symptomatic for ≤2 days; prophylaxis of influenza in patients ≥13 yr.

➦◀ DRUG INTERACTIONS RELATED TO DENTAL THERAPEUTICS
No documented drug-drug interactions. The absence of evidence is not evidence of safety.

ADVERSE EFFECTS
⚠ ORAL: Swelling of tongue.
CNS: Insomnia, vertigo (1%); seizure, confusion.
GI: Nausea (10%); vomiting (9%).
RESP: Bronchitis (2%).

CLINICAL IMPLICATIONS

General
- Determine why drug is being taken. Take precautions to avoid cross-contamination of microorganisms.
- Monitor body temperature and respiratory system to determine infectivity.
- If GI side effects occur, consider semisupine chair position.

Oseum — see calcitonin-salmon
Osiren — see omeprazole
Osteocalcin — see calcitonin-salmon
Osteral — see piroxicam
Otrozol — see metronidazole

---

oxaprozin (ox-uh-PRO-zin)
Daypro
◼✳◼ **Apo-Oxaprozin, Rhoxal-oxaprozin**
Drug Class: Analgesic; NSAID

PHARMACOLOGY

Action
Decreases inflammation, pain, and fever, probably through inhibition of cyclooxygenase activity and prostaglandin synthesis.

Uses
Relief of symptoms of rheumatoid arthritis and osteoarthritis.

➦◀ DRUG INTERACTIONS RELATED TO DENTAL THERAPEUTICS
No documented drug-drug interactions. The absence of evidence is not evidence of safety

ADVERSE EFFECTS
⚠ ORAL: Stomatitis.
CNS: Depression; sedation; somnolence; confusion; disturbed sleep.
GI: Gastric distress; peptic ulcers; occult blood loss; diarrhea, nausea, dyspepsia (9%);

contipation; vomiting; flatulence; anorexia; abdominal distress/cramps/pain; agranulocytosis, leukopenia, thrombocytopenia.

CLINICAL IMPLICATIONS

General

- Determine why drug is being taken. Consider implications of condition on dental treatment.
- *Arthritis*: Consider patient comfort and need for semisupine chair position.
- If GI side effects occur, consider semisupine chair position.
- Blood dyscrasias are rarely reported; anticipate increased bleeding, infection, and poor healing.

Oral Health Education

- Evaluate manual dexterity; consider need for power toothbrush.
- Encourage daily plaque control procedures for effective, nontraumatic self-care.

---

oxazepam (ox-AZE-uh-pam)

Serax

🇨🇦 **Apo-Oxazepam**

Drug Class: Antianxiety; Benzodiazepine

PHARMACOLOGY

Action

Potentiates action of GABA, an inhibitory neurotransmitter, resulting in increased neuronal inhibition and CNS depression, especially in limbic system and reticular formation.

Uses

Control of anxiety, anxiety associated with depression; control of anxiety, tension, agitation, and irritability in elderly; treatment of alcoholic patients with acute tremulousness, inebriation, or anxiety associated with alcohol withdrawal.

➡⬅ DRUG INTERACTIONS RELATED TO DENTAL THERAPEUTICS

No documented drug-drug interactions. The absence of evidence is not evidence of safety.

ADVERSE EFFECTS

⚠ **ORAL:** Dry mouth; gingival pain; salivation; coated tongue; difficulty in swallowing.

CNS: Drowsiness; dizziness; lethargy; vertigo; tremor; fatigue; memory impairment; disorientation; anterograde amnesia; ataxia; hallucinations; restlessness; headache; slurred speech; stupor; euphoria; paradoxical reactions (e.g., anger, hostility, mania, insomnia).

CVS: Bradycardia or tachycardia; hypertension or hypotension; palpitations.

GI: Nausea.

MISC: Dependence/withdrawal syndrome (e.g., confusion, abnormal perception of movement, depersonalization, muscle twitching, psychosis, paranoid delusions, seizures); edema; altered libido; incontinence; fever; menstrual irregularities; blood dyscrasias including agranulocytosis, leukopenia, anemia, thrombocytopenia, others.

CLINICAL IMPLICATIONS

General

- Determine why drug is being taken. Consider implications of condition on dental treatment.

- Determine ability to adapt to stress of dental treatment. Consider short appointments.
- Depressed or anxious patients may neglect self-care. Monitor for plaque control effectiveness.
- Monitor vital signs.
- Chronic dry mouth is possible; anticipate increased caries and candidiasis.
- Blood dyscrasias are rarely reported; anticipate increased bleeding, infection, and poor healing.

Oral Health Education
- Encourage daily plaque control procedures for effective, nontraumatic self-care.
- If chronic dry mouth occurs, recommend home fluoride therapy and use of nonalcoholic oral health care products.

---

oxcarbazepine (ox-kar-BAZE-uh-peen)
Trileptal

Drug Class: Antiepileptic

PHARMACOLOGY
Action
The pharmacological activity is primarily through the 10-monohydroxy metabolite (MHD) of oxcarbazepine, but the exact mechanism is unknown. It may block voltage-sensitive sodium channels resulting in stabilization of hyperexcited neural membranes, inhibition of repetitive neuronal firing, and diminution of propagation of synaptic impulses.

Uses
As monotherapy or adjunctive therapy in the treatment of partial seizures in patients with epilepsy.

➡⬅ DRUG INTERACTIONS RELATED TO DENTAL THERAPEUTICS
No documented drug-drug interactions. The absence of evidence is not evidence of safety.

ADVERSE EFFECTS
⚠ **ORAL:** Dry mouth; toothache; taste disturbance (high doses).

CNS: Ataxia; abnormal coordination; fatigue; asthenia; headache; dizziness; somnolence; anxiety; abnormal gait; insomnia; tremor; amnesia; nervousness; agitation; confusion; speech disorder; aggravated convulsions.

CVS: Chest pain; hypotension (high doses).

GI: Nausea (15% to 29%); vomiting; abdominal pain; anorexia; diarrhea; dyspepsia; constipation; gastritis; rectum hemorrhage.

RESP: Rhinitis; URI; cough; bronchitis; pharyngitis; epistaxis; sinusitis.

MISC: Muscle weakness; back pain; sprains/strains; fever; allergy; weight increase; infection; lymphadenopathy.

CLINICAL IMPLICATIONS
General
- Determine why drug is being taken. Consider implications of condition on dental treatment.
- Determine level of disease control, type and frequency of seizure, and compliance with medication regimen.
- Determine ability to adapt to stress of dental treatment. Consider short appointments.
- If GI side effects occur, consider semisupine chair position.
- Chronic dry mouth is possible; anticipate increased caries and candidiasis.

Oral Health Education
- Determine need for power toothbrush for self-care.
- If chronic dry mouth occurs, recommend home fluoride therapy and use of nonalcoholic oral health care products.

Oxeze Turbuhaler — see formoterol fumarate
Oxicanol — see piroxicam

---

oxidized cellulose

Oxycel: Pads: 3″ × 3″, 8 ply; Pledgets: 2″ × 1″ × 1″; Strips: 18″ × 2″, 4 ply
Surgicel: Strips: 2″ × 14″, 4″ × 8″, 2″ × 3″, ½″ × 2″; Surgical Nu-knit: 1″ × 1″, 3″ × 4″, 6″ × 9″

Drug Class: Hematological agent

PHARMACOLOGY

Action
Forms a matrix for fibrin deposition and propagation of blood clot.

Uses
Hemorrhage: Used adjunctively in surgical procedures to assist in the control of capillary, venous, and small arterial hemorrhage when ligation or other conventional methods of control are impractical or ineffective. Also indicated for use in oral surgery and exodontia.

Contraindications
Packing or wadding as a hemostatic agent; packing or implantation in fractures or laminectomies (it interferes with bone regeneration and can cause cyst formation); control of hemorrhage from large arteries or on nonhemorrhagic serous oozing surfaces since body fluids other than whole blood (e.g., serum) do not react with oxidized cellulose to produce satisfactory hemostatic effects; do not use around the optic nerve and chiasm; do not use as a wrap in vascular surgery because it has a stenotic effect.

Usual Dosage
Local bleeding associated with oral surgical procedures
STRIPS OR PADS
ADULTS AND CHILDREN: Apply strips or pads as a surgical dressing for wounds or over extraction sites (do not place into a socket).

➡️⬅ DRUG INTERACTIONS
No documented drug-drug interactions. The absence of evidence is not evidence of safety.

ADVERSE EFFECTS
MISC: Foreign body reaction.

CLINICAL IMPLICATIONS

General
- Apply by loosely packing against the bleeding surface. Avoid wadding or packing tightly. **Use sparingly.**
- Application of topical thrombin solution to cellulose gauze will inactivate thrombin due to acidity.
- Ensure therapeutic response and decreased bleeding before patient dismissed.

Pregnancy Risk Category: No information available.

Oral Health Education
• Advise patient to report uncontrolled bleeding to dentist.

Oxifungol — see fluconazole
Oxis — see formoterol fumarate

---

oxybutynin Cl (OX-ee-BYOO-tih-nin KLOR-ide)
Ditropan, Ditropan XL, Oxytrol

■✦■ Apo-Oxybutynin, Gen-Oxybutynin, Novo-Oxybutynin, Nu-Oxybutynin, PMS-Oxybutynin

■✦■ Tavor

Drug Class: Antispasmodic, urinary

PHARMACOLOGY

Action
Increases bladder capacity; diminishes frequency of uninhibited contractions of detrusor muscle; and delays initial desire to void.

Uses
Treatment of symptoms of bladder instability associated with voiding in patients with uninhibited and reflex neurogenic bladder (e.g., urinary leakage, dysuria); treatment of overactive bladder with symptoms of urge urinary incontinence, urgency, and frequency (extended release [ER] tablet).

➡◀ DRUG INTERACTIONS RELATED TO DENTAL THERAPEUTICS
No documented drug-drug interactions. The absence of evidence is not evidence of safety.

ADVERSE EFFECTS
⚠ ORAL: ER TABLETS: Dry mouth (60.8%).
IMMEDIATE-RELEASE TABLETS AND SYRUP: Dry mouth.
TRANSDERMAL SYSTEM: Dry mouth.
CNS: ER TABLETS: Somnolence (11.9%); headache (9.8%); dizziness (6.3%); drowsiness, hallucinations, restlessness, insomnia, nervousness, confusion (2% to <5%).
IMMEDIATE-RELEASE TABLETS AND SYRUP: Dizziness; drowsiness; hallucinations; insomnia; restlessness.
TRANSDERMAL SYSTEM: Fatigue; somnolence; headache (>1%).
GI: ER TABLETS: Constipation (13.1%); diarrhea (9.1%); nausea (8.9%); dyspepsia (6.8%); vomiting, decreased GI motility, flatulence, gastroesophageal reflux (2% to <5%).
IMMEDIATE-RELEASE TABLETS AND SYRUP: Constipation; decreased GI motility; nausea.
TRANSDERMAL SYSTEM: Diarrhea, constipation (≥2%); abdominal pain, nausea, flatulence (>1%).
RESP: ER TABLETS: URI, cough, bronchitis (2% to <5%).
MISC: ER TABLETS: Asthenia, pain (6.8%); rhinitis (5.6%); UTI (5.1%); decreased sweating, suppression of lactation, abdominal pain, accidental injury, back pain, flulike syndrome, arthritis (2% to <5%).
IMMEDIATE-RELEASE TABLETS AND SYRUP: Asthenia; impotence; suppression of lactation.
TRANSDERMAL SYSTEM: Flushing, back pain, application site burning (>1%).

CLINICAL IMPLICATIONS

General
• Determine why drug is being taken. Consider implications of condition on dental treatment.

- Chronic dry mouth is possible; anticipate increased caries activity and candidiasis.
- *Appointment planning:* Short appointments are recommended.
- Place on frequent maintenance schedule to avoid periodontal inflammation.

Oral Health Education

- Encourage daily plaque control procedures for effective self-care.
- If chronic dry mouth occurs, recommend home fluoride therapy and use of nonalcoholic oral health care products.

Oxycel — see oxidized cellulose

---

oxycodone HCl (OX-ee-KOE-dohn HIGH-droe-KLOR-ide)

Endocodone, M-oxy, OxyContin, Oxydose, OxyFAST, OxyIR, Percolone, Roxicodone, Roxicodone Intensol

■✦■ Supeudol

Drug Class: Narcotic analgesic
DEA Schedule: Schedule II

PHARMACOLOGY

Action

Relieves pain by stimulating opiate receptors in CNS; may cause respiratory depression, peripheral vasodilation, inhibition of intestinal peristalsis, sphincter of Oddi spasm, stimulation of chemoreceptors that cause vomiting and increased bladder tone.

Uses

Relief of moderate to moderately severe pain.

➡◀ DRUG INTERACTIONS RELATED TO DENTAL THERAPEUTICS

No documented drug-drug interactions. The absence of evidence is not evidence of safety.

ADVERSE EFFECTS

⚠ **ORAL:** Dry mouth; taste disturbance.
CNS: Lightheadedness; dizziness; sedation; disorientation; incoordination.
CVS: Bradycardia (frequent); flushing; tachycardia; arrhythmia; palpitations, hypertension or hypotension; orthostatic hypotension, syncope.
GI: Nausea; vomiting; constipation; abdominal pain.
RESP: Respiratory depression; laryngospasm; depression of cough reflex.
MISC: Tolerance; psychological and physical dependence with long-term use.

CLINICAL IMPLICATIONS

General

- Determine why drug is being taken. Consider implications of condition on dental treatment.
- Monitor vital signs (e.g., BP, pulse, respiration).
- *Postural hypotension:* Monitor BP at the beginning and end of each appointment; anticipate syncope. Have patient sit upright for several min at the end of the dental appointment before dismissing.
- Chronic dry mouth is possible; anticipate increased caries and candidiasis.
- If GI side effects occur, consider semisupine chair position.
- Avoid prescribing opioids for dental pain. Acetaminophen is appropriate if GI bleeding is present.

Oral Health Education

- If chronic dry mouth occurs, recommend home fluoride therapy and use of nonalcoholic oral health care products.

oxycodone HCl/acetaminophen — see acetaminophen/oxycodone HCl
oxycodone HCl/aspirin — see aspirin/oxycodone HCl
oxycodone/ibuprofen — see ibuprofen/oxycodone
OxyContin — see oxycodone HCl
Oxydose — see oxycodone HCl
OxyFAST — see oxycodone HCl
OxyIR — see oxycodone HCl
Oxytrol — see oxybutynin Cl
Ozoken — see omeprazole
Pacerone — see amiodarone
Pacitran — see diazepam
Pactens — see naproxen
Pain Doctor — see capsaicin
Pain-X — see capsaicin
Palafer — see ferrous salts
Palane — see enalapril maleate
Pamelor — see nortriptyline HCl
Panacet 5/500 — see acetaminophen/hydrocodone bitartrate
Panadol — see acetaminophen
Panadol Infants' Drops — see acetaminophen
Panasol 5/500 — see aspirin/hydrocodone bitartrate
Panasol-S — see prednisone
Pandel — see hydrocortisone
Panretin — see alitretinoin
Panto IV — see pantoprazole sodium
Pantoloc — see pantoprazole sodium
Pantomicina — see erythromycin

---

pantoprazole sodium (pahn-TOE-prazz-ole SO-dee-uhm)
Protonix, Protonix IV

▌❋▌ **Panto IV, Pantoloc**

▌❖▌ **Pantozol, Zurcal**

Drug Class: GI; Proton pump inhibitor

PHARMACOLOGY

Action
Suppresses gastric acid secretion by blocking acid (proton) pump within gastric parietal cells.

Uses
ORAL: Short-term (no longer than 8 wk) treatment in the healing and symptomatic relief of erosive esophagitis associated with gastroesophageal reflux disease (GERD); long-term

treatment of pathologic hypersecretory conditions, including Zollinger-Ellison syndrome; maintenance of healing of erosive esophagitis.

IV: Short-term (7- to 10-day) treatment of GERD, as an alternative to oral therapy in patients unable to continue oral pantoprazole; hypersecretory conditions associated with Zollinger-Ellison syndrome or other neoplastic conditions.

➡◀ DRUG INTERACTIONS RELATED TO DENTAL THERAPEUTICS

Ketoconazole or itraconazole: Decreased ketoconazole or itraconazole effect (decreased absorption)
- Avoid concurrent use.

ADVERSE EFFECTS

⚠ ORAL: Increased salivation.

CNS: Headache (9%); insomnia (1%); anxiety, asthenia, increased dizziness, hypertonia (≥1%); anterior ischemic optic neuropathy, confusion, hypokinesia, speech disorder, tinnitus, vertigo.

GI: Diarrhea (6%); flatulence, abdominal pain (4%); nausea, vomiting (2%); eructation (1%); constipation, dyspepsia, gastroenteritis, GI disorder, vomiting (≥1%); pancreatitis.

RESP: Bronchitis, cough, dyspnea, sinusitis, upper respiratory tract infection (≥1%).

MISC: Chest pain, flu-like syndrome, infection, pain (≥1%); anaphylaxis, angioedema, rhabdomyolysis.

CLINICAL IMPLICATIONS

General

- Determine why drug is being taken. Consider implications of condition on dental treatment.
- If patient has GI disease, consider semisupine chair position.
- Drugs that lower acidity in intestinal tract may interfere with absorption of some antibiotics (penicillin, tetracyclines).
- Anticipate chemical erosion of teeth.
- Substernal pain (heartburn) may mimic pain of cardiac origin.
- Use COX inhibitors with caution, as they may exacerbate PUD and GERD.

Oral Health Education

- Inform patient that toothbrushing should not be done after reflux, but to only rinse mouth with water, then use home fluoride product to minimize chemical erosion caries.

Pantozol — see pantoprazole sodium

para-aminosalicylate sodium — see aminosalicylate sodium

Pariet — see rabeprazole sodium

Parlodel — see bromocriptine mesylate

Parnate — see tranylcypromine sulfate

---

paroxetine (puh-ROKS-uh-teen)

(paroxetine mesylate, paroxetine HCl)

Paxil, Paxil CR, Pexeva

■◖■ Aropax

Drug Class: Antidepressant

PHARMACOLOGY

Action

Blocks reuptake of serotonin, enhancing serotonergic function.

Uses

Panic disorder or social anxiety disorder (except Pexeva); major depressive disorder. IMMEDIATE RELEASE ONLY: Obsessive-compulsive disorder (OCD); generalized anxiety disorder (GAD) (except Pexeva); posttraumatic stress disorder (PTSD) (except Pexeva). CONTROLLED RELEASE ONLY: Premenstrual dysphoric disorder (PMDD).

➕ DRUG INTERACTIONS RELATED TO DENTAL THERAPEUTICS

No documented drug-drug interactions. The absence of evidence is not evidence of safety.

ADVERSE EFFECTS

Incidences of adverse reactions are stated in broad ranges because those reported varied depending on the dose or indication.

⚠ ORAL: Dry mouth ((5%); tooth disorder/caries (1%).

CNS: Headache, somnolence, dizziness, insomnia, tremor, nervousness, anxiety, decreased libido ((5%); paresthesia, drugged feeling, confusion, agitation, abnormal dreams, migraine, impaired concentration, depersonalization, myoclonus, amnesia, stimulation, depression, emotional lability, vertigo (1% to 4%); neuroleptic malignant syndrome; extrapyramidal symptoms; status epilepticus; eclampsia.

CVS: Chest pain; palpitations; tachycardia; vasodilation; hypertension.

GI: Nausea, constipation, diarrhea, abdominal pain, decreased appetite (5%); flatulence; oropharynx disorder, dyspepsia, increased appetite, vomiting (1% to 4%).

RESP: Yawn, increased cough (1% to 4%); pulmonary hypertension; allergic alveolitis.

MISC: Asthenia (5%); chest pain, back pain, chills, trauma, allergic reaction, photosensitivity, malaise (1% to 4%); Guillain-Barré syndrome; prolactinemia; galactorrhea; serotonin syndrome; anaphylaxis.

CLINICAL IMPLICATIONS

General

- Determine why drug is being taken. Consider implications of condition on dental treatment.
- Determine ability to adapt to stress of dental treatment. Consider short appointments.
- Depressed or anxious patients may neglect self-care. Monitor for plaque control effectiveness.
- Chronic dry mouth is possible; anticipate increased caries and candidiasis.
- Monitor vital signs.
- If GI side effects occur, consider semisupine chair position.
- Increased photosensitization with dental drugs having photosensitization side effect.

Oral Health Education

- Encourage daily plaque control procedures for effective self-care.
- If chronic dry mouth occurs, recommend home fluoride therapy and use of nonalcoholic oral health care products.

---

paroxetine HCl — see paroxetine

paroxetine mesylate — see paroxetine

PAS — see aminosalicylate sodium

Paser — see aminosalicylate sodium

Patanol — see olopatadine HCl

Paxil — see paroxetine

Paxil CR — see paroxetine

PCE Dispertab — see erythromycin

PediaCare Fever — see ibuprofen

PediaCare Infant's Decongestant — see pseudoephedrine

PediaCare Nasal Decongestant — see pseudoephedrine
Pediaflor — see sodium fluoride
Pediapred — see prednisolone
Pediatric Advil Drops — see ibuprofen
Pediatric Vicks 44d Dry Hacking Cough and Head Congestion —
see dextromethorphan HBr
Pediatrix — see acetaminophen
Pedi-Dri — see nystatin
Penamox — see amoxicillin

penbutolol sulfate (pen-BYOO-toe-lole SULL-fate)
Levatol

Drug Class: Beta-adrenergic blocker

PHARMACOLOGY
Action
Nonselectively blocks beta-adrenergic receptors, primarily affecting the cardiovascular system (e.g., decreased heart rate, decreased cardiac contractility, decreased BP) and lungs (promotes bronchospasm).

Uses
Management of mild to moderate hypertension.

➡◀ DRUG INTERACTIONS RELATED TO DENTAL THERAPEUTICS
COX-1 inhibitors: Decreased antihypertensive effect (decreased prostaglandin synthesis)
 • Monitor blood pressure.
Sympathomimetic amines: Decreased antihypertensive effect (pharmacologic antagonism; unopposed alpha-adrenergic stimulation)
 • Monitor blood pressure.

ADVERSE EFFECTS
⚠ **ORAL:** Dry mouth; taste disturbance; taste loss.
CNS: Dizziness; tiredness; fatigue; headache; insomnia; depression; short-term memory loss; emotional lability.
CVS: Hypotension; bradycardia; arrhythmia; postural hypotension.
MISC: Photosensitivity reactions.
GI: Diarrhea; nausea; dyspepsia.
RESP: Cough; dyspnea; bronchospasm.

CLINICAL IMPLICATIONS
General
• Monitor vital signs (e.g., BP, pulse pressure, rate and rhythm) at each appointment to assess disease control. Do not provide elective dental treatment when BP is ≥180/110 or in the presence of other high-risk CV conditions. Refer to the section entitled "The Patient Taking Cardiovascular Drugs" in Chapter 6: *Clinical Medicine*.
• Chronic dry mouth is possible; anticipate increased caries, candidiasis, and lichenoid mucositis.
• If GI side effects occur, consider semisupine chair position.
• Use local anesthetic agents with vasoconstrictor with caution based on functional capacity of the patient, and use aspirating technique to prevent intravascular injection.
• Beta blockers may mask epinephrine-induced signs and symptoms of hypoglycemia in patients with diabetes.

- Determine ability to adapt to stress of dental treatment. Consider short appointments.
- *Postural hypotension:* Monitor BP at the beginning and end of each appointment; antici-pate syncope. Have patient sit upright for several min at the end of the dental appoint-ment before dismissing.
- Place on frequent maintenance schedule to avoid periodontal inflammation.

Oral Health Education

- Encourage daily plaque control procedures for effective self-care in patient at risk for car-diovascular disease.
- If chronic dry mouth occurs, recommend home fluoride therapy and use of nonalcoholic oral health care products.

 # penciclovir (pen-SICK-low-vihr)

Denavir: Cream: 10 mg/g

Drug Class: Anti-infective, topical; Antiviral

PHARMACOLOGY

Action
Selectively inhibits herpes viral DNA synthesis and replication.

Uses
Treatment of recurrent herpes labialis (cold sores) in adults.

Contraindications
Standard considerations.

Usual Dosage
ADULTS: *Topical:* Apply to lesions q 2 hr while awake for 4 days. Start treatment as early as possible, during the prodrome or when lesions first appear.

➡️⬅️ DRUG INTERACTIONS

No documented drug-drug interactions. The absence of evidence is not evidence of safety.

ADVERSE EFFECTS

⚠️ **ORAL:** Taste alteration.

CLINICAL IMPLICATIONS

General
When prescribed by DDS:
- *Lactation:* Undetermined.
- *Children:* Safety and efficacy not established.
- *Elderly:* Side-effect profile similar to younger patients.
- Assess lesions prior to and daily during therapy.

When prescribed by medical facility:
- Determine why drug is being taken.
- Be aware that herpetic infections are infectious during prodromal, vesicular, and crusting stages.

Pregnancy Risk Category: Category B.

Oral Health Education
When prescribed by DDS:
- Instruct patient to begin treatment as soon as possible, during the prodrome, or as soon as lesions appear.
- Advise patient to apply the medication exactly as directed and to only apply to lesions on the face and lips.

- Advise patient to avoid applying cream to mucous membranes and within or near eyes.
- Advise patient to wash hands before and after applying cream.
- Advise patient to discontinue use and notify health care provider if local irritation develops.
- Advise the patient that the use of additional OTC creams or ointments may delay the healing process or even spread the disease.
- Instruct the patient to notify the health care provider if the symptoms do not improve in 7 days of topical therapy.
- Instruct the patient to apply sufficient ointment to cover all lesions q 2 hr while awake.
- Advise the patient to use a finger cot or glove when applying the ointment to prevent spread of the virus.
- Recommend that toothbrush be replaced following clearance of oral infection.

Penecort — see hydrocortisone

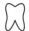 # penicillin V (pen-ih-SILL-in V)

Synonym: phenoxymethyl penicillin; penicillin V potassium

Beepen-VK, Pen-Vee K, Penicillin VK: Tablets: 250, 500 mg; Powder for oral solution: 125 mg/5 mL, 250 mg/5 mL
Veetids: Tablets: 250, 500 mg; Powder for oral solution: 125 mg/5 mL
Veetids '250': Powder for oral solution: 250 mg/5 mL

■✦■ APO-Pen VK, Nadopen-V, Novo-Pen-VK, Nu-Pen-VK, Pen-Vee, PVF K

■❀■ Anapenil, Pen-Vi-K

Drug Class: Antibiotic, penicillin

PHARMACOLOGY

Action
Inhibits mucopeptide synthesis of bacterial cell wall.

Uses
Treatment of upper respiratory tract infections; treatment of pneumococcal, streptococcal, and staphylococcal infections and fusospirochetosis (Vincent infection) of oropharynx caused by susceptible microorganisms.

Unlabeled Uses
Prophylactic treatment of sickle cell anemia in children; treatment of anaerobic infections; treatment of Lyme disease (*Borrelia burgdorferi*).

Contraindications
Hypersensitivity to penicillins. Do not treat severe pneumonia, empyema, bacteremia, pericarditis, meningitis, or purulent or septic arthritis with oral penicillin V during acute stage.

Usual Dosage
ADULTS AND CHILDREN OVER 12 YR: *PO:* 250 to 500 mg qid.

Pharmacokinetics
ABSORP: Oral absorption is 60% to 73%. T_{max} is 0.5 to 1 hr. C_{max} is 2 to 3 mcg/mL.
DIST: Widely distributed to most tissues and body fluids; distribution into CSF is low with noninflamed meninges. Protein binding is 80%. Vd is 0.5 L/kg. Crosses the placenta and distributes into breast milk.
METAB: Hepatic biotransformation is 55%.
EXCRET: Mainly renal (20% to 40% as unchanged). $T_{1/2}$ is 0.5 to 1 hr.
SPECIAL POP: *Renal failure:* For Ccr less than 10 mL/min, $t_{1/2}$ increased to 4.1 hr.

➡← DRUG INTERACTIONS

Allopurinol: Increased incidence of rash (mechanism unknown)
- Monitor clinical status.

ADVERSE EFFECTS

⚠ **ORAL:** Glossitis; dry mouth; black hairy tongue; candidiasis.
CNS: Dizziness; fatigue; insomnia; reversible hyperactivity; neurotoxicity (e.g., lethargy, neuromuscular irritability, hallucinations, convulsions, seizures).
GI: Gastritis; nausea; vomiting; abdominal pain or cramps; epigastric distress; diarrhea or bloody diarrhea; rectal bleeding; flatulence; enterocolitis; pseudomembranous colitis.
MISC: Hypersensitivity reactions (e.g., urticaria, angioneurotic edema, laryngospasm, laryngeal edema, bronchospasm, hypotension, vascular collapse, death, maculopapular to exfoliative dermatitis, vesicular eruptions, erythema multiforme, serum sickness, skin rashes, prostration); vaginitis; hyperthermia.

CLINICAL IMPLICATIONS

General
When prescribed by DDS:
- *Lactation:* Small amount excreted in breast milk. May cause diarrhea, candidiasis, or allergic response in nursing infant.
- *Hypersensitivity:* Reactions range from mild to life threatening. Administer drug with caution to cephalosporin-sensitive patients because of possible cross-reactivity.
- *Renal failure:* Use drug with caution; dosage adjustment may be necessary.
- *Superinfection:* May result in bacterial or fungal overgrowth of nonsusceptible organisms.
- *Pseudomembranous colitis:* May occur because of overgrowth of clostridia.
- *Streptococcal infections:* Therapy must be for a minimum of 10 days.
- *Overdosage:* Neuromuscular hyperexcitability, agitation, confusion, asterixis, hallucinations, stupor, coma, multifocal myoclonus, encephalopathy, hyperkalemia.

When prescribed by medical facility:
- Determine why drug is being taken. Prolonged use of antibiotics may result in bacterial or fungal overgrowth of nonsusceptible microorganisms; anticipate candidiasis.
- If GI side effects occur, consider semisupine chair position.

Pregnancy Risk Category: Category B.

Oral Health Education
When prescribed by DDS:
- Instruct patient to complete entire course of therapy even if feeling better.
- Advise patient to use calibrated measuring device for liquid preparation.
- Instruct penicillin allergic patient to wear Medi-Alert necklace or bracelet.
- Advise patient to use nonhormonal form of contraceptive during penicillin V therapy.
- Inform patient of the signs of hypersensitivity (e.g., skin rash, itching, hives, shortness of breath, wheezing) and other side effects (e.g., black tongue, sore throat, nausea, vomiting, severe diarrhea, fever, swollen joints). Instruct patient to notify health care provider if these symptoms occur.
- Instruct patient to notify health care provider if there is no improvement in symptoms of infection.
- Instruct patient to notify health care provider of signs of superinfection (e.g., vaginitis, black "hairy" tongue).

Penicillin VK — see penicillin V

penicillin V potassium — see penicillin V

Pentasa — see mesalamine

---

pentazocine (pen-TAZ-oh-seen)
Talacen, Talwin, Talwin Compound, Talwin NX
Drug Class: Analgesic, narcotic agonist-antagonist
DEA Schedule: Schedule IV

PHARMACOLOGY

Action
Produces analgesia by an agonistic effect at the kappa opioid receptor. Weakly antagonizes effects of opiates at mu opioid receptor; does not appear to increase biliary tract pressure.

Uses
ORAL AND PARENTERAL FORMS: Management of moderate to severe pain.
PARENTERAL FORM: Preoperative or preanesthetic medication; supplement to surgical anesthesia.

➡◀ DRUG INTERACTIONS RELATED TO DENTAL THERAPEUTICS
No documented drug-drug interactions. The absence of evidence is not evidence of safety.

ADVERSE EFFECTS
⚠ **ORAL:** Dry mouth; taste alteration.
CNS: Lightheadedness; dizziness; euphoria; hallucinations; disorientation; confusion; seizures.
CVS: Hypotension, tachycardia; hypertension.
GI: Nausea.
RESP: Respiratory depression; transient apnea in newborns whose mothers received parenteral pentazocine during labor.
MISC: Anaphylaxis; tolerance; psychological and physical dependence in long-term use.

CLINICAL IMPLICATIONS

General
- Determine why drug is being taken. Consider implications of condition on dental treatment.
- If oral pain requires additional analgesics, consider nonopioid products.
- *When prescribed by DDS:* Short-term use only; there is no justification for long-term use in the management of dental pain.
- *Geriatric patients*: Use lower dose of opioid.
- Chronic dry mouth is possible; anticipate increased caries and candidiasis.
- Monitor vital signs.

Oral Health Education
- If chronic dry mouth occurs, recommend home fluoride therapy and use of nonalcoholic oral health care products.
- *If prescribed by DDS:* Warn patient not to drive, sign important papers, or operate mechanical equipment.

---

 pentobarbital sodium (pen-toe-BAR-bih-tahl SO-dee-uhm)

Nembutal Sodium: Capsules: 50, 100 mg; Suppositories: 30, 60, 120, 200 mg; Elixir: Equivalent to 20 mg/5 mL; Injection: 50 mg/mL

Drug Class: Sedative and hypnotic, barbiturate, short-acting; Anticonvulsant
DEA Schedule: Schedule II

PHARMACOLOGY

Action
Depresses sensory cortex; decreases motor activity; alters cerebellar function; and produces drowsiness, sedation, and hypnosis.

Uses
Sedation; short-term treatment of insomnia; preanesthesia; emergency control of convulsions (parenteral form).

Contraindications
Hypersensitivity to barbiturates; manifest or latent porphyria.

Usual Dosage
Sedation
ADULTS: *PO/PR:* 20 to 30 mg bid to qid.
CHILDREN: *PO/IM:* 2 to 6 mg/kg (max, 100 mg). *IV:* 50 mg.
Pediatric patients unable to take orally or by injection
CHILDREN 12 TO 14 YR (36.4 TO 50 KG): *PR:* 60 or 120 mg.
CHILDREN 5 TO 12 YR (18.2 TO 36.4 KG): *PR:* 60 mg.
CHILDREN 1 TO 4 YR (9 TO 18.2 KG): *PR:* 30 or 60 mg.

Pharmacokinetics
ABSORP: Pentobarbital sodium is absorbed in varying degrees. T_{max} is 15 min (IV), maximal CNS depression.
DIST: Rapidly distributed to all tissues and fluids with high concentration in brain, liver, and kidneys due to lipid solubility. Protein binding is 60% to 70%. Pentobarbital sodium distributes into breast milk.
METAB: Metabolized by hepatic microsomal enzyme system.
EXCRET: Urine (very little unchanged); less commonly in the feces. The $t_{1/2}$ is 15 to 50 hr.
ONSET: Immediate following IV administration.
DURATION: 3 to 4 hr.

➡️⬅️ DRUG INTERACTIONS
Alcohol: Decreased sedative effect with long-term alcohol abuse (increased metabolism)
  • Avoid concurrent use.
Beta-adrenergic blockers: Decreased beta-blocker effect (increased metabolism)
  • Avoid concurrent use.
Nortriptyline: Decreased antidepressant effect (increased metabolism)
  • Avoid concurrent use.
Quinidine: Decreased quinidine effect (increased metabolism)
  • Avoid concurrent use.

ADVERSE EFFECTS
CVS: Bradycardia; hypotension; syncope.
CNS: Drowsiness; agitation; confusion; headache; hyperkinesia; ataxia; CNS depression; paradoxical excitement; nightmares; psychiatric disturbances; hallucinations; insomnia; dizziness.
GI: Nausea; vomiting; constipation.
RESP: Hypoventilation; apnea; laryngospasm; bronchospasm.
MISC: Hypersensitivity reactions (e.g., angioedema, rashes, exfoliative dermatitis); fever; injection site reactions (e.g., local pain, thrombophlebitis).

CLINICAL IMPLICATIONS
General
When prescribed or used by DDS:
  • *Lactation:* Excreted in breast milk.
  • *Children:* May respond with excitement rather than depression.
  • *Elderly:* More sensitive to drug effects; dosage reduction is required.
  • *Renal failure:* Use drug with caution; dosage reduction may be required.
  • *Hepatic failure:* Use drug with caution; dosage reduction may be required.
  • Monitor blood pressure, pulse, and respiration.
  • *Dependence:* Tolerance or psychological and physical dependence may occur with continued use.

- *IV administration:* Do not exceed maximal IV rate; respiratory depression, apnea, and hypotension may result. Parenteral solutions are highly alkaline; extravasation may cause tissue damage and necrosis. Inadvertent intra-arterial injection may lead to arterial spasm, thrombosis, and gangrene.
- *Seizure disorders:* Status epilepticus may result from abrupt discontinuation.
- *Overdosage:* CNS and respiratory depression, Cheyne-Stokes respiration, areflexia, constriction of pupils, oliguria, tachycardia, hypotension, lowered body temperature, coma, apnea, circulatory collapse, respiratory arrest, death.

Pregnancy Risk Category: Category D.

Oral Health Education

When prescribed or used by DDS:

- Warn patient that medication may be habit forming and for this reason it is important to take medicine exactly as directed. Taking too little or too much can have serious complications.
- Instruct patient to report the following symptoms to health care provider: nausea, vomiting, drowsiness, dizziness, fever, sore throat, mouth sores, easy bleeding, bruising, skin irritation, or exaggerated sunburn.
- Caution patient to avoid intake of alcoholic beverages or other CNS depressants.
- Advise patient that drug may cause drowsiness, and to use caution while driving or performing other tasks requiring mental alertness.

Pentrexyl — see ampicillin

Pen-Vee — see penicillin V

Pen-Vee K — see penicillin V

Pen-Vi-K — see penicillin V

Pepcid — see famotidine

Pepcid AC — see famotidine

Pepcidine — see famotidine

Pepcid IV — see famotidine

Pepcid RPD — see famotidine

Pepevit — see niacin

Pepto-Bismol — see bismuth subsalicylate

Pepto-Bismol Maximum Strength — see bismuth subsalicylate

Pepto Diarrhea Control — see loperamide HCl

Percocet — see acetaminophen/oxycodone HCl

Percocet-Demi — see acetaminophen/oxycodone HCl

Percodan — see aspirin/oxycodone HCl

Percolone — see oxycodone HCl

---

pergolide mesylate (PURR-go-lide MEH-sih-LATE)

Permax

Drug Class: Antiparkinson

PHARMACOLOGY

Action

Directly stimulates postsynaptic dopamine receptors in nigrostriatal system.

Uses

Adjunctive treatment to levodopa-carbidopa in management of Parkinson disease.

➡️⬅️ DRUG INTERACTIONS RELATED TO DENTAL THERAPEUTICS

No documented drug-drug interactions. The absence of evidence is not evidence of safety.

ADVERSE EFFECTS

⚠️ **ORAL:** Dry mouth (3.7%).

CNS: Dyskinesia (62.4%); dizziness (19.1%); hallucinations (13.8%); dystonia (11.6%); confusion (11.1%); somnolence (10.1%); insomnia (7.9%); anxiety (6.4%); personality disorder; psychosis; extrapyramidal syndrome; incoordination; akinesia; hypertonia; neuralgia; akathisia.

CVS: Postural hypotension (9%), vasodilation, palpitations, hypotension, syncope, chest pain (>2%); hypertension, arrhythmia (1%).

GI: Nausea (24.3%); constipation (10.6%); diarrhea (6.4%); dyspepsia (6.4%); anorexia (4.8%); vomiting (2.7%); abdominal pain (5.8%).

RESP: Rhinitis (12.2%); dyspnea (4.8%); epistaxis; hiccups.

MISC: Pain (7%); accidental injury; flu-like syndrome; chills; peripheral edema (7.4%); facial edema; edema; weight gain; anemia; bursitis; myalgia; twitching; infection.

CLINICAL IMPLICATIONS

General

- Determine why drug is being taken. Consider implications of condition on dental treatment.
- Extrapyramidal behaviors associated with Parkinson disease can complicate access to oral cavity and complicate oral procedures.
- Chronic dry mouth is possible; anticipate increased caries and candidiasis.
- If GI side effects occur, consider semisupine chair position.
- Monitor vital signs.
- *Postural hypotension*: Monitor BP at the beginning and end of each appointment; anticipate syncope. Have patient sit upright for several min at the end of the dental appointment before dismissing.

Oral Health Education

- Evaluate manual dexterity; consider need for power toothbrush.
- If chronic dry mouth occurs, recommend home fluoride therapy and use of nonalcoholic oral health care products.

Peridex — see chlorhexidine gluconate

---

perindopril erbumine (per-IN-doe prill ehr-BYOO-meen)

Aceon

■✚■ **Coversyl**

Drug Class: Antihypertensive; Angiotensin-converting enzyme (ACE) inhibitor

PHARMACOLOGY

Action

Competitively inhibits angiotensin I–converting enzyme, resulting in prevention of angiotensin I conversion to angiotensin II, a potent vasoconstrictor that also stimulates aldosterone release. Clinical consequences are a decrease in BP, reduced sodium resorption, and potassium retention.

Uses

Treatment of essential hypertension.

➡️⬅️ DRUG INTERACTIONS RELATED TO DENTAL THERAPEUTICS

COX-1 inhibitors: Decreased antihypertensive effect (decreased prostaglandin synthesis)
- Monitor blood pressure.

ADVERSE EFFECTS
⚠ **ORAL:** Dry mouth (1%).
CNS: Dizziness (8%); cerebrovascular accident (0.2%).
CVS: Chest pain; palpitations.
GI: Dyspepsia (2%).
RESP: Cough (12%); pulmonary fibrosis (<0.1%).
MISC: Back pain (6%); viral infection, upper extremity pain, hypertonia (3%); fever (2%); angioedema (0.1%); anaphylactoid reactions.

CLINICAL IMPLICATIONS
General
- Monitor vital signs (e.g., BP, pulse pressure, rate, and rhythm) at each appointment to assess disease control. Do not provide elective dental treatment when BP is ≥180/110 or in the presence of other high-risk CV conditions. Refer to the section entitled "The Patient Taking Cardiovascular Drugs" in Chapter 6: *Clinical Medicine*.
- Use local anesthetic agents with vasoconstrictor with caution based on functional capacity of the patient, and use aspirating technique to prevent intravascular injection.
- If coughing is problematic, consider semisupine chair position for treatment.
- Susceptible patients with DM may experience severe recurrent hypoglycemia.
- *Postural hypotension:* Monitor BP at the beginning and end of each appointment; anticipate syncope. Have patient sit upright for several min at the end of the dental appointment before dismissing.
- Determine ability to adapt to stress of dental treatment. Consider short appointments.
- Place on frequent maintenance schedule to avoid periodontal inflammation.
- Chronic dry mouth is possible; anticipate increased caries activity and candidiasis.

Oral Health Education
- Encourage daily plaque control procedures for effective self-care in patient at risk for cardiovascular disease.
- If chronic dry mouth occurs, recommend home fluoride therapy and use of nonalcoholic oral health care products.

PerioChip — see chlorhexidine gluconate
PerioGard — see chlorhexidine gluconate
Periostat — see doxycycline hyclate
Permax — see pergolide mesylate
Perphenazine — see perphenazine

---

perphenazine (per-FEN-uh-zeen)
Perphenazine
◼✦◼ **Apo-Perphenazine**

◼◼ **Leptopsique**

Drug Class: Antipsychotic, phenothiazine; Antiemetic

PHARMACOLOGY
Action
Effects apparently caused by postsynaptic dopamine receptor blockade in CNS.

Uses
Management of psychotic disorders; treatment of schizophrenia; control of severe nausea/vomiting in adults.

➡◀ DRUG INTERACTIONS RELATED TO DENTAL THERAPEUTICS

No documented drug-drug interactions. The absence of evidence is not evidence of safety.

ADVERSE EFFECTS

⚠ **ORAL:** Tardive dyskinesia; tongue ache (unspecified).

CNS: Lightheadedness, faintness, dizziness; pseudoparkinsonism; dystonia; dyskinesia, motor restlessness; oculogyric crisis; dystonias; hyperreflexia; drowsiness, fatigue; headache; abnormalities of the cerebrospinal fluid proteins; paradoxical excitement or exacerbation of psychotic symptoms; catatonic-like states; weakness; tremor; paranoid reactions; lethargy; seizures; hyperactivity; nocturnal confusion; bizarre dreams; vertigo; insomnia.

CVS: Pulse rate changes.

GI: Dyspepsia; adynamic ileus (may result in death); nausea; vomiting; constipation.

RESP: Laryngospasm; bronchospasm; dyspnea.

MISC: Increases in appetite and weight; polydipsia; increased prolactin levels; photophobia.

CLINICAL IMPLICATIONS

General

- Determine why drug is being taken. Consider implications of condition on dental treatment.
- Depressed or anxious patients may neglect self-care. Monitor for plaque control effectiveness.
- Place on frequent maintenance schedule to avoid periodontal inflammation.
- Extrapyramidal behaviors can complicate performance of oral procedures. If present, consult with MD to consider medication changes.
- *Photophobia:* Direct dental light out of patient's eyes and offer dark glasses for comfort.
- Monitor vital signs.
- If GI side effects occur, consider semisupine chair position.

Oral Health Education

- Evaluate manual dexterity; consider need for power toothbrush.
- Encourage daily plaque control procedures for effective self-care.

Persantine — see dipyridamole

Pertussin CS — see dextromethorphan HBr

Pertussin ES — see dextromethorphan HBr

Pestarin — see rifampin

Pexeva — see paroxetine

Pharmaflur — see sodium fluoride

Pharmaflur 1.1 — see sodium fluoride

Pharmaflur df — see sodium fluoride

Phenaphen w/Codeine No. 3 — see acetaminophen/codeine phosphate

Phenaphen w/Codeine No. 4 — see acetaminophen/codeine phosphate

---

phenelzine sulfate (FEN-uhl-zeen SULL-fate)

Nardil

Drug Class: Antidepressant, MAO inhibitor

PHARMACOLOGY

Action

Phenelzine blocks activity of enzyme MAO, thereby increasing monoamine (e.g., epinephrine, norepinephrine, serotonin) concentrations in CNS.

Uses

Treatment of atypical ("nonendogenous" or "neurotic") depression; management of depression in patients unresponsive to other antidepressant drugs.

Unlabeled Uses

Treatment of bulimia; treatment of cocaine addiction; control of panic disorder with agoraphobia.

➦← DRUG INTERACTIONS RELATED TO DENTAL THERAPEUTICS

Tramadol: Increased risk of serotonin syndrome (reduced reuptake)
  • Avoid concurrent use.
Sympathomimetic amines: Severe hypertension (additive)
  • Monitor blood pressure.

ADVERSE EFFECTS

⚠ **ORAL:** Dry mouth.

CNS: Dizziness; headache; sleep disturbances; tremors; hyperflexemia; manic symptoms; convulsions; toxic delirium; coma.

CVS: Postural hypotension, tachycardia, palpitations, syncope.

GI: Constipation; nausea; GI disturbances; anorexia.

MISC: Transient respiratory and circulatory depression after electroconvulsive therapy; agranulocytosis, thrombocytopenia, leukopenia (<1%).

CLINICAL IMPLICATIONS

General

• Determine why drug is being taken. Consider implications of condition on dental treatment.
• Depressed or anxious patients may neglect self-care. Monitor for plaque control effectiveness.
• Determine ability to adapt to stress of dental treatment. Consider short appointments.
• Chronic dry mouth is possible; anticipate increased caries and candidiasis.
• *Postural hypotension*: Monitor BP at the beginning and end of each appointment; anticipate syncope. Have patient sit upright for several min at the end of the dental appointment before dismissing.
• Monitor vital signs.
• Blood dyscrasias are rarely reported; anticipate increased bleeding, infection, and poor healing.
• Place patient on frequent maintenance schedule to avoid periodontal inflammation.

Oral Health Education

• Evaluate manual dexterity; consider need for power toothbrush.
• Encourage daily plaque control procedures for effective self-care.
• If chronic dry mouth occurs, recommend home fluoride therapy and use of nonalcoholic oral health care products.

Phenergan — see promethazine HCl

---

phenobarbital (fee-no-BAR-bih-tahl)

(phenobarbital sodium)

Bellatal, Luminal Sodium, Solfoton

Drug Class: Sedative and hypnotic; Barbiturate; Anticonvulsant

DEA Schedule: Schedule IV

PHARMACOLOGY

Action

Depresses sensory cortex; decreases motor activity; alters cerebellar function; and produces drowsiness, sedation, and hypnosis.

Uses

Short-term treatment of insomnia; long-term treatment of generalized tonic-clonic and cortical focal seizures; emergency control of acute convulsions; preanesthetic sedation.

Unlabeled Uses

Treatment of febrile seizures in children; treatment and prevention of hyperbilirubinemia in newborns; management of chronic cholestasis.

➡️⬅️ DRUG INTERACTIONS RELATED TO DENTAL THERAPEUTICS

Acetaminophen: Acetaminophen hepatotoxicity (mechanism unknown)
- Avoid concurrent use.

Clonazepam: Decreased clonazepam effect (increased metabolism)
- Monitor clinical status.

Metronidazole: Decreased metronidazole effect (increased metabolism)
- Avoid concurrent use.

Doxycycline: Decreased doxycycline effect (increased metabolism)
- Avoid concurrent use.

ADVERSE EFFECTS

CNS: Drowsiness; agitation; confusion; anxiety; headache; hyperkinesia; ataxia; CNS depression; paradoxical excitement; nightmares; psychiatric disturbances; hallucinations; insomnia; dizziness.

CVS: Bradycardia, hypotension, syncope (1%).

GI: Nausea; vomiting; constipation.

RESP: Hypoventilation; apnea; laryngospasm; bronchospasm.

MISC: Hypersensitivity reactions (e.g., angioedema, rashes, exfoliative dermatitis); fever; injection site reactions (e.g., local pain, thrombophlebitis).

CLINICAL IMPLICATIONS

General

- Determine why drug is being taken. Consider implications of condition on dental treatment.
- Determine ability to adapt to stress of dental treatment. Consider short appointments.
- *Seizures:* Determine level of disease control, type and frequency of seizure, and compliance with medication regimen.
- Depressed or anxious patients may neglect self-care. Monitor for plaque control effectiveness.
- Monitor vital signs.

Oral Health Education

- Encourage daily plaque control procedures for effective self-care.

---

phenobarbital sodium — see phenobarbital
phenoxymethyl penicillin — see penicillin V

---

phentermine HCl (FEN-ter-meen HIGH-droe-KLOR-ide)

Adipex-P, Ionamin, Obe-Nix 30, Phentermine HCl, Phentermine Resin

◼️◼️◼️ Ifa Reduccing S

Drug Class: CNS stimulant; Anorexiant

PHARMACOLOGY

Action

May stimulate satiety center in brain, causing appetite suppression.

Uses

Short-term (i.e., no longer than a few weeks) adjunct to diet plan to reduce weight.

➜← DRUG INTERACTIONS RELATED TO DENTAL THERAPEUTICS

Pilocarpine: Increased myopia (mechanism unknown)
 • Monitor clinical status.

ADVERSE EFFECTS

⚠ **ORAL:** Dry mouth; unpleasant taste.

CNS: Overstimulation; restlessness; dizziness; insomnia; euphoria; dysphoria; tremor; headache; psychotic episodes.

CVS: Palpitations; tachycardia; arrhythmias; cardiac valve disease; hypertension.

MISC: Bone marrow depression; agranulocytosis; leukopenia.

GI: Diarrhea; constipation.

RESP: Primary pulmonary hypertension.

CLINICAL IMPLICATIONS

General

• Determine why drug is being taken. Consider implications of condition on dental treatment.
• Monitor vital signs (e.g., BP, pulse pressure, rate, and rhythm) at each appointment to assess disease control. Do not provide elective dental treatment when BP is ≥180/110 or in the presence of other high-risk CV conditions. Refer to the section entitled "The Patient Taking Cardiovascular Drugs" in Chapter 6: *Clinical Medicine*.
• Determine whether antibiotic prophylaxis is indicated before beginning dental treatment involving significant bleeding.
• *Antibiotic prophylaxis:* Inquire whether antibiotic was taken, when it was taken, and what dosage was taken; record in dental record.
• Chronic dry mouth is possible; anticipate increased caries and candidiasis.
• Blood dyscrasias rarely reported; anticipate increased bleeding, infection, and poor healing.
• *Valvular heart disease:* Serious regurgitant cardiac valvular disease has been reported with concurrent use of phentermine and fenfluramine or dexfenfluramine. Determine whether the combination drug regimen was used; if so, has echocardiogram examination been completed to determine valve disease?

Oral Health Education

• Encourage daily plaque control procedures for effective, nontraumatic self-care.
• If chronic dry mouth occurs, recommend home fluoride therapy and nonalcoholic oral health care products.
• *Antibiotic prophylaxis:* Inform patient that antibiotic needs to be taken 1 hr before dental appointment according to prescription instructions.

Phentermine Resin — see phentermine HCl

---

phenytoin (FEN-ih-toe-in)

(phenytoin sodium)

Dilantin, Dilantin Infatab, Dilantin Kapseals, Dilantin-125

▮✦▮ **Dilantin-30 Pediatric**

▮✦▮ **Epamin, Fenidantoin, Fenitron, Hydantoina**

Drug Class: Anticonvulsant, hydantoin

PHARMACOLOGY

Action

Appears to act at motor cortex in inhibiting spread of seizure activity. Possibly works by promoting sodium efflux from neurons, thereby stabilizing threshold against hyperexcitability. Also decreases post-tetanic potentiation at synapse.

Uses

Control of grand mal and psychomotor seizures; prevention and treatment of seizures occurring during or after neurosurgery; control of grand mal type of status epilepticus (parenteral administration).

Unlabeled Uses

Control of arrhythmias (particularly cardiac glycoside-induced arrhythmias); control of convulsions in severe preeclampsia; treatment of trigeminal neuralgia (tic douloureux), recessive dystrophic epidermolysis bullosa, and junctional epidermolysis bullosa.

➡️⬅ DRUG INTERACTIONS RELATED TO DENTAL THERAPEUTICS

Acetaminophen: Possible increased acetaminophen toxicity (enzyme induction)
 • Avoid concurrent use.
Fluconazole: Phenytoin toxicity (decreased metabolism)
 • Avoid concurrent use.
Metronidazole: Possible phenytoin toxicity (decreased metabolism)
 • Avoid concurrent use.
Doxycycline: Decreased doxycycline effect (increased metabolism)
 • Avoid concurrent use.

ADVERSE EFFECTS

⚠ **ORAL:** Gingival hyperplasia (30%); taste perversion.

CNS: Nystagmus; ataxia; dysarthria; slurred speech; mental confusion; dizziness; insomnia; transient nervousness; motor twitching; diplopia; fatigue; irritability; drowsiness; depression; numbness; tremor; headache; choreoathetosis (IV use).

GI: Nausea; vomiting; diarrhea; constipation.

RESP: Pharyngitis; sinusitis; cough.

MISC: Coarsening of facial features; lip enlargement; Peyronie disease; polyarthropathy; hyperglycemia; weight gain; chest pain; IgA depression; fever; photophobia; gynecomastia; periarteritis nodosa; pulmonary fibrosis; tissue injury at injection site; lymph node hyperplasia; hypothyroidism; photophobia; blood dyscrasias, some fatal.

CLINICAL IMPLICATIONS

General

• Determine why drug is being taken. Consider implications of condition on dental treatment.
• Determine level of disease control, type and frequency of seizure, and patient's compliance with medication regimen.
• Place on frequent maintenance schedule to avoid periodontal inflammation associated with gingival hyperplasia.
• Blood dyscrasias rarely reported; anticipate increased bleeding, infection, and poor healing.
• Monitor vital signs.

Oral Health Education

• Evaluate manual dexterity; consider need for power toothbrush.
• Encourage daily plaque control procedures for effective self-care. Strict plaque control may slow rate of gingival enlargement.

---

phenytoin sodium — see phenytoin

Phos-Flur — see sodium fluoride

Phyllocontin — see aminophylline

Phyllocontin-350 — see aminophylline

Pilocar — see pilocarpine HCl

pilocarpine HCl (pie-low-CAR-peen HIGH-droe-KLOR-ide)

Salagen: Tablets: 5 mg
Adsorbocarpine, Akarpine, Isopto-Carpine, Ocusert Pilo-20, Ocusert Pilo-40, Pilocar, Pilopine HS, Piloptic-1, Piloptic-1/2, Piloptic-2, Piloptic-3, Piloptic-4, Piloptic-6, Pilostat

▌✦▐ Minims-Pilocarpine

▌✦▐ Pilogrin

Drug Class: Ophthalmic; Antiglaucoma; Mouth and throat product

PHARMACOLOGY

Action

OPHTHALMIC: Decreases intraocular pressure (IOP) by constricting pupil and stimulating ciliary muscles to open trabecular meshwork spaces and facilitate outflow of aqueous humor.
ORAL (PO): Stimulates exocrine glands including mucous cells of respiratory tract and salivary glands in oral cavity.

Uses

OPHTHALMIC: Treatment of chronic simple glaucoma, chronic angle-closure glaucoma, acute angle-closure glaucoma, pre- and postoperative management of intraocular tension, treatment of mydriasis.
ORAL (PO): Treatment of xerostomia in patients with malfunctioning salivary glands because of radiotherapy for cancer of head and neck, relief of dry mouth in patients with Sjögren syndrome.

Unlabeled Uses

Relief of dry mouth in patients with graft-vs-host disease (PO).

Contraindications

Hypersensitivity; conditions in which cholinergic effects such as constriction are undesirable. Oral use also contraindicated in uncontrolled asthma, acute iritis, narrow-angle glaucoma, acute inflammatory disease of anterior segment of eye.

Usual Dosage

ADULTS: *PO:* Titrate dosage based on therapeutic response and tolerance. To reduce the incidence and severity of side effects, use the lowest effective dose. Do not exceed a maximum of 10 mg/dose.
Radiation-induced xerostomia
ADULTS: *PO:* 5 mg tid. If no response, increase dose to 10 mg tid. Continue uninterrupted for at least 12 wk before assessing for full therapeutic benefit.
Sjögren syndrome
ADULTS: *PO:* 5 mg qid. Continue uninterrupted for at least 6 wk before assessing for full therapeutic benefit.

Pharmacokinetics

ABSORP: T_{max} is 0.85 to 1.25 hr. C_{max} is 15 to 41 ng/mL. AUC is 33 to 108 hr ng/mL. High-fat meals decrease the rate of absorption.
METAB: Limited information available; however, it is thought to occur at neuronal synapses and probably in plasma.
EXCRET: Urine (as unchanged pilocarpine, minimal active/inactive degradation products). $T_{1/2}$ is 0.76 to 1.35 hr.
ONSET: 20 min.

PEAK: 1 hr.

DURATION: 3 to 5 hr.

SPECIAL POP: *Gender:* Elderly women had C_{max} and AUC approximately twice that of elderly or young men.

➡◀ DRUG INTERACTIONS

Sympathomimetic amines: Increased myopia (mechanism unknown)
* Monitor clinical status.

ADVERSE EFFECTS

⚠ **ORAL:** Excessive salivation.

CVS: Transient hypertension; tachycardia; edema; palpitations.

MISC: OPHTH: Stinging, burning of eyes.

CNS: Chills; headache; dizziness; asthenia.

GI: Excessive salivation; nausea; vomiting; diarrhea dyspepsia; abdominal pain.

RESP: Bronchial spasm; pulmonary edema; rhinitis; sinusitis; pharyngitis; increased coughing; increased airway resistance; bronchial smooth muscle tone; bronchial secretions.

CLINICAL IMPLICATIONS

General
When prescribed by DDS:
* *Lactation:* Undetermined.
* *Children:* Safety and efficacy not established.
* *Elderly:* Elderly patients also may be at increased risk for certain adverse effects during therapy, including diarrhea, urinary frequency, and dizziness.
* *Special risk:* Use oral pilocarpine with caution in acute cardiac failure, bronchial asthma, peptic ulcer, hypertension, hyperthyroidism, retinal disease, GI or biliary tract spasm or obstruction, urinary tract obstruction, Parkinson disease, angina pectoris, MI, chronic bronchitis, chronic obstructive pulmonary disease, underlying psychiatric disorders.
* *Overdosage:* Salivation, lacrimation, nausea, vomiting, diarrhea, cramping, sweating, frequent urination, bradycardia, asystole, death (PO).

When prescribed by medical facility:
* Determine why drug is being taken. Consider implications of condition on dental treatment.
* *Ophthalmic doseform:* Direct dental light out of patient's eyes and offer dark glasses for comfort.
* *PO doseform:* Monitor vital signs.

Pregnancy Risk Category: Category C.

Oral Health Education
When prescribed by DDS:
* Explain that long-term therapy may be required.
* Advise patients to drink additional water or noncaffeinated fluids during therapy.
* Tell patients using oral form to report the following symptoms to health care provider: sweating, nausea, nasal congestion, chills, flushing, frequent urination, dizziness, weakness, headache, indigestion, tearing, diarrhea, fluid retention.

Pilogrin — see pilocarpine HCl

Pilopine HS — see pilocarpine HCl

Piloptic-1/2 — see pilocarpine HCl

Piloptic-1 — see pilocarpine HCl

Piloptic-2 — see pilocarpine HCl

Piloptic-3 — see pilocarpine HCl

Piloptic-4 — see pilocarpine HCl

Piloptic-6 — see pilocarpine HCl
Pilostat — see pilocarpine HCl

pimecrolimus (pim-eh-CROW-lih-muss)
Elidel

Drug Class: Immunomodulator, topical

PHARMACOLOGY

Action
Mechanism in atopic dermatitis is not known; however, pimecrolimus inhibits T-cell activation by blocking the transcription of early cytokines.

Uses
Short-term and intermittent long-term treatment of mild to moderate atopic dermatitis in nonimmunocompromised patients.

➡◆ DRUG INTERACTIONS RELATED TO DENTAL THERAPEUTICS
No documented drug-drug interactions. The absence of evidence is not evidence of safety.

ADVERSE EFFECTS

CNS: Headache.
GI: Gastroenteritis; upper abdominal pain; vomiting; diarrhea; nausea.
RESP: URI; pneumonia; bronchitis; aggravated asthma; sinus congestion; asthma; cough.
MISC: Bacterial infection; folliculitis; herpes simplex; chicken pox; pyrexia; flu-like symptoms; hypersensitivity; back pain; arthralgia; increased malignancies.

CLINICAL IMPLICATIONS

General
- *Viral infections:* The topical ointment may be associated with increased risk of varicella zoster virus infection (chicken pox or shingles), herpes simplex virus infection, or eczema herpeticum.
- This drug is associated with causing an increased risk for malignancies. Complete a thorough head and neck cancer examination.

pindolol (PIN-doe-lahl)
Visken

■✦■ **Alti-Pindolol, APO-Pindol, Gen-Pindolol, Novo-Pindol, Nu-Pindol, PMS-Pindolol**

Drug Class: Beta-adrenergic blocker

PHARMACOLOGY

Action
Nonselectively blocks beta receptors, which primarily affect heart (slows rate), vascular musculature (decreases blood pressure), and lungs (reduces function).

Uses
Management of mild to moderate hypertension.

➡◆ DRUG INTERACTIONS RELATED TO DENTAL THERAPEUTICS
COX-1 inhibitors: Decreased antihypertensive effect (decreased prostaglandin synthesis)
- Monitor blood pressure.

Sympathomimetic amines: Decreased antihypertensive effect (pharmacological antagonism; unopposed alpha-adrenergic stimulation)
- Monitor blood pressure.

ADVERSE EFFECTS

⚠ **ORAL:** Dry mouth; taste disturbance, taste loss.

CNS: Depression; visual disturbances; short-term memory loss; dizziness.

CVS: Hypotension; bradycardia; arrhythmia; postural hypotension.

MISC: Photosensitivity reactions.

GI: Nausea; vomiting; diarrhea.

RESP: Wheezing; bronchospasm; difficulty breathing (at higher doses).

CLINICAL IMPLICATIONS

General

- Monitor vital signs (e.g., BP, pulse pressure, rate, and rhythm) at each appointment to assess disease control. Do not provide elective dental treatment when BP is ≥180/110 or in the presence of other high-risk CV conditions. Refer to the section entitled "The Patient Taking Cardiovascular Drugs" in Chapter 6: *Clinical Medicine*.
- Chronic dry mouth is possible; anticipate increased caries, candidiasis, and lichenoid mucositis.
- If GI side effects occur, consider semisupine chair position.
- Use local anesthetic agents with vasoconstrictor with caution based on functional capacity of the patient and use aspirating technique to prevent intravascular injection.
- Beta blockers may mask epinephrine-induced signs and symptoms of hypoglycemia in patient with diabetes.
- Determine ability to adapt to stress of dental treatment. Consider short appointments.
- Place on frequent maintenance schedule to avoid periodontal inflammation.
- *Postural hypotension:* Monitor BP at the beginning and end of each appointment; anticipate syncope. Have patient sit upright for several min at the end of the dental appointment before dismissing.

Oral Health Education

- Encourage daily plaque control procedures for effective self-care in patient at risk for cardiovascular disease.
- If chronic dry mouth occurs, recommend home fluoride therapy and use of nonalcoholic oral health care products.

Pink Bismuth — see bismuth subsalicylate

---

pioglitazone (pye-oh-GLI-ta-zone)

Actos

Drug Class: Antidiabetic, thiazolidinedione

PHARMACOLOGY

Action

Increases insulin sensitivity in muscle and adipose tissue and inhibits hepatic gluconeogenesis.

Uses

Patients with type 2 diabetes, as an adjunct to diet and exercise; may also be used in conjunction with a sulfonylurea, metformin, or insulin when diet, exercise, and a single agent alone does not result in adequate glycemic control in patients with type 2 diabetes mellitus.

➡◀ DRUG INTERACTIONS RELATED TO DENTAL THERAPEUTICS

No documented drug-drug interactions. The absence of evidence is not evidence of safety.

ADVERSE EFFECTS

⚠ **ORAL:** Tooth disorder (unspecified) (5.3%).

CNS: Headache (9%).

RESP: URI (13%); sinusitis (6%).
MISC: Myalgia, edema (5%).

CLINICAL IMPLICATIONS
General
- Determine degree of disease control and current blood sugar levels. Goals should be <120 mg/dL and A_{1C} <7%. A_{1C} levels ≥8% indicate significant uncontrolled diabetes.
- The routine use of antibiotics in the dental management of diabetic patients is not indicated; however, antibiotic therapy in patients with poorly controlled diabetes has been shown to improve disease control and improve response after periodontal debridement.
- Monitor blood pressure because hypertension and dyslipidemia (CAD) are prevalent in diabetes mellitus.
- Monitor vital signs (e.g., BP, pulse pressure, rate, and rhythm) at each appointment to assess disease control. Do not provide elective dental treatment when BP ≥180/110 or in presence of other high-risk CV conditions. Refer to the section entitled "The Patient Taking Cardiovascular Drugs" in Chapter 6: *Clinical Medicine*.
- *Loss of blood sugar control:* Certain medical conditions (e.g., surgery, fever, infection, trauma) and drugs (e.g., corticosteroids) affect glucose control. In these situations, it may be necessary to seek medical consultation before surgical procedures.
- Obtain patient history regarding diabetic ketoacidosis or hypoglycemia with current drug regimen; combination therapy with insulin or oral sulfonylureas can result in hypoglycemia.
- *Insulin or oral sulfonylurea drug combinations*: Observe for signs of hypoglycemia (e.g., confusion, argumentativeness, perspiration, altered consciousness). Be prepared to treat hypoglycemic reactions with oral glucose or sucrose.
- Ensure that patient has taken medication and eaten meal.
- Determine ability to adapt to stress of dental treatment. Consider short, morning appointments.
- Medical consult advised if fasting blood glucose is <70 mg/dL (hypoglycemic risk) or >200 mg/dL (hyperglycemic crisis risk).
- Place patient on frequent maintenance schedule to avoid periodontal inflammation.

Oral Health Education
- Encourage daily plaque control procedures for effective self-care in patient at risk for cardiovascular disease.

---

piperazine estrone sulfate — see estropipate

---

pirbuterol acetate (pihr-BYOO-tuh-role ASS-uh-TATE)
Maxair Autohaler

Drug Class: Bronchodilator; Sympathomimetic

PHARMACOLOGY
Action
Produces bronchodilation by relaxing bronchial smooth muscle through beta-2 receptor stimulation.

Uses
Prevention and treatment of reversible bronchospasm associated with asthma or other obstructive pulmonary diseases.

➡◀ DRUG INTERACTIONS RELATED TO DENTAL THERAPEUTICS
No documented drug-drug interactions. The absence of evidence is not evidence of safety.

ADVERSE EFFECTS
⚠ **ORAL:** Dry mouth; throat irritation (unspecified); unpleasant taste.
CNS: Tremor; anxiety; confusion; fatigue; dizziness; nervousness; headache; weakness; hyperactivity/hyperkinesia/excitement; insomnia.

CVS: Palpitations; tachycardia.
GI: GI distress; diarrhea; nausea/vomiting.
RESP: Cough.
MISC: Flushing; anorexia/appetite loss; taste/smell change.

CLINICAL IMPLICATIONS

General
- Determine why drug is being taken. Consider implications of condition on dental treatment.
- Monitor vital signs (e.g., BP, pulse rate) and respiratory function. Uncontrolled disease characterized by wheezing and coughing.
- Acute bronchoconstriction can occur during dental treatment; have bronchodilator inhaler available.
- Ensure that bronchodilator inhaler is present at each dental appointment.
- Be aware that sulfites in local anesthetic with vasoconstrictor can precipitate acute asthma attack in susceptible patients.
- Inhalants can dry oral mucosa; anticipate candidiasis, increased calculus, plaque levels, and increased caries.

Oral Health Education
- Rinse mouth with water after bronchodilator use to prevent dryness.
- If chronic dry mouth occurs, recommend home fluoride therapy and use of nonalcoholic oral health care products.

Piroxan — see piroxicam

Piroxen — see piroxicam

---

piroxicam (pihr-OX-ih-kam)

Feldene

■✷■ **Alti-Piroxicam, Apo-Piroxicam, Gen-Piroxicam, Novo-Pirocam, Nu-Pirox**

■☙■ **Androxicam, Artinor, Artyflam, Brexicam, Citoken, Dixonal, Dolzycam, Facicam, Flogosan, Osteral, Oxicanol, Piroxan, Piroxen, Rogal**

Drug Class: Analgesic; NSAID

PHARMACOLOGY

Action
Decreases inflammation, pain, and fever, probably through inhibition of COX activity and prostaglandin synthesis.

Uses
Treatment of acute or long-term use of rheumatoid arthritis and osteoarthritis.

Unlabeled Uses
Symptomatic relief of primary dysmenorrhea, pain, sunburn, juvenile rheumatoid arthritis.

➡◀ DRUG INTERACTIONS RELATED TO DENTAL THERAPEUTICS

No documented drug-drug interactions. The absence of evidence is not evidence of safety.

ADVERSE EFFECTS

⚠ **ORAL:** Dry mouth, stomatitis, glossitis (<1%).
CNS: Headache; malaise; somnolence; vertigo; depression; insomnia; nervousness.
MISC: Anemia; increased bleeding time (1% to 10%); agranulocytosis; thrombocytopenia; leukopenia (<1%).
GI: Epigastric distress; nausea; vomiting; anorexia; constipation; stomatitis; abdominal discomfort; diarrhea; flatulence; abdominal pain; indigestion; toxicity (e.g., bleeding, ulceration, perforation); heartburn; dyspepsia; anorexia.
RESP: Bronchospasm; laryngeal edema; dyspnea; hemoptysis; shortness of breath.

CLINICAL IMPLICATIONS

General
- Determine why drug is being taken. Consider implications of condition on dental treatment.
- *Arthritis*: Consider patient comfort and need for semisupine chair position.
- Chronic dry mouth is possible; anticipate increased caries activity and candidiasis.
- If GI side effects occur, consider semisupine chair position.
- Blood dyscrasias are rarely reported; anticipate increased bleeding, infection, and poor healing.

Oral Health Education
- Evaluate manual dexterity; consider need for power toothbrush.
- If chronic dry mouth occurs, recommend home fluoride therapy and use of nonalcoholic oral health care products.

Pisacaina — see lidocaine HCl

Plaquenil — see hydroxychloroquine sulfate

Plasil — see metoclopramide

Plavix — see clopidogrel

Plendil — see felodipine

PMS-Atenolol — see atenolol

PMS-Bethanechol — see bethanechol chloride

PMS-Bromocriptine — see bromocriptine mesylate

PMS-Buspirone — see buspirone HCl

PMS-Captopril — see captopril

PMS-Carbamazepine CR — see carbamazepine

PMS-Cefaclor — see cefaclor

PMS-Chloral Hydrate — see chloral hydrate

PMS-Clonazepam — see clonazepam

PMS-Desipramine — see desipramine HCl

PMS-Dexamethasone — see dexamethasone

PMS-Diclofenac — see diclofenac

PMS-Diclofenac SR — see diclofenac

PMS-Diphenhydramine — see diphenhydramine HCl

PMS-Erythromycin — see erythromycin

PMS-Fenofibrate Micro — see fenofibrate

PMS-Fluoxetine — see fluoxetine HCl

PMS-Fluphenazine Decanoate — see fluphenazine

PMS-Fluvoxamine — see fluvoxamine maleate

PMS-Gabapentin — see gabapentin

PMS-Gemfibrozil — see gemfibrozil

PMS-Glyburide — see glyburide

PMS-Haloperidol LA — see haloperidol

PMS-Hydromorphone — see hydromorphone HCl

PMS-Hydroxyzine — see hydroxyzine

PMS-Indapamide — see indapamide
PMS-Ipratropium — see ipratropium bromide
PMS-Isoniazid — see isoniazid
PMS-Lithium Carbonate — see lithium
PMS-Lithium Citrate — see lithium
PMS-Loperamide Hydrochloride — see loperamide HCl
PMS-Mefenamic Acid — see mefenamic acid
PMS-Metformin — see metformin HCl
PMS-Methylphenidate — see methylphenidate HCl
PMS-Metoprolol-B — see metoprolol
PMS-Minocycline — see minocycline HCl
PMS-Nizatidine — see nizatidine
PMS-Nortriptyline — see nortriptyline HCl
PMS-Nystatin — see nystatin
PMS-Oxybutynin — see oxybutynin Cl
PMS-Pindolol — see pindolol
PMS-Ranitidine — see ranitidine HCl
PMS-Salbutamol Respirator Solution — see albuterol
PMS-Sotalol — see sotalol HCl
PMS-Sucralfate — see sucralfate
PMS-Tamoxifen — see tamoxifen citrate
PMS-Temazepam — see temazepam
PMS-Terazosin — see terazosin
PMS-Terbinafine — see terbinafine
PMS-Ticlopidine — see ticlopidine HCl
PMS-Timolol — see timolol maleate
PMS-Trazodone — see trazodone HCl
PMS-Valproic Acid — see valproic acid and derivatives
Pneumomist — see guaifenesin
Point-Two — see sodium fluoride
Polocaine — see mepivacaine HCl
Polocaine MPF — see mepivacaine HCl
Polocaine with Levonordefrin — see mepivacaine HCl

polyethylene glycol (peg) (poli-ETH-uh-leen GLI-cawl)
MiraLax
Drug Class: Bowel evacuant
PHARMACOLOGY
Action
Acts as an osmotic agent by causing water to be retained with the stool.
Uses
Treatment of occasional constipation; use should be limited to ≤14 days.

➤◀ DRUG INTERACTIONS RELATED TO DENTAL THERAPEUTICS

No documented drug-drug interactions. The absence of evidence is not evidence of safety.

ADVERSE EFFECTS

GI: Nausea; abdominal bloating; cramping; flatulence; diarrhea; excessive stool frequency.

CLINICAL IMPLICATIONS

General
- Determine why drug is being taken. Consider implications of condition on dental treatment.
- If GI side effects occur, consider semisupine chair position.

Polymox — see amoxicillin

Ponstan — see mefenamic acid

Ponstel — see mefenamic acid

Posipen — see dicloxacillin sodium

Potasalan — see potassium products

---

potassium products (poe-TASS-ee-uhm)

Cena-K, Effer-K, Gen-K, K + 10, K + 8, K + Care, K + Care ET, K Lyte, K Lyte DS, K Lyte/Cl, K Lyte/Cl 50, Kaon, Kaon Cl-10, Kaon-Cl, Kaon-Cl 20%, Kay Ciel, Kaylixir, K-Dur 10, K-Dur 20, K-G Elixir, K-Lor, Klor-Con, Klor-Con 10, Klor-Con 8, Klor-Con M10, Klor-Con M15, Klor-Con M20, Klor-Con/25, Klor-Con/EF, Klorvess, Klorvess, Klotrix, Kolyum, K-Tab, K-vescent Potassium Chloride, Micro-K Extencaps, Micro-K LS, Potasalan, Rum-K, Ten-K, Tri-K, Twin-K

■✽■ **APO-K, K-10 Solution, Kaoch, Kaochlor-20 Concentrate, K-Lor**

Drug Class: Electrolyte

PHARMACOLOGY

Action
Major intracellular cation; essential in maintaining acid-base balance and isotonicity within cells. Functions in muscle contraction, nerve impulse transmission, gastric secretion, renal function, and metabolism.

Uses
Treatment of hypokalemia; prevention of potassium depletion in certain conditions. Parenterally, as prophylaxis or treatment of moderate to severe potassium loss when oral therapy is not adequate or feasible.

Unlabeled Uses
Treatment of thallium poisoning; with anticholinesterase agents in myasthenia gravis.

➤◀ DRUG INTERACTIONS RELATED TO DENTAL THERAPEUTICS

No documented drug-drug interactions. The absence of evidence is not evidence of safety.

ADVERSE EFFECTS

GI: Abdominal discomfort or distention; GI obstruction; bleeding; ulceration or perforation; nausea; vomiting; flatulence.

MISC: Hyperkalemia (symptoms may include paresthesia of extremities; listlessness; confusion; weak or heavy limbs; flaccid paralysis; hypotension; arrhythmias; heart block; cardiac arrest; prolonged QT interval; wide QRS complex; peaked T waves; ST depression).

CLINICAL IMPLICATIONS

General
- Determine why drug is being taken. Consider implications of condition on dental treatment.
- If GI side effects occur, consider semisupine chair position.
- Monitor vital signs.

Povidine — see povidone iodine
Povidine-Iodine — see povidone iodine

---

 povidone iodine (POE-vih-dohn EYE-uh-dine)

Betadine: Aerosol: 5%; Gel (vaginal): 10%; Ointment: 10%; Skin cleanser, foam: 7.5%; Solution: 10%; Solution, swab aid: 10%; Solution, swab sticks: 10%; Surgical scrub: 7.5%
Betagen: Ointment: 1/5 available iodine; Solution: 10%; Surgical scrub: 7.5%
Biodine Topical: Solution: 1% iodine
Etodine: Ointment: 1% available iodine
Minidyne: Solution: 10%
Povidine: Ointment: 10%; Solution: 10%; Surgical scrub: 5.5%
Povidine-Iodine: Ointment: 10%; Liquid: 10%; Solution: 10%; Spray: 10%

█✦█ Proviodine

██✦█ Isodine, Yodine

Drug Class: Anti-infective, topical

PHARMACOLOGY

Action
Broad-spectrum antimicrobial agent.

Uses
Topical application for the treatment or prevention of infection with susceptible microorganisms.

Contraindications
Allergy to iodine.

Usual Dosage
Infection
SCRUB, OINTMENT, OR SOLUTION
ADULTS AND CHILDREN: Apply as needed for treatment or prevention.

➡◀ DRUG INTERACTIONS
No documented drug-drug interactions. The absence of evidence is not evidence of safety.

ADVERSE EFFECTS
⚠ ORAL: Mucous membrane discoloration, irritation; taste disturbance.

CLINICAL IMPLICATIONS

General
- Assess patient for allergy to seafood; if reaction is positive, do not use.
- Do not apply to areas of rash, abrasion, or stomatitis due to risk of systemic absorption.
- Store in tight container; out of light.

Pregnancy Risk Category: Category D.

Pramidal — see loperamide HCl

pramipexole dihydrochloride (pram-ih-PEX-ole DIE-HIGH-droe-KLOR-ide)

Mirapex

Drug Class: Anti-Parkinson, non-ergot dopamine receptor agonist

PHARMACOLOGY

Action
Stimulates dopamine receptors in the corpus striatum, relieving parkinsonian symptoms.

Uses
Treatment of the signs and symptoms of idiopathic Parkinson disease. May be used in conjunction with L-dopa.

➡◀ DRUG INTERACTIONS RELATED TO DENTAL THERAPEUTICS
No documented drug-drug interactions. The absence of evidence is not evidence of safety.

ADVERSE EFFECTS
⚠ **ORAL:** Dry mouth.
CNS: Dizziness; somnolence; headache; confusion; hallucinations; abnormal dreams; tremor; insomnia; aggravated Parkinson disease; dyskinesia; hypokinesia; hypesthesia; amnesia; extrapyramidal syndrome; abnormal thinking; hypertonia; akathisia; dystonia; delusions; paranoid reactions.
GI: Nausea (28%); dyspepsia; constipation (14%); anorexia; dysphagia.
RESP: Dyspnea; pneumonia.
MISC: Asthenia; edema; malaise; injury; fever; weight decrease; myoclonus.

CLINICAL IMPLICATIONS

General
- Extrapyramidal behaviors associated with Parkinson disease can complicate access to oral cavity and complicate oral procedures.
- Chronic dry mouth is possible; anticipate increased caries and candidiasis.
- If GI side effects occur, consider semisupine chair position.
- Place on frequent maintenance schedule to avoid periodontal inflammation.

Oral Health Education
- Evaluate manual dexterity; consider need for power toothbrush.
- If chronic dry mouth occurs, recommend home fluoride therapy and use of nonalcoholic oral health care products.

Pramotil — see metoclopramide

Prandase — see acarbose

Prandin — see repaglinide

Pravachol — see pravastatin sodium

Pravacol — see pravastatin sodium

---

pravastatin sodium (PRUH-vuh-stuh-tin SO-dee-uhm)
Pravachol

■✦■ **Apo-Pravastatin, Nu-Pravastatin**

■✦■ **Pravacol**

Drug Class: Antihyperlipidemic, HMG-CoA reductase inhibitor

PHARMACOLOGY

Action

Increases rate at which body removes cholesterol from blood and reduces production of cholesterol in body by inhibiting enzyme that catalyzes early rate-limiting step in cholesterol synthesis.

Uses

As an adjunct to diet for reduction of elevated total and LDL cholesterol, apolipoprotein B, and triglyceride levels, and to increase HDL cholesterol in patients with primary hypercholesterolemia and mixed dyslipidemia (Frederickson types IIa and IIb); as adjunctive therapy to diet for treatment of patients with elevated serum triglyceride levels (Frederickson type IV); treatment of primary dysbetalipoproteinemia (Frederickson type III) in patients who do not respond adequately to diet; treatment for hypercholesterolemic patients without clinically evident coronary heart disease (CHD) to reduce risk of MI or CV mortality with no increase in death from noncardiovascular causes; treatment of patients with clinically evident CHD to reduce risk of total mortality by reducing coronary death, MI and those undergoing myocardial revascularization procedures, stroke, and stroke/transient ischemic attack and slow progression of coronary arteriosclerosis.

➡◄ DRUG INTERACTIONS RELATED TO DENTAL THERAPEUTICS

No documented drug-drug interactions. The absence of evidence is not evidence of safety.

ADVERSE EFFECTS

CNS: Headache; dizziness.

CVS: Arrhythmia; palpitation; postural hypotension; syncope; vasodilation.

GI: Nausea; vomiting; diarrhea; abdominal pain; constipation; flatulence; heartburn; dyspepsia; pancreatitis.

RESP: Common cold; rhinitis; cough; influenza.

MISC: Localized pain; myalgia; myopathy; rhabdomyolysis; fatigue; paresthesia; peripheral neuropathy. An apparent hypersensitivity syndrome has been reported rarely that has included one or more of the following features: anaphylaxis; angioedema; lupus erythematous–like syndrome; polymyalgia rheumatica; vasculitis; purpura; thrombocytopenia; leukopenia; hemolytic anemia; positive antinuclear antibodies; increase in erythrocyte sedimentation rate; arthritis; arthralgia; urticaria; asthenia; photosensitivity; fever; chills; flushing; malaise; dyspnea; toxic epidermal necrolysis; erythema multiforme, including Stevens-Johnson syndrome.

CLINICAL IMPLICATIONS

General

- High LDL cholesterol concentration is the major cause of atherosclerosis, which leads to CAD (e.g., angina, MI); determine degree of CV health and ability to withstand stress of dental treatment.
- Monitor vital signs (e.g., BP, pulse pressure, rate, and rhythm) at each appointment to assess disease control. Do not provide elective dental treatment when BP is ≥180/110 or in the presence of other high-risk CV conditions. Refer to the section entitled "The Patient Taking Cardiovascular Drugs" in Chapter 6: *Clinical Medicine*.
- Use local anesthetic agents with vasoconstrictor with caution based on functional capacity of the patient, and use aspirating technique to prevent intravascular injection.
- *Postural hypotension:* Monitor BP at the beginning and end of each appointment; anticipate syncope. Have patient sit upright for several min at the end of the dental appointment before dismissing.
- If GI side effects occur, consider semisupine chair position.

Oral Health Education

- Encourage daily plaque control procedures for effective self-care in patient at risk for cardiovascular disease.

Prazidec — see omeprazole
Prazolit — see omeprazole

prazosin HCl (PRAY-zoe-sin HIGH-droe-KLOR-ide)

Minipress

■✦■ **Alti-Prazosi, APO-Prazo, Novo-Prazin, Nu-Prazo**

■◣■ **Minipres, Sinozzard**

Drug Class: Antihypertensive; Antiadrenergic, peripherally acting

PHARMACOLOGY

Action

Selectively blocks postsynaptic alpha-1 adrenergic receptors, resulting in dilation of arterioles and veins.

Uses

Treatment of hypertension.

➡✦ DRUG INTERACTIONS RELATED TO DENTAL THERAPEUTICS

No documented drug-drug interactions. The absence of evidence is not evidence of safety.

ADVERSE EFFECTS

⚠ **ORAL:** Dry mouth.

CNS: Depression; dizziness (10%); weakness (6.5%); nervousness; paresthesia; asthenia; drowsiness; headache.

CVS: Palpitations (5%); postural hypotension, hypotension, syncope (1% to 4%); tachycardia.

GI: Nausea (5%); vomiting (1% to 4%); diarrhea; constipation; abdominal discomfort or pain.

RESP: Dyspnea.

MISC: Arthralgia; edema; fever.

CLINICAL IMPLICATIONS

General

- Monitor vital signs (e.g., BP, pulse pressure, rate, and rhythm) at each appointment to assess disease control. Do not provide elective dental treatment when BP is ≥180/110 or in the presence of other high-risk CV condition. Refer to the section entitled "The Patient Taking Cardiovascular Drugs" in Chapter 6: *Clinical Medicine*.
- Use local anesthetic agents with vasoconstrictor with caution based on functional capacity of the patient, and use aspiration technique to prevent intravascular injection.
- Determine ability to adapt to stress of dental treatment. Consider short appointments.
- *Postural hypotension*: Monitor BP at the beginning and end of each appointment; anticipate syncope. Have patient sit upright for several min at the end of the dental appointment before dismissing.
- Chronic dry mouth is possible; anticipate increased caries, candidiasis, and lichenoid mucositis.
- If GI side effects occur, consider semisupine chair position.

Oral Health Education

- Encourage daily plaque control procedures for effective self-care in patient at risk for cardiovascular disease.
- If chronic dry mouth occurs, recommend home fluoride therapy and use of nonalcoholic oral health care products.

Precaptil — see captopril
Precose — see acarbose

Predalone 50 — see prednisolone
Predcor-50 — see prednisolone
Pred Forte — see prednisolone
Pred Mild — see prednisolone
Prednicen-M — see prednisone
Prednidib — see prednisone
Prednisol TBA — see prednisolone

prednisolone (pred-NISS-oh-lone)

(prednisolone tebutate, prednisolone sodium phosphate, prednisolone acetate)

AK-Pred, Delta-Cortef, Econopred, Econopred Plus, Hydeltrasol, Inflamase Forte, Inflamase Mild, Key-Pred 25, Key-Pred 50, Key-Pred-SP, Pediapred, Pred Forte, Pred Mild, Predalone 50, Predcor-50, Prednisol TBA, Prelone

■✦■ **Minims Prednisolone, Novo-Prednisolone**

■✦■ **Fisopred, Sophipren Ofteno**

Drug Class: Corticosteroid

PHARMACOLOGY

Action

Intermediate-acting glucocorticoid that depresses formation, release, and activity of endogenous mediators of inflammation, including prostaglandins, kinins, histamine, liposomal enzymes, and the complement system; also modifies body's immune response.

Uses

ORAL/PARENTERAL ADMINISTRATION: Endocrine disorders: Rheumatic disorders; collagen diseases; dermatological diseases; allergic and inflammatory ophthalmic processes; respiratory diseases; hematological disorders; neoplastic diseases; edematous states caused by nephrotic syndrome; GI diseases; multiple sclerosis; tuberculous meningitis; trichinosis with neurological or myocardial involvement.

INTRA-ARTICULAR OR SOFT TISSUE ADMINISTRATION: Short-term adjunctive therapy of synovitis of osteoarthritis, rheumatoid arthritis, bursitis, acute gouty arthritis, epicondylitis, acute nonspecific tenosynovitis, post-traumatic osteoarthritis.

INTRALESIONAL ADMINISTRATION: Treatment of the following lesions: Keloids; localized hypertrophic, infiltrated, inflammatory lesions of lichen planus, psoriatic plaques, granuloma annulare, lichen simplex chronicus; discoid lupus erythematosus; necrobiosis lipoidica diabeticorum; alopecia areata; cystic tumors of aponeurosis or tendon.

OPHTHALMIC ADMINISTRATION: Treatment of steroid-responsive inflammatory conditions of palpebral and bulbar conjunctiva, lid, cornea, and anterior segment of globe.

Unlabeled Uses

Adjunctive therapy for tuberculous pleurisy.

➔◆ DRUG INTERACTIONS RELATED TO DENTAL THERAPEUTICS

COX-1 inhibitors: Increased risk of peptic ulcers (additive)
• Avoid concurrent use.
Midazolam: Possible decreased midazolam effect (Increased metabolism)
• Monitor clinical status.

Metronidazole: Possible decreased metronidazole effect (increased metabolism)
- Avoid concurrent use.

ADVERSE EFFECTS

⚠ **ORAL:** Ulcerative esophagitis; masked infection; impaired wound healing.

CNS: Convulsions; pseudotumor cerebri (i.e., increased intracranial pressure with papilledema); vertigo; headache; neuritis; paresthesias; psychosis.

GI: Pancreatitis; abdominal distention; nausea; vomiting; increased appetite and weight gain; peptic ulcer with perforation and hemorrhage; small and large bowel perforation.

MISC: Musculoskeletal effects (e.g., weakness, myopathy, muscle mass loss, tendon rupture, osteoporosis, aseptic necrosis of femoral and humoral heads, spontaneous fractures); endocrine abnormalities (e.g., menstrual irregularities, cushingoid state, growth suppression in children, sweating, decreased carbohydrate tolerance, hyperglycemia, glycosuria, increased insulin or sulfonylurea requirements in diabetic patients, hirsutism); anaphylactoid or hypersensitivity reactions; aggravation or masking of infections; fatigue; insomnia. With intra-articular administration: osteonecrosis; tendon rupture; infection; skin atrophy; postinjection flare; hypersensitivity; facial flushing; hypokalemic syndrome (irregular heartbeat, muscle cramps, weakness).

CLINICAL IMPLICATIONS

General

- Determine why drug is being taken. Consider implications of condition on dental treatment.
- Despite the anticipated perioperative physiological stress (i.e., minor surgical stress), patients undergoing dental care under local anesthesia should take only their usual daily glucocorticoid dose before dental intervention. No supplementation is justified.
- Anticipate oral candidiasis when steroids are used.
- Be aware that signs of bacterial oral infection may be masked and anticipate oral candidiasis.
- Place on frequent maintenance schedule to avoid periodontal inflammation.
- Anticipate addisonian or cushingoid complications affecting the head and neck area.
- Monitor blood pressure and pulse.
- Patient may be high-risk candidates for pathological fractures or jaw fractures during extractions.
- Monitor pulse characteristics.

Oral Health Education

- Encourage daily plaque control procedures for effective self-care.

---

prednisolone acetate — see prednisolone

prednisolone sodium phosphate — see prednisolone

prednisolone tebutate — see prednisolone

---

 prednisone (PRED-nih-sone)

Deltasone: Tablets: 2.5, 5, 10, 20, 50 mg; Tablets
Liquid Pred: Syrup: 5 mg/5 mL
Meticorten: Tablets: 1 mg
Orasone: Tablets: 1, 5, 10, 20, 50 mg
Panasol-S: Tablets: 1 mg
Prednicen-M: Tablets: 5 mg
Prednisone Intensol Concentrate: Oral solution: 5 mg/mL
Sterapred: Tablets: 5 mg
Sterapred DS: Tablets: 10 mg

■✦■ **Alti-Prednisone, Apo-Prednisone, Jaa Prednisone**

■↩■ **Meticorten, Prednidib**

Drug Class: Corticosteroid

PHARMACOLOGY

Action

Intermediate-acting glucocorticoid that depresses formation, release, and activity of endogenous mediators of inflammation, including prostaglandins, kinins, histamine, liposomal enzymes, and complement system. Also modifies body's immune response.

Uses

Endocrine disorders; rheumatic disorders; collagen diseases; dermatological diseases; allergic states; allergic and inflammatory ophthalmic processes; respiratory diseases; hematological disorders; neoplastic diseases; edematous states (because of nephrotic syndrome); GI diseases; multiple sclerosis; tuberculous meningitis; trichinosis with neurological or myocardial involvement.

Unlabeled Uses

COPD; Duchenne muscular dystrophy; Graves ophthalmopathy.

Contraindications

Systemic fungal infections; administration of live virus vaccines.

Usual Dosage

ADULTS: *PO:* 5 to 60 mg/day.

Pharmacokinetics

ABSORP: Rapid, almost complete.
DIST: Crosses placenta.
METAB: Mainly hepatic, also renal and in the tissue. Prednisone is inactive and rapidly metabolized to active prednisolone.
EXCRET: Renal. Plasma $t_{1/2}$ is 3.4 to 3.8 hr.
PEAK: 1 to 2 hr.
DURATION: 1.25 to 1.5 days.

➡◀ DRUG INTERACTIONS

Albuterol or fenoterol: Hypokalemia (additive)
• Monitor vital signs.
Antacids: Decreased oral prednisone effect (decreased absorption)
• Administer as far apart as possible.
Bupropion: Increased risk of seizure (additive proconvulsant)
• Monitor clinical status.
Chlorambucil: Possible increased risk of seizure (additive proconvulsant)
• Monitor clinical status.
COX-1 inhibitors: Increased risk of peptic ulcer disease (additive)
• Avoid concurrent use.
Fluoroquinolones: Possible increased risk of Achilles tendon disorder (mechanism unknown)
• Assess risk/benefit.
Itraconazole or ketoconazole: Possible prednisone toxicity (decreased metabolism)
• Monitor clinical status.
Metronidazole: Decreased metronidazole effect (increased metabolism)
• Avoid concurrent use.
Omeprazole: Decreased prednisone effect (mechanism unknown)
• Monitor clinical status.
Rifampin: Marked decreased in prednisone effect (increased metabolism)
• Avoid concurrent use.
Thiazide diuretics: Increased potassium loss (additive)
• Monitor vital signs.

ADVERSE EFFECTS

⚠ **ORAL:** Ulcerative esophagitis; masked infection; impaired wound healing.

CVS: Thromboembolism or fat embolism; thrombophlebitis; necrotizing angiitis; cardiac arrhythmias or ECG changes; syncopal episodes; hypertension; myocardial rupture; CHF.

CNS: Convulsions; pseudotumor cerebri (increased intracranial pressure with papilledema); vertigo; headache; neuritis/paresthesias; psychosis.

GI: Pancreatitis; abdominal distention; nausea; vomiting; increased appetite and weight gain; peptic ulcer with perforation and hemorrhage; small and large bowel perforation.

MISC: Musculoskeletal effects (e.g., muscle weakness, steroid myopathy, muscle mass loss, tendon rupture, osteoporosis, aseptic necrosis of femoral and humeral heads, spontaneous fractures, including vertebral compression fractures and pathological fracture of long bones); endocrine abnormalities (e.g., menstrual irregularities, cushingoid state, growth suppression in children secary to adrenocortical and pituitary unresponsiveness, increased sweating, decreased carbohydrate tolerance, hyperglycemia, glycosuria, increased insulin or sulfonylurea requirements in patients with diabetes, negative nitrogen balance because of protein catabolism, hirsutism); anaphylactoid/hypersensitivity reactions; aggravation or masking of infections; malaise; fatigue; insomnia.

CLINICAL IMPLICATIONS

General

- Determine why drug is being taken. Consider implications of condition on dental treatment.
- Anticipate oral candidiasis when steroids are used.
- Be aware that signs of bacterial oral infection may be masked and anticipate oral candidiasis.
- Place on frequent maintenance schedule to avoid periodontal inflammation.
- Anticipate addisonian or cushingoid complications affecting the head and neck area.
- Monitor blood pressure and pulse.
- Patient may be high-risk candidate for pathological fractures or jaw fractures during extractions.
- Monitor pulse characteristics.
- Despite the anticipated perioperative physiological stress (i.e., minor surgical stress), patients undergoing dental care under local anesthesia should take only their usual daily glucocorticoid dose before dental intervention. No supplementation is justified.

When prescribed by DDS:

- *Lactation:* Excreted in breast milk.
- *Elderly:* May require lower doses.
- *Hypersensitivity:* May occur, including anaphylaxis.
- *Renal failure:* Use with caution; monitor renal function.
- *Adrenal suppression:* Prolonged therapy may lead to HPA suppression.
- *Cardiovascular effects:* Use drug with great caution in patients who have suffered recent MI.
- *Hepatitis:* Drug may be harmful in patients with chronic active hepatitis positive for hepatitis B surface antigen.
- *Immunosuppression:* Do not administer live virus vaccines during treatment.
- *Infections:* May mask signs of infection. May decrease host-defense mechanisms to prevent dissemination of infection.
- *Ocular effects:* Use systemic drug cautiously in ocular herpes simplex because of possible corneal perforation.
- *Ophthalmic use:* Prolonged use may result in glaucoma, cataracts, or other complications.
- *Peptic ulcer:* May contribute to peptic ulceration, especially with large doses.
- *Stress:* Increased dosage of rapidly acting corticosteroid may be needed before, during, and after stressful situations.
- *Withdrawal:* Abrupt discontinuation may result in adrenal insufficiency.
- *Overdosage:* Cushingoid changes, moonfaced, striae, central obesity, hirsutism, acne, ecchymoses, hypertension, osteoporosis, myopathy, sexual dysfunction, diabetes mellitus, hyperlipidemia, peptic ulcer, GI bleeding, increased susceptibility to infection, electrolyte and fluid imbalance, psychosis.

Pregnancy Risk Category: Category C.

Oral Health Education

When prescribed by DDS:
- Advise patient to take single daily doses or alternate day doses in morning (before 9 AM) and to take multiple doses at evenly spaced intervals throughout day.
- Instruct patient to take medication with meals or snack to avoid GI irritation.
- Caution patient not to discontinue drug suddenly to avoid withdrawal syndrome. Explain that dosage will be tapered slowly (until 5 mg/day or less) before stopping.
- Warn patient to avoid people with known viral infections, particularly chickenpox or measles, and to inform health care provider if exposure occurs.
- Explain that patient should not receive live virus vaccinations.
- Instruct patients with diabetes to monitor blood glucose closely.
- Advise patient to notify health care providers of drug regimen before any surgical procedure, emergency treatment, immunization, or skin test.
- Tell patient to carry medical identification card at all times describing medication being taken.
- Tell patient about symptoms of adrenal insufficiency (e.g., fever, myalgia, malaise, anorexia, nausea, orthostatic hypotension, dizziness, fainting) and need to report these symptoms to health care provider immediately.
- Instruct patient to report the following symptoms to health care provider: black tarry stools, vomiting of blood, menstrual irregularities, unusual weight gain, swelling of lower extremities, puffy face, muscle weakness, prolonged sore throat, fever, or cold.

Prednisone Intensol Concentrate — see prednisone

Prelone — see prednisolone

Premarin — see estrogens, conjugated or esterified

Premarin IV — see estrogens, conjugated or esterified

Premphase — see estrogens, conjugated/medroxyprogesterone acetate

Prempro — see estrogens, conjugated/medroxyprogesterone acetate

Presoken — see diltiazem HCl

Presoquim — see diltiazem HCl

Prevacid — see lansoprazole

Prevacid I.V. — see lansoprazole

Prevalite — see cholestyramine

Prevex B — see betamethasone

Prevex HC — see hydrocortisone

PreviDent — see sodium fluoride

PreviDent Plus — see sodium fluoride

PreviDent 5000 Plus — see sodium fluoride

PreviDent Rinse — see sodium fluoride

Priftin — see rifapentine

---

 prilocaine HCl (PRILL-oh-cane HIGH-droe-KLOR-ide)

Citanest Forte with Epinephrine: Injection: 4% with 1:200,000 epinephrine
Citanest Plain 4% Injection: Injection: 4% plain

Drug Class: Injectable local anesthetic; Amide

PHARMACOLOGY

Action

Inhibits sodium ion fluxes across membrane to block nerve action potential.

Uses

For local anesthesia by nerve block or infiltration in dental procedures.

Contraindications

Hypersensitivity to local anesthetics or any components of the products, para-aminobenzoic acid (esters only) or parabens; congenital or idiopathic methemoglobinemia; spinal and caudal anesthesia in septicemia, existing neurological disease, spinal deformities, and severe hypertension, hemorrhage, shock, or heart block.

Usual Dosage

Local anesthesia in association with dental procedures

ADULTS AND CHILDREN: *IV:* 8 mg/kg of body weight not to exceed 600 mg.

Pharmacokinetics

METAB: Liver.

EXCRET: Kidney.

ONSET: 2 to 10 min.

DURATION: 2 to 4 hr.

SPECIAL POP: *Elderly:* Repeated doses may cause accumulation of the drug or its metabolites or slow metabolic degradation; give reduced doses.

➡️⬅️ DRUG INTERACTIONS

Intercurrent use: Mixtures of local anesthetics are sometimes employed to compensate for the slower onset of one drug and the shorter duration of action of the sec drug. Toxicity is probably additive with mixtures of local anesthetics, but some experiments suggest synergisms. Exercise caution regarding toxic equivalence when mixtures of local anesthetics are employed. Some preparations contain vasoconstrictors. Keep this in mind when using concurrently with other drugs that may interact with vasoconstrictors

Sedatives: If employed to reduce patient apprehension during dental procedures, use reduced doses, since local anesthetics used in combination with CNS depressants may have additive effects. Give young children minimal doses of each agent.

Sulfonamides: The para-aminobenzoic acid metabolite of procaine inhibits the action of sulfonamides. Therefore, do not use procaine in any condition in which a sulfonamide drug is employed.

Trimethoprim-sulfamethoxazole: Methemoglobinemia (additive)
  • Avoid concurrent use.

ADVERSE EFFECTS

⚠ **ORAL:** Trismus; tingling.

CNS: Convulsions, loss of consciousness (overdose).

CVS: Myocardial depression, cardiac arrest, dysrhythmias, bradycardia.

RESP: Status asthmaticus, respiratory arrest, anaphylaxis (allergy).

MISC: May produce dose-dependent methemoglobinemia. Although methemoglobin values of < 20% do not generally produce any clinical symptoms, evaluate the appearance of cyanosis at 2 to 4 hr following administration in terms of the patient's overall status.

CLINICAL IMPLICATIONS

General

  • *Lactation:* Safety for use during lactation has not been established.
  • Use the lowest dosage that results in effective anesthesia to avoid high plasma levels and serious adverse effects. Inject slowly, with frequent aspirations before and during the injection, to avoid intravascular injection. Perform syringe aspirations before and dur-

ing each supplemental injection in continuous (intermittent) catheter techniques. During the administration of epidural anesthesia, it is recommended that a test dose be administered initially and that the patient be monitored for CNS toxicity and cardiovascular toxicity, as well as for signs of unintended intrathecal administration, before proceeding.

- *Inflammation or sepsis:* Use local anesthetic procedures with caution when there is inflammation or sepsis in the region of proposed injection.
- *CNS toxicity:* Monitor cardiovascular and respiratory vital signs and state of consciousness after each injection. Restlessness, anxiety, incoherent speech, lightheadedness, numbness, and tingling of the mouth and lips, metallic taste, tinnitus, dizziness, blurred vision, tremors, twitching, depression, or drowsiness may be early signs of CNS toxicity.
- *Malignant hyperthermia:* Many drugs used during anesthesia are considered potential triggering agents for familial malignant hyperthermia. It is not known whether local anesthetics may trigger this reaction and the need for supplemental general anesthesia cannot be predicted in advance; therefore, have a standard protocol for management available.
- *Vasoconstrictors:* Use solutions containing a vasoconstrictor with caution and in carefully circumscribed quantities in areas of the body supplied by end arteries or having otherwise compromised blood supply (e.g., digits, nose, external ear, penis). Use with extreme caution in patients whose medical history and physical evaluation suggest the existence of hypertension, peripheral vascular disease, arteriosclerotic heart disease, cerebral vascular insufficiency, or heart block; these individuals may exhibit exaggerated vasoconstrictor response. Serious dose-related cardiac arrhythmias may occur if preparations containing a vasoconstrictor such as epinephrine are employed in patients during or following the administration of potent inhalation agents.

Pregnancy Risk Category: Category B.

Oral Health Education

- Advise the patient to exert caution to avoid inadvertent trauma to the lips, tongue, cheek, mucosae, or soft palate when these structures remain anesthetized. The ingestion of food should therefore be postponed until normal function returns.
- Advise the patient to consult the dentist if anesthesia persists or a rash develops.

---

prilocaine/lidocaine HCl — see lidocaine HCl/prilocaine
Prilosec — see omeprazole
Prilosec OTC — see omeprazole
Primatene Mist — see epinephrine

---

primidone (PRIM-ih-dohn)
Mysoline

■✚■ Apo-Primidone, Sertan

Drug Class: Anticonvulsant

PHARMACOLOGY

Action

Primidone and its metabolites (e.g., phenobarbital and phenylethylmalonamide) have anticonvulsant activity, raising seizure threshold and altering seizure patterns.

Uses

Control of grand mal, psychomotor, or focal epileptic seizures; may control grand mal seizures refractory to other anticonvulsants.

Unlabeled Uses

Treatment of benign familial tremor (essential tremor).

➡️⬅️ DRUG INTERACTIONS RELATED TO DENTAL THERAPEUTICS
No documented drug-drug interactions. The absence of evidence is not evidence of safety.

ADVERSE EFFECTS
CNS: Ataxia; vertigo; fatigue; hyperirritability; emotional disturbances; drowsiness; personality deterioration; mood changes; paranoia.
GI: Nausea; anorexia; vomiting.
MISC: Granulocytopenia; agranulocytosis; megaloblastic anemia.

CLINICAL IMPLICATIONS
General
- Determine why drug is being taken. Consider implications of condition on dental treatment.
- Determine level of disease control, type and frequency of seizure, and compliance with medication regimen.
- Determine ability to adapt to stress of dental treatment. Consider short appointments.
- Blood dyscrasias are rarely reported; anticipate increased bleeding, infection, and poor healing.
- Place on frequent maintenance schedule to avoid periodontal inflammation.

Oral Health Education
- Encourage daily plaque control procedures for effective, nontraumatic self-care.

Principen — see ampicillin
Prinivil — see lisinopril
Pro-Banthine — see propantheline bromide

---

probenecid (pro-BEN-uh-sid)
Probenecid
■✦■ **Benuryl**

■◆■ **Benecid**

Drug Class: Uricosuric

PHARMACOLOGY
Action
Inhibits tubular reabsorption of urate, thus increasing urinary excretion of uric acid. Inhibits tubular secretion of most penicillin and cephalosporin antibiotics.

Uses
Treatment of hyperuricemia associated with gout and gouty arthritis; adjunctive therapy with penicillins or cephalosporins to elevate and prolong serum levels.

➡️⬅️ DRUG INTERACTIONS RELATED TO DENTAL THERAPEUTICS
Acetaminophen: Possible acetaminophen toxicity (decreased metabolism)
- Avoid concurrent use.

COX-1 inhibitors: Possible COX-1 inhibitor toxicity (decreased excretion)
- Monitor clinical status.

Midazolam: Shortened induction of midazolam anesthesia (displacement from protein binding)
- Monitor clinical status.

ADVERSE EFFECTS
⚠️ **ORAL:** Gingival pain.
CNS: Headaches; dizziness.

GI: Anorexia; nausea; GI distress; vomiting.

MISC: Hypersensitivity reactions; anaphylaxis; fever; flushing; exacerbation of gout; uric acid stones; costovertebral pain.

CLINICAL IMPLICATIONS

General

- Determine why drug is being taken. Consider implications of condition on dental treatment.
- Avoid prescribing aspirin products that antagonize probenecid.
- If GI side effects occur, consider semisupine chair position.
- *Gout*: Consider semisupine chair position for patient comfort.
- Patient may experience unilateral or bilateral TMJ pain (gouty arthritis) associated with acute exacerbation of gout.

---

procainamide HCl (pro-CANE-uh-mide HIGH-droe-KLOR-ide)

Procanbid, Pronestyl, Pronestyl-SR

■✦■ **Apo-Procainamide, Procan SR**

Drug Class: Antiarrhythmic

PHARMACOLOGY

Action

Increases effective refractory period of atria and bundle of His-Purkinje system; reduces impulse conduction velocity and myocardial excitability in atria, Purkinje fibers, and ventricles.

Uses

Treatment of documented ventricular arrhythmias that are considered life threatening.

➡✦ DRUG INTERACTIONS RELATED TO DENTAL THERAPEUTICS

No documented drug-drug interactions. The absence of evidence is not evidence of safety.

ADVERSE EFFECTS

⚠ **ORAL:** Bitter taste.

CNS: Dizziness; weakness; depression; psychosis with hallucinations.

GI: Nausea; vomiting; anorexia; abdominal pain.

MISC: Lupus erythematosus–like syndrome; blood dyscrasias (neutropenia, agranulocytosis, thrombocytopenia, hemolytic anemia).

CLINICAL IMPLICATIONS

General

- Determine why drug is being taken. Consider implications of condition on dental treatment.
- Monitor vital signs (e.g., BP, pulse pressure, rate, and rhythm) at each appointment to assess disease control. Do not provide elective dental treatment when BP is ≥180/110 or in the presence of other high-risk CV conditions. Refer to the section entitled "The Patient Taking Cardiovascular Drugs" in Chapter 6: *Clinical Medicine*.
- Use local anesthetic agents with vasoconstrictor with caution based on functional capacity of the patient, and use aspirating technique to prevent intravascular injection.
- Place patient on frequent maintenance schedule to avoid periodontal inflammation.
- Determine ability to adapt to stress of dental treatment. Consider short appointments.
- Blood dyscrasias are rarely reported; anticipate increased bleeding, infection, and poor healing.

Oral Health Education
- Encourage daily plaque control procedures for effective self-care in patient at risk for cardiovascular disease.

Procanbid — see procainamide HCl
Procan SR — see procainamide HCl
Procardia — see nifedipine
Procardia XL — see nifedipine
Procef — see cefprozil
Procephal — see erythromycin
Procrit — see epoetin alfa
Proctocort — see hydrocortisone
ProctoCream-HC — see hydrocortisone
Profenid — see ketoprofen
Prograf — see tacrolimus
Proken M — see metoprolol
Prolaken — see metoprolol
Prolixin Decanoate — see fluphenazine

---

promethazine HCl (pro-METH-uh-zeen HIGH-droe-KLOR-ide)
Phenergan
Drug Class: Antihistamine; Antiemetic; Antivertigo

PHARMACOLOGY

Action
Competitively antagonizes histamine at H_1 receptor sites. Produces sedative and antiemetic effects.

Uses
ORAL/RECTAL: Temporary relief of runny nose and sneezing from common cold; symptomatic relief of perennial and seasonal allergic rhinitis, vasomotor rhinitis, allergic conjunctivitis, allergic and nonallergic pruritus, mild, uncomplicated skin manifestations of urticaria and angioedema; amelioration of allergic reactions to blood or plasma; treatment of dermographism; adjunctive therapy in anaphylactic reactions; preoperative, postoperative, obstetric sedation; prevention and control of nausea and vomiting associated with certain types of anesthesia and surgery; adjunctive therapy with analgesics for postoperative pain; sedation and relief of apprehension; induction of light sleep; active and prophylactic treatment of motion sickness.
INJECTION: Amelioration of allergic reactions to blood or plasma; adjunct to epinephrine and other standard measures after acute symptoms of anaphylaxis have been controlled; uncomplicated allergic conditions of the immediate type when other therapy is impossible or contraindicated; sedation and relief of apprehension and inducement of light sleep from which patient can be easily aroused; active treatment of motion sickness; prevention and control of nausea and vomiting associated with certain types of anesthesia and surgery; adjunct to analgesics for control of postoperative pain; preoperative, postoperative, and obstetric (during labor) sedation; intravenously in special surgical situations (e.g., repeated bronchoscopy, ophthalmic surgery, poor-risk patients with reduced amounts of meperidine or other narcotic analgesic as an adjunct to anesthesia and analgesia).

➔◆ DRUG INTERACTIONS RELATED TO DENTAL THERAPEUTICS

No documented drug-drug interactions. The absence of evidence is not evidence of safety.

ADVERSE EFFECTS

⚠ **ORAL:** Dry mouth; tardive dyskinesia (dose related).

CNS: Drowsiness; sedation; dizziness; faintness; disturbed coordination; extrapyramidal effects (usually dose related and include three forms: pseudoparkinsonism, akathisia, dystonias); adverse behavioral effects; abnormal movements; hyperexcitability.

GI: Epigastric distress; nausea; vomiting; diarrhea; constipation.

RESP: Thickening of bronchial secretions; chest tightness; wheezing; respiratory depression; asthma; apnea.

MISC: Hypersensitivity reactions; photosensitivity; elevated prolactin levels; neuroleptic malignant syndrome; angioneurotic edema.

CLINICAL IMPLICATIONS

General

- Determine why drug is being taken. Consider implications of condition on dental treatment.
- Chronic dry mouth is possible; anticipate increased caries and candidiasis.
- If GI or respiratory side effects occur, consider semisupine chair position.
- Extrapyramidal behaviors can complicate performance of oral procedures. If present, consult with MD to consider medication changes.

Oral Health Education

- Evaluate manual dexterity; consider need for power toothbrush.
- If chronic dry mouth occurs, recommend home fluoride therapy and use of nonalcoholic oral health care products.

Pronaxil — see naproxen

Pronestyl — see procainamide HCl

Pronestyl-SR — see procainamide HCl

Prontofort — see tramadol HCl

---

propafenone (proe-pa-FEEN-one)

Rythmol

■◆■ **Nistaken, Norfenon**

Drug Class: Antiarrhythmic

PHARMACOLOGY

Action

Reduces fast inward current carried by sodium ion in the Purkinje fibers and, to a lesser extent, myocardial fibers.

Uses

IMMEDIATE RELEASE (IR): Prolong time to recurrence of paroxysmal atrial fibrillation/flutter or paroxysmal supraventricular tachycardia associated with disabling symptoms in patients without structural heart disease; treatment of ventricular arrhythmias (e.g., sustained ventricular tachycardia [VT]) that are life threatening.

EXTENDED RELEASE (ER): Prolong time to recurrence of symptomatic atrial fibrillation in patients with structural heart disease.

➔◆ DRUG INTERACTIONS RELATED TO DENTAL THERAPEUTICS

Lidocaine: CNS toxicity (additive)
- Minimize lidocaine dosage and monitor clinical status.

ADVERSE EFFECTS

⚠ **ORAL:** Unusual taste (9%); dry mouth (2%).

CNS: Dizziness (13%); fatigue (6%); headache (5%); insomnia, anorexia, anxiety, ataxia (2%); drowsiness, tremor (1%).

CVS: AV block, first degree (4.5 %); conduction delay; palpitations.

GI: Nausea and vomiting (11%); constipation (7%); diarrhea, dyspepsia (3%); abdominal pain, cramps (2%); flatulence (1%).

MISC: Dyspnea (5%); edema, diaphoresis (1%); blood dyscrasias (agranulocytosis, thrombocytopenia, granulocytopenia, anemia); increased bleeding time.

CLINICAL IMPLICATIONS

General

- Monitor vital signs (e.g., BP, pulse pressure, rate, and rhythm) at each appointment to assess disease control. Do not provide elective dental treatment when BP is ≥180/110 or in the presence of other high-risk CV conditions. Refer to the section entitled "The Patient Taking Cardiovascular Drugs" in Chapter 6: *Clinical Medicine*.
- Use local anesthetic agents with vasoconstrictor with caution based on functional capacity of the patient and use aspirating technique to prevent intravascular injection.
- Determine ability to adapt to stress of dental treatment. Consider short appointments.
- Chronic dry mouth is possible; anticipate increased caries and candidiasis.
- If GI side effects occur, consider semisupine chair position.
- Blood dyscrasias are rarely reported; anticipate increased bleeding, infection, and poor healing.

Oral Health Education

- Encourage daily plaque control procedures for effective self-care in patient at risk for cardiovascular disease.
- If chronic dry mouth occurs, recommend home fluoride therapy and use of nonalcoholic oral health care products.

Propanthel — see propantheline bromide

---

propantheline bromide (pro-PAN-thuh-leen BROE-mide)

Pro-Banthine

■✦■ **Propanthel**

Drug Class: Anticholinergic; Antispasmodic

PHARMACOLOGY

Action

Exerts anticholinergic effects, resulting in GI smooth muscle relaxation and diminished volume and acidity of GI secretions.

Uses

Adjunctive therapy in treatment of peptic ulcer.

Unlabeled Uses

Treatment of secretory and spastic disorders of GI tract, biliary tract, urinary tract, and bladder.

➡◀ DRUG INTERACTIONS RELATED TO DENTAL THERAPEUTICS

No documented drug-drug interactions. The absence of evidence is not evidence of safety.

ADVERSE EFFECTS

⚠ **ORAL:** Dry mouth; altered taste perception.
CNS: Headache; flushing; nervousness; drowsiness; weakness; dizziness; confusion; insomnia; fever; mental confusion or excitement; restlessness; tremor.
CVS: Palpitations; bradycardia; tachycardia (high doses).
GI: Nausea; vomiting; dysphagia; heartburn; constipation; bloated feeling; paralytic ileus.
MISC: Suppression of lactation; decreased sweating; photophobia.

CLINICAL IMPLICATIONS

General

- Determine why drug is being taken. Consider implications of condition on dental treatment.
- Anticholinergics have strong xerostomic effects. Anticipate increased caries and candidiasis.
- Substernal pain (heartburn) may mimic pain of cardiac origin.
- Use COX inhibitors with caution because they may exacerbate PUD and GERD.
- Monitor vital signs.
- *Photophobia:* Direct dental light out of patient's eyes, and offer dark glasses for comfort.

Oral Health Education

- If chronic dry mouth occurs, recommend home fluoride therapy and use of nonalcoholic oral health care products.

Propecia — see finasteride

Propeshia — see finasteride

---

 propofol (PRO-puh-FOLE)

Diprivan: Injection: 10 mg/mL

■ Fresofol, Recofol

Drug Class: General anesthetic

PHARMACOLOGY

Action

Produces sedation/hypnosis rapidly (within 40 sec) and smoothly with minimal excitation; decreases intraocular pressure and systemic vascular resistance; rarely is associated with malignant hyperthermia and histamine release; suppresses cardiac output and respiratory drive.

Uses

Induction and maintenance of anesthesia in adults; induction anesthesia in children at least 3 yr old; maintenance anesthesia in pediatric patients at least 2 mo old; initiation and maintenance of monitored anesthesia care sedation in adults; sedation in intubated or respiratory-controlled adult ICU patients.

Contraindications

Situations in which general anesthesia or sedation are contraindicated.

Usual Dosage

Sedation

ADULTS UNDER 55 YR: *IV:* Initiation 100 to 150 mcg/kg/min (6 to 9 mg/kg/hr) for 3 to 5 min (preferred method) or slow injection of 0.5 mg/kg over 3 to 5 min; follow by maintenance infusion. For maintenance, use 25 to 75 mcg/kg/min (1.5 to 4.5 mg/kg/hr) (preferred method) or incremental bolus doses of 10 to 20 mg.
ELDERLY, DEBILITATED, OR ASA III/IV: *IV:* Initiation same as adults; not as rapid bolus. For maintenance, use 20% reduction of adult dose; avoid rapid bolus doses.

Pharmacokinetics

ABSORP: Rapidly and extensively distributed. Vd is approximately 60 L/kg (10-day infusion), highly lipophilic. Crosses blood brain barrier and placenta; distributes into breast milk. Protein binding is 95% to 99%.

METAB: Liver conjugation to inactive metabolites.

EXCRET: 50% of dose is excreted in the kidney (metabolites). Clearance is 23 to 50 mL/kg/min. Terminal $t_{1/2}$ is 1 to 3 days (10-day infusion). $T_{1/2}$ of rapid distribution is 2 to 4 min. $T_{1/2}$ of slower distribution is 30 to 64 min.

ONSET: Rapid onset, usually within 40 sec from start of injection.

DURATION: 3 to 5 min (single bolus).

SPECIAL POP: *Elderly:* With increasing age, the dosage requirement decreases because of occurrence of higher peak plasma concentrations.

➡◆ DRUG INTERACTIONS

Atropine: Reduced heart rate (mechanism unknown)
- Monitor clinical status.

Midazolam: Prolonged midazolam effect (decreased metabolism)
- Monitor clinical status.

Clonidine: Possible propofol toxicity (additive)
- Decreased propofol dose and monitor clinical status.

Maprotiline: Possible increased risk of seizure (additive proconvulsant effect)
- Use with caution.

INCOMPATIBILITIES: For IV, do not mix with other therapeutic agents prior to administration. Avoid mixing blood or plasma in same IV catheter.

ADVERSE EFFECTS

CVS: Myocardial ischemia; hypotension; bradycardia; decreased cardiac output; hypertension (especially in children).

CNS: Amorous behavior; movement hypotonia; hallucinations; neuropathy; opisthotonos.

RESP: Apnea; cough; respiratory acidosis during weaning.

MISC: Asthenia; burning, stinging, or pain at injection site; fever.

CLINICAL IMPLICATIONS

General

When used by DDS:
- *Lactation:* Excreted in breast milk.
- *Special risk:* Use lower induction and maintenance doses in elderly, debilitated, and ASA III/IV patients, and monitor continuously for sign of hypotension or bradycardia. Use with caution in patients with lipid metabolism disorders, because propofol is an emulsion. Epileptic patients may be at risk of convulsions during recovery phase. Avoid significant decreases in mean arterial pressure and cerebral perfusion in patients with increased intracranial pressure or impaired cerebral circulation.
- *Anaphylaxis:* Has occurred rarely; relationship to drug has not been established.
- *Overdosage:* Cardiorespiratory and cardiovascular depression.

Pregnancy Risk Category: Category B.

Oral Health Education
- Advise patient that mental alertness, coordination, and physical dexterity may be impaired for some time after administration.

---

propoxyphene — see propoxyphene HCl

propoxyphene/acetaminophen — see acetaminophen/propoxyphene

---

propoxyphene HCl (pro-POX-ee-feen HIGH-droe-KLOR-ide)

Synonyms: propoxyphene, propoxyphene napsylate

Darvon Pulvules, Darvon-N

■✦■ 642
Drug Class: Narcotic analgesic
DEA Schedule: Schedule IV

PHARMACOLOGY

Action
Relieves pain by stimulating opiate receptors in CNS; also causes respiratory depression, peripheral vasodilation, inhibition of intestinal peristalsis, sphincter of Oddi spasm, stimulation of chemoreceptors that cause vomiting and increased bladder tone.

Uses
Relief of mild to moderate pain.

➡◀ DRUG INTERACTIONS RELATED TO DENTAL THERAPEUTICS
Alprazolam: Possible alprazolam toxicity (decreased metabolism)
• Avoid concurrent use.

ADVERSE EFFECTS
⚠ **ORAL:** Dry mouth.
CNS: Lightheadedness; dizziness; sedation; disorientation; incoordination; paradoxical excitement; hallucinations; euphoria; dysphoria; insomnia.
CVS: Hypotension; tachycardia; vasodilation; orthostatic hypotension.
GI: Nausea; vomiting; constipation; abdominal pain.
RESP: Depression of cough reflex.
MISC: Tolerance; psychological and physical dependence with chronic use; weakness.

CLINICAL IMPLICATIONS

General
• Determine why drug is being taken. Consider implications of condition on dental treatment.
• Monitor vital signs.
• *Postural hypotension:* Monitor BP at the beginning and end of each appointment; anticipate syncope. Have patient sit upright for several min at the end of the dental appointment before dismissing.
• Chronic dry mouth is possible; anticipate increased caries and candidiasis.
• If GI side effects occur, consider semisupine chair position.
• If oral pain requires additional analgesics, consider nonopioid products.

Oral Health Education
• If chronic dry mouth occurs, recommend home fluoride therapy and use of nonalcoholic oral health care products.

---

propoxyphene HCl/acetaminophen — see acetaminophen/propoxyphene
propoxyphene napsylate/acetaminophen — see acetaminophen/propoxyphene

---

propranolol HCl (pro-PRAN-oh-lahl HIGH-droe-KLOR-ide)
Inderal, Inderal LA, InnoPran XL, Propranolol Intensol
■✦■ APO-Propranolol, Detensol, Nu-Propranolol

■✦■ Inderalici
Drug Class: Beta-adrenergic blocker

PHARMACOLOGY

Action
Blocks beta receptors, primarily affecting the CV system (decreased heart rate, decreased cardiac contractility, decreased BP) and lungs (promotes bronchospasm).

Uses

Angina pectoris (except InnoPran XL); cardiac arrhythmias (except sustained release); essential tremor (except sustained release); hypertension; hypertrophic subaortic stenosis (except InnoPran XL); migraine prophylaxis (except InnoPran XL); MI (except sustained release); pheochromocytoma (except sustained release).

➜⬅ DRUG INTERACTIONS RELATED TO DENTAL THERAPEUTICS

COX-1 inhibitors: Decreased antihypertensive effect (decreased prostaglandin synthesis)
- Monitor blood pressure.

Diazepam: Possible diazepam toxicity (decreased metabolism)
- Avoid concurrent used.

Lidocaine: Lidocaine toxicity (decreased metabolism)
- Minimize lidocaine dosage and monitor clinical status.

Sympathomimetic amines: Decreased antihypertensive effect (pharmacological antagonism; unopposed alpha-adrenergic stimulation)
- Monitor blood pressure.

ADVERSE EFFECTS

⚠ **ORAL:** Dry mouth.

CNS: Bizarre dreams; decreased performance on neuropsychometric tests; depression; dizziness; emotional lability; fatigue; hallucinations; insomnia; lethargy; short-term memory loss; sleep disturbances; slightly clouded sensorium; tiredness; weakness.

CVS: Bradycardia; arrhythmia; chest pain; hypotension or hypertension; orthostatic hypotension.

GI: Dyspepsia; nausea; vomiting; diarrhea; epigastric distress; abdominal cramping; constipation; mesenteric arterial thrombosis; ischemic colitis.

RESP: Wheezing; dyspnea; bronchospasm; difficulty breathing.

MISC: Decreased exercise tolerance; hypersensitivity, including anaphylactic/anaphylactoid reactions; increased sensitivity to cold (e.g., Raynaud phenomenon); oculomucocutaneous reactions; pharyngitis; agranulocytosis; erythematous rash; fever; laryngospasm; respiratory distress; psoriasis-like eruptions; skin necrosis; systemic lupus erythematosus; blood dyscrasias (e.g., thrombocytopenia, leukopenia, agranulocytosis, anemia, others).

CLINICAL IMPLICATIONS

General

- Monitor vital signs (e.g., BP, pulse pressure, rate and rhythm) at each appointment to assess disease control. Do not provide elective dental treatment when BP is ≥180/110 or in the presence of other high-risk CV conditions. Refer to the section entitled "The Patient Taking Cardiovascular Drugs" in Chapter 6: *Clinical Medicine*.
- Use local anesthetic agents with vasoconstrictor with caution based on functional capacity of the patient and use aspirating technique to prevent intravascular injection.
- Determine ability to adapt to stress of dental treatment. Consider short appointments.
- *Postural hypotension*: Monitor BP at the beginning and end of each appointment; anticipate syncope. Have patient sit upright for several min at the end of the dental appointment before dismissing.
- Beta blockers may mask epinephrine-induced signs and symptoms of hypoglycemia in patients with diabetes.
- Chronic dry mouth is possible; anticipate increased caries and candidiasis.
- If GI side effects occur, consider semisupine chair position.
- Blood dyscrasias are rarely reported; anticipate increased bleeding, infection, and poor healing.
- Place on frequent maintenance schedule to avoid periodontal inflammation.

Oral Health Education

- Encourage daily plaque control procedures for effective self-care in patient at risk for cardiovascular disease.
- If chronic dry mouth occurs, recommend home fluoride therapy and use of nonalcoholic oral health care products.

Propranolol Intensol — see propranolol HCl

propylthiouracil (pro-puhl-thigh-oh-YOU-rah-sill)

Synonym: PTU

■✦■ **Propyl-Thyracil**

Drug Class: Antithyroid

PHARMACOLOGY

Action

Inhibits synthesis of thyroid hormones.

Uses

Long-term therapy of hyperthyroidism; amelioration of hyperthyroidism in preparation for subtotal thyroidectomy or radioactive iodine therapy; when thyroidectomy is contraindicated or not advisable.

Unlabeled Uses

Management of alcoholism-related liver disease.

➡✦ DRUG INTERACTIONS RELATED TO DENTAL THERAPEUTICS

No documented drug-drug interactions. The absence of evidence is not evidence of safety.

ADVERSE EFFECTS

⚠ ORAL: Taste loss.

CNS: Paresthesias; neuritis; headache; vertigo; drowsiness; neuropathies; CNS stimulation; depression.

GI: Nausea; vomiting; epigastric distress.

MISC: Abnormal hair loss; arthralgia; myalgia; edema; lymphadenopathy; drug fever; interstitial pneumonitis; insulin autoimmune syndrome (hypoglycemia); hypoprothrombinemia, increased bleeding, agranulocytosis, leukopenia, granulocytopenia.

CLINICAL IMPLICATIONS

General

- Be aware that uncontrolled hyperthyroid disease poses a risk for cardiovascular events during dental treatment.
- Monitor blood pressure and pulse rate to determine degree of thyroid disease control.
- Use local anesthetic agents with a vasoconstrictor with caution. Thyroid hormones and epinephrine are synergistic; use aspiration technique.
- Blood dyscrasias are rarely reported; anticipate increased bleeding, infection, and poor healing.

Oral Health Education

- Encourage daily plaque control procedures for effective, nontraumatic self-care.

Propyl-Thyracil — see propylthiouracil
Proquin XR — see ciprofloxacin
Proscar — see finasteride
ProStep — see nicotine
Protonix — see pantoprazole sodium
Protonix IV — see pantoprazole sodium
Protopic — see tacrolimus
Protostat — see metronidazole

Proventil — see albuterol

Proventil HFA — see albuterol

Provera — see medroxyprogesterone acetate

Provigil — see modafinil

Proviodine — see povidone iodine

Prozac — see fluoxetine HCl

Prozac Weekly — see fluoxetine HCl

Pseudo — see pseudoephedrine

pseudoephedrine (SUE-doe-eh-FED-rin)

Synonym: d-isoephedrine

Allermed, Cenafed, Children's Congestion Relief, Children's Silfedrine, Congestion Relief, Decofed Syrup, Defed-60, Dorcol Children's Decongestant, Dynafed Pseudo, Genaphed, Halofed, Mini Thin Pseudo, PediaCare Infant's Decongestant, PediaCare Nasal Decongestant, Pseudo, Pseudo-Gest, Seudotabs, Sinustop Pro, Sudafed, Sudafed 12 Hour Caplets, Sudex, Triaminic AM Decongestant Formula, Triaminic Infant Oral Decongestant Drops

■✦■ Balminil Decongestant Syrup, Benylin Decongestant, Contac Cold 12 Hour Non-Drowsy, Eltor 120, Pseudofrin, Sudafed Decongestant 12 Hour, Sudafed Decongestant Children's, Sudafed Decongestant Extra Strength, Triaminic Pediatric

■✦■ Lertamine-D

Drug Class: Nasal decongestant

PHARMACOLOGY

Action

Causes vasoconstriction and subsequent shrinkage of nasal mucous membranes by alpha-adrenergic stimulation, promoting nasal drainage.

Uses

Relief of nasal or eustachian tube congestion.

➜✦ DRUG INTERACTIONS RELATED TO DENTAL THERAPEUTICS

Pilocarpine: Increased myopia (mechanism unknown)
- Monitor clinical status.

ADVERSE EFFECTS

⚠ ORAL: Dry mouth.
CNS: Nervousness; excitability; dizziness; tremor; insomnia; restlessness; depression.
CVS: Arrhythmia; tachycardia; palpitations; bradycardia; transient hypertension.
GI: Anorexia; nausea; vomiting.
MISC: Leukopenia; agranulocytosis; thrombocytopenia; photophobia.

CLINICAL IMPLICATIONS

General

- Determine why drug is being taken. Consider implications of condition on dental treatment.
- Chronic dry mouth is possible; anticipate increased caries and candidiasis.
- Monitor vital signs.
- Blood dyscrasias are rarely reported; anticipate increased bleeding, infection, and poor healing.
- Monitor for respiratory effects; consider semisupine chair position.

Oral Health Education
- If chronic dry mouth occurs, recommend home fluoride therapy and use of nonalcoholic oral health care products.

---

pseudoephedrine HCl/cetirizine HCl — see cetirizine HCl/ pseudoephedrine HCl

pseudoephedrine HCl/fexofenadine HCl — see fexofenadine HCl/ pseudoephedrine HCl

Pseudofrin — see pseudoephedrine

Pseudo-Gest — see pseudoephedrine

pseudomonic acid A — see mupirocin

Psorcon E — see diflorasone diacetate

PTU — see propylthiouracil

Pulmicort Nebuamp — see budesonide

Pulmicort Respules — see budesonide

Pulmicort Turbuhaler — see budesonide

Pulsol — see enalapril maleate

PVF K — see penicillin V

---

pyrazinamide (peer-uh-ZIN-uh-mide)
Pyrazinamide

■✦■ Tebrazid

■✦■ Braccoprial

Drug Class: Anti-infective; Antitubercular

PHARMACOLOGY

Action
Pyrazine analog of nicotinamide may be bacteriostatic or bactericidal against *Mycobacterium tuberculosis*.

Uses
Initial treatment of active tuberculosis in adults and selected children when combined with other antituberculosis agents.

➡◆ DRUG INTERACTIONS RELATED TO DENTAL THERAPEUTICS
No documented drug-drug interactions. The absence of evidence is not evidence of safety.

ADVERSE EFFECTS
GI: Nausea; vomiting; anorexia.
MISC: Arthralgia and myalgia; hypersensitivity reactions (e.g., urticaria, pruritus); fever; thrombocytopenia; photosensitivity.

CLINICAL IMPLICATIONS

General
- Determine why drug is being taken (prevention or treatment). Consider implications of condition on dental treatment.
- Order complete medical consult to ensure noninfectious state exists before providing dental treatment.

- *For dental emergencies:* Follow special precautions to minimize disease transmission (particulate respirators) or refer patient to a hospital-based dental facility.
- Blood dyscrasias are rarely reported; anticipate increased bleeding.

Questran — see cholestyramine
Questran Light — see cholestyramine

quetiapine fumarate (cue-TIE-ah-peen FEW-mah-rate)
Seroquel

Drug Class: Atypical antipsychotic

PHARMACOLOGY
Action
Has antipsychotic effects, apparently caused by dopamine and serotonin receptor blockade in the CNS.

Uses
Treatment of schizophrenia; short-term treatment of acute manic episodes associated with bipolar I disorder, as either monotherapy or adjunct therapy to lithium or divalproex.

➡◀ DRUG INTERACTIONS RELATED TO DENTAL THERAPEUTICS
No documented drug-drug interactions. The absence of evidence is not evidence of safety.

ADVERSE EFFECTS
⚠ ORAL: Dry mouth (19%); tardive dyskinesia.
CNS: Somnolence (34%); headache (21%); agitation (20%); dizziness (11%); tremor (8%); anxiety (4%); hypertonia, dysarthria (≥1%).
CVS: Postural hypotension, hypotension, tachycardia (7%).
GI: Constipation (10%); abdominal pain (7%); vomiting (6%); dyspepsia (5%); gastroenteritis (2%); anorexia (≥1%).
RESP: Increased cough, dyspnea (≥1%); rhinitis (3%).
MISC: Asthenia (10%); pain (7%); back pain (5%); fever (2%); flulike syndrome (≥1%); leukopenia (>1%) anaphylaxis.

CLINICAL IMPLICATIONS
General
- Determine why drug is being taken. Consider implications of condition on dental treatment.
- Monitor blood pressure, pulse, and respiration.
- Determine ability to adapt to stress of dental treatment. Consider short appointments.
- Depressed or anxious patients may neglect self-care. Monitor for plaque control effectiveness.
- Chronic dry mouth is possible; anticipate increased caries and candidiasis.
- *Postural hypotension*: Monitor BP at the beginning and end of each appointment; anticipate syncope. Have patient sit upright for several min at the end of the dental appointment before dismissing.
- If GI side effects occur, consider semisupine chair position.
- If blood dyscrasias are reported, anticipate increased infection and poor healing.

Oral Health Education
- If chronic dry mouth occurs, recommend home fluoride therapy and use of nonalcoholic oral health care products.
- Evaluate manual dexterity; consider need for power toothbrush.
- Encourage daily plaque control procedures for effective self-care.

Quibron-T Dividose — see theophylline
Quibron-T/SR Dividose — see theophylline

Quimocyclar — see tetracycline HCl
Quinaglute Dura-Tabs — see quinidine
Quinalan — see quinidine

---

quinapril HCl (KWIN-uh-PRILL HIGH-droe-KLOR-ide)
Accupril

■◆■ **Acupril**

Drug Class: Antihypertensive; Angiotensin-converting enzyme (ACE) inhibitor

PHARMACOLOGY
Action
Competitively inhibits angiotensin I-converting enzyme, resulting in prevention of angiotensin I conversion to angiotensin II, a potent vasoconstrictor that also stimulates aldosterone release. Clinical consequences are decreased BP, reduced sodium resorption, and potassium retention.

Uses
Treatment of hypertension; adjunctive therapy of CHF.

➡️◀ DRUG INTERACTIONS RELATED TO DENTAL THERAPEUTICS
COX-1 inhibitors: Decreased antihypertensive effect (decreased prostaglandin synthesis)
- Monitor blood pressure.

ADVERSE EFFECTS
⚠️ **ORAL:** Dry mouth (1%).
CNS: Dizziness (8%); headache (6%); fatigue (3%).
CVS: Chest pain, hypotension (3%); tachycardia, palpitations, orthostatic hypotension (1%).
GI: Nausea, vomiting, diarrhea (2%); abdominal pain (1%).
RESP: Cough (4%).
MISC: Back pain (1%); angioedema (0.1%); anaphylactoid reactions.

CLINICAL IMPLICATIONS
General
- Monitor vital signs (e.g., BP, pulse pressure, rate, and rhythm) at each appointment to assess disease control. Do not provide elective dental treatment when BP is ≥180/110 or in the presence of other high-risk CV conditions. Refer to the section entitled "The Patient Taking Cardiovascular Drugs" in Chapter 6: *Clinical Medicine.*
- Use local anesthetic agents with vasoconstrictor with caution based on functional capacity of the patient, and use aspirating technique to prevent intravascular injection.
- Determine ability to adapt to stress of dental treatment. Consider short appointments.
- *Postural hypotension:* Monitor BP at the beginning and end of each appointment; anticipate syncope. Have patient sit upright for several min at the end of the dental appointment before dismissing.
- If coughing is problematic, consider semisupine chair position for treatment.
- Susceptible patient with DM may experience severe recurrent hypoglycemia.
- Chronic dry mouth is possible; anticipate increased caries, candidiasis, and lichenoid mucositis.
- Place on frequent maintenance schedule to avoid periodontal inflammation.

Oral Health Education
- Encourage daily plaque control procedures for effective self-care in patient at risk for cardiovascular disease.

quinidine (KWIN-ih-deen)

(quinidine gluconate, quinidine polygalacturonate, quinidine sulfate)

Cardioquin, Quinaglute Dura-Tabs, Quinalan, Quinora

❚✸❚ Apo-Quinidine, Biquin Durules

❚✦❚ Quini Durules

Drug Class: Antiarrhythmic

PHARMACOLOGY

Action

Depresses myocardial excitability, conduction velocity, and contractility; prolongs effective refractory period and increases conduction time; has indirect anticholinergic effects; may decrease vagal tone at low doses, paradoxically increasing conduction through the AV node.

Uses

Treatment of premature atrial, atrioventricular junctional, and ventricular contractions; treatment of paroxysmal supraventricular tachycardia, paroxysmal atrioventricular junctional rhythm, atrial flutter, paroxysmal and chronic atrial fibrillation, and paroxysmal ventricular tachycardia not associated with complete heart block; maintenance therapy after electrical conversion of atrial fibrillation or flutter.

QUINIDINE GLUCONATE (IV ADMINISTRATION): Treatment of life-threatening *Plasmodium falciparum* malaria.

➦← DRUG INTERACTIONS RELATED TO DENTAL THERAPEUTICS

Ketoconazole or itraconazole: Possible quinidine toxicity (decreased metabolism)
 • Avoid concurrent use.

Aspirin: Increased bleeding (additive antiplatelet effect)
 • Avoid concurrent use.

Codeine: Absence of codeine analgesia (blocked conversion to morphine in rapid metabolizers)
 • Monitor analgesic effect.

ADVERSE EFFECTS

CNS: Headache; fever; vertigo; excitement; confusion; delirium; syncope.

CVS: Arrhythmia; tachycardia; hypotension.

GI: Nausea; vomiting; anorexia; abdominal pain; diarrhea.

MISC: Lupus erythematosus–like syndrome; cinchonism (i.e., headache, tinnitus, nausea, photophobia, deafness, dizziness, vertigo, lightheadedness); hypersensitivity reactions; arthralgia; photosensitivity; myalgia; blood dyscrasias (e.g., acute hemolytic anemia, hypoprothrombinemia, thrombocytopenia, agranulocytosis, neutropenia, leukocytosis).

CLINICAL IMPLICATIONS

General

 • Determine why drug is being taken. Consider implications of condition on dental treatment.
 • Monitor vital signs (e.g., BP, pulse pressure, rate and rhythm) at each appointment to assess disease control. Do not provide elective dental treatment when BP is ≥180/110 or in the presence of other high-risk CV conditions. Refer to the section entitled "The Patient Taking Cardiovascular Drugs" in Chapter 6: *Clinical Medicine.*
 • Use local anesthetic agents with vasoconstrictor with caution based on functional capacity of the patient and use aspirating technique to prevent intravascular injection.
 • Determine ability to adapt to stress of dental treatment. Consider short appointments.
 • *Photophobia:* Direct dental light out of patient's eyes and offer dark glasses for comfort.

- Blood dyscrasias are rarely reported; anticipate increased bleeding, infection, and poor healing.
- If GI side effects occur, consider semisupine chair position.

Oral Health Education
- Encourage daily plaque control procedures for effective self-care in patient at risk for cardiovascular disease.

---

quinidine gluconate — see quinidine
quinidine polygalacturonate — see quinidine
quinidine sulfate — see quinidine
Quini Durules — see quinidine
Quinine-Odan — see quinine sulfate

---

quinine sulfate (KWIE-nine SULL-fate)
Quinine sulfate
■✦■ Quinine-Odan

Drug Class: Anti-infective; Antimalarial

PHARMACOLOGY
Action
Causes pH elevation in intracellular organelles of parasites; also has skeletal muscle relaxant effects and cardiovascular effects similar to those of quinidine.

Uses
Treatment of chloroquine-resistant falciparum malaria; alternative treatment for chloroquine-sensitive strains of *P. falciparum*, *P. malariae*, *P. ovale*, and *P. vivax*.

Unlabeled Uses
Prevention and treatment of nocturnal recumbency leg cramps.

➡✦ DRUG INTERACTIONS RELATED TO DENTAL THERAPEUTICS
No documented drug-drug interactions. The absence of evidence is not evidence of safety.

ADVERSE EFFECTS
CNS: Vertigo; dizziness; headache; fever; apprehension; restlessness; confusion; syncope; excitement; delirium; hypothermia; seizures.
CVS: Anginal symptoms; syncope.
GI: Nausea; vomiting; diarrhea; epigastric pain.
MISC: Cinchonism (i.e., headache, tinnitus, nausea, diarrhea, disturbed vision, skin, CV and CNS symptoms at very high doses); hypersensitivity (i.e., rash, pruritus, flushing, sweating, facial edema, asthmatic symptoms).

CLINICAL IMPLICATIONS
General
- Determine why drug is being taken. Consider implications of condition on dental treatment.
- Monitor respiration, blood pressure, and pulse.

Quinoflox — see ciprofloxacin
Quinora — see quinidine
Quixin — see levofloxacin
QVAR — see beclomethasone dipropionate

rabeprazole sodium (ra-BE-pray-zole SO-dee-uhm)

AcipHex

■✦■ **Pariet**

Drug Class: GI; Proton pump inhibitor

PHARMACOLOGY

Action

Suppresses gastric acid secretion by blocking acid (proton) pump within gastric parietal cells.

Uses

Short-term treatment in healing and symptomatic relief of duodenal ulcers and erosive or ulcerative GERD; maintaining healing and reducing relapse rates of heartburn symptoms in patients with GERD; treatment of daytime and nighttime heartburn and other symptoms associated with GERD; long-term treatment of pathological hypersecretory conditions, including Zollinger-Ellison syndrome and in combination with amoxicillin and clarithromycin to eradicate *Helicobacter pylori*.

➼← DRUG INTERACTIONS RELATED TO DENTAL THERAPEUTICS

Ketoconazole: Possible reduced ketoconazole effect (decreased absorption)
 • Avoid concurrent use.

ADVERSE EFFECTS

⚠ **ORAL:** Dry mouth; mouth ulceration; stomatitis; gingivitis; glossitis; esophagitis.

CNS: Headache (2%); insomnia; anxiety; dizziness; depression; nervousness; somnolence; hypertonia; neuralgia; vertigo; convulsion; abnormal dreaming; decreased libido; neuropathology; paresthesia; tremor; delirium; disorientation.

GI: Diarrhea; nausea; abdominal pain; vomiting; dyspepsia; flatulence; constipation; eructation; gastroenteritis; rectal hemorrhage; melena; anorexia; dysphagia; increased appetite; abnormal stools; proctitis; colitis; pancreatitis; cholelithiasis; cholecystitis.

RESP: Dyspnea; asthma; epistaxis; laryngitis; hiccups; hyperventilation; interstitial pneumonia.

MISC: Asthenia; fever; allergic reaction; chills; malaise; substernal chest pain; neck rigidity; photosensitivity reaction; myalgia; arthritis; leg cramps; bone pain; arthrosis; bursitis; anaphylaxis; angioedema; coma; hyperammonemia; rhabdomyolysis; sudden death.

CLINICAL IMPLICATIONS

General

 • If patient has GI disease, consider semisupine chair position.
 • Use COX inhibitors with caution, they may exacerbate PUD and GERD.
 • Drugs that lower acidity in intestinal tract may interfere with absorption of some antibiotics (penicillin, tetracyclines).
 • Anticipate chemical erosion of teeth.
 • Substernal pain (heartburn) may mimic pain of cardiac origin.

Oral Health Education

 • Inform patient that toothbrushing should not be done after reflux, but to only rinse mouth with water, then use home fluoride product to minimize chemical erosion-related caries.

Racovel — see levodopa/carbidopa

raloxifene hydrochloride (ral-OX-ih-FEEN HIGH-droe-KLOR-ide)

Evista

Drug Class: Selective estrogen receptor modulator

PHARMACOLOGY

Action

The biological actions of raloxifene are mediated largely through binding to estrogen receptors, which results in activation of certain estrogenic pathways and blockade of others. Raloxifene decreases resorption of bone and reduced biochemical markers of bone turnover to the premenopausal range. Effects on bone are manifested as reductions in the serum and urine levels of bone turnover markers, decreases in bone resorption based on radiocalcium kinetics studies, increases in bone mineral density, and decreases in incidence of fractures. Raloxifene also affects lipid metabolism, decreasing total and LDL cholesterol levels, but does not increase triglyceride levels or change total HDL cholesterol levels.

Uses

For the prevention and treatment of osteoporosis in postmenopausal women.

➡◀ DRUG INTERACTIONS RELATED TO DENTAL THERAPEUTICS

No documented drug-drug interactions. The absence of evidence is not evidence of safety.

ADVERSE EFFECTS

CNS: Migraine; depression; insomnia.
GI: Nausea; dyspepsia; vomiting; flatulence; gastroenteritis; abdominal pain.
RESP: Cough; pneumonia.
MISC: Infection; flu-like syndrome; leg cramps; chest pain; fever; weight gain; edema; arthralgia; myalgia; arthritis; hot flashes.

CLINICAL IMPLICATIONS

General

- Determine why drug is being taken. Consider implications of condition on dental treatment.
- Patient may be at high risk for pathological fractures or jaw fractures during extractions.
- If GI side effects occur, consider semisupine chair position.

Ramace — see ramipril

---

ramipril (ruh-MIH-prill)

Altace

■ ■ **Ramace, Tritace**

Drug Class: Antihypertensive; Angiotensin-converting enzyme (ACE inhibitor)

PHARMACOLOGY

Action

Competitively inhibits angiotensin I–converting enzyme, resulting in prevention of angiotensin I conversion to angiotensin II, a potent vasoconstrictor. Clinical consequences include decrease in BP and indirect (by inhibiting aldosterone) decrease in sodium and fluid retention and increase in diuresis.

Uses

Treatment of hypertension; for otherwise stable patients who have demonstrated clinical signs of CHF within the first few days after sustaining acute MI; reduce risk of MI, stroke, or death from CV causes in patients at high risk.

➡◀ DRUG INTERACTIONS RELATED TO DENTAL THERAPEUTICS

COX-1 inhibitors: Reduced antihypertensive effect (reduced prostaglandin synthesis)
- Monitor blood pressure.

ADVERSE EFFECTS

⚠ **ORAL:** Dry mouth (<1%).
CNS: Dizziness (4%).
CVS: Hypotension (11%); orthostatic hypotension (2%).
GI: Nausea, vomiting (2%); diarrhea (1%).
RESP: Cough (8%).
MISC: Angioedema (0.3%); anaphylactoid reactions.

CLINICAL IMPLICATIONS

General

- Monitor vital signs (e.g., BP, pulse pressure, rate, and rhythm) at each appointment to assess disease control. Do not provide elective dental treatment when BP is ≥180/110 or in the presence of other high-risk CV conditions. Refer to the section entitled "The Patient Taking Cardiovascular Drugs" in Chapter 6: *Clinical Medicine*.
- Use local anesthetic agents with vasoconstrictor with caution based on functional capacity of the patient and use aspirating technique to prevent intravascular injection.
- Determine ability to adapt to stress of dental treatment. Consider short appointments.
- If coughing is problematic, consider semisupine chair position for treatment.
- Susceptible patient with DM may experience severe recurrent hypoglycemia.
- Chronic dry mouth is possible; anticipate increased caries, candidiasis, and lichenoid mucositis.
- Place patient on frequent maintenance schedule to avoid periodontal inflammation.

Oral Health Education

- Encourage daily plaque control procedures for effective self-care in patient at risk for CV disease.
- If chronic dry mouth occurs, recommend home fluoride therapy and use of nonalcoholic oral health care products.

---

ranitidine HCl (ran-EYE-tih-DEEN HIGH-droe-KLOR-ide)

Zantac, Zantac 75, Zantac EFFERdose

■✦■ **Alti-Ranitidine HCl, Apo-Ranitidine, Novo-Ranitidine, Nu-Ranit, PMS-Ranitidine, ratio-Ranitidine, Rhoxal-ranitidine**

Drug Class: Histamine H_2 antagonist

PHARMACOLOGY

Action

Reversibly and competitively blocks histamine at H_2 receptors, particularly those in gastric parietal cells, leading to inhibition of gastric acid secretion.

Uses

Treatment and maintenance of duodenal ulcer; management of GERD (including erosive or ulcerative disease); short-term treatment of benign gastric ulcer; treatment of pathological hypersecretory conditions (Zollinger-Ellison).

Unlabeled Uses

Prevention of upper GI bleeding; treatment of aspiration pneumonia; stress ulcer; and gastric NSAID damage. Used as a part of a multidrug regimen to eradicate *Helicobacter pylori* in the treatment of peptic ulcer; protection against aspiration of acid during anesthesia; prevention of gastroduodenal mucosal damage that may be associated with long-term NSAIDs; to control acute upper GI bleeding; prevention of stress ulcers.

➤◀ DRUG INTERACTIONS RELATED TO DENTAL THERAPEUTICS

Ketoconazole or itraconazole: Reduced ketoconazole or itraconazole effect (decreased absorption)
- Avoid concurrent use.

Bupivacaine: Possible bupivacaine toxicity (decreased metabolism)
  • Avoid concurrent use.

ADVERSE EFFECTS

CNS: Headache; somnolence; fatigue; dizziness; hallucinations; depression; insomnia.

GI: Nausea; vomiting; abdominal discomfort; diarrhea; constipation; pancreatitis.

MISC: Hypersensitivity reactions; thrombocytopenia; granulocytopenia; agranulocytosis.

CLINICAL IMPLICATIONS

General
  • Determine why drug is being taken. Consider implications of condition on dental treatment.
  • If patient has GI disease, consider semisupine chair position.
  • Drugs that lower acidity in intestinal tract may interfere with absorption of some antibiotics (e.g., penicillin, tetracyclines).
  • Anticipate chemical erosion of teeth.
  • Substernal pain (heartburn) may mimic pain of cardiac origin.
  • Use COX inhibitors with caution, they may exacerbate PUD and GERD.

Oral Health Education
  • Inform patient that toothbrushing should not be done after reflux, but to only rinse mouth with water, then use home fluoride product to minimize chemical erosion–related caries.

Rastinon — see tolbutamide

ratio-Alprazolam — see alprazolam

ratio-Amiodarone — see amiodarone

ratio-Amoxi Clav — see amoxicillin/clavulanate potassium

ratio-Atenolol — see atenolol

ratio-Azathioprine — see azathioprine

ratio-Buspirone — see buspirone HCl

ratio-Captopril — see captopril

ratio-Clindamycin — see clindamycin

ratio-Clonazepam — see clonazepam

ratio-Codeine — see codeine phosphate

ratio-Cyclobenzaprine — see cyclobenzaprine HCl

ratio-Desipramine — see desipramine HCl

ratio-Dexamethasone — see dexamethasone

ratio-Diltiazem CD — see diltiazem HCl

ratio-Doxazosin — see doxazosin mesylate

ratio-Doxycycline — see doxycycline hyclate

ratio-Famotidine — see famotidine

ratio-Flunisolide — see flunisolide

ratio-Fluoxetine — see fluoxetine HCl

ratio-Flurbiprofen — see flurbiprofen

ratio-Fluvoxamine — see fluvoxamine maleate

ratio-Glyburide — see glyburide

ratio-Haloperidol — see haloperidol

ratio-Indomethacin — see indomethacin
ratio-Ipratropium — see ipratropium bromide
ratio-Ipratropium UDV — see ipratropium bromide
ratio-Lovastatin — see lovastatin
ratio-Metformin — see metformin HCl
ratio-Methotrexate — see methotrexate
ratio-Methylphenidate — see methylphenidate HCl
ratio-Minocycline — see minocycline HCl
ratio-Morphine SR — see morphine sulfate
ratio-MPA — see medroxyprogesterone acetate
ratio-Nadolol — see nadolol
ratio-Naproxen — see naproxen
ratio-Nortriptyline — see nortriptyline HCl
ratio-Nystatin — see nystatin
ratio-Oxycocet — see acetaminophen/oxycodone HCl
ratio-Oxycodan — see aspirin/oxycodone HCl
ratio-Ranitidine — see ranitidine HCl
ratio-Salbutamol — see albuterol
ratio-Sertraline — see sertraline HCl
ratio-Sotalol — see sotalol HCl
ratio-Sulfasalazine — see sulfasalazine
ratio-Terazosin — see terazosin
ratio-Timolol — see timolol maleate
ratio-Topilene — see betamethasone
ratio-Topisone — see betamethasone
ratio-Trazodone — see trazodone HCl
ratio-Valproic — see valproic acid and derivatives
Raxedin — see loperamide HCl
Reactine — see cetirizine
Rebetol — see ribavirin
Recofol — see propofol
Reductil — see sibutramine HCl
Redutemp — see acetaminophen
Regaine — see minoxidil
Reglan — see metoclopramide
Relafen — see nabumetone
Relenza — see zanamivir
Relifex — see nabumetone
Relpax — see eletriptan hydrobromide
Remeron — see mirtazapine

Remicade — see infliximab

Reminyl — see galantamine HBr

Renedil — see felodipine

Renitec — see enalapril maleate

Renova — see tretinoin

repaglinide (reh-PAG-lih-nide)

Prandin

█✦█ **GlucoNorm**

Drug Class: Antidiabetic, meglitinide

PHARMACOLOGY

Action

Decreases blood glucose by stimulating insulin release from the pancreas.

Uses

Adjunct to diet and exercise to lower blood glucose in patients with type 2 diabetes mellitus whose hyperglycemia cannot be controlled by diet and exercise alone. Can be used with metformin or thiazolidinediones (such as rosiglitazone) when hyperglycemia cannot be controlled by exercise, diet, and monotherapy with metformin, sulfonylureas, repaglinide, or thiazolidinediones.

➡◀ DRUG INTERACTIONS RELATED TO DENTAL THERAPEUTICS

Clarithromycin: Increased risk of hypoglycemia (decreased metabolism)
 • Avoid concurrent use.

ADVERSE EFFECTS

⚠ **ORAL:** Tooth disorder (unspecified) (2%).

CNS: Headache (11%).

CVS: Chest pain, angina (3%).

GI: Diarrhea, nausea (5%); dyspepsia (4%); constipation, vomiting (3%); pancreatitis.

RESP: URI (16%); sinusitis, bronchitis (6%).

MISC: Paresthesia (3%); allergy (2%).

CLINICAL IMPLICATIONS

General

• Determine degree of disease control and current blood sugar levels. Goals should be <120 mg/dL and A1C <7%. A1C levels ≥8% indicate significant uncontrolled diabetes.
• The routine use of antibiotics in the dental management of diabetic patients is not indicated; however, antibiotic therapy in patients with poorly controlled diabetes has been shown to improve disease control and improve response after periodontal debridement.
• Monitor blood pressure as hypertension and dyslipidemia (CAD) are prevalent in diabetes mellitus.
• Monitor vital signs (e.g., BP, pulse pressure, rate, and rhythm) at each appointment to assess disease control. Do not provide elective dental treatment when BP is ≥180/110 or in presence of other high-risk CV conditions. Refer to the section entitled "The Patient Taking Cardiovascular Drugs" in Chapter 6: *Clinical Medicine*.
• *Loss of blood sugar control:* certain medical conditions (e.g., surgery, fever, infection, trauma) and drugs (such as corticosteroids) affect glucose control. In these situations, it may be necessary to seek medical consultation before surgical procedures.
• Obtain patient history regarding diabetic ketoacidosis or hypoglycemia with current drug regimen.
• Observe for signs of hypoglycemia (e.g., confusion, argumentative state, perspiration, altered consciousness). Be prepared to treat hypoglycemic reactions with oral glucose or sucrose.

- Ensure patient has taken medication and eaten meal.
- Determine ability to adapt to stress of dental treatment. Consider short, morning appointments.
- Medical consult advised if fasting blood glucose is <70 mg/dL (hypoglycemic risk) or >200 mg/dL (hyperglycemic crisis risk).
- *If insulin is used:* Consider time of peak hypoglycemic effect.
- If GI or respiratory side effects occur, consider semisupine chair position.
- Place patient on frequent maintenance schedule to avoid periodontal inflammation.

Oral Health Education
- Encourage daily plaque control procedures for effective self-care.

Requip — see ropinirole HCl

Rescriptor — see delavirdine mesylate

Restasis — see cyclosporine

Restoril — see temazepam

Retard — see etodolac

Retin-A — see tretinoin

Retin-A Micro — see tretinoin

Retisol-A — see tretinoin

Retrovir — see zidovudine

Retrovir AZT — see zidovudine

Revatio — see sildenafil citrate

ReVia — see naltrexone HCl

Reyataz — see atazanavir sulfate

R-Gel — see capsaicin

Rheumatrex Dose Pack — see methotrexate

Rhinocort Aqua — see budesonide

Rhinocort Turbuhaler — see budesonide

Rhodacine — see indomethacin

Rhodis — see ketoprofen

Rhodis-EC — see ketoprofen

Rhodis SR — see ketoprofen

Rho-Salbutamol — see albuterol

Rhotral — see acebutolol HCl

Rhovai — see ketoprofen

Rhoxal-amiodarone — see amiodarone

Rhoxal-atenolol — see atenolol

Rhoxal-clonazepam — see clonazepam

Rhoxal-clozapine — see clozapine

Rhoxal-cyclosporine — see cyclosporine

Rhoxal-diltiazem CD — see diltiazem HCl

Rhoxal-famotidine — see famotidine

Rhoxal-fluoxetine — see fluoxetine HCl

Rhoxal-loperamide — see loperamide HCl

Rhoxal-metformin — see metformin HCl
Rhoxal-metformin FC — see metformin HCl
Rhoxal-minocycline — see minocycline HCl
Rhoxal-nabumetone — see nabumetone
Rhoxal-oxaprozin — see oxaprozin
Rhoxal-ranitidine — see ranitidine HCl
Rhoxal-salbutamol — see albuterol
Rhoxal-sotalol — see sotalol HCl
Rhoxal-ticlopidine — see ticlopidine HCl
Rhoxal-timolol — see timolol maleate
Rhoxal-valproic — see valproic acid and derivatives
Rhoxal-valproic EC — see valproic acid and derivatives

---

ribavirin (rye-buh-VIE-rin)

Copegus, Rebetol, Virazole

■◆■ **Vilona, Vilona Pediatrica, Virazide**

Drug Class: Anti-infective; Antiviral

PHARMACOLOGY

Action
Has antiviral inhibitory activity against respiratory syncytial virus (RSV), influenza virus, and herpes simplex virus. Exact mechanism is unknown.

Uses
AEROSOL: Treatment of carefully selected hospitalized infants and young children with severe lower respiratory tract infections caused by RSV.
CAPSULE: In combination with recombinant interferon alfa-2b injection for the treatment of chronic hepatitis C in patients with compensated liver disease previously untreated with alpha interferon or who have relapsed after alpha interferon therapy.
TABLET: In combination with peginterferon alfa-2a for the treatment of adults with chronic hepatitis C virus infection who have compensated liver disease and have not been previously treated with interferon alpha.

➡◀ DRUG INTERACTIONS RELATED TO DENTAL THERAPEUTICS
No documented drug-drug interactions. The absence of evidence is not evidence of safety.

ADVERSE EFFECTS
⚠ ORAL: Dry mouth (4% to 7%, tablet or capsule, injection).

CNS: Headache, dizziness, insomnia, irritability, depression, emotional lability, impaired concentration, nervousness, fatigue (capsules).

GI: Nausea, anorexia, dyspepsia, vomiting (capsules).

RESP: Worsening of respiratory status, bacterial pneumonia, pneumothorax, apnea, ventilator dependence (aerosol); dyspnea (capsules).

MISC: Myalgia, arthralgia, musculoskeletal pain, rigors, fever, flu-like symptoms, asthenia, chest pain (capsules); neutropenia, thrombocytopenia (peg-interferon injection); anemia (capsule).

CLINICAL IMPLICATIONS
General
- Determine why drug is being taken. Consider implications of condition on dental treatment. Coinfection with HIV and HBV may be present.
- This drug is used in combination with peg-interferon alpha-2a and adverse drug effects represent the drug combination.
- Consider medical consult to determine disease control and influence on dental treatment.
- Chronic dry mouth is possible; anticipate increased caries and candidiasis.
- Consider semisupine chair position if respiratory side effects are present.
- Blood dyscrasias rarely reported; anticipate increased bleeding, infection, and poor healing.

Oral Health Education
- If chronic dry mouth occurs, recommend home fluoride therapy and use of nonalcoholic oral health care products.

riboflavin (RYE-boh-FLAY-vin)
Synonym: vitamin B2

Riboflavin

Drug Class: Vitamin

PHARMACOLOGY
Action
Converted in body to coenzyme necessary in oxidation reduction. Also necessary in maintaining integrity of RBCs.

Uses
Prevention and treatment of riboflavin deficiency.

➡️⬅️ DRUG INTERACTIONS RELATED TO DENTAL THERAPEUTICS
No documented drug-drug interactions. The absence of evidence is not evidence of safety.

ADVERSE EFFECTS
No adverse effects are reported with this drug; not toxic to humans due to limited absorption from GI tract.

CLINICAL IMPLICATIONS
General
- Determine why drug is being taken. Consider implications of condition on dental treatment.

Ridaura — see auranofin
Ridene — see nicardipine HCl
Ridenol — see acetaminophen

rifabutin (RIFF-uh-BYOO-tin)
Mycobutin

Drug Class: Anti-infective; Antitubercular

PHARMACOLOGY
Action
Inhibits DNA-dependent RNA polymerase in susceptible strains of bacteria.

Uses

Prevention of disseminated *Mycobacterium avium* complex disease in patients with advanced HIV infection.

▶◀ DRUG INTERACTIONS RELATED TO DENTAL THERAPEUTICS

Clarithromycin: Increased rifabutin toxicity (decreased metabolism) and decreased clarithromycin effect (increased metabolism)
- Avoid concurrent use.

ADVERSE EFFECTS

⚠ **ORAL:** Discolored saliva, sputum; taste disturbance (3%).

CNS: Asthenia; headache; insomnia.

GI: Anorexia; diarrhea; dyspepsia; abdominal pain; eructation; flatulence; nausea; vomiting.

MISC: Myalgia; fever; discolored tears or skin; neutropenia.

CLINICAL IMPLICATIONS

General

- Determine why drug is being taken (prevention or treatment). Consider implications of condition on dental treatment.
- Complete medical consult to ensure noninfectious state exists before providing dental treatment.
- *For dental emergencies:* Follow special precautions to minimize disease transmission (particulate respirators) or refer patient to a hospital-based dental facility.
- If GI side effects occur, consider semisupine chair position.
- Blood dyscrasias rarely reported; anticipate increased infection and poor healing.

Oral Health Education

- Encourage daily plaque control procedures for effective, nontraumatic self-care.

Rifadin — see rifampin

---

rifampin (RIFF-am-pin)

Rifadin, Rimactane

■✦■ **Rofact**

■▦■ **Pestarin, Rimactan**

Drug Class: Anti-infective; Antitubercular

PHARMACOLOGY

Action

Inhibits DNA-dependent RNA polymerase in susceptible strains of bacteria.

Uses

Adjunctive treatment of tuberculosis; short-term management to eliminate meningococci from nasopharynx in *Neisseria meningitidis* carriers.

Unlabeled Uses

Treatment of infections caused by *Staphylococcus aureus* and *S. epidermidis*; treatment of gram-negative bacteremia in infancy; treatment of *Legionella*; management of leprosy; prophylaxis of *Haemophilus influenzae* meningitis.

▶◀ DRUG INTERACTIONS RELATED TO DENTAL THERAPEUTICS

Fluconazole, ketoconazole, or itraconazole: Decreased fluconazole, ketoconazole, or itraconazole effect (increased metabolism)
- Avoid concurrent use.

Diazepam, triazolam, or midazolam: Possible decreased oral or IV diazepam or triazolam and decreased oral triazolam effect (increased metabolism)
- Monitor clinical status.

Prednisone or prednisolone: Marked decreased in prednisone or prednisolone effect (increased metabolism)
- Avoid concurrent use.

Codeine: Possible decreased analgesia (mechanism unknown)
- Avoid concurrent use.

Doxycycline: Possible decreased doxycycline effect (increased metabolism)
- Avoid concurrent use.

ADVERSE EFFECTS
⚠ **ORAL:** Sore mouth and tongue.

CNS: Headache; drowsiness; fatigue; dizziness; inability to concentrate; mental confusion; generalized numbness; behavioral changes; myopathy.

CVS: Decrease in blood pressure; shock.

GI: Heartburn; epigastric distress; anorexia; nausea; vomiting; gas; cramps; diarrhea; pseudomembranous colitis; pancreatitis.

RESP: Shortness of breath; wheezing.

MISC: Ataxia; muscular weakness; pain in extremities; osteomalacia; myopathy; menstrual disturbances; fever; elevations in BUN; elevated serum uric acid; possible immunosuppression; abnormal growth of lung tumors; reduced 25-hydroxycholecalciferol levels; edema of face and extremities; discoloration of body fluids; leukopenia, thrombocytopenia, hemolytic anemia (dose related).

CLINICAL IMPLICATIONS
General
- Determine why drug is being taken (prevention or treatment). Consider implications of condition on dental treatment.
- Complete medical consult to ensure noninfectious state exists before providing dental treatment.
- *For dental emergencies:* Follow special precautions to minimize disease transmission (particulate respirators) or refer patient to a hospital-based dental facility.
- Monitor vital signs.
- Blood dyscrasias rarely reported; anticipate increased bleeding, infection, and poor healing.

Oral Health Education
- Encourage daily plaque control procedures for effective, nontraumatic self-care.

---

rifapentine (RIFF-ah-pen-teen)
Priftin
Drug Class: Anti-infective; Antitubercular

PHARMACOLOGY
Action
Inhibits DNA-dependent RNA polymerase in susceptible strains of *Mycobacterium tuberculosis*. Bactericidal for intracellular and extracellular *M. tuberculosis* organisms.

Uses
Treatment of pulmonary tuberculosis in conjunction with one or more other antituberculosis drugs to which the isolate is susceptible.

➡◀ DRUG INTERACTIONS RELATED TO DENTAL THERAPEUTICS
No documented drug-drug interactions. The absence of evidence is not evidence of safety.

ADVERSE EFFECTS
The following adverse reactions were reported in patients receiving rifapentine combination therapy and occurred in at least 1% of the patients.

CNS: Headache; dizziness.

GI: Anorexia; nausea; vomiting; dyspepsia; diarrhea; hemoptysis.

MISC: Arthralgia; pain; hyperuricemia; blood dyscrasias (1.1% to 5%, leukopenia, neutropenia, thrombocytosis, anemia).

CLINICAL IMPLICATIONS

General

- Determine why drug is being taken (prevention or treatment). Consider implications of condition on dental treatment.
- Complete medical consult to ensure noninfectious state exists before providing dental treatment.
- *For dental emergencies:* Follow special precautions to minimize disease transmission (particulate respirators) or refer patient to a hospital-based dental facility.
- If GI side effects occur, consider semisupine chair position.
- Blood dyscrasias rarely reported; anticipate increased bleeding, infection, and poor healing.

Oral Health Education

- Encourage daily plaque control procedures for effective, nontraumatic self-care.

Rimactan — see rifampin

Rimactane — see rifampin

---

rimantadine HCl (rih-MAN-tuh-deen HIGH-droe-KLOR-ide)

Flumadine

Drug Class: Anti-infective; Antiviral

PHARMACOLOGY

Action

Inhibits viral replication cycle in various strains of influenza A virus.

Uses

ADULTS: Prophylaxis and treatment of infection caused by various strains of influenza A virus.

CHILDREN: Prophylaxis against influenza A virus.

➡️⬅️ DRUG INTERACTIONS RELATED TO DENTAL THERAPEUTICS

No documented drug-drug interactions. The absence of evidence is not evidence of safety.

ADVERSE EFFECTS

⚠️ **ORAL:** Dry mouth; taste disturbance.

CNS: Insomnia; dizziness; headache; nervousness; asthenia; impaired concentration.

GI: Nausea; vomiting; anorexia; abdominal pain.

CLINICAL IMPLICATIONS

General

- Determine why drug is being taken. Consider implications of condition on dental treatment. Take precautions to avoid cross-contamination of microorganisms.

Riomet — see metformin HCl

Riopan — see magaldrate

---

risedronate sodium (riss-ED-row-nate SO-dee-uhm)

Actonel

Drug Class: Hormone; Bisphosphonate

PHARMACOLOGY

Action

Inhibits normal and abnormal bone resorption.

Uses

Treatment of osteoporosis in postmenopausal women; prevention of osteoporosis in post-menopausal women at risk of developing osteoporosis; prevention and treatment of gluco-corticoid-induced osteoporosis in men and women; treatment of Paget disease of the bone.

➜◄ DRUG INTERACTIONS RELATED TO DENTAL THERAPEUTICS

No documented drug-drug interactions. The absence of evidence is not evidence of safety.

ADVERSE EFFECTS

⚠ **ORAL:** Pharyngitis (5.8%).

CNS: Headache; dizziness.

CVS: Hypertension (10%), chest pain (2.5% to 5%).

GI: Diarrhea; abdominal pain; nausea; constipation; belching; colitis; dysphagia; esophagitis; esophageal ulcers; gastric ulcer.

RESP: Bronchitis.

MISC: Flu-like syndrome; chest pain; asthenia; neoplasm; arthralgia; bone pain; leg cramps; myasthenia; peripheral edema; anemia, ecchymosis (2.4% to 4.3%).

CLINICAL IMPLICATIONS

General

- Determine why drug is being taken. Consider implications of condition on dental treatment.
- Patient may be high-risk candidates for pathological fractures or jaw fractures during extractions.
- Osteonecrosis of the jaw is reported; consider this adverse drug effect when osteolytic disease is suspected.
- If GI side effects occur, consider semisupine chair position.
- Monitor vital signs.
- Blood dyscrasias rarely reported; anticipate increased bleeding, infection, and poor healing.

Oral Health Education

- Encourage daily plaque control procedures for effective, nontraumatic self-care.

Risperdal — see risperidone
Risperdal Consta — see risperidone
Risperdal M-TAB — see risperidone

---

risperidone (RISS-PER-ih-dohn)

Risperdal, Risperdal Consta, Risperdal M-TAB

Drug Class: Atypical antipsychotic, benzisoxazole

PHARMACOLOGY

Action

Has antipsychotic effect, apparently caused by dopamine and serotonin receptor blocking in CNS.

Uses

Treatment of schizophrenia; short-term treatment of acute manic or mixed episodes associated with bipolar disorder (oral only) as either monotherapy or adjunct therapy to lithium or valproate.

➡️⬅️ DRUG INTERACTIONS RELATED TO DENTAL THERAPEUTICS

No documented drug-drug interactions. The absence of evidence is not evidence of safety.

ADVERSE EFFECTS

⚠️ **ORAL:** LONG-ACTING INJECTION: Dry mouth (7%); toothache (3%); increased saliva, tooth disorder (2%).
ORAL: Salivation (2%); dry mouth (1%); toothache (2%).

CNS: LONG-ACTING INJECTION: Headache (22%); insomnia (16%); dizziness (11%); parkinsonism (10%); akathisia (9%); hallucinations (7%); somnolence (6%); suicide attempts (4%); abnormal thinking, tremor (3%); abnormal dreaming, hypoesthesia (2%); agitation, anxiety, psychosis, depression, paranoid reaction, delusion, apathy, hypertonia, dystonia (≥1%).
ORAL: Extrapyramidal symptoms (up to 34%); insomnia, agitation (26%); headache (22%); anxiety (20%); dizziness (11%); somnolence (8%); aggressive reaction (3%); increased dream activity, diminished sexual desire, nervousness, increased sleep duration (≥1%); sleepiness, increased duration of sleep, parkinsonism, extrapyramidal symptoms, asthenia, lassitude, increased fatigability (dose related); mania, Parkinson disease aggravation.

CVS: Tachycardia (3% to 5%).

GI: LONG-ACTING INJECTION: Dyspepsia, constipation, diarrhea (5%).
ORAL: Constipation (13%); dyspepsia (10%); vomiting (7%); nausea (6%); abdominal pain (4%); anorexia, (≥1%); intestinal obstruction.

RESP: Coughing (5%); pharyngitis, upper respiratory tract infection, sinusitis (3%); dyspnea (1%); apnea, pulmonary embolism.

MISC: LONG-ACTING INJECTION: Pain (10%); leg pain, myalgia (4%); peripheral edema (3%); syncope (2%); fever (1%); arthralgia, skeletal pain, injection site pain, asthenia, chest pain (≥1%).
ORAL: Chest pain, fever, arthralgia (3%); back pain (2%); increased prolactin levels; anaphylactic reaction; angioedema; pancreatitis; sudden unexpected death.

CLINICAL IMPLICATIONS

General
- Determine why drug is being taken. Consider implications of condition on dental treatment.
- Determine ability to adapt to stress of dental treatment. Consider short appointments.
- Depressed or anxious patients may neglect self-care. Monitor for plaque control effectiveness.
- Extrapyramidal behaviors can complicate performance of oral procedures. If present, consult with MD to consider medication changes.
- Chronic dry mouth is possible; anticipate increased caries activity and candidiasis.
- Monitor respiration and pulse.

Oral Health Education
- Encourage daily plaque control procedures for effective self-care.
- Evaluate manual dexterity; consider need for power toothbrush.
- If chronic dry mouth occurs, recommend home fluoride therapy and use of nonalcoholic oral health care products.

Ritalin — see methylphenidate HCl

Ritalin LA — see methylphenidate HCl

Ritalin-SR — see methylphenidate HCl
Ritmolol — see metoprolol

ritonavir (rih-TON-a-veer)
Norvir

Drug Class: Antiretroviral, protease inhibitor

PHARMACOLOGY
Action
Inhibits HIV protease, the enzyme required to form functional proteins in HIV-infected cells.

Uses
Treatment of HIV infections in combination with other antiretroviral agents.

➡◀ DRUG INTERACTIONS RELATED TO DENTAL THERAPEUTICS
Ketoconazole or itraconazole: Possible ritonavir, ketoconazole, or itraconazole toxicity (mutually decreased metabolism)
- Avoid concurrent use.

Diazepam, alprazolam midazolam, or triazolam: Possible diazepam, alprazolam, midazolam, or triazolam toxicity (decreased metabolism)
- Monitor clinical status.

Clarithromycin: Increased toxicity (decreased metabolism)
- Avoid concurrent use.

ADVERSE EFFECTS
⚠ **ORAL:** Circumoral paresthesia; throat irritation; taste perversion.

CNS: Headache; malaise; paresthesia; dizziness; insomnia; somnolence; abnormal thinking; depression; anxiety.

CVS: Syncope; vasodilation.

GI: Anorexia; constipation; diarrhea; dyspepsia; flatulence; nausea; vomiting; abdominal pain.

MISC: Asthenia; fever; myalgia.

CLINICAL IMPLICATIONS
General
- Determine why drug is being taken. Consider implications of condition on dental treatment.
- Antibiotic prophylaxis should be considered when <500 PMN/mm^3 are reported; elective dental treatment should be delayed until blood values improve above this level.
- This drug is frequently prescribed in combination with one or more other antiviral agents. Side effects of all agents must be considered during the drug review process.
- Consider medical consult to determine disease control and influence on dental treatment.
- Anticipate oral candidiasis when HIV disease is reported.
- Monitor vital signs.
- If GI side effects occur, consider semisupine chair position.
- Place on frequent maintenance schedule to avoid periodontal inflammation.

Oral Health Education
- Encourage daily plaque control procedures for effective self-care.

Rivanase AQ — see beclomethasone dipropionate

rivastigmine tartrate (riv-vah-STIGG-meen TAR-trate)

Exelon

Drug Class: Cholinesterase inhibitor

PHARMACOLOGY

Action
Unknown; however, may increase acetylcholine by inhibiting acetylcholinesterase, thereby increasing cholinergic function.

Uses
Treatment of mild to moderate dementia of the Alzheimer type.

➡⬅ DRUG INTERACTIONS RELATED TO DENTAL THERAPEUTICS

No documented drug-drug interactions. The absence of evidence is not evidence of safety.

ADVERSE EFFECTS

⚠ **ORAL:** Taste loss.

CNS: Dizziness; headache; insomnia; confusion; depression; anxiety; somnolence; hallucination; tremor; aggression; vertigo; agitation; nervousness; delusion; paranoid reaction; abnormal gait; ataxia; paresthesia; convulsions.

CVS: Hypertension (3%).

GI: Nausea; vomiting; anorexia; diarrhea; dyspepsia; abdominal pain; constipation; hemorrhoids; flatulence; eructation; fecal incontinence; gastritis.

RESP: URI; bronchoconstriction.

MISC: Asthenia; accidental trauma; fatigue; malaise; flu-like syndrome; back pain; arthralgia; pain; bone fracture; infection; arthritis; leg cramps; myalgia; fever; edema; allergy; hot flashes; anemia; epistaxis; thrombocytopenia; leukocytosis.

CLINICAL IMPLICATIONS

General
- Patient may experience hypotension or hypertension. Monitor vital signs at each appointment; anticipate syncope.
- Ensure that caregiver is present at every dental appointment and understands informed consent.
- If GI or musculoskeletal side effects occur, consider semisupine chair position.
- Blood dyscrasias rarely reported; anticipate increased bleeding, infection, and poor healing.

Oral Health Education
- Teach caregiver to assist patient with oral self-care practices.
- Evaluate manual dexterity; consider need for power toothbrush.

Rivotril — see clonazepam

---

rizatriptan (rye-zah-TRIP-tan)

Maxalt, Maxalt-MLT

▌✦▐ Maxalt RPD

Drug Class: Analgesic; Migraine

PHARMACOLOGY

Action
Binds to serotonin 1_B and 1_D receptors in intracranial arteries leading to vasoconstriction and subsequent relief of migraine headache.

Uses

Treatment of acute migraine attacks with or without aura.

➤← DRUG INTERACTIONS RELATED TO DENTAL THERAPEUTICS

No documented drug-drug interactions. The absence of evidence is not evidence of safety.

ADVERSE EFFECTS

⚠ **ORAL:** Thirst, tongue edema; dry mouth (3%); dysgeusia; tightness, pain, or pressure of neck, throat, or jaw.

CNS: Dizziness (9%); somnolence (8%); paresthesia (4%); headache (2%); hypesthesia, decreased mental acuity, euphoria, tremor (≥1%).

CVS: Palpitation.

GI: Nausea (6%); diarrhea, vomiting (≥1%).

RESP: Dyspnea (≥1%).

MISC: Asthenia, fatigue (7%); atypical sensations (5%); pain, tightness, pressure, or heaviness of chest, localized pain (3%); regional tightness, pressure, or heaviness (2%); warm or cold sensations (≥1%); hypersensitivity (including angioedema), wheezing, or toxic epidermal necrolysis.

CLINICAL IMPLICATIONS

General

- Monitor vital signs (e.g., BP and pulse). Drugs for prevention are sympatholytic; drugs for treatment of acute attack are sympathomimetic.
- This drug is taken to relieve symptoms of acute migraine attack. It is unlikely that dental treatment will be sought. Side effects are not lasting and should not complicate oral health care.

RMS — see morphine sulfate

Roaccutan — see isotretinoin

Robaxin — see methocarbamol

Robaxin-750 — see methocarbamol

Robitussin — see guaifenesin

Robitussin Children's — see dextromethorphan HBr

Robitussin Cough Calmers — see dextromethorphan HBr

Robitussin Extra Strength — see guaifenesin

Robitussin Honey Cough DM — see dextromethorphan HBr

Robitussin Pediatric — see dextromethorphan HBr

Rocaltrol — see calcitriol

Rofact — see rifampin

Rogaine — see minoxidil

Rogal — see piroxicam

Romazicon — see flumazenil

Romilar — see dextromethorphan HBr

Romir — see captopril

---

ropinirole HCl (row-PIN-ih-role HIGH-droe-KLOR-ide)

Requip

Drug Class: Antiparkinson, non-ergot dopamine receptor agonist

PHARMACOLOGY

Action
Stimulates dopamine receptors in the corpus striatum, relieving parkinsonian symptoms.

Uses
Treatment of the signs and symptoms of idiopathic Parkinson disease. May be used in conjunction with L-dopa.

➤◄ DRUG INTERACTIONS RELATED TO DENTAL THERAPEUTICS
No documented drug-drug interactions. The absence of evidence is not evidence of safety.

ADVERSE EFFECTS
⚠ **ORAL:** Dry mouth (5%); increased salivation (with dopamine).

CNS: Dizziness; somnolence; headache; confusion; hallucinations; abnormal dreams; tremor; anxiety; insomnia; aggravated Parkinson disease; hyperkinesia; hypokinesia; dyskinesia; paresthesia; vertigo; amnesia; impaired concentration.

CVS: Syncope (12%); orthostatic symptoms (6%), hypotension (2%); tachycardia; hypertension (5%); atrial fibrillation, extrasystoles.

GI: Nausea; vomiting; dyspepsia; constipation; abdominal pain; anorexia; diarrhea; flatulence; dysphagia.

RESP: Bronchitis; dyspnea; pneumonia.

MISC: Fatigue; viral infection; pain; asthenia; edema; chest pain; malaise; yawning; arthralgia; falls; injury.

CLINICAL IMPLICATIONS

General
- Determine why drug is being taken. Consider implications of condition on dental treatment.
- Extrapyramidal behaviors associated with Parkinson disease can complicate access to oral cavity and complicate oral procedures.
- Chronic dry mouth is possible; anticipate increased caries and candidiasis.
- *Postural hypotension:* Monitor BP at the beginning and end of each appointment; anticipate syncope. Have patient sit upright for several min at the end of the dental appointment before dismissing.
- Monitor blood pressure and pulse.
- Place on frequent maintenance schedule to avoid periodontal inflammation.

Oral Health Education
- Evaluate manual dexterity; consider need for power toothbrush.
- If chronic dry mouth occurs, recommend home fluoride therapy and use of nonalcoholic oral health care products.

---

rosiglitazone maleate (roe-sih-GLIH-tah-sone MAL-ee-ate)
Avandia

Drug Class: Antidiabetic, thiazolidinedione

PHARMACOLOGY

Action
Increases insulin sensitivity; improves sensitivity to insulin in muscles, adipose tissue; inhibits hepatic gluconeogenesis.

Uses
Improves glycemic control of type 2 diabetes mellitus as monotherapy and as an adjunct to diet and exercise; in combination with metformin, insulin, or a sulfonylurea when diet,

exercise, and a single agent does not result in adequate glycemic control in patients with type 2 diabetes mellitus.

➜◀ DRUG INTERACTIONS RELATED TO DENTAL THERAPEUTICS

No documented drug-drug interactions. The absence of evidence is not evidence of safety.

ADVERSE EFFECTS

CNS: Headache (6%); fatigue (4%).
GI: Diarrhea (2%).
RESP: URI (10%).
MISC: Injury (8%); edema (5%); back pain (4%).
POSTMARKETING: Adverse reactions potentially related to volume expansion (e.g., CHF, pulmonary edema, pleura effusions).

CLINICAL IMPLICATIONS

General

- Determine degree of disease control and current blood sugar levels. Goals should be <120 mg/dL and A1C <7%. A1C levels ≥8% indicate significant uncontrolled diabetes.
- The routine use of antibiotics in the dental management of diabetic patients is not indicated; however, antibiotic therapy in patients with poorly controlled diabetes has been shown to improve disease control and improve response after periodontal debridement.
- Monitor blood pressure as hypertension and dyslipidemia (CAD) are prevalent in diabetes mellitus.
- Monitor vital signs (e.g., BP, pulse pressure, rate, and rhythm) at each appointment to assess disease control. Do not provide elective dental treatment when BP is ≥180/110 or in the presence of other high-risk CV conditions. Refer to the section entitled "The Patient Taking Cardiovascular Drugs" in Chapter 6: *Clinical Medicine*.
- *Loss of blood sugar control:* Certain medical conditions (e.g., surgery, fever, infection, trauma) and drugs (such as corticosteroids) affect glucose control. In these situations, it may be necessary to seek medical consultation before surgical procedures.
- Obtain patient history regarding diabetic ketoacidosis or hypoglycemia with current drug regimen.
- Determine ability to adapt to stress of dental treatment. Consider short, morning appointments.
- Place on frequent maintenance schedule to avoid periodontal inflammation.

Oral Health Education

- Explain role of diabetes in periodontal disease and the need to maintain effective plaque control and disease control.
- Advise patient to bring data on blood sugar values and A1C levels to dental appointments.
- Encourage daily plaque control procedures for effective self-care in patient at risk for CV disease.

---

rosiglitazone maleate/metformin HCl (roe-sih-GLIH-tah-sone MAL-ee-ate/met-FORE-min HIGH-droe-KLOR-ide)

Synonym: metformin HCl/rosiglitazone maleate

Avandamet

Drug Class: Antidiabetic combination, thiazolidinedione and biguanide

PHARMACOLOGY

Action

ROSIGLITAZONE: Increases insulin sensitivity.
METFORMIN: Decreases blood glucose by reducing hepatic glucose production, increases peripheral glucose uptake and utilization, and may decrease intestinal absorption of glucose.

Uses

As an adjunct to diet and exercise to improve glycemic control in patients with type 2 diabetes mellitus who are already treated with combination rosiglitazone and metformin or who are not adequately controlled on metformin alone.

➡️⬅️ DRUG INTERACTIONS RELATED TO DENTAL THERAPEUTICS

No documented drug-drug interactions. The absence of evidence is not evidence of safety.

ADVERSE EFFECTS

CNS: Headache, fatigue (≥5%).

GI: Diarrhea (≥5%).

RESP: URI, pulmonary edema, pleural effusions (≥5%).

MISC: Injury, back pain, viral infection, arthralgia, edema (≥5%).

CLINICAL IMPLICATIONS

General

- Determine degree of disease control and current blood sugar levels. Goals should be <120 mg/dL and A1C <7%. A1C levels ≥8% indicate significant uncontrolled diabetes.
- The routine use of antibiotics in the dental management of diabetic patients is not indicated; however, antibiotic therapy in patients with poorly controlled diabetes has been shown to improve disease control and improve response after periodontal debridement.
- Monitor blood pressure as hypertension and dyslipidemia (CAD) are prevalent in DM.
- Monitor vital signs (e.g., BP, pulse pressure, rate, and rhythm) at each appointment to assess disease control. Do not provide elective dental treatment when BP is ≥180/110 or in the presence of other high-risk CV conditions. Refer to the section entitled "The Patient Taking Cardiovascular Drugs" in Chapter 6: *Clinical Medicine*.
- *Loss of blood sugar control:* Certain medical conditions (e.g., surgery, fever, infection, trauma) and drugs (such as corticosteroids) affect glucose control. In these situations, it may be necessary to seek medical consultation before surgical procedures.
- Obtain patient history regarding diabetic ketoacidosis or hypoglycemia with current drug regimen.
- Determine ability to adapt to stress of dental treatment. Consider short, morning appointments.
- Place on frequent maintenance schedule to avoid periodontal inflammation.

Oral Health Education

- Explain role of diabetes in periodontal disease and the need to maintain effective plaque control and disease control.
- Advise patient to bring data on blood sugar values and A1C levels to dental appointments.
- Encourage daily plaque control procedures for effective self-care in patient at risk for CV disease.

---

rosuvastatin calcium (row-SEU-vah-stat-in KAL-see-uhm)

Crestor

Drug Class: Antihyperlipidemic; HMG-CoA reductase inhibitor

PHARMACOLOGY

Action

Inhibits HMG-CoA reductase, the rate-limiting enzyme that converts 3-hydroxy-3-methyl-glutaryl coenzyme A to mevalonate, a precursor of cholesterol.

Uses

As an adjunct to diet to reduce elevated total cholesterol (C), LDL-C, non–HDL-C, Apo B, and TG levels and to increase HDL-C in patients with primary hypercholesterolemia and mixed dyslipidemia; as an adjunct to diet for the treatment of patients with elevated serum triglyceride levels; to reduce LDL-C, total-C, and Apo B in patients with homozygous familial hypercholesterolemia as an adjunct to other lipid-lowering treatments or if such treatments are not available.

➜← DRUG INTERACTIONS RELATED TO DENTAL THERAPEUTICS

No documented drug-drug interactions. The absence of evidence is not evidence of safety.

ADVERSE EFFECTS

⚠ **ORAL:** Periodontal abscess, tooth disorder (1%).

CNS: Headache (6%); dizziness, insomnia, hypertonia, paresthesia, depression (≥2%); anxiety, vertigo, neuralgia (≥1%).

CVS: Hypertension (≥2%).

GI: Diarrhea, dyspepsia, nausea (3%); constipation, gastroenteritis (≥2%); vomiting, flatulence, gastritis (≥1%).

RESP: Bronchitis, increased cough (≥2%); dyspnea, pneumonia, asthma (≥1%).

MISC: Back pain (3%); flu-like syndrome (2%); abdominal pain, accidental injury, chest pain, infection, pain (≥2%); pelvic pain, neck pain (≥1%).

CLINICAL IMPLICATIONS

General

- High LDL cholesterol concentration is the major cause of atherosclerosis which leads to CAD (angina, MI); determine degree of CV health and ability to withstand stress of dental treatment.
- Monitor vital signs (e.g., BP, pulse pressure, rate, and rhythm) at each appointment to assess disease control. Do not provide elective dental treatment when BP is ≥180/110 or in the presence of other high-risk CV conditions. Refer to the section entitled "The Patient Taking Cardiovascular Drugs" in Chapter 6: *Clinical Medicine*.
- Use local anesthetic agents with vasoconstrictor with caution based on functional capacity of the patient and use aspirating technique to prevent intravascular injection.
- If GI or musculoskeletal side effects occur, consider semisupine chair position.

Oral Health Education

- Encourage daily plaque control procedures for effective self-care in patient at risk for CV disease.

Rowasa — see mesalamine

Roxanol — see morphine sulfate

Roxanol 100 — see morphine sulfate

Roxanol Rescudose — see morphine sulfate

Roxanol T — see morphine sulfate

Roxanol UD — see morphine sulfate

Roxicet — see acetaminophen/oxycodone HCl

Roxicet 5/500 — see acetaminophen/oxycodone HCl

Roxicodone — see oxycodone HCl

Roxicodone Intensol — see oxycodone HCl

Roxilox — see acetaminophen/oxycodone HCl

Roxiprin — see narcotic analgesic combinations

Rum-K — see potassium products

Rythmodan — see disopyramide phosphate

Rythmodan-LA — see disopyramide phosphate

Rythmol — see propafenone

S2 — see epinephrine

saccharate — see amphetamine and dextroamphetamine

Salagen — see pilocarpine HCl

Salazopyrin — see sulfasalazine

Salazopyrin Desensitizing Kit — see sulfasalazine

Salazopyrin EN-tabs — see sulfasalazine

Salbulin — see albuterol

Salbutalan — see albuterol

---

salmeterol (sal-MEET-ah-rahl)

Serevent Diskus

■■■ **Zamtirel**

Drug Class: Bronchodilator; Sympathomimetic

PHARMACOLOGY

Action
Produces bronchodilation by relaxing bronchial smooth muscle through beta-2 receptor stimulation.

Uses
Maintenance treatment of asthma and prevention of bronchospasm with reversible obstructive airway disease; prevention of exercise-induced bronchospasm; maintenance treatment of bronchospasm associated with COPD (including emphysema and chronic bronchitis).

➔◆ DRUG INTERACTIONS RELATED TO DENTAL THERAPEUTICS
No documented drug-drug interactions. The absence of evidence is not evidence of safety.

ADVERSE EFFECTS
⚠ **ORAL:** Dental pain, oral candidiasis, throat dryness, irritation (1% to 3%)

CNS: Headache (28%); tremor (4%); dizziness/giddiness, nervousness, malaise/fatigue (3%); anxiety, insomnia, migraine, paresthesia, sleep disturbance (1% to 3%).

CVS: Increased blood pressure; palpitations; tachycardia.

GI: Diarrhea (5%); stomachache (4%); nausea, viral gastroenteritis, vomiting, abdominal pain, dyspepsia, gastric pain, gastric upset, constipation, heartburn (1% to 3%).

RESP: URI (14%); bronchitis, cough, tracheitis (7%); lower respiratory infection, chest congestion (4%); asthma, common cold, influenza (3%); acute bronchitis, dyspnea, pneumonia, wheezing (1% to 3%); serious exacerbations of asthma (some fatal); laryngeal spasm; irritation or swelling (including stridor or choking); oropharyngeal irritation.

MISC: Influenza (5%); fever, body pain, chest discomfort, pain, edema, hyperglycemia, swelling (1% to 3%).

CLINICAL IMPLICATIONS

General
- Determine why drug is being taken. Consider implications of condition on dental treatment.
- Monitor vital signs (e.g., BP, pulse rate, respiratory rate and function); uncontrolled disease characterized by wheezing and coughing.
- Acute bronchoconstriction can occur during dental treatment; have bronchodilator inhaler available.
- Ensure that bronchodilator inhaler is present at each dental appointment.

- Be aware that sulfites in local anesthetic with vasoconstrictor can precipitate acute asthma attack in susceptible individuals.
- If GI or respiratory side effects occur, consider semisupine chair position.
- Chronic dry mouth is possible; anticipate increased caries and candidiasis.

Oral Health Education
- If chronic dry mouth occurs, recommend home fluoride therapy and use of nonalcoholic oral health care products.

---

salmeterol/fluticasone propionate — see fluticasone propionate/salmeterol

Salmonine — see calcitonin-salmon

Salofalk — see mesalamine

Sal-Tropine — see atropine

Sandimmune — see cyclosporine

---

saquinavir mesylate (sack-KWIN-uh-vihr MEH-sih-LATE)
Fortovase, Invirase

▌✦▌ Fortovase Roche

Drug Class: Antiretroviral, protease inhibitor

PHARMACOLOGY

Action
Inhibits HIV protease, the enzyme required to form functional proteins in HIV-infected cells.

Uses
Treatment of advanced HIV infection. Saquinavir is given in combination with nucleoside analogs (such as zidovudine).

➡◀ DRUG INTERACTIONS RELATED TO DENTAL THERAPEUTICS

Fluconazole, ketoconazole, or itraconazole: Possible saquinavir toxicity (inhibition of P-glycoprotein; decreased metabolism)
- Avoid concurrent use.

Midazolam: Prolonged midazolam effect (decreased metabolism)
- Monitor clinical status.

Clarithromycin: Increased clarithromycin toxicity (decreased metabolism)
- Avoid concurrent use.

ADVERSE EFFECTS

CNS: Paresthesia; numbness; confusion; seizures; headache; depression; insomnia; anxiety; libido disorder.

GI: Diarrhea; abdominal pain and discomfort; nausea; dyspepsia; flatulence; vomiting; constipation; intestinal obstruction.

MISC: Ataxia; fatigue; pain weakness; ascites; pancreatitis; drug fever; intracranial hemorrhage; hemolytic anemia; thrombocytopenia.

CLINICAL IMPLICATIONS

General
- Determine why drug is being taken. Consider implications of condition on dental treatment.
- This drug is frequently prescribed in combination with one or more other antiviral agents. Side effects of all agents must be considered during the drug review process.
- Antibiotic prophylaxis should be considered when <500 PMN/mm³ are reported; elective dental treatment should be delayed until blood values are above this level.

- Consider medical consult to determine disease control and influence on dental treatment.
- Anticipate oral candidiasis when HIV disease is reported.
- Place on frequent maintenance schedule to avoid periodontal inflammation.
- If GI side effects occur, consider semisupine chair position.
- Blood dyscrasias rarely reported; anticipate increased bleeding, infection, and poor healing.

Oral Health Education
- Encourage daily plaque control procedures for effective self-care because HIV infection reduces host resistance.

Sarafem — see fluoxetine HCl

Sarna HC — see hydrocortisone

Scalpicin — see hydrocortisone

Scopace — see scopolamine HBr

---

scopolamine HBr (skoe-PAHL-uh-meen HIGH-droe-BRO-mide)
Synonym: hyoscine HBr

Isopto Hyoscine, Scopace

█✦█ Transderm-V

Drug Class: Antiemetic; Antivertigo; Anticholinergic

PHARMACOLOGY
Action
Competitively inhibits action of acetylcholine at muscarinic receptors. Principal effects are on iris and ciliary body (pupil dilations and blurred vision), secretory glands (dry mouth), drowsiness, euphoria, fatigue, decreased nausea, and vomiting.

Uses
Accomplishment of cycloplegia and mydriasis for diagnostic procedures and for preoperative and postoperative states in treatment of iridocyclitis (ophthalmic use); prevention of nausea and vomiting associated with motion sickness (transdermal); preanesthetic sedation and obstetric amnesia in conjunction with analgesics and to calm delirium (parenteral).

➡✦ DRUG INTERACTIONS RELATED TO DENTAL THERAPEUTICS
No documented drug-drug interactions. The absence of evidence is not evidence of safety.

ADVERSE EFFECTS
⚠ ORAL: Dry mouth.
CNS: Drowsiness; disorientation; delirium.
RESP: Decreased respiratory rate.
MISC: Sensitivity to light.

CLINICAL IMPLICATIONS
General
- Chronic dry mouth is possible; anticipate increased caries and candidiasis.
- Direct dental light out of patient's eyes and offer dark glasses for comfort.

Oral Health Education
- If chronic dry mouth occurs, recommend home fluoride therapy and use of nonalcoholic oral health care products.

Scot-Tussin Allergy — see diphenhydramine HCl
Scot-Tussin DM Cough Chasers — see dextromethorphan HBr
Scot-Tussin Expectorant — see guaifenesin
Sectral — see acebutolol HCl
Sedalito — see acetaminophen
Selectadril — see metoprolol
Selectofen — see diclofenac
Selectofur — see furosemide
Selegil — see metronidazole

selegiline HCl (seh-LEH-jih-leen HIGH-droe-KLOR-ide)
Synonym: L-deprenyl

Carbex, Eldepryl

 Apo-Selegiline, Gen-Selegiline, Novo-Selegiline, Nu-Selegiline

Niar

Drug Class: Antiparkinson

PHARMACOLOGY
Action
Selective type B monoamine oxidase (MAO) inhibitor thought to increase dopaminergic activity. MAO enzyme breaks down catecholamines and serotonin. Selegiline may also interfere with dopamine reuptake at synapse.

Uses
Adjunct to levodopa/carbidopa in idiopathic Parkinson disease, postencephalitic parkinsonism/symptomatic parkinsonism.

➔← DRUG INTERACTIONS RELATED TO DENTAL THERAPEUTICS
Tramadol: Increased risk of serotonin syndrome (reduced reuptake of monoamines)
 • Avoid concurrent use.
Sympathomimetic amines: Severe hypertension (additive)
 • Monitor blood pressure.

ADVERSE EFFECTS
⚠ **ORAL:** Dry mouth.

CNS: Dizziness; lightheadedness; fainting; confusion; hallucinations; vivid dreams; headache; anxiety; tension; insomnia; lethargy; depression; loss of balance; delusions; dyskinesias; increased akinetic involuntary movements; bradykinesia; chorea.

CVS: Palpitations; orthostatic hypotension; hypotension and hypertension; arrhythmia, tachycardia and bradycardia.

GI: Nausea; abdominal pain; diarrhea.

MISC: Generalized ache; leg pain; low back pain; weight loss.

CLINICAL IMPLICATIONS
General
• Determine why drug is being taken. Consider implications of condition on dental treatment.
• Extrapyramidal behaviors associated with Parkinson disease can complicate access to oral cavity and complicate oral procedures.
• If GI side effects occur, consider semisupine chair position.

- Chronic dry mouth is possible; anticipate increased caries and candidiasis.
- Monitor vital signs.
- *Postural hypotension:* Monitor BP at the beginning and end of each appointment; antici-
pate syncope. Have patient sit upright for several min at the end of the dental appoint-
ment before dismissing.
- Place on frequent maintenance schedule to avoid periodontal inflammation.

Oral Health Education
- Evaluate manual dexterity; consider need for power toothbrush.
- If chronic dry mouth occurs, recommend home fluoride therapy and use of nonalcoholic
oral health care products.

Seloken — see metoprolol

Selopres — see metoprolol

Sensibit — see loratadine

Sensorcaine — see bupivacaine

Sensorcaine MPF — see bupivacaine

Sensorcaine-MPF Spinal — see bupivacaine

Septocaine — see articaine HCl

Septra — see trimethoprim/sulfamethoxazole

Septra DS — see trimethoprim/sulfamethoxazole

Septra Injection — see trimethoprim/sulfamethoxazole

Septra IV — see trimethoprim/sulfamethoxazole

Serax — see oxazepam

Serevent Diskus — see salmeterol

Serocryptin — see bromocriptine mesylate

Seromycin Pulvules — see cycloserine

Seropram — see citalopram

Seroquel — see quetiapine fumarate

Sertan — see primidone

---

sertraline HCl (SIR-truh-leen HIGH-droe-KLOR-ide)
Zoloft

■✦■ Apo-Sertraline, Novo-Sertraline, ratio-Sertraline

■■■ Altruline

Drug Class: Antidepressant

PHARMACOLOGY

Action
Selectively blocks reuptake of serotonin, enhancing serotonergic function.

Uses
Treatment of major depression; treatment of obsessions and compulsions in patients with
obsessive-compulsive disorder (OCD), as defined in the DSM-III-R; treatment of panic disorder with or without agoraphobia, as defined in DSM-IV; posttraumatic stress disorder

(PTSD); treatment of premenstrual dysphoric disorder, treatment of social anxiety disorder (social phobia).

➤← DRUG INTERACTIONS RELATED TO DENTAL THERAPEUTICS

Oxycodone: Possible increased risk of serotonin syndrome (mechanism unknown)
- Monitor clinical status.

Tramadol: Increased risk of seizure and/or serotonin syndrome (additive)
- Avoid concurrent risk.

ADVERSE EFFECTS

⚠ **ORAL:** Dry mouth; tooth disorder/caries; dysphagia.

CNS: Agitation; anxiety; nervousness; headache; insomnia; dizziness; tremor; fatigue; tingling; diminished sensation; twitching; hypertonia; decreased concentration; confusion; somnolence; depression; decreased libido; agitation; emotional lability; vertigo; hypesthesia; apathy; hypokinesia/hyperkinesia; abnormal dreams; manic reaction.

CVS: Palpitations; chest pain.

GI: Nausea; diarrhea; anorexia; vomiting; flatulence; constipation; abdominal pain; increased appetite; dyspepsia; gastroenteritis; melena.

RESP: URI; pharyngitis; sinusitis; increased cough; dyspnea; bronchitis; rhinitis; epistaxis.

MISC: Muscle pain; weight loss or gain; myalgia; arthralgia; asthenia; fever; allergy/allergic reaction; chills; back pain; malaise; edema; yawning; photosensitivity; agranulocytosis; aplastic anemia; leukopenia; thrombocytopenia.

CLINICAL IMPLICATIONS

General
- Determine why drug is being taken. Consider implications of condition on dental treatment.
- Determine ability to adapt to stress of dental treatment. Consider short appointments.
- Depressed or anxious patients may neglect self-care. Monitor for plaque control effectiveness.
- Chronic dry mouth is possible; anticipate increased caries and candidiasis.
- Monitor vital signs.
- If GI side effects occur, consider semisupine chair position.
- Increased photosensitization with dental drugs having photosensitization side effect.
- Blood dyscrasias rarely reported; anticipate increased bleeding, infection, and poor healing.

Oral Health Education
- Encourage daily plaque control procedures for effective, nontraumatic self-care.
- If chronic dry mouth occurs, recommend home fluoride therapy and use of nonalcoholic oral health care products.

Servamox — see amoxicillin

Servamox Clv — see amoxicillin/clavulanate potassium

Servizol — see metronidazole

Serzone — see nefazodone HCl

Serzone-5HT2 — see nefazodone HCl

Seudotabs — see pseudoephedrine

---

sibutramine HCl (sih-BYOO-trah-meen HIGH-droe-KLOR-ide)
Meridia

■◄■ **Reductil**

Drug Class: CNS stimulant; Anorexiant

PHARMACOLOGY

Action
Inhibits reuptake of norepinephrine, serotonin, and dopamine. May stimulate satiety center in brain, causing appetite suppression.

Uses
As an adjunct to a reduced calorie diet for the management of obesity, including weight loss and maintenance of weight loss. Recommended for patients with an initial body mass index >30 kg/m² or >27 kg/m² in the presence of other risk factors (e.g., hypertension, diabetes, dyslipidemia).

➡◀ DRUG INTERACTIONS RELATED TO DENTAL THERAPEUTICS

Ketoconazole or itraconazole: Possible sibutramine toxicity (decreased metabolism)
- Avoid concurrent use.

Sympathomimetic amines: Possible hypertension (additive)
- Monitor blood pressure.

ADVERSE EFFECTS

⚠ **ORAL:** Tooth disorder, thirst; dry mouth (17.2%); taste perversion.

CNS: Headache; migraine; dizziness; nervousness; anxiety; depression; paresthesia; somnolence; CNS stimulation; emotional lability; agitation; hypertonia; abnormal thinking; insomnia.

CVS: Hypertension; tachycardia, vasodilation, palpitation.

GI: Abdominal pain; anorexia; constipation; increased appetite; nausea; dyspepsia; gastritis; vomiting; rectal disorder; diarrhea; flatulence; gastroenteritis.

RESP: Cough; bronchitis; dyspnea.

MISC: Back, chest, or neck pain; flu-like syndrome; accidental injury; asthenia; allergic reactions; edema; arthralgia; myalgia; tenosynovitis; fever; leg cramps; ecchymosis, reduced platelet function.

CLINICAL IMPLICATIONS

General
- Determine why drug is being taken. Consider implications of condition on dental treatment (e.g., hypertension, dyslipidemia, increased risk for diabetes).
- Monitor vital signs.
- If GI side effects occur, consider semisupine chair position.
- Chronic dry mouth is possible; anticipate increased caries activity and candidiasis.
- Anticipate increased bleeding, small risk of reduced platelet function.

Oral Health Education
- Encourage daily plaque control procedures for effective self-care in patient at risk for cardiovascular disease.
- If chronic dry mouth occurs, recommend home fluoride therapy and use of nonalcoholic oral health care products.

Sigafam — see famotidine

Siladryl — see diphenhydramine HCl

---

sildenafil citrate (sill-DEN-ah-fil SIGH-trayt)

Revatio, Viagra

Drug Class: Agent for impotence; Antihypertensive

PHARMACOLOGY

Action
Enhances the effect of nitric oxide by inhibiting phosphodiesterase type 5 in the corpus cavernosum of the penis. This results in vasodilation, increased inflow of blood into the corpora cavernosa, and ensuing penile erection upon sexual stimulation.

Uses

Treatment of impotence related to erectile dysfunction of the penis; treatment of pulmonary arterial hypertension.

➡️⬅️ DRUG INTERACTIONS RELATED TO DENTAL THERAPEUTICS

No documented drug-drug interactions. The absence of evidence is not evidence of safety.

ADVERSE EFFECTS

⚠️ **ORAL:** Stomatitis, dry mouth, gingivitis (>2%).

CNS: Headache (16%); dizziness (2%); ataxia, hypertonia, neuralgia, paresthesia, tremor, vertigo, depression, insomnia, somnolence, migraine, neuropathy, abnormal dreams, decreased reflexes, hypesthesia (>2%); seizure, anxiety (postmarketing).

GI: Dyspepsia (7%); diarrhea (3%); vomiting, glossitis, colitis, dysphagia, gastritis, gastroenteritis, esophagitis, rectal hemorrhage (>2%).

RESP: Asthma, dyspnea, laryngitis, pharyngitis, sinusitis, bronchitis, increased sputum, increased cough (>2%).

MISC: Face edema, photosensitivity, shock, asthenia, pain, chills, accidental falls, abdominal pain, allergic reaction, chest pain, accidental injury (>2%).

CLINICAL IMPLICATIONS

General

- Concurrent administration with nitroglycerin may lead to severe hypotension. Avoid concurrent use.
- Monitor vital signs from cardiovascular effects.
- The short half-life of sildenafil reduces treatment related risks of the drug effects.

Silphen DM — see dextromethorphan HBr

Siltussin SA — see guaifenesin

Simply Sleep — see diphenhydramine HCl

---

simvastatin (SIM-vuh-STAT-in)

Zocor

Drug Class: Antihyperlipidemic; HMG-CoA reductase inhibitor

PHARMACOLOGY

Action

Increases rate at which body removes cholesterol from blood and reduces production of cholesterol by inhibiting enzyme that catalyzes early rate-limiting step in cholesterol synthesis.

Uses

Adjunct to diet for reducing elevated total cholesterol and LDL cholesterol levels in patients with primary hypercholesterolemia (types IIa and IIb) when response to diet and other nonpharmacological measures alone are inadequate; to reduce the risk of stroke or transient ischemic attack.

Unlabeled Uses

Lower elevated cholesterol levels in patients with heterozygous familial hypercholesterolemia, familial combined hyperlipidemia, diabetic dyslipidemia in type 2 diabetic patients, hyperlipidemia secary to nephrotic syndrome, and homozygous familial hypercholesterolemia in patients who have defective, rather than absent, LDL receptors.

➔◀ DRUG INTERACTIONS RELATED TO DENTAL THERAPEUTICS

Fluconazole, ketoconazole, or itraconazole: Rhabdomyolysis (decreased metabolism)
- Avoid concurrent use.

Clarithromycin: Rhabdomyolysis (decreased metabolism)
- Avoid concurrent use.

ADVERSE EFFECTS

⚠ **ORAL:** Taste disturbance.

CNS: Headache; asthenia; paresthesia; peripheral neuropathy.

GI: Nausea; vomiting; diarrhea; abdominal pain; constipation; flatulence; dyspepsia; pancreatitis.

RESP: URI.

MISC: Myopathy; rhabdomyolysis; fatigue. Apparent hypersensitivity syndrome has been reported rarely that has included one or more of the following features: anaphylaxis; angioedema; lupus erythematous–like syndrome; polymyalgia rheumatica; vasculitis; purpura; thrombocytopenia; leukopenia; hemolytic anemia; positive antinuclear antibody; erythrocyte sedimentation rate increase; arthritis; arthralgia; urticaria; asthenia; photosensitivity; fever; chills; flushing; malaise; dyspnea; toxic epidermal necrolysis; erythema multiforme, including Stevens-Johnson syndrome.

CLINICAL IMPLICATIONS

General
- High LDL cholesterol concentration is the major cause of atherosclerosis which leads to CAD (angina, MI); determine degree of CV health and ability to withstand stress of dental treatment.
- Monitor vital signs (e.g., BP, pulse pressure, rate, and rhythm) at each appointment to assess disease control. Do not provide elective dental treatment when BP is ≥180/110 or in the presence of other high-risk CV conditions. Refer to the section entitled "The Patient Taking Cardiovascular Drugs" in Chapter 6: *Clinical Medicine.*
- If GI side effects occur, consider semisupine chair position.
- Blood dyscrasias rarely reported; anticipate increased bleeding, infection, and poor healing.

Oral Health Education
- Encourage daily plaque control procedures for effective self-care in patient at risk for CV disease.

Sinaplin — see ampicillin

Sinedol — see acetaminophen

Sinedol 500 — see acetaminophen

Sinemet 10/100 — see levodopa/carbidopa

Sinemet 25/100 — see levodopa/carbidopa

Sinemet 25/250 — see levodopa/carbidopa

Sinemet CR — see levodopa/carbidopa

Sinequan — see doxepin HCl

Sinestron — see lorazepam

Singulair — see montelukast sodium

Sinozzard — see prazosin HCl

Sinumist-SR Capsulets — see guaifenesin

Sinustop Pro — see pseudoephedrine

Siquial — see fluoxetine HCl

Sirdalud — see tizanidine HCl

Skelaxin — see metaxalone
Sleep-Eze 3 — see diphenhydramine HCl
Sleepwell 2-nite — see diphenhydramine HCl
Slo-bid Gyrocaps — see theophylline
Slo-Niacin — see niacin
Slo-Phyllin — see theophylline
Slow-FE — see ferrous salts
Snoozefast — see diphenhydramine HCl

---

 sodium fluoride (SO-dee-uhm FLUR-ide)

Synonym: fluoride sodium

ACT: OTC Rinse: 0.02% (from 0.05% sodium fluoride)
Denta 5000 Plus: Cream: 1.1%
DentaGel 1.1%: Gel: 1.1%
EtheDent: Cream: 1.1%; Tablets, Chewable: 0.25 mg, 0.5 mg (from 1.1 mg sodium fluoride), 1 mg (from 2.2 mg sodium fluoride)
Fluoride: Tablets: 1 mg (from 2.2 mg sodium fluoride)
Fluoride Loz: Lozenges: 1 mg (from 2.2 mg sodium fluoride)
Fluorigard: Rinse: 0.02% (from 0.05% sodium fluoride)
Fluorinse: Rinse: 0.09% (from 0.2% sodium fluoride)
Fluoritab: Drops: 0.25 mg per drop (from ~ 0.275 mg sodium fluoride); Tablets, Chewable: 0.5 mg (from 1.1 mg sodium fluoride)
Flura: Tablets: 1 mg (from 2.2 mg sodium fluoride)
Flura-Loz: Lozenges: 1 mg (from 2.2 mg sodium fluoride)
Gel-Kam: Gel: 0.1% (from 0.4% stannous fluoride); Rinse: 0.04%
Gel-Tin: Gel: 0.1% (from 0.4% stannous fluoride)
Karidium: Tablets, chewable: 1 mg (from 2.2 mg sodium fluoride)
Karigel, Karigel-N: Gel: 0.5% (from 1.1% sodium fluoride)
Luride: Drops: 0.5 mg per mL (from 1.1 mg sodium fluoride); Gel: 1.2% (from sodium fluoride and hydrogen fluoride)
Luride Lozi-Tabs: Tablets, Chewable: 0.25 mg, 0.5 mg (from 1.1 mg sodium fluoride), 1 mg (from 2.2 mg sodium fluoride)
Luride-SF Lozi-Tabs: Tablets, Chewable: 1 mg (from 2.2 mg sodium fluoride)
MouthKote F/R: Rinse: 0.04%
NeutraGard Advanced: Gel: 1.1%
Pediaflor: Drops: 0.5 mg per mL (from 1.1 mg sodium fluoride)
Pharmaflur, Pharmaflur df: Tablets, Chewable: 1 mg (from 2.2 mg sodium fluoride)
Pharmaflur 1.1: Tablets, Chewable: 0.5 mg (from 1.1 mg sodium fluoride)
Phos-Flur: Solution: 0.2 mg per mL (from 0.44 mg sodium fluoride)
Point-Two: Rinse: 0.09% (from 0.2% sodium fluoride)
PreviDent: Gel: 0.5% (from 1.1% sodium fluoride)
PreviDent Plus: Gel: 1.2% (from sodium fluoride and hydrogen fluoride)
PreviDent 5000 Plus: Cream: 1.1%
PreviDent Rinse: Rinse: 0.2% neutral sodium fluoride
Sodium Fluoride: Drops: 0.125 mg per drop (from ~ 0.275 mg sodium fluoride), 0.5 mg per mL (from 1.1 mg sodium fluoride); Tablets, Chewable: 0.25 mg, 1 mg (from 2.2 mg sodium fluoride)

Stannous Fluoride: Gel: 0.4%; Rinse concentrate: 0.63%
Stop: Gel: 0.1% (from 0.4% stannous fluoride)
Thera-Flur, Thera-Flur-N: Gel-Drops: 0.5% (from 1.1% sodium fluoride)

Drug Class: Dental anticaries agent

PHARMACOLOGY

Action

Combines with hydroxyapatite to form fluorapatite, which is less soluble in acidic environment.

Uses

For prevention of dental caries.

Unlabeled Uses

Sodium fluoride may be effective in treating osteoporosis. Doses (as fluoride) up to 60 mg daily or more are used in conjunction with calcium supplements, vitamin D, or estrogen. However, large doses may result in a higher frequency of side effects. Some data suggest that doses <50 mg/day are efficacious with fewer adverse reactions. No commercially available products contain high sodium fluoride doses for this use; therefore, a large number of tablets would be required to obtain this dosage. Fluoride supplementation is not recommended for the prophylaxis of osteoporosis due to the potential for increased incidence of fractures.

Contraindications

When the fluoride content of drinking water exceeds 0.7 ppm; low sodium or sodium-free diets; hypersensitivity to fluoride.

Do not use 1-mg tablets in children younger than 3 yr old or when the drinking water fluoride content is 0.3 ppm or higher. Do not use 1-mg/5-mL rinse (as a supplement) in children younger than 6 yr old.

Usual Dosage

Prevention of dental caries

SOLUTION, GEL (CREAM), OR TABLET (2.2 mg of sodium fluoride is equivalent to 1 mg of fluoride ion)

ADULTS: *Dental rinse or gel (cream):* Rinse or brush with 10 mL daily and spit out after use.
CHILDREN: *Oral (tablets or drops)*
  Fluoride in drinking water <0.3 ppm
    YOUNGER THAN 6 MO OF AGE: None
    6 MO TO 3 YR: 0.25 mg
    3 YR TO 6 YR: 0.5 mg
    OLDER THAN 6 YR: 1.0 mg
  Fluoride in drinking water 0.3 to 0.7 ppm
    Younger than 6 mo: None
    6 MO TO 3 YR: 0.125 mg
    3 YR TO 6 YR: 0.25 mg
    OLDER THAN 6 YR: 0.5 mg
CHILDREN AGES 6 TO 12: *Dental rinse or gel (cream):* Rinse or brush with 5 to 10 mL daily and spit out after rinsing or brushing.

Pharmacokinetics

ABSORP: Well absorbed.
DIST: Distributed to calcified tissues (bone and enamel).
EXCRET: Urine, feces, breast milk; crosses placenta.

➡◀ DRUG INTERACTIONS

Antacids (magnesium-, aluminum-, and calcium-containing formulations): Decreased efficacy of fluoride (decreased absorption)
  • Avoid concurrent use.

Milk: Decreased efficacy of fluoride (decreased absorption)
- Avoid concurrent use.

ADVERSE EFFECTS

Oral: Mottled enamel (overdose).

MISC: Gastric distress; headache; weakness. Rinses and gels containing stannous fluoride may produce surface staining of the teeth; this does not occur with nonstannous fluoride topical preparations. Acidulated fluoride may dull porcelain and composite restorations.

ACUTE OVERDOSE: Back tarry stools, bloody vomitus, diarrhea, decreased respiration, increased salivation, watery eyes.

CHRONIC OVERDOSE: Hypocalcemia, tetany, respiratory arrest, constipation, loss of appetite, nausea, vomiting, weight loss.

CLINICAL IMPLICATIONS

General

- Follow manufacturer's instructions for application; tell patient not to swallow fluoride.
- Determine fluoride concentration in water supply, then calculate dosage.
- The use of fluoride supplements is not recommended when community drinking water contains at least 0.6 ppm fluoride or in children older than age 16 yr.
- Recommended doses should not be exceeded because dental fluorosis and osseous changes may occur.
- To reduce risk of accidental overdosage, ADA recommends that a limit of 264 mg sodium fluoride be dispensed in prepackaged containers.
- Tablets may be chewed; do not swallow whole; may be given with juice.
- *Tablets and drops:* Milk and other dairy products may decrease absorption of sodium fluoride; avoid simultaneous ingestion.
- Monitor children using gel or rinse; not to be swallowed.

Pregnancy Risk Category: No information available.

Oral Health Education

- *Rinses and gels:* Rinses and gels are most effective immediately after brushing or flossing and just prior to sleep. Expectorate any excess. Do not swallow. Do not eat, drink, or rinse mouth for 30 min after application.
- Notify dentist if tooth enamel becomes discolored.
- Tell parent to store product out of children's reach to prevent excessive ingestion.

Treatment of acute overdose:
- Gastric lavage with calcium chloride or calcium hydroxide solution.
- Maintain high urine output.
- Take child to hospital emergency room.

---

sodium valproate — see valproic acid and derivatives
Solaraze — see diclofenac
Solarcaine Aloe Extra Burn Relief — see lidocaine HCl
Solarcaine Medicated First-Aid Spray — see benzocaine
Solciclina — see amoxicillin
Solfoton — see phenobarbital
Solu-Cortef — see hydrocortisone
Solu-Medrol — see methylprednisolone
Solurex — see dexamethasone
Solurex LA — see dexamethasone
Soma — see carisoprodol

Sominex — see diphenhydramine HCl
Sophipren Ofteno — see prednisolone
Sophixin — see ciprofloxacin
Sorbitrate — see isosorbide dinitrate
Soriatane — see acitretin
Sotacor — see sotalol HCl

---

sotalol HCl (SOTT-uh-lahl HIGH-droe-KLOR-ide)

Betapace AF, Betapace

■✦■ Sotacor, Rhoxal-sotalol, ratio-Sotalol, PMS-Sotalol, Nu-Sotalol, Novo-Sotalol, Gen-Sotalol, Apo-Sotalol

Drug Class: Beta-adrenergic blocker

PHARMACOLOGY

Action
Blocks beta receptors, which primarily affect heart (slows rate), vascular musculature (decreases blood pressure), and lungs (reduces function).

Uses
BETAPACE: Management or prevention of life-threatening ventricular arrhythmias.
BETAPACE AF: Maintenance of normal sinus rhythm in patients with highly symptomatic atrial fibrillation/atrial flutter.

➡✦ DRUG INTERACTIONS RELATED TO DENTAL THERAPEUTICS

COX-1 inhibitors: Decreased antihypertensive effect (decreased prostaglandin synthesis)
 • Monitor blood pressure.
Sympathomimetic amines: Decreased antihypertensive effect (pharmacological antagonism)
 • Monitor blood pressure.

ADVERSE EFFECTS

⚠ **ORAL:** Dry mouth; taste disturbance; mouth ulceration.
CNS: Depression; dizziness; headache; lethargy; paresthesias; vivid dreams.
CVS: Bradycardia; ventricular arrhythmia; syncope.
RESP: Bronchospasm; difficulty breathing; wheezing.
GI: Anorexia; constipation; diarrhea; dyspepsia; flatulence; nausea; vomiting.
MISC: Agranulocytosis; thrombocytopenia; leukopenia or leukocytosis; anemia; other blood dyscrasias.

CLINICAL IMPLICATIONS

General
 • Monitor vital signs (e.g., BP, pulse pressure, rate, and rhythm) at each appointment to assess disease control. Do not provide elective dental treatment when BP is ≥180/110 or in the presence of other high-risk CV conditions. Refer to the section entitled "The Patient Taking Cardiovascular Drugs" in Chapter 6: *Clinical Medicine*.
 • Use local anesthetic agents with vasoconstrictor with caution based on functional capacity of the patient and use aspirating technique to prevent intravascular injection.
 • Determine ability to adapt to stress of dental treatment. Consider short appointments.
 • Place patient on frequent maintenance schedule to avoid periodontal inflammation.
 • Chronic dry mouth is possible; anticipate increased caries, candidiasis, and lichenoid mucositis.
 • Beta blockers may mask epinephrine-induced signs and symptoms of hypoglycemia in patients with diabetes.
 • Blood dyscrasias rarely reported; anticipate increased bleeding, infection, and poor healing.

Oral Health Education
- Encourage daily plaque control procedures for effective self-care in patient at risk for cardiovascular disease.
- If chronic dry mouth occurs, recommend home fluoride therapy and use of nonalcoholic oral health care products.

---

sparfloxacin (spar-FLOX-ah-sin)
Zagam

Drug Class: Antibiotic, fluoroquinolone

PHARMACOLOGY
Action
Interferes with microbial DNA synthesis.

Uses
Treatment of community acquired pneumonia or bacterial exacerbation of chronic bronchitis caused by susceptible organisms.

➦✦ DRUG INTERACTIONS RELATED TO DENTAL THERAPEUTICS
Corticosteroids: Possible increased risk of Achilles tendon disorder (mechanism unknown)
- Consider risk/benefit.

Oral Health Education
- If chronic dry mouth occurs, recommend home fluoride therapy and use of nonalcoholic oral health care products.

Spectracef — see cefditoren pivoxil

---

spironolactone (SPEER-oh-no-LAK-tone)
Spironolactone, Aldactone

∎✦∎ Novo-Spirozine, Novo-Spiroton

Drug Class: Diuretic, potassium-sparing

PHARMACOLOGY
Action
Competitively inhibits aldosterone in distal tubules, resulting in increased excretion of sodium and water and decreased excretion of potassium.

Uses
Short-term preoperative treatment of primary hyperaldosteronism; long-term maintenance therapy for idiopathic hyperaldosteronism; management of edematous conditions in CHF, cirrhosis and nephrotic syndrome; management of essential hypertension; treatment of hypokalemia.

Unlabeled Uses
Treatment of hirsutism; relief of premenstrual syndrome symptoms; short-term treatment of familial male precocious puberty; and short-term treatment of acne vulgaris.

➦✦ DRUG INTERACTIONS RELATED TO DENTAL THERAPEUTICS
No documented drug-drug interactions. The absence of evidence is not evidence of safety.

ADVERSE EFFECTS
⚠ **ORAL:** Dry mouth; thirst.
CNS: Drowsiness; lethargy; headache; mental confusion; ataxia.
GI: Cramping; diarrhea; gastric bleeding; gastric ulceration; gastritis; vomiting.

MISC: Gynecomastia; irregular menses or amenorrhea; postmenopausal bleeding; hirsutism; deepening of voice; drug fever; agranulocytosis.

CLINICAL IMPLICATIONS

General
- Determine why drug is being taken. Consider implications of condition on dental treatment.
- Determine ability to adapt to stress of dental treatment. Consider short appointments.
- Monitor vital signs (e.g., BP, pulse pressure, rate, and rhythm) at each appointment to assess disease control. Do not provide elective dental treatment when BP is ≥180/110 or in the presence of other high-risk CV conditions. Refer to the section entitled "The Patient Taking Cardiovascular Drugs" in Chapter 6: *Clinical Medicine*.
- Use local anesthetic agents with vasoconstrictor with caution based on functional capacity of the patient and use aspirating technique to prevent intravascular injection.
- Chronic dry mouth is possible; anticipate increased caries, candidiasis, and lichenoid mucositis.
- Place patient on frequent maintenance schedule to avoid periodontal inflammation.
- Blood dyscrasias rarely reported; anticipate increased infection and poor healing.

Oral Health Education
- Encourage daily plaque control procedures for effective self-care in patient at risk for cardiovascular disease.
- If chronic dry mouth occurs, recommend home fluoride therapy and use of nonalcoholic oral health care products.

Sporanox — see itraconazole

S-P-T — see thyroid, desiccated

S-T Cort — see hydrocortisone

Stagesic — see acetaminophen/hydrocodone bitartrate

Stannous Fluoride — see sodium fluoride

Starlix — see nateglinide

Statex — see morphine sulfate

---

stavudine (STAV-yoo-deen)

Zerit, Zerit XR

Drug Class: Antiretroviral, nucleoside reverse transcriptase inhibitor

PHARMACOLOGY

Action
Inhibits replication of HIV.

Uses
For the treatment of HIV-1 infection in combination with other antiretroviral agents.

➡️⬅️ DRUG INTERACTIONS RELATED TO DENTAL THERAPEUTICS

No documented drug-drug interactions. The absence of evidence is not evidence of safety.

ADVERSE EFFECTS

CNS: Peripheral neuropathy; headache; insomnia.
GI: Pancreatitis (may be fatal); diarrhea; nausea and vomiting; abdominal pain; anorexia.
MISC: Allergic reaction; chills/fever; myalgia.

CLINICAL IMPLICATIONS

General
- Determine why drug is being taken. Consider implications of condition on dental treatment.

- This drug is frequently prescribed in combination with one or more other antiviral agents. Side effects of all agents must be considered during the drug review process.
- Antibiotic prophylaxis should be considered when <500 PMN/mm^3 are reported; elective dental treatment should be delayed until blood values are above this level.
- Consider medical consult to determine disease control and influence on dental treatment.
- Anticipate oral candidiasis when HIV disease is reported.
- Place patient on frequent maintenance schedule to avoid periodontal inflammation.
- If GI side effects occur, consider semisupine chair position.

Oral Health Education
- Encourage daily plaque control procedures for effective self-care because HIV infection reduces host resistance.

STCC-Fluoxetine — see fluoxetine HCl

Sterapred — see prednisone

Sterapred DS — see prednisone

Stieva-A — see tretinoin

St. Joseph Adult Chewable Aspirin — see aspirin

St. Joseph Cough Suppressant — see dextromethorphan HBr

Stop — see sodium fluoride

stradiol cypionate — see estradiol

Strattera — see atomoxetine

Suboxone — see buprenorphine HCl/naloxone HCl

Subutex — see buprenorphine HCl

---

sucralfate (sue-KRAL-fate)
Carafate

■✦■ **PMS-Sucralfate, Nu-Sucralfate, Novo-Sucralfate**

■✦■ **Antepsin**

Drug Class: GI

PHARMACOLOGY

Action
Adheres to ulcer in acidic gastric juice, forming protective layer that serves as barrier against acid, bile salts, and enzymes present in stomach and duodenum.

Uses
Short-term treatment of duodenal ulcer; maintenance therapy of duodenal ulcer (tablets only).

Unlabeled Uses
Treatment of gastric ulcers; reflux and peptic esophagitis; treatment of NSAID- or aspirin-induced GI symptoms and mucosal damage; prevention of stress ulcers and GI bleeding in critically ill patients; treatment of oral and esophageal ulcers caused by radiation, chemotherapy, and sclerotherapy; treatment of oral ulcerations and dysphagia in patients with epidermolysis bullosa.

�➤ DRUG INTERACTIONS RELATED TO DENTAL THERAPEUTICS

Ketoconazole: Decreased ketoconazole effect (decreased absorption)
- Avoid concurrent use.

ADVERSE EFFECTS

⚠ **ORAL:** Dry mouth.
CNS: Dizziness; insomnia; vertigo; headache.
GI: Constipation (2%); diarrhea; nausea; vomiting; indigestion; flatulence.
MISC: Back pain.

CLINICAL IMPLICATIONS

General

- If patient has GI disease, consider semisupine chair position.
- Use COX inhibitors with caution; they may exacerbate PUD and GERD.
- Chronic dry mouth is possible; anticipate increased caries and candidiasis.

Sucrets 4-hr Cough — see dextromethorphan HBr

Sucrets Cough Control — see dextromethorphan HBr

Sudafed — see pseudoephedrine

Sudafed 12 Hour Caplets — see pseudoephedrine

Sudafed Decongestant 12 Hour — see pseudoephedrine

Sudafed Decongestant Children's — see pseudoephedrine

Sudafed Decongestant Extra Strength — see pseudoephedrine

Sudex — see pseudoephedrine

Suiflox — see ciprofloxacin

Sular — see nisoldipine

sulfamethoxazole/trimethoprim — see trimethoprim/sulfamethoxazole

---

sulfasalazine (SULL-fuh-SAL-uh-zeen)

Azulfidine EN-tabs, Azulfidine

■✦■ **Salazopyrin EN-tabs, Salazopyrin Desensitizing Kit, Salazopyrin, ratio-Sulfasalazine**

Drug Class: Anti-infective, sulfonamide

PHARMACOLOGY

Action

Competitively antagonizes paraaminobenzoic acid (PABA), an essential component in folic acid synthesis.

Uses

Treatment of ulcerative colitis; rheumatoid arthritis and juvenile rheumatoid arthritis (enteric-coated tablets).

Unlabeled Uses

Treatment of ankylosing spondylitis, collagenous colitis, Crohn disease, psoriasis, psoriatic arthritis.

➡✦ DRUG INTERACTIONS RELATED TO DENTAL THERAPEUTICS

No documented drug-drug interactions. The absence of evidence is not evidence of safety.

ADVERSE EFFECTS

CNS: Headache; insomnia; peripheral neuropathy; depression; convulsions.
GI: Nausea; vomiting; abdominal pain; diarrhea; anorexia; pancreatitis; impaired folic acid absorption; pseudomembranous enterocolitis.
RESP: Pulmonary infiltrates.

MISC: Drug fever; chills; pyrexia; arthralgia; myalgia; periarteritis nodosum; lupus erythematosus phenomenon.

CLINICAL IMPLICATIONS
General
- Determine why drug is being taken. Consider implications of condition on dental treatment.
- *Arthritis:* Consider patient comfort and need for semisupine chair position.
- If GI side effects occur, consider semisupine chair position.

Oral Health Education
- Evaluate manual dexterity; consider need for power toothbrush.

Sulfatrim — see trimethoprim/sulfamethoxazole

---

sulfisoxazole (sull-fih-SOX-uh-zole)
Gantrisin Pediatric

Drug Class: Anti-infective, sulfonamide

PHARMACOLOGY
Action
Exerts bacteriostatic action by competing with paraaminobenzoic acid (PABA), an essential component in folic acid synthesis, thus preventing synthesis of folic acid, needed by bacteria for growth.

Uses
ORAL: Treatment of UTI, chancroid, inclusion conjunctivitis, malaria, meningitis caused by *Haemophilus influenzae* or meningococci, nocardiosis, acute otitis media, toxoplasmosis, and trachoma.

OPHTHALMIC: Treatment of conjunctivitis, corneal ulcer, and superficial ocular infections, adjunct to systemic sulfonamide therapy of trachoma.

Unlabeled Uses
ORAL: Treatment of recurrent otitis media.

➡️⬅ DRUG INTERACTIONS RELATED TO DENTAL THERAPEUTICS
No documented drug-drug interactions. The absence of evidence is not evidence of safety.

ADVERSE EFFECTS
CNS: Headache; peripheral neuropathy; depression; convulsions; dizziness; ataxia.
GI: Nausea; vomiting; abdominal pain; diarrhea; anorexia; pancreatitis; impaired folic acid absorption; pseudomembranous enterocolitis.
RESP: Pulmonary infiltrates.
MISC: Drug fever; chills; pyrexia; arthralgia; myalgia; periarteritis nodosum; lupus erythematosus phenomenon. Hypersensitivity reactions may present as erythema multiforme of Stevens-Johnson type, generalized skin eruptions, allergic myocarditis, epidermal necrolysis with or without corneal damage, urticaria, serum sickness; pruritus, exfoliative dermatitis, anaphylactoid reactions, periorbital edema, photosensitization, arthralgia, and transient pulmonary changes with eosinophilia and decreased pulmonary function.

CLINICAL IMPLICATIONS
General
- Determine why drug is being taken. Take precautions to avoid cross-contamination of microorganisms.
- If oral infection occurs that requires antibiotic therapy, select an appropriate product from a different class of anti-infectives.

sulindac (sull-IN-dak)

Clinoril

◼◆◼ Nu-Sulindac, Novo-Sundac, APO-Sulin

◼◆◼ Copal, Kenalin

Drug Class: Analgesic; NSAID

PHARMACOLOGY

Action

Decreases inflammation, pain, and fever, probably through inhibition of cyclooxygenase activity and prostaglandin synthesis.

Uses

Treatment of acute and chronic rheumatoid arthritis and osteoarthritis, ankylosing spondylitis, acute gouty arthritis, acute painful shoulder, tendinitis, bursitis.

Unlabeled Uses

Treatment of juvenile rheumatoid arthritis and sunburn.

➡◆ DRUG INTERACTIONS RELATED TO DENTAL THERAPEUTICS

No documented drug-drug interactions. The absence of evidence is not evidence of safety.

ADVERSE EFFECTS

⚠ **ORAL:** Stomatitis; dry mucous membranes.

CNS: Dizziness; headaches; nervousness; anxiety; vertigo; lightheadedness; drowsiness; somnolence; tiredness; insomnia; depression; psychic disturbances; seizures; syncope; aseptic meningitis.

GI: Peptic ulceration; GI bleeding; GI pain; dyspepsia; nausea; vomiting; diarrhea; constipation; pancreatitis; flatulence; anorexia; GI cramps; abdominal distress.

RESP: Bronchospasm; laryngeal edema; rhinitis, dyspnea, pharyngitis; hemoptysis; shortness of breath.

CLINICAL IMPLICATIONS

General

- Determine why drug is being taken. Consider implications of condition on dental treatment.
- *Arthritis:* Consider patient comfort and need for semisupine chair position.
- If GI side effects occur, consider semisupine chair position.
- Chronic dry mouth is possible; anticipate increased caries and candidiasis.

Oral Health Education

- Evaluate manual dexterity; consider need for power toothbrush.
- If chronic dry mouth occurs, recommend home fluoride therapy and use of nonalcoholic oral health care products.

---

sumatriptan (SUE-muh-TRIP-tan)

Imitrex

◼◆◼ Imigran

Drug Class: Analgesic; Migraine

PHARMACOLOGY

Action

Selective agonist for vascular serotonin (5-HT) receptor subtype, causing vasoconstriction of cranial arteries.

Uses

Acute treatment of migraine attacks with/without aura; treatment of acute cluster headaches (injection only).

➡◆ DRUG INTERACTIONS RELATED TO DENTAL THERAPEUTICS

No documented drug-drug interactions. The absence of evidence is not evidence of safety.

ADVERSE EFFECTS

⚠ **ORAL:** Mouth or tongue discomfort (5%); jaw discomfort (2%), dry mouth.

CNS: Dizziness/vertigo (12%); paresthesia (5%); drowsiness/sedation, malaise or fatigue (3%); headache (2%); anxiety (1%); phonophobia, photophobia (≥1%); vasculitis; cerebrovascular accident; dysphasia; subarachnoid hemorrhage; panic disorder.

GI: Nausea, vomiting (4% [14% intranasal]); abdominal discomfort, dysphagia (1%); diarrhea, gastric symptoms (≥1%); ischemic colitis with rectal bleeding.

RESP: Bronchospasm (1%); dyspnea (≥1%).

MISC: Tingling (14%); warm/hot sensation (11%); burning sensation (8%); feeling of heaviness or pressure (7%); feeling of tightness, numbness (5%); tightness in chest, cold sensation (3%); pressure in chest, feeling strange, head tightness, pain (2%).

CLINICAL IMPLICATIONS

General

- Determine why drug is being taken. Consider implications of condition on dental treatment.
- Monitor vital signs (e.g., BP and pulse). Drugs for prevention are sympatholytic; drugs for treatment of acute attack are sympathomimetic.
- *Photophobia:* Direct dental light out of patient's eyes and offer dark glasses for comfort.
- Chronic dry mouth is possible; anticipate increased caries and candidiasis.

Oral Health Education

- If chronic dry mouth occurs, recommend home fluoride therapy and use of nonalcoholic oral health care products.

Sumycin 250 — see tetracycline HCl

Sumycin 500 — see tetracycline HCl

Sumycin Syrup — see tetracycline HCl

Supeudol — see oxycodone HCl

Suppress — see dextromethorphan HBr

Supradol — see naproxen

Suprax — see cefixime

Surgicel — see oxidized cellulose

Sustiva — see efavirenz

Sydolil — see ergotamine tartrate

Sylphen Cough — see diphenhydramine HCl

Symmetrel — see amantadine HCl

Synalgos-DC — see narcotic analgesic combinations

Syngestal — see norethindrone acetate

synthetic conjugated estrogens — see estrogens, synthetic conjugated, a or b

Synthroid — see levothyroxine sodium

Syscor — see nisoldipine

Systen — see estradiol

T3 — see liothyronine sodium
T4 — see levothyroxine sodium
Tac-3 — see triamcinolone

---

tacrine HCl (TAK-reen HIGH-droe-KLOR-ide)

Synonyms: tetrahydroaminoacridine; THA

Cognex

Drug Class: Reversible cholinesterase inhibitor

PHARMACOLOGY

Action
Believed to inhibit (reversibly) cholinesterase in CNS, leading to increased concentrations of acetylcholine.

Uses
Treatment of mild to moderate dementia of Alzheimer type.

➡◀ DRUG INTERACTIONS RELATED TO DENTAL THERAPEUTICS
No documented drug-drug interactions. The absence of evidence is not evidence of safety.

ADVERSE EFFECTS
⚠ **ORAL:** Glossitis, dry mouth, stomatitis (1%); salivation.

CNS: Dizziness (12%); headache (11%); agitation, confusion (7%); ataxia, insomnia (6%); depression, fatigue, somnolence (4%); abnormal thinking, anxiety (3%); tremor, hallucinations, hostility (2%); convulsions, vertigo, syncope, hyperkinesias, paresthesia, nervousness (≥1%).

CVS: Hypotension, hypertension (>1%); atrial fibrillation; palpitation.

GI: Nausea/vomiting (28%); diarrhea (16%); dyspepsia, anorexia (9%); abdominal pain (8%); flatulence, constipation (4%).

RESP: Coughing, URI (3%); bronchitis, pneumonia, dyspnea (≥1%).

MISC: Elevated transaminases (29%); chest pain (4%); back pain, asthenia, purpura (2%); chills, fever, malaise, peripheral edema (≥1%).

CLINICAL IMPLICATIONS

General
- Patient may experience hypotension or hypertension. Monitor vital signs at each appointment; anticipate syncope.
- Ensure that caregiver is present at every dental appointment and understands informed consent.
- Place on frequent maintenance schedule to avoid periodontal inflammation.
- If GI side effects occur, consider semisupine chair position.
- Chronic dry mouth is possible; anticipate increased caries and candidiasis.

Oral Health Education
- Teach caregiver to assist patient with oral self-care practices.
- If chronic dry mouth occurs, recommend home fluoride therapy and use of nonalcoholic oral health care products.
- Evaluate manual dexterity; consider need for power toothbrush.

---

tacrolimus (tack-CROW-lih-muss)

(FK506)

Prograf, Protopic

Drug Class: Immunosuppressive

PHARMACOLOGY

Action

Suppresses cell-mediated immune reactions and some humoral immunity, but exact mechanism is not known.

Uses

PO AND IV: Prophylaxis of organ rejection in patients receiving allogenic liver or kidney transplants. Used in conjunction with adrenal corticosteroids.
TOPICAL: Atopic dermatitis.

Unlabeled Uses

Prophylaxis of rejection for patients receiving kidney, bone marrow, cardiac, pancreas, pancreatic island cell, and small bowel transplantation.

➡⬅ DRUG INTERACTIONS RELATED TO DENTAL THERAPEUTICS

Fluconazole, ketoconazole, or itraconazole: Possible tacrolimus toxicity (decreased metabolism)
  • Avoid concurrent use.
Clarithromycin: Tacrolimus toxicity (decreased metabolism)
  • Avoid concurrent use.
Metronidazole: Possible tacrolimus toxicity (decreased metabolism)
  • Avoid concurrent use.

ADVERSE EFFECTS

CNS: Headache; insomnia; anxiety; paresthesia; tremor, weakness, abnormal dreams, agitation, confusion (oral and IV); depression, dizziness, migraine, neuritis (topical).
CVS: Chest pain, hypertension (47% to 56%); hyperkalemia (45%); postural hypotension (3% to 15%).
GI: Diarrhea; nausea; constipation; anorexia; vomiting; abdominal pain; dyspepsia, gastroenteritis, gastritis (topical).
RESP: Dyspnea; pleural effusion, atelectasis (oral and IV); increased cough, asthma, bronchitis, pneumonia, hypoxia, lung disorder (topical).
MISC: Fever; pain; back pain; ascites (oral and IV); flu-like symptoms, allergic reaction, infection, accidental injury, lack of drug effect, lymphadenopathy, face edema, hyperesthesia, varicella zoster/herpes zoster, asthenia, periodontal abscess, myalgia, cyst, arthralgia, arthritis, anaphylactoid reaction, angioedema, breast pain, cheilitis, chills, dehydration, epistaxis, exacerbation of untreated area, hernia, malaise, neck pain, photosensitivity (topical); anemia (5% to 47%); thrombocytopenia (14% to 24%); leukocytosis.

CLINICAL IMPLICATIONS

General

  • Determine why drug is being taken. Consider implications of condition on dental treatment.
  • Consider medical consult to determine disease control and influence on dental treatment.
  • Blood dyscrasias reported; anticipate increased bleeding, infection, and poor healing.
  • *Postural hypotension:* Monitor BP at the beginning and end of each appointment; anticipate syncope. Have patient sit upright for several min at the end of the dental appointment before dismissing.
  • If GI side effects occur, consider semisupine chair position.

Oral Health Education

  • Determine need for power toothbrush for self-care.
  • Encourage daily plaque control procedures for effective self-care.

tadalafil (tah-DAH-lah-fil)
Cialis
Drug Class: Agent for impotence

PHARMACOLOGY
Action
Enhances the effect of nitric oxide at the nerve ending and endothelial cells in the corpus cavernosum by inhibiting phosphodiesterase type 5 in the corpus cavernosum of the penis. This results in vasodilation, increased inflow of blood into the corporus cavernosum, and ensuing penile erection upon sexual stimulation.

Uses
Treatment of erectile dysfunction.

➜← DRUG INTERACTIONS RELATED TO DENTAL THERAPEUTICS
No documented drug-drug interactions. The absence of evidence is not evidence of safety.

ADVERSE EFFECTS
⚠ **ORAL:** Dry mouth, dysphagia, esophagitis (<2%).
CNS: Headache (15%); fatigue, dizziness, hypesthesia, insomnia, paresthesia, somnolence, vertigo (<2%).
CVS: Hypotension; vasodilation.
GI: Dyspepsia (10%); diarrhea (<2%).
RESP: Epistaxis, pharyngitis (<2%).
MISC: Back pain (6%); limb pain, flushing (3%); asthenia, face edema, pain (<2%).

CLINICAL IMPLICATIONS
General
- Concurrent administration with nitroglycerin may lead to severe hypotension. Avoid concurrent use.
- Tadalafil is long-acting; monitor vital signs for cardiovascular effects.
- Chronic dry mouth is possible; anticipate increased caries activity and candidiasis.
- *For back pain:* Consider semisupine chair position for patient comfort.

Tafil — see alprazolam

Tagamet — see cimetidine

Tagamet HB — see cimetidine

Talacen — see pentazocine

Talpramin — see imipramine HCl

Talwin — see pentazocine

Talwin Compound — see pentazocine

Talwin NX — see pentazocine

Tambocor — see flecainide acetate

Tamiflu — see oseltamivir phosphate

Tamofen — see tamoxifen citrate

Tamoxan — see tamoxifen citrate

---

tamoxifen citrate (ta-MOX-ih-fen SI-trait)
Nolvadex
■✦■ **Apo-Tamox, Gen-Tamoxifen, Nolvadex-D, Novo-Tamoxifen, PMS-Tamoxifen, Tamofen**

■◢■ **Bilem, Cryoxifeno, Tamoxan, Taxus, Tecnofen**

Drug Class: Antiestrogen hormone

PHARMACOLOGY

Action

A nonsteroidal agent with antiestrogenic properties.

Uses

Breast carcinoma in women; metastatic breast carcinoma in men and women; reduction in risk of breast cancer in high-risk women; lower risk of invasive breast cancer in women with ductal carcinoma in situ.

Unlabeled Uses

Mastalgia; decreasing the size and pain of gynecomastia; McCune-Albright syndrome in female pediatric patients (in combination with other agents).

➡️⬅️ DRUG INTERACTIONS RELATED TO DENTAL THERAPEUTICS

No documented drug-drug interactions. The absence of evidence is not evidence of safety.

ADVERSE EFFECTS

⚠ **ORAL:** Taste disturbance; food distaste.

CNS: Headache; dizziness; depression.

GI: Moderate to low potential for nausea and vomiting.

MISC: At doses of 40 mg/day, tamoxifen has increased the risk of endometrial cancer; hot flashes.

CLINICAL IMPLICATIONS

General

- Determine why drug is being taken. Consider implications of condition on dental treatment.
- Consider medical consult to determine disease control and influence on dental treatment.

Oral Health Education

- Encourage daily plaque control procedures for effective self-care.

---

tamsulosin HCl (tam-SOO-loe-sin HIGH-droe-KLOR-ide)

Flomax

Drug Class: Antiadrenergic, peripherally acting

PHARMACOLOGY

Action

Selectively blocks alpha$_1$-adrenergic receptors causing relaxation of prostate smooth muscle resulting in an increase in urinary flow rate and a reduction in symptoms of BPH.

Uses

Treatment of signs and symptoms of benign prostatic hyperplasia.

➡️⬅️ DRUG INTERACTIONS RELATED TO DENTAL THERAPEUTICS

No documented drug-drug interactions. The absence of evidence is not evidence of safety.

ADVERSE EFFECTS

⚠ **ORAL:** Tooth disorder (2%).

CNS: Headache (21%); dizziness (17%); somnolence (4%); decreased libido (2%); insomnia (1%).

CVS: Chest pain (4%).

GI: Diarrhea (6%); nausea (4%).
RESP: Increased cough (5%); sinusitis (4%).
MISC: Infection (11%); asthenia (9%); back pain (8%).

CLINICAL IMPLICATIONS
General
• If respiratory or musculoskeletal side effects occur, consider semisupine chair position.

Tandax — see naproxen
Tapanol Extra Strength — see acetaminophen
Tapanol Regular Strength — see acetaminophen
Tapazole — see methimazole
Taro-Carbamazepine — see carbamazepine
Taro-Sone — see betamethasone
Taro-Warfarin — see warfarin
Tasmar — see tolcapone
Tavanic — see levofloxacin
Tavist — see clemastine fumarate
Tavist Allergy — see clemastine fumarate
Tavist ND — see loratadine
Tavor — see oxybutynin Cl
Taxus — see tamoxifen citrate
Taziken — see terbutaline sulfate
Taztia XT — see diltiazem HCl
Tebrazid — see pyrazinamide
Tecnofen — see tamoxifen citrate
Tegretol — see carbamazepine
Tegretol XR — see carbamazepine
Teladar — see betamethasone

---

telithromycin (tel-ITH-roe-MY-sin)
Ketek
Drug Class: Antibiotic

PHARMACOLOGY
Action
Interferes with microbial protein synthesis.

Uses
Treatment of acute bacterial exacerbation of chronic bronchitis, acute bacterial sinusitis, and community-acquired pneumonia caused by strains of susceptible organisms.

➼← DRUG INTERACTIONS RELATED TO DENTAL THERAPEUTICS
No documented drug-drug interactions. The absence of evidence is not evidence of safety.

ADVERSE EFFECTS
⚠ **ORAL:** Dry mouth; oral candidiasis; glossitis; stomatitis.

CNS: Headache (6%); dizziness (4%); somnolence, insomnia, vertigo, increased sweating, fatigue (<2%).

GI: Diarrhea (11%); nausea (8%); vomiting (3%); loose stools, dysgeusia (2%); abdominal distension, dyspepsia, GI upset, flatulence, constipation, gastroenteritis, gastritis, anorexia, watery stools, abdominal pain, upper abdominal pain (<2%).

MISC: Allergy, including face edema, angioedema, anaphylaxis.

CLINICAL IMPLICATIONS
General
- Determine why drug is being taken. Take precautions to avoid cross-contamination of microorganisms.
- If oral infection occurs that requires antibiotic therapy, select an appropriate product from a different class of anti-infectives.
- Prolonged use of antibiotics may result in bacterial or fungal overgrowth of nonsusceptible microorganisms; anticipate candidiasis.
- Chronic dry mouth is possible; anticipate increased caries and candidiasis.
- If GI side effects occur, consider semisupine chair position.

Oral Health Education
- If chronic dry mouth occurs, recommend home fluoride therapy and use of nonalcoholic oral health care products.

---

telmisartan (tell-mih-SAHR-tan)
Micardis

Drug Class: Antihypertensive; Angiotensin II antagonist

PHARMACOLOGY
Action
Antagonizes the effect of angiotensin II (vasoconstriction and aldosterone secretion) by blocking the angiotensin II (AT_1 receptor) in vascular smooth muscle and the adrenal gland, producing decreased BP.

Uses
Treatment of hypertension.

➡️⬅ DRUG INTERACTIONS RELATED TO DENTAL THERAPEUTICS
No documented drug-drug interactions. The absence of evidence is not evidence of safety.

ADVERSE EFFECTS
⚠ **ORAL:** Dry mouth.
GI: Diarrhea (3%).
RESP: URI (7%).
CVS: Palpitation.
MISC: Back pain (3%).

CLINICAL IMPLICATIONS
General
- Monitor vital signs (e.g., BP, pulse pressure, rate, and rhythm) at each appointment to assess disease control. Do not provide elective dental treatment when BP is ≥180/110 or in the presence of other high-risk CV conditions. Refer to the section entitled "The Patient Taking Cardiovascular Drugs" in Chapter 6: *Clinical Medicine*.
- Use local anesthetic agents with vasoconstrictor with caution based on functional capacity of the patient and use aspirating technique to prevent intravascular injection.
- Determine ability to adapt to stress of dental treatment. Consider short appointments.
- Chronic dry mouth is possible; anticipate increased caries, candidiasis, and lichenoid mucositis.
- Place on frequent maintenance schedule to avoid periodontal inflammation.

Oral Health Education
- Encourage daily plaque control procedures for effective self-care in patient at risk for CV disease.
- If chronic dry mouth occurs, recommend home fluoride therapy and use of nonalcoholic oral health care products.

temazepam (tem-AZE-uh-pam)

Restoril

■✦■ **Apo-Temazepam, Gen-Temazepam, Novo-Temazepam, Nu-Temazepam, PMS-Temazepam**

Drug Class: Sedative; Hypnotic; Benzodiazepine
DEA Schedule: Schedule IV (Canada: Schedule F)

PHARMACOLOGY

Action
Potentiates action of GABA (gamma-aminobutyric acid), an inhibitory neurotransmitter, resulting in increased neuronal inhibition and CNS depression, especially in limbic system and reticular formation.

Uses
Short-term management of insomnia.

➜◆ DRUG INTERACTIONS RELATED TO DENTAL THERAPEUTICS
No documented drug-drug interactions. The absence of evidence is not evidence of safety.

ADVERSE EFFECTS
⚠ **ORAL:** Taste alteration; dry mouth.
CNS: Drowsiness; dizziness; lethargy; confusion; euphoria; weakness; falling; ataxia; hallucinations; paradoxical reactions (e.g., excitement, agitation); headache; memory impairment.
CVS: Palpitation; tachycardia.
GI: Anorexia; diarrhea; abdominal cramping; constipation; nausea; vomiting.
MISC: Tolerance; physical and psychological dependence; slurred speech; elevated AST, ALT, bilirubin; leukopenia; granulocytopenia.

CLINICAL IMPLICATIONS

General
- Chronic dry mouth is possible; anticipate increased caries activity and candidiasis.
- Monitor vital signs.
- Blood dyscrasias rarely reported; anticipate increased infection and poor healing.

Oral Health Education
- If chronic dry mouth occurs, recommend home fluoride therapy and use of nonalcoholic oral health care products.

Temgesic — see buprenorphine HCl

Temovate — see clobetasol propionate

Temovate Emollient — see clobetasol propionate

Temperal — see acetaminophen

Tempra — see acetaminophen

Tempra 1 — see acetaminophen

Tempra 2 Syrup — see acetaminophen

Tempra 3 — see acetaminophen

Tenex — see guanfacine HCl
Ten-K — see potassium products

---

tenofovir disoproxil fumarate (teh-NOE-fo-veer DIE-so-prox-ill FYU-mah-rate)

Viread

Drug Class: Antiretroviral, nucleotide analog reverse transcriptase inhibitor

PHARMACOLOGY

Action

Tenofovir disoproxil fumarate is a prodrug of tenofovir, which inhibits the activity of HIV reverse transcriptase by competing with deoxyadenosine 5'-triphosphate and by DNA chain termination after incorporation into DNA.

Uses

Treatment of HIV-1 infection in combination with other antiretroviral agents.

➜ DRUG INTERACTIONS RELATED TO DENTAL THERAPEUTICS

No documented drug-drug interactions. The absence of evidence is not evidence of safety.

ADVERSE EFFECTS

CNS: Asthenia (11%); headache, depression (8%); peripheral neuropathy (5%); insomnia (4%); dizziness (3%).

GI: Diarrhea (16%); nausea (11%); abdominal pain, vomiting (7%); anorexia, dyspepsia, flatulence (4%); pancreatitis.

RESP: Pneumonia (3%), dyspnea (postmarketing).

MISC: Pain (12%); fever (4%); chest pain (3%).

CLINICAL IMPLICATIONS

General

- Determine why drug is being taken. Consider implications of condition on dental treatment.
- Consider medical consult to determine disease control and influence on dental treatment.
- This drug is frequently prescribed in combination with one or more other antiviral agents. Side effects of all agents must be considered during the drug review process.
- Antibiotic prophylaxis should be considered when <500 PMN/mm^3 are reported; elective dental treatment should be delayed until blood values are above this level.
- Anticipate oral candidiasis when HIV disease is reported.
- Place on frequent maintenance schedule to avoid periodontal inflammation.

Oral Health Education

- Encourage daily plaque control procedures for effective self-care because HIV infection reduces host resistance.

Tenormin — see atenolol
Teolong — see theophylline
Tequin — see gatifloxacin

---

terazosin (ter-AZE-oh-sin)

Hytrin

■✦■ **Apo-Terazosin, Novo-Terazosin, Nu-Terazosin, PMS-Terazosin, ratio-Terazosin**

■◆■ Adecur

Drug Class: Antihypertensive; Antiadrenergic, peripherally acting

PHARMACOLOGY

Action

Selectively blocks postsynaptic alpha$_1$-adrenergic receptors, resulting in dilation of arteries and veins.

Uses

Management of hypertension and symptomatic BPH.

➡◆ DRUG INTERACTIONS RELATED TO DENTAL THERAPEUTICS

No documented drug-drug interactions. The absence of evidence is not evidence of safety.

ADVERSE EFFECTS

⚠ **ORAL:** Dry mouth.

CNS: Dizziness; nervousness; paresthesia; somnolence; anxiety; headache; insomnia; weakness; drowsiness.

CVS: Postural hypotension (4%).

GI: Nausea; vomiting; diarrhea; constipation; abdominal discomfort or pain; flatulence.

RESP: Dyspnea; bronchitis; bronchospasm; flu-like symptoms; increased cough.

MISC: Shoulder, neck, back, or extremity pain; arthralgia; edema; fever; weight gain; thrombocytopenia.

CLINICAL IMPLICATIONS

General

- Monitor vital signs (e.g., BP, pulse pressure, rate, and rhythm) at each appointment to assess disease control. Do not provide elective dental treatment when BP is ≥180/110 or in the presence of other high-risk CV conditions. Refer to the section entitled "The Patient Taking Cardiovascular Drugs" in Chapter 6: *Clinical Medicine*.
- Use local anesthetic agents with vasoconstrictor with caution based on functional capacity of the patient and use aspirating technique to prevent intravascular injection.
- Determine ability to adapt to stress of dental treatment. Consider short appointments.
- *Postural hypotension:* Monitor BP at the beginning and end of each appointment; anticipate syncope. Have patient sit upright for several min at the end of the dental appointment before dismissing.
- Chronic dry mouth is possible; anticipate increased caries and candidiasis.
- Blood dyscrasias rarely reported; anticipate increased bleeding.
- If musculoskeletal pain occurs, consider semisupine chair position for patient comfort.

Oral Health Education

- Encourage daily plaque control procedures for effective self-care in patient at risk for CV disease.
- If chronic dry mouth occurs, recommend home fluoride therapy and use of nonalcoholic oral health care products.

---

terbinafine (TER-bin-a-feen)

Lamisil, Lamisil AT

■✶■ Apo-Terbinafine, Gen-Terbinafine, Novo-Terbinafine, PMS-Terbinafine

Drug Class: Anti-infective; Antifungal

PHARMACOLOGY

Action

Inhibits squalene epoxidase, resulting in ergosterol deficiency and a corresponding accumulation of squalene within the fungal cell leading to fungal cell death.

Uses

Treatment of onychomycosis caused by dermatophytes.

TOPICAL: Interdigital tinea pedis, tinea cruris, or tinea corporis caused by *Epidermophyton floccosum*, *Trichophyton mentagrophytes*, or *T. rubrum*.

Unlabeled Uses

Cutaneous candidiasis, pityriasis (tinea) versicolor (topical).

➜◀ DRUG INTERACTIONS RELATED TO DENTAL THERAPEUTICS

No documented drug-drug interactions. The absence of evidence is not evidence of safety.

ADVERSE EFFECTS

⚠ ORAL: Taste disturbance.

GI: Abdominal pain; diarrhea; dyspepsia; flatulence; nausea.

MISC: Headache; liver enzyme abnormalities; visual disturbance.

CLINICAL IMPLICATIONS

General

• If GI side effects occur, consider semisupine chair position.

---

terbutaline sulfate (ter-BYOO-tuh-leen SULL-fate)

Brethaire, Brethine, Bricanyl

■✚■ **Bricanyl Turbuhaler**

■◆■ **Taziken**

Drug Class: Bronchodilator; Sympathomimetic

PHARMACOLOGY

Action

Produces bronchodilation by relaxing bronchial smooth muscle through beta$_2$-receptor stimulation.

Uses

Treatment of reversible bronchospasm associated with asthma, bronchitis, and emphysema.

➜◀ DRUG INTERACTIONS RELATED TO DENTAL THERAPEUTICS

No documented drug-drug interactions. The absence of evidence is not evidence of safety.

ADVERSE EFFECTS

⚠ ORAL: Taste disturbance.

CNS: Stimulation; tremor; dizziness; nervousness; drowsiness; headache; weakness.

CVS: Palpitations (23%); tachycardia, chest tightness, arrhythmia; ECG changes (e.g., sinus pause, atrial premature beats, AV block, ventricular premature beats, ST–T-wave depression, T-wave inversion, sinus bradycardia, atrial escape beat with aberrant conduction); increased heart rate.

GI: Nausea; vomiting; GI distress.

RESP: Dyspnea.

MISC: Flushing; sweating; muscle cramps; hypersensitivity vasculitis; muscle cramps; central stimulations; pain at injection site; elevations in liver enzymes; seizures; hypersensitivity vasculitis.

CLINICAL IMPLICATIONS

General

• Determine why drug is being taken. Consider implications of condition on dental treatment.

- Be aware that sulfites in local anesthetic with vasoconstrictor can precipitate acute asthma attack in susceptible individuals.
- Monitor vital signs (e.g., BP, pulse rate, respiratory rate and function); uncontrolled disease characterized by wheezing and coughing.
- Acute bronchoconstriction can occur during dental treatment, have bronchodilator inhaler available.
- Ensure that bronchodilator inhaler is present at each dental appointment.

Oral Health Education
- Request patient bring bronchodilator inhaler to each dental appointment.

teriparatide (TEH-rih-PAR-ah-TIDE)
Forteo
Drug Class: Parathyroid hormone

PHARMACOLOGY
Action
Regulates bone metabolism, renal tubular reabsorption of calcium and phosphate, and intestinal calcium reabsorption.

Uses
Treatment of postmenopausal women with osteoporosis who are at high risk for fracture (i.e., history of osteoporotic fracture); increase bone mass in men with primary or hypogonadal osteoporosis who are at high risk of fracture (i.e., history of osteoporotic fracture).

➔◆ DRUG INTERACTIONS RELATED TO DENTAL THERAPEUTICS
No documented drug-drug interactions. The absence of evidence is not evidence of safety.

ADVERSE EFFECTS
⚠ **ORAL:** Tooth disorder (unspecified).
CNS: Dizziness; headache; insomnia; depression; vertigo.
CVS: Postural hypotension.
GI: Nausea; constipation; dyspepsia; diarrhea; vomiting; GI disorder.
RESP: Rhinitis; increased cough; pharyngitis; pneumonia; dyspnea.
MISC: Arthralgia; leg cramp; pain; asthenia; neck pain.

CLINICAL IMPLICATIONS
General
- Determine why drug is being taken. Consider implications of condition on dental treatment.
- Patient may be high-risk candidate for pathological fractures or jaw fractures during extractions.
- *Postural hypotension:* Monitor BP at the beginning and end of each appointment; anticipate syncope. Have patient sit upright for several min at the end of the dental appointment before dismissing.

Termizol — see ketoconazole
Terranumonyl — see tetracycline HCl
Tetra-Atlantis — see tetracycline HCl

⬜ tetracaine HCl (TEH-trah-cane HIGH-droe-KLOR-ide)

Cepacol Viractin: Cream: 2%; Gel: 2%
■✦■ **Ametop**
Drug Class: Local anesthetic, topical, ester type

PHARMACOLOGY
Action
Blocks sodium ion influx into neurons preventing depolarization of nerve fibers.

Uses
Skin disorders: For topical anesthesia in local skin disorders, including pruritus and pain due to minor burns, skin manifestations of systemic disease (e.g., chickenpox), prickly heat, abrasions, sunburn, plant poisoning, insect bites, eczema; local analgesia on normal, intact skin.

Mucous membranes: For local anesthesia of accessible mucous membranes, including oral, nasal, and laryngeal mucous membranes; respiratory or urinary tracts. Also for the treatment of pruritus ani, pruritus vulvae, and hemorrhoids.

Contraindications
Hypersensitivity to any component of these products; ophthalmic use.

Usual Dosage
Painful oral mucosal lesions
2% CREAM OR GEL
ADULTS AND CHILDREN: Apply topically 3 to 4 times daily.

➡◀ DRUG INTERACTIONS
No documented drug-drug interactions. The absence of evidence is not evidence of safety.

ADVERSE EFFECTS
⚠ ORAL: Stinging; burning; numbness.

CLINICAL IMPLICATIONS
General
• Topical anesthetics may impair swallowing and enhance danger of aspiration. Do not ingest food for 1 hr after anesthetic use in mouth or throat. This is particularly important in children because of their frequency of eating.
• Limit area of application; avoid using spray form of product due to risk of toxicity.

Pregnancy Risk Category: Category C.
Oral Health Education
• Do not ingest food for 1 hr following use of oral topical anesthetic preparations in the mouth or throat. Topical anesthesia may impair swallowing, thus enhancing the danger of aspiration.
• Numbness of the tongue or buccal mucosa may increase the danger of biting trauma. Do not eat or chew gum while the mouth or throat area is anesthetized.

---

tetracycline HCl (teh-truh-SIGH-kleen HIGH-droe-KLOR-ide)

Sumycin 250: Tablets: 250 mg
Sumycin 500: Tablets: 500 mg
Sumycin Syrup: Oral Suspension: 125 mg per 5 mL
■✦■ **Apo-Tetra, Novo-Tetra, Nu-Tetra**

■✦■ **Acromicina, Ambotetra, Quimocyclar, Terranumonyl, Tetra-Atlantis, Zorbenal-G**

Drug Class: Antibiotic, tetracycline

PHARMACOLOGY

Action
Inhibits bacterial protein synthesis.

Uses
Treatment of infections caused by susceptible strains of gram-positive and gram-negative bacteria; treatment of *Rickettsia*, *Mycoplasma pneumoniae*; chlamydial infections including treatment of trachoma; adjunctive treatment in severe acne; treatment of susceptible infections when penicillins are contraindicated; adjunctive treatment of acute intestinal amebiasis; treatment of nongonococcal urethritis caused by *Ureaplasma urealyticum*; treatment of relapsing fever due to *Borrelia recurrentis*.

Contraindications
Hypersensitivity to tetracyclines or any component.

Usual Dosage
ADULTS: *PO:* Usual dose: 1 to 2 g/day in two or four equal doses.
    MILD TO MODERATE INFECTIONS: 500 mg bid or 250 mg qid.
    SEVERE INFECTIONS: 500 mg qid.
CHILDREN OLDER THAN 8 YR: *PO:* 25 to 50 mg/kg/day in four equally divided doses.

Pharmacokinetics
ABSORP: Tetracycline is adequately, but incompletely, absorbed from the GI tract.
DIST: Tetracycline is about 65% bound to plasma proteins (short-acting). The protein binding for intermediate and long-acting analogs is usually greater. Penetration into most body fluids and tissues is excellent. Tetracycline is distributed in varying degrees in liver, bile, lung, kidney, prostate, urine, CSF, synovial fluid, mucosa of the maxillary sinus, brain, sputum, and bone. Tetracycline crosses the placenta and enters fetal circulation and amniotic fluid.
METAB: Tetracycline is concentrated by the liver in the bile.
EXCRET: Tetracycline is excreted in both urine and feces at high concentrations in a biologically active form.
SPECIAL POP: *Renal failure:* Because renal clearance is by glomerular filtration, excretion is significantly affected by the state of renal function.

➡️⬅️ DRUG INTERACTIONS

Antacids: Decreased oral tetracycline effect (decreased absorption)
- Avoid concurrent use.

Antiseptics, mercurial (contact lens cleansing solutions): Conjunctivitis (mechanism unknown)
- Avoid concurrent use.

Atovaquone: Decreased atovaquone effect (decreased metabolism)
- Avoid concurrent use.

Bismuth subsalicylate: Decreased tetracycline effect (decreased absorption)
- Avoid concurrent use.

Digoxin: Possible digoxin toxicity (decreased metabolism)
- Avoid concurrent use.

Iron: Decreased tetracycline effect (decreased absorption)
- Administer 3 hr apart.

Kaolin or kaolin-pectin: Decreased tetracycline effect (decreased absorption)
- Avoid concurrent use.

Lithium: Lithium toxicity (decreased renal excretion)
- Monitor clinical status.

Molindone: Decreased tetracycline effect (decreased absorption)
- Administer 2 hr apart.

Risperidone: Possible decreased risperidone effect (mechanism unknown)
- Monitor clinical status.

Zinc: Decreased tetracycline effect (decreased absorption)
- Avoid concurrent use.

ADVERSE EFFECTS

⚠ **ORAL:** Black hairy tongue; dysphagia; glossitis; stomatitis; sore throat.
CVS: Pericarditis (as component of hypersensitivity reaction).
CNS: Dizziness; headache.
GI: Diarrhea; nausea; vomiting; abdominal pain or discomfort; bulky, loose stools; anorexia; hoarseness; enterocolitis; inflammatory lesions; epigastric distress.
MISC: Hypersensitivity, including anaphylaxis.

CLINICAL IMPLICATIONS

General

When prescribed by DDS:

* *Lactation:* Excreted in breast milk.
* *Children:* Avoid in children younger than 8 yr of age because abnormal bone formation and discoloration of teeth may occur.
* *Renal failure:* Excessive accumulation may occur in patients with renal impairment, resulting in possible liver toxicity; dosage reduction may be required.
* *Superinfection:* Prolonged use may result in bacterial or fungal overgrowth.
* *Pseudomembranous colitis:* Consider in patients in whom diarrhea develops.
* *Pseudotumor cerebri (benign intracranial hypertension):* Reported in adults. Usual manifestations are headache and blurred vision.
* *Sensitivity reactions:* Because sensitivity reactions are more likely to occur in persons with a history of allergy, hay fever, or urticaria, the preparation should be used with caution in such individuals. Cross-sensitization among the various tetracyclines is extremely common.
* *Overdosage:* Nausea, vomiting, headache, increased intracranial pressure, skin pigmentation.

When prescribed by medical facility:

* Determine why drug is being taken. If oral infection occurs that requires antibiotic therapy, select an appropriate product from a different class of anti-infectives.
* Prolonged use of antibiotics may result in bacterial or fungal overgrowth of nonsusceptible microorganisms; anticipate candidiasis.

Pregnancy Risk Category: Category D. Avoid during pregnancy.

Oral Health Education

When prescribed by DDS:

* Ensure patient knows how to take the drug, how long it should be taken and to immediately report adverse effects (e.g., rash, difficult breathing, diarrhea, GI upset). See Chapter 4: *Medical Management of Odontogenic Infections.*
* Explain name, dose, action, and potential side effects of drug.
* Review dosing schedule and prescribed length of therapy with patient. Advise patient that dose, dosing frequency, and duration of therapy are dependent on site and cause of infection.
* Inform patient that antibacterial drug regimens must be followed to completion.
* Instruct patient using capsules or tablets to take prescribed dose with a full glass of water to reduce risk of esophageal irritation or ulceration.
* Instruct patient or caregiver using oral suspension to measure and administer prescribed dose using dosing spoon, dosing syringe, or medicine cup.
* Advise patient to take prescribed dose at least 2 hr before or after meals.
* Advise patient to take 2 hr before or after antacids containing aluminum, calcium, or magnesium or preparations containing iron or zinc, milk, or other dairy products.
* Instruct patient to complete entire course of therapy, even if symptoms of infection disappear.
* Advise patient to discontinue therapy and contact health care provider immediately if skin rash, hives, itching, shortness of breath, or headache and blurred vision occur.
* Advise patient that medication may cause photosensitivity (sensitivity to sunlight) and to avoid unnecessary exposure to sunlight or tanning lamps, to use sunscreens, and to wear protective clothing to avoid photosensitivity reactions.
* Caution women taking oral contraceptives that tetracycline may make birth control pills less effective and to use nonhormonal forms of contraception during treatment.

- Advise women to notify health care provider if pregnant, planning to become pregnant, or breast feeding.
- Caution patient that drug may cause dizziness, lightheadedness, or feeling of a whirling motion and to use caution while driving or performing other hazardous tasks until tolerance is determined.
- Advise patient to report following signs of superinfection to health care provider: black furry tongue, white patches in mouth, foul-smelling stools, or vaginal itching or discharge.
- Warn patient that diarrhea containing blood or pus may be a sign of a serious disorder and to seek medical care if noted and not treat at home.
- Caution patient to not take any prescription or OTC medications, dietary supplements, or herbal preparations unless advised by health care provider.
- Advise patient to discard any unused tetracycline by the expiration date noted on the label.
- Advise patient that follow-up examinations and laboratory tests may be required to monitor therapy and to keep appointments.

---

tetrahydroaminoacridine — see tacrine HCl

Teveten — see eprosartan mesylate

Texacort — see hydrocortisone

Texate — see methotrexate

T-Gesic — see acetaminophen/hydrocodone bitartrate

THA — see tacrine HCl

Thalitone — see chlorthalidone

Theo-24 — see theophylline

Theochron — see theophylline

Theo-Dur — see theophylline

Theolair — see theophylline

---

theophylline (thee-AHF-ih-lin)

Accurbron, Asmalix, Bronkodyl, Elixomin, Elixophyllin, Lanophyllin, Quibron-T Dividose, Quibron-T/SR Dividose, Slo-bid Gyrocaps, Slo-Phyllin, Theo-24, Theochron, Theo-Dur, Theolair, T-Phyl, Uni-Dur, Uniphyl

■✦■ Apo-Theo LA, Novo-Theophyl SR

■▪■ Teolong

Drug Class: Bronchodilator; Xanthine derivative

PHARMACOLOGY

Action
Relaxes bronchial smooth muscle and stimulates central respiratory drive.

Uses
Prevention or treatment of reversible bronchospasm associated with asthma or COPD.

Unlabeled Uses
Treatment of apnea and bradycardia of prematurity; reduction of essential tremor.

➡✦ DRUG INTERACTIONS RELATED TO DENTAL THERAPEUTICS

Diazepam, alprazolam, or midazolam: Decreased diazepam, alprazolam, or midazolam effect (pharmacological antagonism)
- Avoid concurrent use.

Clarithromycin or azithromycin: Possible theophylline toxicity (decreased metabolism)
- Avoid concurrent use.

Sympathomimetic amines: Arrhythmias (mechanism unknown)
- Monitor clinical status.

ADVERSE EFFECTS
CNS: Irritability; headache; insomnia; muscle twitching; seizures.
CVS: Hypotension; cardiac arrhythmia; tachycardia (high doses).
GI: Nausea; vomiting; gastroesophageal reflux; epigastric pain.
RESP: Tachypnea; respiratory arrest.
MISC: Fever; flushing; hyperglycemia; inappropriate antidiuretic hormone secretion; sensitivity reactions (e.g., exfoliative dermatitis, urticaria).

CLINICAL IMPLICATIONS
General
- Monitor vital signs (e.g., BP, pulse rate, respiratory rate and function); uncontrolled disease characterized by wheezing and coughing.
- Acute bronchoconstriction can occur during dental treatment; have bronchodilator inhaler available.
- Ensure that bronchodilator inhaler is present at each dental appointment.
- Be aware that sulfites in local anesthetic with vasoconstrictor can precipitate acute asthma attack in susceptible individuals.

Oral Health Education
- Request patient bring bronchodilator inhaler to each dental appointment.

---

theophylline ethylenediamine — see aminophylline

Thera-Flur — see sodium fluoride

Thera-Flur-N — see sodium fluoride

Theraflu Thin Strips Multisymptom — see diphenhydramine HCl

Theramycin Z — see erythromycin

---

thioridazine HCl (THIGH-oh-RID-uh-zeen HIGH-droe-KLOR-ide)
Thioridazine HCl, Mellaril

▮✳▮ **Apo-Thioridazine**

▮◆▮ **Melleril**

Drug Class: Antipsychotic, phenothiazine

PHARMACOLOGY
Action
Effects apparently caused by dopamine receptor blocking in CNS.

Uses
Management of schizophrenia.

➡◆ DRUG INTERACTIONS RELATED TO DENTAL THERAPEUTICS
No documented drug-drug interactions. The absence of evidence is not evidence of safety.

ADVERSE EFFECTS
⚠ **ORAL:** Dry mouth; tardive dyskinesia.
CNS: Pseudoparkinsonism; dystonias; motor restlessness; headache; weakness; tremor; fatigue; slurring; insomnia; vertigo; seizures; drowsiness; paradoxical excitement; headache; confusion.
CVS: Hypotension.
GI: Dyspepsia; constipation; adynamic ileus; nausea; vomiting; diarrhea.
RESP: Laryngospasm; respiratory depression; bronchospasm; dyspnea.

MISC: Increase in appetite and weight; polydipsia; neuroleptic malignant syndrome; allergy (e.g., fever, laryngeal edema, angioneurotic edema, asthma); elevated prolactin levels; agranulocytosis; leukopenia; anemia; thrombocytopenia.

CLINICAL IMPLICATIONS

General

- Clients with psychological disease may present with behavior management problems.
- Depressed or anxious patients may neglect self-care. Monitor for plaque control effectiveness.
- Extrapyramidal behaviors can complicate performance of oral procedures. If present, consult with MD to consider medication changes.
- Determine ability to adapt to stress of dental treatment. Consider short appointments.
- Place patient on frequent maintenance schedule to avoid periodontal inflammation.
- Chronic dry mouth is possible; anticipate increased caries and candidiasis.
- If GI side effects occur, consider semisupine chair position.
- Monitor vital signs.
- Blood dyscrasias rarely reported; anticipate increased bleeding, infection, and poor healing.

Oral Health Education

- Encourage daily plaque control procedures for effective self-care.
- Evaluate manual dexterity; consider need for power toothbrush.
- If chronic dry mouth occurs, recommend home fluoride therapy and use of nonalcoholic oral health care products.

---

thiothixene (THIGH-oh-THIX-een)

Navane

Drug Class: Antipsychotic, thioxanthene

PHARMACOLOGY

Action

Produces antipsychotic effects apparently because of dopamine receptor blocking in CNS.

Uses

Management of schizophrenia.

➡◀ DRUG INTERACTIONS RELATED TO DENTAL THERAPEUTICS

No documented drug-drug interactions. The absence of evidence is not evidence of safety.

ADVERSE EFFECTS

⚠ **ORAL:** Dry mouth; tardive dyskinesia.

CNS: Extrapyramidal symptoms (e.g., pseudoparkinsonism, akathisia, dystonias); drowsiness; insomnia; restlessness; agitation; seizures; paradoxical exacerbation of psychotic symptoms.

CVS: Hypotension, tachycardia.

GI: Anorexia; diarrhea; nausea; vomiting; constipation.

RESP: Laryngospasm; bronchospasm; increased depth of respiration.

MISC: Hypoglycemia; hyperglycemia; glycosuria; polydipsia; increase in appetite and weight; peripheral edema; elevated prolactin levels; increased sweating; photosensitivity.

CLINICAL IMPLICATIONS

General

- Patients with psychological disease may present with behavior management problems.
- Depressed or anxious patients may neglect self-care. Monitor for plaque control effectiveness.
- Extrapyramidal behaviors can complicate performance of oral procedures. If present, consult with MD to consider medication changes.
- Determine ability to adapt to stress of dental treatment. Consider short appointments.

- Place on frequent maintenance schedule to avoid periodontal inflammation.
- Chronic dry mouth is possible; anticipate increased caries and candidiasis.
- If GI side effects occur, consider semisupine chair position.
- Monitor vital signs.

Oral Health Education
- Encourage daily plaque control procedures for effective self-care.
- Evaluate manual dexterity; consider need for power toothbrush.
- If chronic dry mouth occurs, recommend home fluoride therapy and use of nonalcoholic oral health care products.

Thorazine — see chlorpromazine HCl
Thyrar — see thyroid, desiccated

---

thyroid, desiccated (THIGH-royd, DESS-ih-KATE-uhd)
Synonym: thyroid USP

Armour Thyroid, S-P-T, Thyrar, Thyroid Strong

Drug Class: Thyroid

PHARMACOLOGY
Action
Increases metabolic rate of body tissues.

Uses
Replacement or supplemental therapy in hypothyroidism; thyroid-stimulating hormone suppression in thyroid cancer, nodules, goiters, and enlargement in chronic thyroiditis; diagnostic agent to differentiate suspected hyperthyroidism from euthyroidism.

➔← DRUG INTERACTIONS RELATED TO DENTAL THERAPEUTICS
No documented drug-drug interactions. The absence of evidence is not evidence of safety.

ADVERSE EFFECTS
CNS: Tremors; headache; nervousness; insomnia.
GI: Diarrhea; vomiting.
MISC: Hypersensitivity; weight loss; sweating; heat intolerance; fever. Adverse reactions generally indicate hyperthyroidism caused by therapeutic overdosage.

CLINICAL IMPLICATIONS
General
- Determine why drug is being taken. Consider implications of condition on dental treatment.
- *Hypothyroidism:* Oral health care has no contraindications when the disease is controlled with medication.
- Monitor blood pressure and pulse rate to determine degree of thyroid disease control.
- Avoid prescribing CNS depressant drugs to the patient with uncontrolled hypothyroid disease.

Oral Health Education
- Determine need for power toothbrush for self-care.

Thyroid Strong — see thyroid, desiccated
thyroid USP — see thyroid, desiccated
Thyrolar 1/4 — see liotrix
Thyrolar 1/2 — see liotrix
Thyrolar 1 — see liotrix

Thyrolar 2 — see liotrix

Thyrolar 3 — see liotrix

tiagabine HCl (TIE-egg-un-bine HIGH-droe-KLOR-ide)

Gabitril Filmtabs

Drug Class: Anticonvulsant

PHARMACOLOGY

Action

Mechanism unknown; may block gamma-aminobutyric acid (GABA) uptake into presynaptic neurons, allowing more GABA to be available for binding with the GABA receptor of post-synaptic cells.

Uses

Adjunctive treatment in treatment of partial seizures.

➡◀ DRUG INTERACTIONS RELATED TO DENTAL THERAPEUTICS

No documented drug-drug interactions. The absence of evidence is not evidence of safety.

ADVERSE EFFECTS

⚠ **ORAL:** Mouth ulceration; gingivitis.

CNS: Dizziness; lightheadedness; somnolence; nervousness; irritability; agitation; hostility; language problem; tremor; abnormal gait; ataxia; abnormal thinking; concentration/attention difficulty; depression; confusion; insomnia; speech disorder; difficulty with memory; paresthesia; emotional lability.

CVS: Vasodilation.

GI: Nausea; abdominal pain; diarrhea; vomiting; increased appetite.

MISC: Asthenia; lack of energy; pain; cough; myasthenia; accidental injury; infection; flu-like syndrome; myalgia; urinary tract infection.

CLINICAL IMPLICATIONS

General

- Determine why drug is being taken. Consider implications of condition on dental treatment.
- Determine level of disease control, type and frequency of seizure, and compliance with medication regimen.
- Determine ability to adapt to stress of dental treatment. Consider short appointments.

Oral Health Education

- Evaluate manual dexterity; consider need for power toothbrush.

Tiamol — see fluocinonide

Tiazac — see diltiazem HCl

Ticlid — see ticlopidine HCl

---

ticlopidine HCl (tie-KLOE-pih-DEEN HIGH-droe-KLOR-ide)

Ticlid

■✚■ **Apo-Ticlopidine, Gen-Ticlopidine, Nu-Ticlopidine, PMS-Ticlopidine, Rhoxal-ticlopidine**

Drug Class: Antiplatelet

PHARMACOLOGY

Action

Produces time- and dose-dependent inhibition of both platelet aggregation and release of platelet granule constituents as well as prolongation of bleeding time; interferes with platelet membrane function by inhibiting platelet-fibrinogen binding and subsequent platelet-platelet interactions.

Uses

Reduction of risk of thrombotic stroke in patients who have experienced stroke precursors and in patients who have suffered thrombotic stroke. Reserved for patients intolerant to aspirin because of greater risk of adverse reactions.

Unlabeled Uses

Improved walking distance in intermittent claudication; vascular improvement in chronic arterial occlusion; reduced incidence of neurological deficit in subarachnoid hemorrhage; reduced incidence of vascular occlusion in uremic patients with arteriovenous shunts or fistulas; control of platelet count in open heart surgery; decreased graft occlusion in coronary artery bypass grafts; reduced degree of proteinuria and hematuria in primary glomerulonephritis; reduced incidence, duration, and severity of infarctive crises in sickle cell disease.

DRUG INTERACTIONS RELATED TO DENTAL THERAPEUTICS

No documented drug-drug interactions. The absence of evidence is not evidence of safety.

ADVERSE EFFECTS

⚠ **ORAL:** Increased bleeding.

CNS: Headache; peripheral neuropathy; dizziness.

GI: Diarrhea; nausea; fullness; dyspepsia; GI pain; purpura; vomiting; flatulence; anorexia.

MISC: Weakness; pain; allergic pneumonitis; systemic lupus erythematosus; arthropathy; myositis; hyponatremia; aplastic anemia; hepatic necrosis; peptic ulcer; renal failure; sepsis; angioedema; hepatocellular jaundice; neutropenia; agranulocytosis; thrombocytopenia; leukopenia.

CLINICAL IMPLICATIONS

General

- Determine why drug is being taken. Consider implications of condition on dental treatment.
- Determine bleeding time before completing procedures that may result in significant bleeding. Safe levels are <20 min.
- Monitor frequently to ensure adequate clotting during treatment that involves bleeding.
- If uncontrolled bleeding develops, use hemostatic agents and positive pressure to induce hemostasis. Do not dismiss patient until bleeding is controlled.
- Blood dyscrasias rarely reported; anticipate increased bleeding, infection, and poor healing.

Oral Health Education

- Encourage daily plaque control procedures for effective self-care in patient at risk for CV disease.

Tikosyn — see dofetilide

Tilade — see nedocromil sodium

Tilazem — see diltiazem HCl

---

timolol maleate (TI-moe-lahl MAL-ee-ate)

Betimol, Blocadren, Istalol, Timoptic, Timoptic Ocudose, Timoptic-XE

Apo-Timol, Apo-Timop, Gen-Timolol, Novo-Timol Tablets, Nu-Timolol, PMS-Timolol, ratio-Timolol, Rhoxal-timolol

Drug Class: Beta-adrenergic blocker

PHARMACOLOGY

Action
Blocks beta-receptors, which primarily affect heart (slows rate), vascular musculature (decreases BP), and lungs (reduces function). Reduces elevated and normal intraocular pressure (IOP) via decreasing production of aqueous humor or increasing flow.

Uses
Treatment of hypertension, alone or in combination with other agents; reduction of risk of reinfarction post-MI; migraine prophylaxis; treatment of elevated IOP in chronic open-angle glaucoma, ocular hypertension, aphakic glaucoma patients, patients with secary glaucoma, and in patients with elevated IOP who need ocular pressure lowered.

➡️⬅️ DRUG INTERACTIONS RELATED TO DENTAL THERAPEUTICS

COX-1 inhibitors: Decreased antihypertensive effect (decreased prostaglandin synthesis)
 • Monitor blood pressure.
Sympathomimetic amines: Decreased antihypertensive effect (pharmacological antagonism)
 • Monitor blood pressure.

ADVERSE EFFECTS
⚠ **ORAL:** Dry mouth; taste disturbance; stomatitis.
CNS: Dizziness; depression; lethargy; headache; insomnia; anxiety; tremor; paresthesia.
CVS: Bradycardia; arrhythmia.
GI: Abdominal pain; diarrhea; nausea.
RESP: Wheezing; cough; breathing difficulties, especially in asthmatic patients or patients with COPD.
MISC: Joint pain; muscle cramps.

CLINICAL IMPLICATIONS

General
• Determine why drug is being taken. Consider implications of condition on dental treatment.
• Monitor vital signs (e.g., BP, pulse pressure, rate, and rhythm) at each appointment to assess disease control. Do not provide elective dental treatment when BP is ≥180/110 or in presence of other high-risk CV conditions. Refer to the section entitled "The Patient Taking Cardiovascular Drugs" in Chapter 6: *Clinical Medicine*.
• Use local anesthetic agents with vasoconstrictor with caution based on functional capacity of the patient and use aspirating technique to prevent intravascular injection.
• Determine ability to adapt to stress of dental treatment. Consider short appointments.
• Place patient on frequent maintenance schedule to avoid periodontal inflammation.
• Chronic dry mouth is possible; anticipate increased caries, candidiasis, and lichenoid mucositis.
• Beta blockers may mask epinephrine-induced signs and symptoms of hypoglycemia in patients with diabetes.
• Blood dyscrasias rarely reported; anticipate increased bleeding, infection, and poor healing.

Oral Health Education
• Encourage daily plaque control procedures for effective self-care in patient at risk for CV disease.
• If chronic dry mouth occurs, recommend home fluoride therapy and use of nonalcoholic oral health care products.

Timoptic — see timolol maleate

Timoptic Ocudose — see timolol maleate

Timoptic-XE — see timolol maleate

Tiniazol — see ketoconazole

Tirocal — see calcitriol
Tiroidine — see levothyroxine sodium

tizanidine HCl (tye-ZAN-i-deen HIGH-droe-KLOR-ide)
Zanaflex

██ Sirdalud

Drug Class: Skeletal muscle relaxant, centrally acting

PHARMACOLOGY

Action
Unknown; may increase presynaptic inhibition of motor neurons.

Uses
Acute and intermittent management of increased muscle tone associated with spasticity.

➡️⬅️ DRUG INTERACTIONS RELATED TO DENTAL THERAPEUTICS
No documented drug-drug interactions. The absence of evidence is not evidence of safety.

ADVERSE EFFECTS
⚠️ **ORAL:** Dry mouth (49%).
CNS: Somnolence; dizziness; dyskinesia; nervousness; depression; anxiety; paresthesia.
CVS: Orthostatic hypotension (1%).
GI: Constipation; vomiting; abdominal pain; diarrhea; dyspepsia.
RESP: Sinusitis; pneumonia; bronchitis.
MISC: Asthenia; increased spasm or tone; flu-like syndrome; infection; speech disorder; myasthenia; back pain; fever; allergic reaction; malaise; abscess; neck pain; cellulitis.

CLINICAL IMPLICATIONS

General
- Determine why drug is being taken. Consider implications of condition on dental treatment.
- *Postural hypotension:* Monitor BP at the beginning and end of each appointment; anticipate syncope. Have patient sit upright for several min at the end of the dental appointment before dismissing.
- *For back pain:* Consider semisupine chair position for patient comfort.
- Chronic dry mouth is possible; anticipate increased caries and candidiasis.

Oral Health Education
- If chronic dry mouth occurs, recommend home fluoride therapy and use of nonalcoholic oral health care products.
- Determine need for power toothbrush for self-care.

TMP-SMZ — see trimethoprim/sulfamethoxazole
Tofranil — see imipramine HCl
Tofranil-PM — see imipramine HCl

tolazamide (tole-AZE-uh-mid)
Tolinase

Drug Class: Antidiabetic, sulfonylurea

PHARMACOLOGY

Action
Decreases blood glucose by stimulating release of insulin from pancreas.

Uses
Adjunct to diet to lower blood glucose in patients with type 2 diabetes mellitus whose hyperglycemia cannot be controlled by diet alone.

Unlabeled Uses

Temporary adjunct to insulin therapy in selected patients with type 2 diabetes mellitus to improve diabetic control.

➜✦ DRUG INTERACTIONS RELATED TO DENTAL THERAPEUTICS

No documented drug-drug interactions. The absence of evidence is not evidence of safety.

ADVERSE EFFECTS

⚠ **ORAL:** Taste alteration; thirst.

CNS: Dizziness; vertigo.

CVS: Hypertension; syncope.

GI: Nausea; epigastric fullness; heartburn; cholestatic jaundice.

MISC: Disulfiram-like reaction; weakness; paresthesia; fatigue; malaise; leukopenia; thrombocytopenia; agranulocytosis; hemolytic anemia.

CLINICAL IMPLICATIONS

General

- Determine degree of disease control and current blood sugar levels. Goals should be <120 mg/dL and A1C <7%. A1C levels ≥8% indicate significant uncontrolled diabetes.
- The routine use of antibiotics in the dental management of diabetic patients is not indicated; however, antibiotic therapy in patients with poorly controlled diabetes has been shown to improve disease control and improve response after periodontal debridement.
- Monitor blood pressure because hypertension and dyslipidemia (CAD) are prevalent in DM.
- *Loss of blood sugar control:* Certain medical conditions (e.g., surgery, fever, infection, trauma) and drugs (e.g., corticosteroids) affect glucose control. In these situations, it may be necessary to seek medical consultation before surgical procedures.
- Obtain patient history regarding diabetic ketoacidosis or hypoglycemia with current drug regimen.
- Observe for signs of hypoglycemia (e.g., confusion, argumentativeness, perspiration, altered consciousness). Be prepared to treat hypoglycemic reactions with oral glucose or sucrose.
- Ensure patient has taken medication and eaten meal.
- Monitor vital signs (e.g., BP, pulse pressure, rate, and rhythm) at each appointment to assess disease control. Do not provide elective dental treatment when BP is ≥180/110 or in presence of other high-risk CV conditions. Refer to the section entitled "The Patient Taking Cardiovascular Drugs" in Chapter 6: *Clinical Medicine*.
- Determine ability to adapt to stress of dental treatment. Consider short, morning appointments.
- Medical consult advised if fasting blood glucose is <70 mg/dL (hypoglycemic risk) or >200 mg/dL (hyperglycemic crisis risk).
- *If insulin is used:* Consider time of peak hypoglycemic effect.
- If GI side effects occur, consider semisupine chair position.
- Blood dyscrasias rarely reported; anticipate increased bleeding, infection, and poor healing.
- Place patient on frequent maintenance schedule to avoid periodontal inflammation.

Oral Health Education

- Encourage daily plaque control procedures for effective, nontraumatic self-care.
- Explain role of diabetes in periodontal disease and the need to maintain effective plaque control and disease control.
- Advise patient to bring data on blood sugar values and A1C levels to dental appointments.

---

tolbutamide (tole-BYOO-tuh-mide)

Orinase, Orinase Diagnostic

■✦■ Apo-Tolbutamide, Novo-Butamide

■✦■ Artosin, Diaval, Rastinon

Drug Class: Antidiabetic, sulfonylurea

PHARMACOLOGY
Action
Decreases blood glucose by stimulating release of insulin from the pancreas.
Uses
ORAL FORM: Adjunct to diet to lower blood glucose in patients with type 2 diabetes mellitus whose hyperglycemia cannot be controlled by diet alone.

IV FORM (TOLBUTAMIDE SODIUM): Aid in diagnosis of pancreatic islet cell adenoma.

➡️⬅️ DRUG INTERACTIONS RELATED TO DENTAL THERAPEUTICS
No documented drug-drug interactions. The absence of evidence is not evidence of safety.

ADVERSE EFFECTS
⚠️ **ORAL:** Taste alteration; thirst.
CNS: Dizziness; vertigo.
CVS: Hypertension; syncope.
GI: Nausea; epigastric fullness; heartburn.
MISC: Disulfiram-like reaction; weakness; paresthesia; fatigue; malaise; slight burning sensation along course of vein during IV injection; thrombophlebitis with thrombosis of injected vein; leukopenia; thrombocytopenia; agranulocytosis; hemolytic anemia.

CLINICAL IMPLICATIONS
General
- Determine degree of disease control and current blood sugar levels. Goals should be <120 mg/dL and A1C <7%. A1C levels ≥8% indicate significant uncontrolled diabetes.
- The routine use of antibiotics in the dental management of diabetic patients is not indicated; however, antibiotic therapy in patients with poorly controlled diabetes has been shown to improve disease control and improve response following periodontal debridement.
- Monitor blood pressure because hypertension and dyslipidemia (CAD) are prevalent in DM.
- *Loss of blood sugar control:* certain medical conditions (e.g., surgery, fever, infection, trauma) and drugs (such as corticosteroids) affect glucose control. In these situations, it may be necessary to seek medical consultation before surgical procedures.
- Obtain patient history regarding diabetic ketoacidosis or hypoglycemia with current drug regimen.
- Observe for signs of hypoglycemia (e.g., confusion, argumentativeness, perspiration, altered consciousness). Be prepared to treat hypoglycemic reactions with oral glucose or sucrose.
- Ensure patient has taken medication and eaten meal.
- Monitor vital signs (e.g., BP, pulse pressure, rate, and rhythm) at each appointment to assess disease control. Do not provide elective dental treatment when BP is ≥180/110 or in presence of other high-risk CV conditions. Refer to the section entitled "The Patient Taking Cardiovascular Drugs" in Chapter 6: *Clinical Medicine*.
- Determine ability to adapt to stress of dental treatment. Consider short, morning appointments.
- Medical consult advised if fasting blood glucose is <70 mg/dL (hypoglycemic risk) or >200 mg/dL (hyperglycemic crisis risk).
- If insulin is used: consider time of peak hypoglycemic effect.
- If GI side effects occur, consider semisupine chair position.
- Blood dyscrasias rarely reported; anticipate increased bleeding, infection, and poor healing.
- Place patient on frequent maintenance schedule to avoid periodontal inflammation.

Oral Health Education
- Encourage daily plaque control procedures for effective, nontraumatic self-care.
- Explain role of diabetes in periodontal disease and the need to maintain effective plaque control and disease control.
- Advise patient to bring data on blood sugar values and A1C levels to dental appointments.

tolcapone (TOLE-kah-pone)

Tasmar

Drug Class: Antiparkinson

PHARMACOLOGY

Action

The exact mechanism of action is unknown. Inhibits catechol-*O*-methyl transferase (COMT), thus blocking the degradation of catechols including dopamine and levodopa. This may lead to more sustained levels of dopamine and consequently a more prolonged antiparkinsonian effect.

Uses

As an adjunct to levodopa/carbidopa for the management of signs and symptoms of Parkinson disease.

➡️⬅️ DRUG INTERACTIONS RELATED TO DENTAL THERAPEUTICS

No documented drug-drug interactions. The absence of evidence is not evidence of safety.

ADVERSE EFFECTS

⚠️ **ORAL:** Dry mouth (6%).

CNS: Sleep disorder; excessive dreaming; somnolence; confusion; dizziness; headache; hallucination; dyskinesia; dystonia; fatigue; balance loss; hyperkinesia; paresthesia; hypokinesia; agitation; irritability; mental deficiency; hyperactivity; panic reaction; euphoria; hypertonia.

CVS: Orthostatic hypotension; chest pain; hypotension.

GI: Nausea; diarrhea; vomiting; constipation; abdominal pain; dyspepsia; flatulence.

RESP: URI; dyspnea; sinus congestion.

MISC: Muscle cramps; anorexia; falling; increased sweating; rhabdomyolysis; stiffness; arthritis; neck pain; influenza; burning; malaise; fever.

CLINICAL IMPLICATIONS

General

- Determine why drug is being taken. Consider implications of condition on dental treatment.
- Extrapyramidal behaviors associated with Parkinson disease can complicate access to oral cavity and complicate oral procedures.
- Chronic dry mouth is possible; anticipate increased caries and candidiasis.
- Monitor vital signs.
- *Postural hypotension:* Monitor BP at the beginning and end of each appointment; anticipate syncope. Have patient sit upright for several min at the end of the dental appointment before dismissing.
- If GI side effects occur, consider semisupine chair position.
- Place on frequent maintenance schedule to avoid periodontal inflammation.

Oral Health Education

- Evaluate manual dexterity; consider need for power toothbrush.
- If chronic dry mouth occurs, recommend home fluoride therapy and use of nonalcoholic oral health care products.

Tolectin 200 — see tolmetin sodium

Tolectin 600 — see tolmetin sodium

Tolinase — see tolazamide

tolmetin sodium (TOLE-mee-tin SO-dee-uhm)
Tolectin 200, Tolectin 600

Drug Class: Analgesic; NSAID

PHARMACOLOGY

Action
Decreases inflammation, pain, and fever, probably through inhibition of COX activity and prostaglandin synthesis.

Uses
Treatment of chronic and acute rheumatoid arthritis and osteoarthritis and juvenile rheumatoid arthritis.

➡← DRUG INTERACTIONS RELATED TO DENTAL THERAPEUTICS
No documented drug-drug interactions. The absence of evidence is not evidence of safety.

ADVERSE EFFECTS
⚠ **ORAL:** Glossitis; stomatitis; mouth ulcers.
CNS: Dizziness; drowsiness; lightheadedness; confusion; increased sweating; vertigo; headache; nervousness; migraine; anxiety; aggravated Parkinson disease or epilepsy; paresthesia; peripheral neuropathy; myalgia; fatigue; asthenia; depression.
CVS: Hypertension.
MISC: Agranulocytosis; thrombocytopenia; hemolytic anemia.
GI: Nausea; dyspepsia; abdominal pain or discomfort; flatulence; diarrhea; constipation; vomiting; gastritis; anorexia; peptic ulcer; GI distress.
RESP: Bronchospasm; laryngeal edema; rhinitis; dyspnea; pharyngitis; hemoptysis; shortness of breath.

CLINICAL IMPLICATIONS

General
- Determine why drug is being taken. Consider implications of condition on dental treatment.
- *Arthritis:* Consider patient comfort and need for semisupine chair position.
- Monitor vital signs.
- If GI side effects occur, consider semisupine chair position.
- Blood dyscrasias rarely reported; anticipate increased bleeding, infection, and poor healing.

Oral Health Education
- Evaluate manual dexterity; consider need for power toothbrush.

tolterodine tartrate (tole-THE-roe-deen TAR-trait)
Detrol, Detrol LA

■✦■ **Unidet**

■◔■ **Detrusitol**

Drug Class: Urinary tract product; Muscarinic antagonist

PHARMACOLOGY

Action
Antagonizes muscarinic receptor, which mediates urinary bladder contraction and salivation.

Uses
Treatment of overactive bladder with symptoms of urinary frequency, urgency, or urge incontinence.

➡️⬅️ DRUG INTERACTIONS RELATED TO DENTAL THERAPEUTICS

No documented drug-drug interactions. The absence of evidence is not evidence of safety.

ADVERSE EFFECTS

⚠️ **ORAL:** Dry mouth (37%).

CNS: Headache; somnolence; paresthesia, nervousness (immediate-release); dizziness, anxiety (extended-release).

GI: Constipation; abdominal pain; dyspepsia; flatulence, vomiting, nausea (immediate-release).

RESP: Bronchitis; coughing.

MISC: Chest pain; infection; fungal infection; falls (immediate-release); fatigue (extended-release).

CLINICAL IMPLICATIONS

General

- Determine why drug is being taken. Consider implications of condition on dental treatment.
- Anticholinergics have strong xerostomic effects. Anticipate increased caries and candidiasis.

Oral Health Education

- If chronic dry mouth occurs, recommend home fluoride therapy and use of nonalcoholic oral health care products.

Tonocalcin — see calcitonin-salmon

Topamax — see topiramate

Top-Dal — see loperamide HCl

Topicort — see desoximetasone

Topicort LP — see desoximetasone

Topilene — see betamethasone

---

topiramate (toe-PEER-ah-mate)

Topamax

Drug Class: Anticonvulsant

PHARMACOLOGY

Action

Precise mechanism is unknown but topiramate may block repetitively elicited action potentials, affect ability of chloride ion to move into neurons, and antagonize an excitatory amino acid receptor.

Uses

Adjunctive therapy for partial onset seizures; primary generalized tonic-clonic seizures; seizures associated with Lennox-Gastaut syndrome.

➡️⬅️ DRUG INTERACTIONS RELATED TO DENTAL THERAPEUTICS

No documented drug-drug interactions. The absence of evidence is not evidence of safety.

ADVERSE EFFECTS

⚠️ **ORAL:** Dry mouth (4%); gingivitis; candidiasis; taste perversion.

CNS: Dizziness (32%); fatigue (30%); somnolence (29%); psychomotor slowing (21%); nervousness, paresthesia (19%); ataxia (16%); difficulty with memory, confusion, difficulty with concentration (14%); speech disorders/related speech problems, depression (13%); nystagmus (11%); language problems (10%); tremor, mood problems (9%); abnormal coordination

(4%); agitation, aggressive reaction, apathy, emotional lability, abnormal gait (3%); hypesthesia, depersonalization, decreased libido, involuntary muscle contractions, stupor, vertigo (2%); hypertonia, hallucination, euphoria, psychosis, headache, anxiety, convulsions, insomnia, suicide attempt (≥1%).

GI: Nausea, anorexia (12%); dyspepsia, abdominal pain (7%); constipation, gastroenteritis (2%); GI disorder (1%); diarrhea, vomiting (≥1%).

RESP: Rhinitis (7%); sinusitis (6%); dyspnea (2%); coughing, URI (≥1%).

MISC: Asthenia (6%); back pain (5%); chest pain, flu-like symptoms, leg pain (4%); myalgia, epistaxis, hot flashes, infection, viral infection, allergy (2%); fever, pain (≥1%); edema; body odor, rigors, skeletal pain (1%); pancreatitis.

CLINICAL IMPLICATIONS
General
- Determine why drug is being taken. Consider implications of condition on dental treatment.
- Determine ability to adapt to stress of dental treatment. Consider short appointments.
- Determine level of disease control, type and frequency of seizures, and compliance with medication regimen.
- If GI side effects occur, consider semisupine chair position.
- Chronic dry mouth is possible; anticipate increased caries and candidiasis.

Oral Health Education
- Evaluate manual dexterity; consider need for power toothbrush.
- If chronic dry mouth occurs, recommend home fluoride therapy and use of nonalcoholic oral health care products.

Toprol XL — see metoprolol

Topsyn — see fluocinonide

Toradol — see ketorolac tromethamine

Toradol I — see ketorolac tromethamine

---

torsemide (TORE-suh-MIDE)
Demadex

Drug Class: Loop diuretic

PHARMACOLOGY
Action
Inhibits sodium/potassium/chloride carrier system in ascending loop of Henle, resulting in increased urinary excretion of sodium, chloride, and water. Does not significantly alter glomerular filtration rate, renal plasma flow, or acid-base balance.

Uses
Management of edema associated with CHF, cirrhosis, and renal disease; treatment of hypertension.

➡◀ DRUG INTERACTIONS RELATED TO DENTAL THERAPEUTICS
No documented drug-drug interactions. The absence of evidence is not evidence of safety.

ADVERSE EFFECTS
CNS: Headache; dizziness; asthenia; insomnia; nervousness; syncope.
CVS: Hypotension; tachycardia.
GI: Diarrhea; constipation; nausea; dyspepsia; GI hemorrhage; rectal bleeding.
RESP: Rhinitis; cough increase.
MISC: Arthralgia; myalgia; photosensitivity; hypokalemia.

CLINICAL IMPLICATIONS

General

- Determine why drug is being taken. Consider implications of condition on dental treatment.
- Monitor vital signs (e.g., BP, pulse pressure, rate, and rhythm) at each appointment to assess disease control. Do not provide elective dental treatment when BP is ≥180/110 or in the presence of other high-risk CV conditions. Refer to the section entitled "The Patient Taking Cardiovascular Drugs" in Chapter 6: *Clinical Medicine*.
- Determine ability to adapt to stress of dental treatment. Consider short appointments.
- Use local anesthetic agents with vasoconstrictor with caution based on functional capacity of the patient and use aspirating technique to prevent intravascular injection.
- Monitor pulse rhythm to assess for electrolyte imbalance.
- Place patient on frequent maintenance schedule to avoid periodontal inflammation.

Oral Health Education

- Encourage daily plaque control procedures for effective self-care in patient at risk for CV disease.

T-Phyl — see theophylline

Tradol — see tramadol HCl

tramadol HCl/acetaminophen — see acetaminophen/tramadol HCl

---

 tramadol HCl (TRAM-uh-dole HIGH-droe-KLOR-ide)

Ultram: Tablets: 50 mg

▮▬▮ Nobligan, Prontofort, Tradol

Drug Class: Analgesic

PHARMACOLOGY

Action

Binds to certain opioid receptors and inhibits reuptake of norepinephrine and serotonin; exact mechanism of action unknown.

Uses

Relief of moderate to moderately severe pain.

Contraindications

Acute intoxication with alcohol, hypnotics, centrally acting analgesics, opioids, or psychotropic agents.

Usual Dosage

ADULTS AND CHILDREN 16 YR AND OLDER: *PO:* Start with 25 mg/day in the morning and titrate in 25-mg increments as separate doses q 3 days to reach 100 mg/day (25 mg qid). Thereafter, increase the dose by 50 mg as tolerated q 3 days to reach 200 mg/day (50 mg qid). After titration, administer 50 to 100 mg q 4 to 6 hr as needed for pain relief (max, 400 mg/day).

ELDERLY (OVER 65 YR): *PO:* Start with low end of dosing (max, 300 mg/day in patients 75 yr and older).

RENAL IMPAIRMENT (CCR LESS THAN 30 ML/MIN): *PO:* Increase the dosing interval to 12 hr (max, 200 mg/day).

HEPATIC IMPAIRMENT: *PO:* 50 mg q 12 hr.

Pharmacokinetics

ABSORP: Mean absolute bioavailability of tramadol is 75%. Food has no effect. T_{max} is 2 to 3 hr. Steady-state plasma concentration of both tramadol and the metabolite are achieved within 2 days.

DIST: Tramadol is 20% protein bound and is independent of concentrations up to 10 mcg/mL. Vd is approximately 2.7 L/kg. Tramadol follows linear kinetics.

METAB: There is no evidence of self-induction. Production of M1 (metabolite) is dependent on cytochrome P450 CYP2D6. The O-demethylated metabolite is M1. Tramadol is extensively metabolized after administration. The major metabolic pathway is N- and O-demethylation and glucuronidation or sulfation in liver.

EXCRET: 30% of a dose is excreted in urine unchanged; 60% is excreted as metabolites. The $t_{1/2}$ is 6.3 hr for tramadol and 7.4 hr for the metabolite.

ONSET: The onset of action is 1 hr.

PEAK: Time to peak effect is 2 to 3 hr.

SPECIAL POP: *Renal failure:* In patients with renal impairment, there is a decreased rate and extent of excretion of tramadol and M1. In patients with Ccr less than 30 mL/min, dose adjustment is recommended.

Hepatic failure: Metabolism of tramadol and M1 is reduced in patients with advanced cirrhosis. In all patients with cirrhosis, dose adjustment is recommended.

Elderly: In patients older than 75 yr, dose adjustment is recommended.

➡◀ DRUG INTERACTIONS

Warfarin: Bleeding into skin (mechanism unknown)
- Avoid concurrent use.

Antidepressants, tricyclic: Increased risk of seizure (additive proconvulsants)
- Avoid concurrent use.

Carbamazepine: Decreased tramadol effect (increased metabolism)
- Avoid concurrent use.

Citalopram: Increased risk of seizure (additive proconvulsants)
- Avoid concurrent use.

Fluoxetine: Increased risk of seizure (additive proconvulsants)
- Avoid concurrent use.

Fluvoxamine: Increased risk of seizure (additive proconvulsants)
- Avoid concurrent use.

Monoamine oxidase inhibitors: Increased risk of serotonin syndrome (reduced uptake of monoamines)
- Avoid concurrent use.

Olanzapine: Possible increased risk of serotonin syndrome (mechanism unknown)
- Monitor clinical status.

Ondansetron: Possible decreased tramadol analgesia (antagonism at serotonin receptors)
- Monitor clinical status.

Paroxetine: Increased risk of seizure (additive proconvulsants)
- Avoid concurrent use.

Sertraline: Serotonin syndrome (additive serotonergic effect)
- Avoid concurrent use.

Increased risk of seizure (additive proconvulsants)
- Avoid concurrent use.

ADVERSE EFFECTS

⚠ **ORAL:** Dry mouth (10%).

CVS: Vasodilation (5%); orthostatic hypotension (1%); tachycardia.

CNS: Dizziness/vertigo; headache; somnolence; stimulation; anxiety; confusion; coordination disturbances; euphoria; nervousness; sleep disorder; seizures.

GI: Nausea; diarrhea; constipation; vomiting; dyspepsia; abdominal pain; anorexia; flatulence.

MISC: Asthenia; hypertonia.

CLINICAL IMPLICATIONS

General
- Chronic dry mouth is possible; anticipate increased caries and candidiasis.
- Monitor vital signs.

- *Postural hypotension:* Monitor BP at the beginning and end of each appointment; anticipate syncope. Have patient sit upright for several min at the end of the dental appointment before dismissing.

When prescribed by DDS:
- Short-term use only; there is no justification for long-term use in the management of dental pain.
- *Lactation:* Excreted in breast milk.
- *Children:* Not recommended for children younger than 16 yr.
- *Elderly:* In elderly patients older than 75 yr, concentrations may be slightly elevated; may have less ability to tolerate adverse effects; use reduced dosage.
- *Hypersensitivity:* Serious and, rarely, fatal anaphylactoid reactions may occur.
- *Renal failure:* Dosage adjustments may be required.
- *Hepatic failure:* Dosage adjustments may be required in patients with cirrhosis.
- *CNS depressants:* Use with caution and reduce dosage when administering to patients receiving CNS depressants or SSRIs.
- *Drug abuse:* May induce psychic and physical dependence of the morphine type. Do not use in opioid dependent patients.
- *MAO inhibitors (e.g., isocarboxazid):* Use with great caution in patients taking MAO inhibitors.
- *Opioid dependence:* Not recommended for patients who are opioid dependent; use caution when administering to patients who have recently received substantial amounts of opioids.
- *Respiratory depression:* Use with caution.
- *Seizures:* Seizures may occur within the recommended dosage range.
- *Withdrawal:* If tramadol is discontinued abruptly, withdrawal symptoms may occur.
- *Overdosage:* Respiratory depression, seizures, vomiting.

Pregnancy Risk Category: Category C.

Oral Health Education
- If chronic dry mouth occurs, recommend home fluoride therapy and use of nonalcoholic oral health care products.

When prescribed by DDS:
- Warn patient not to drink alcoholic products while taking the drug.
- Inform patient not to drive, sign important papers, or operate mechanical equipment while taking drug.
- May produce sedation and interfere with eye-hand coordination and the ability to operate mechanical equipment.
- Instruct patient to take the prescribed dose at the recommended intervals.
- Inform patient to check with health care provider first before taking any OTC or prescription medications, including analgesics.
- Have patient report any serious side effects to health care provider.
- Advise patient not to wait until pain level is high to self-medicate, because drug will not be as effective.
- Advise patient to avoid using alcohol or other CNS depressants (e.g., sleeping pills).
- Advise the patient that this medication may cause drowsiness and to use caution while driving or using heavy equipment or performing other tasks requiring mental alertness.
- Advise patient to notify health care provider if the pain is not relieved by the medication at the prescribed dosage.

Trandate — see labetalol HCl

---

trandolapril (tran-DOE-lah-prill)

Mavik

■▶■ Gopten

Drug Class: Antihypertensive; Angiotensin converting enzyme (ACE) inhibitor

PHARMACOLOGY

Action
Reduces the formation of the vasopressor hormone angiotensin II by inhibiting ACE. Results in decreased BP and reduced sodium reabsorption and potassium retention.

Uses
HEART FAILURE POST-MI/LEFT VENTRICULAR DYSFUNCTION POST-MI: For stable patients who have evidence of left ventricular systolic dysfunction (identified by wall motion abnormalities) or who are symptomatic from CHF within the first few days after sustaining acute MI. HYPERTENSION: Treatment of hypertension either alone or in combination with other antihypertensive drugs.

➤◀ DRUG INTERACTIONS RELATED TO DENTAL THERAPEUTICS

COX-1 inhibitors: Decreased antihypertensive effect (decreased prostaglandin synthesis)
- Monitor blood pressure.

ADVERSE EFFECTS
CNS: Dizziness (23%).
CVS: Bradycardia; hypotension; syncope.
GI: Dyspepsia (6%); gastritis (4%); diarrhea (1%).
RESP: Cough (35%).
MISC: Asthenia (3%); angioedema (0.13%); anaphylactoid reactions; leukopenia; thrombocytopenia.

CLINICAL IMPLICATIONS

General
- Monitor vital signs (e.g., BP, pulse pressure, rate, and rhythm) at each appointment to assess disease control. Do not provide elective dental treatment when BP is ≥180/110 or in the presence of other high-risk CV conditions. Refer to the section entitled "The Patient Taking Cardiovascular Drugs" in Chapter 6: *Clinical Medicine.*
- Use local anesthetic agents with vasoconstrictors with caution based on functional capacity of the patient and use aspirating technique to prevent intravascular injection.
- Determine ability to adapt to stress of dental treatment. Consider short appointments.
- If coughing is problematic, consider semisupine chair position for treatment.
- Susceptible patient with DM may experience severe recurrent hypoglycemia.
- *Postural hypotension:* Monitor BP at the beginning and end of each appointment; anticipate syncope. Have patient sit upright for several min at the end of the dental appointment before dismissing.
- Place on frequent maintenance schedule to avoid periodontal inflammation.
- Blood dyscrasias rarely reported; anticipate increased bleeding, infection, and poor healing.

Oral Health Education
- Encourage daily plaque control procedures for effective self-care in patient at risk for CV disease.

---

 tranexamic acid (tran-ex-AM-ik AS-id)

Cyklokapron: Injection: 100 mg per mL; Tablets: 500 mg
Drug Class: Hematological agent

PHARMACOLOGY

Action
Exerts an antifibrinolytic effect by reversibly blocking the lysine-binding sites on plasminogen molecules.

Uses

Hemorrhage: For short-term use (from 2 to 8 days) in hemophilia patients to reduce or prevent hemorrhage, and to reduce the need for replacement therapy during and following tooth extraction.

Unlabeled Uses

Topically as a mouthwash to reduce bleeding after oral surgery in patients receiving anticoagulant therapy. The drug also inhibits induced hyperfibrinolysis during thrombolytic treatment with plasminogen activators.

Tranexamic acid has been used for many hemostatic purposes including prevention of bleeding after surgery or trauma (e.g., tonsillectomy and adenoidectomy, prostatic surgery, cervical conization), and to prevent rebleeding of subarachnoid hemorrhage.

It has also been used to treat primary or IUD-induced menorrhalgia, gastric and intestinal hemorrhage, recurrent epistaxis, and hereditary angioneurotic edema.

Contraindications

Acquired defective color vision: Prohibits measuring one end-point of toxicity.

Subarachnoid hemorrhage: Cerebral edema and cerebral infarction may be caused by tranexamic acid in patients with subarachnoid hemorrhage.

Usual Dosage

Hemophilia

INJECTABLE OR ORAL FORMULATION

ADULTS: Immediately before surgery, substitution therapy is given with tranexamic acid, 10 mg/kg IV. After surgery, give 25 mg/kg orally 3 to 4 times daily for 2 to 8 days. *Alternative:* Give 25 mg/kg orally, 3 to 4 times per day beginning 1 day prior to surgery.

Oral mucosal or alveolar bleeding

INJECTABLE FORMULATION USED AS A RINSE

Tranexamic acid mouthwash is not commercially available in Canada or the United States; it can be extemporaneously prepared by compounding pharmacist using the commercial tablets or injection. Because stability data for aqueous solution are lacking, compounded solutions should be freshly prepared.

ADULTS AND CHILDREN: Rinse with 5 mL 4 times a day as needed to control bleeding; expectorate, do not swallow.

Pharmacokinetics

ABSORP: Bioavailability 30% to 50%.

DIST: Low protein binding (<3%).

METAB: Little metabolism.

EXCRET: Kidney.

PEAK: 3 hr.

➜← DRUG INTERACTIONS

Retinoic acid: Fatal thromboembolism (mechanism unknown)
- Avoid concurrent use.

ADVERSE EFFECTS

CNS: IV: Giddiness.

CVS: IV: Hypotension has been observed when IV injection is too rapid. Do not inject more rapidly than 1 mL/min; this reaction has not been reported with oral use.

GI: TAB: Nausea, vomiting, and diarrhea occur, but disappear when dosage is reduced.

CLINICAL IMPLICATIONS

General

- *Lactation:* Tranexamic acid is present in breast milk at 1% of the corresponding serum levels. Exercise caution when administering during lactation.

Pregnancy Risk Category: Category B.

Transderm-Nitro — see nitroglycerin
Transderm-V — see scopolamine HBr
trans-retinoic acid — see tretinoin
Tranxene — see clorazepate dipotassium
Tranxene-SD — see clorazepate dipotassium
Tranxene-SD Half Strength — see clorazepate dipotassium
Tranxene T-tab — see clorazepate dipotassium

tranylcypromine sulfate (tran-ill-SIP-row-meen SULL-fate)

Parnate

Drug Class: Antidepressant, MAO inhibitor

PHARMACOLOGY

Action

Tranylcypromine blocks activity of enzyme MAO, thereby increasing monoamine (e.g., epinephrine, norepinephrine, serotonin) concentrations in CNS.

Uses

Treatment of reactive depression.

Unlabeled Uses

Bulimia; treatment of panic disorders with associated agoraphobia.

➔⬅ DRUG INTERACTIONS RELATED TO DENTAL THERAPEUTICS

Tramadol: Increased risk of serotonin syndrome (reduced uptake of monoamines)
- Avoid concurrent use.

Sympathomimetic amines: Severe hypertension (additive)
- Monitor blood pressure.

ADVERSE EFFECTS

⚠ **ORAL:** Dry mouth.

CNS: Dizziness; headache; sleep disturbances; tremors; hyperreflexion; manic symptoms; muscle twitching; convulsions; vertigo; confusion; memory impairment; toxic delirium; hypomania; coma.

CVS: Postural hypotension, syncope, tachycardia, palpitation.

GI: Constipation; nausea; diarrhea; anorexia; abdominal pain.

MISC: Edema, weight gain, chills; anemia, agranulocytosis, leukopenia, thrombocytopenia.

CLINICAL IMPLICATIONS

General

- Determine why drug is being taken. Consider implications of condition on dental treatment.
- Determine ability to adapt to stress of dental treatment. Consider short appointments.
- Depressed or anxious patients may neglect self-care. Monitor for plaque control effectiveness.
- Monitor vital signs.
- *Postural hypotension:* Monitor BP at the beginning and end of each appointment; anticipate syncope. Have patient sit upright for several min at the end of the dental appointment before dismissing.
- If GI side effects occur consider semisupine chair position.

Oral Health Education

- If chronic dry mouth occurs, recommend home fluoride therapy and use of nonalcoholic oral health care products.
- Encourage daily plaque control procedures for effective, nontraumatic self-care.

trazodone HCl (TRAY-zoe-dohn HIGH-droe-KLOR-ide)

Desyrel, Desyrel Dividose

■✦■ **Alti-Trazodone, Alti-Trazodone Dividose, Apo-Trazodone, Apo-Trazodone D, Gen-Trazodone, Novo-Trazodone, Nu-Trazodone, Nu-Trazodone-D, PMS-Trazodone, ratio-Trazodone**

Drug Class: Antidepressant

PHARMACOLOGY

Action
Undetermined; may affect serotonin uptake at presynaptic neuronal membrane.

Uses
Treatment of depression.

Unlabeled Uses
Treatment of neurogenic pain, aggression, panic disorder, cocaine withdrawal.

➡️◀ DRUG INTERACTIONS RELATED TO DENTAL THERAPEUTICS
No documented drug-drug interactions. The absence of evidence is not evidence of safety.

ADVERSE EFFECTS
⚠ **ORAL:** Dry mouth (34%); unpleasant taste.

CNS: Anger; hostility; nightmares/vivid dreams; confusion; disorientation; decreased concentration; dizziness; drowsiness; excitement; fatigue; headache; insomnia; impaired memory; nervousness; tingling; tremors; convulsions; incoordination; paresthesia; agitation; anxiety; grand mal seizures; hallucinations/delusions.

CVS: Hypotension, syncope; cardiac arrest; cardiospasm; cerebrovascular accident.

GI: Abdominal/gastric disorders; nausea; vomiting; diarrhea; constipation; flatulence.

MISC: Hypersensitivity reaction (e.g., skin conditions, edema, rash, itching, purpura); muscle aches and pains; decreased appetite; sweating; changes in weight; malaise; allergic skin condition/edema; nasal/sinus congestion; akathisia; allergic reaction; alopecia; anemia; aphasia; apnea; ataxia; chills; cholestasis; clitorism; diplopia; extrapyramidal symptoms; hematuria; hemolytic anemia; hirsutism; hyperbilirubinemia.

CLINICAL IMPLICATIONS

General
- Determine why drug is being taken. Consider implications of condition on dental treatment.
- Determine ability to adapt to stress of dental treatment. Consider short appointments.
- Depressed or anxious patients may neglect self-care. Monitor for plaque control effectiveness.
- Monitor vital signs.
- *Postural hypotension:* Monitor BP at the beginning and end of each appointment; anticipate syncope. Have patient sit upright for several min at the end of the dental appointment before dismissing.
- Chronic dry mouth is possible; anticipate increased caries and candidiasis.
- If GI side effects occur, consider semisupine chair position.
- Blood dyscrasias rarely reported; anticipate increased bleeding, infection, and poor healing.

Oral Health Education
- If chronic dry mouth occurs, recommend home fluoride therapy and use of nonalcoholic oral health care products.
- Encourage daily plaque control procedures for effective, nontraumatic self-care.

Trecator — see ethionamide
Trecator-SC — see ethionamide

tretinoin (TREH-tih-NO-in)

Synonym: rans-retinoic acid; vitamin A aci

Avita, Renova, Retin-A, Retin-A Micro, Vesanoid

■✦■ **Retisol-A, Stieva-A**

Drug Class: Retinoids

PHARMACOLOGY

Action

TOPICAL: Decreases cohesiveness and stimulates mitotic activity and turnover of follicular epithelial cells, resulting in decreased formation and increased extrusion of comedones. PO: Induces maturation of acute promyelocytic leukemia cells. When given PO, time to reach peak concentration is between 1 and 2 hr. Tretinoin is more than 95% bound in plasma, predominantly to albumin. CYP450 enzymes have been implicated in the oxidative metabolism of tretinoin.

Uses

Topical treatment of acne vulgaris; as an adjunctive agent for use in the mitigation of fine wrinkles, mottled hyperpigmentation, and tactile roughness of facial skin. PO treatment for acute promyelocytic leukemia.

Unlabeled Uses

Treatment of skin cancer; various dermatological conditions including lamellar ichthyosis, warts, and Darier disease.

➡◀ DRUG INTERACTIONS RELATED TO DENTAL THERAPEUTICS

No documented drug-drug interactions. The absence of evidence is not evidence of safety.

ADVERSE EFFECTS

⚠ **ORAL:** Dry mouth and lips; mucositis.

CNS: Fatigue; weakness; headache; fever; malaise; dizziness; anxiety; paresthesia; insomnia; depression; confusion; agitation; hallucination; severe headache may be more common in children; cerebral hemorrhage; intracranial hypertension; pseudotumor cerebri.

CVS: Arrhythmia (23%); hypotension (14%); hypertension (11%); cardiac failure (6%).

GI: Nausea and vomiting; elevated LFTs; GI hemorrhage; abdominal pain; diarrhea; anorexia; constipation; dyspepsia.

RESP: Upper and lower respiratory tract disorders; dyspnea; pleural effusion.

MISC: Retinoic acid-acute promyelocytic leukemia syndrome, characterized by fever, dyspnea, weight gain, radiographic pulmonary infiltrates, and pleural or pericardial effusions; infections; photosensitivity.

CLINICAL IMPLICATIONS

General

- Determine why drug is being taken. Consider implications of condition on dental treatment.
- Consider medical consult to determine disease control and influence on dental treatment.
- Monitor blood pressure and pulse (capsules).
- Advise products for palliative relief of oral manifestations (e.g., stomatitis, mucositis, xerostomia, etc.)

- Chronic dry mouth is possible; anticipate increased caries and candidiasis.
- Do not prescribe drugs with the potential for additive photosensitivity, risk of phototoxicity (cream).

Oral Health Education

- If chronic dry mouth occurs, recommend home fluoride therapy and use of nonalcoholic oral health care products.

Trexall — see methotrexate

Triacet — see triamcinolone

Triam Forte — see triamcinolone

---

triamcinolone (TRY-am-SIN-oh-lone)
(triamcinolone acetonide, triamcinolone diacetate, triamcinolone hexacetonide)

Aristocort: Tablets: 4 mg; Ointment: 0.1%; Cream: 0.025, 0.1, 0.5%
Aristocort A: Ointment: 0.1%; Cream: 0.025, 0.1, 0.5%
Aristocort Intralesional: Injection: 25-mg/mL suspension
Aristospan Intra-articular: Injection: 20-mg/mL suspension
Aristospan Intralesional: Injection: 5-mg/mL suspension
Azmacort: Aerosol: 100 mcg/actuation (Inhaler contains 60 mg)
Kenalog: Ointment: 0.025, 0.1%; Cream: 0.025, 0.5%; Aerosol: 2 sec. Spray
Kenalog-10: Injection: 10-mg/mL suspension
Kenalog-40, Amcort, Cinacort, Triam Forte, Trilone, Tristoject: Injection: 40-mg/mL suspension
Kenalog-H, Triacet, Triderm: Cream: 0.1%
Kenalog in Orabase: Paste: 0.1%
Nasacort AQ: Spray: 55 mcg/actuation
Nasacort HFA: Aerosol: 55 mcg/actuation
Tac-3: Injection: 3-mg/mL suspension

🔳🍁🔳 **Aristospan, Oracort, Aristocort Parenteral, Aristocort Syrup**

🔳🍁🔳 **Kenacort, Ledercort, Triamsicort, Zamacort**

Drug Class: Corticosteroid

PHARMACOLOGY

Action
Anti-inflammatory effect by depressing formation, release, and activity of endogenous mediators of inflammation including prostaglandins, kinins, histamine, liposomal enzymes, and complement system. Also modifies body's immune response.

Uses
PO/IM/IV administration: Replacement therapy in endocrine disorders; adjunctive therapy for short-term administration in rheumatic disorders; maintenance therapy or control of exacerbation of collagen diseases; treatment of dermatological diseases; control of allergic states; management of allergic and inflammatory ophthalmic processes; treatment of respiratory diseases, including pulmonary emphysema and diffuse interstitial pulmonary fibrosis; treatment of selected hematological disorders; palliative management of selective neoplastic diseases; induction of diuresis in edematous states caused by nephrotic syndrome or refractory CHF, and in ascites caused by cirrhosis; control of exacerbation in selected GI diseases (e.g., inflammatory bowel disease); control of exacerbation of multiple sclerosis; adjunctive treatment of tuberculous meningitis; treatment of trichinosis with neurologic or myocardial involvement; management of postoperative dental inflammatory reactions.
Intra-articular or soft tissue administration: Short-term adjunctive therapy in synovitis of os-

teoarthritis, rheumatoid arthritis, bursitis, acute gouty arthritis, epicondylitis, acute nonspecific tenosynovitis, posttraumatic osteoarthritis.

Intralesional administration: Management of keloids; treatment of localized hypertrophic, infiltrated, inflammatory lesions of lichen planus, psoriatic plaques, granuloma annulare, lichen simplex chronicus; treatment of discoid lupus erythematosus, necrobiosis lipoidica diabeticorum, alopecia areata, cystic tumors of aponeurosis or tendon.

Topical application: Relief of inflammatory and pruritic manifestations of corticosteroid-responsive dermatoses.

Oral inhalation: Maintenance treatment of asthma as prophylactic therapy; use in asthma patients requiring systemic corticosteroid administration.

Intranasal administration: Relief of seasonal and perennial allergic rhinitis symptoms.

Contraindications

Systemic fungal infections; IM use in idiopathic thrombocytopenic purpura; administration of live virus vaccines; topical monotherapy in primary bacterial infections; topical use on face, groin, or axilla; oral inhalation as primary treatment for status asthmaticus or other acute episodes of asthma; intranasal administration in untreated localized infections involving nasal mucosa.

Usual Dosage

TRIAMCINOLONE
ADULTS: *PO:* 4 to 100 mg/day.
CHILDREN: *PO:* 0.117 to 1.66 mg/kg/day.

TRIAMCINOLONE ACETONIDE
ADULTS AND CHILDREN: *Topical:* Apply sparingly bid to qid.

➜← DRUG INTERACTIONS

No documented drug-drug interactions (topical use). The absence of evidence is not evidence of safety.

ADVERSE EFFECTS

⚠ **ORAL:** Dry mouth, throat; oral candidiasis (inhalation); stinging (cream); masking of infection.

CVS: Edema; thromboembolism or fat embolism; thrombophlebitis; necrotizing angiitis; cardiac arrhythmias or ECG changes; syncopal episodes; hypertension; myocardial rupture; CHF.

CNS: Convulsions; pseudotumor cerebri; vertigo; headache; neuritis; paresthesias; psychosis.

GI: Pancreatitis; nausea; vomiting; increased appetite and weight gain; peptic ulcer; bowel perforation.

RESP: Wheezing (oral).

MISC: Musculoskeletal effects (e.g., weakness, myopathy, muscle mass loss, osteoporosis, spontaneous fractures); endocrine abnormalities (e.g., menstrual irregularities, cushingoid state, growth suppression in children, sweating, decreased carbohydrate tolerance or hyperglycemia, glycosuria, increased insulin or sulfonylurea requirements in diabetic patients, hirsutism); anaphylactoid or hypersensitivity reactions; aggravation or masking of infections; osteonecrosis, tendon rupture, infection, skin atrophy, postinjection flare, hypersensitivity, facial flushing (intra-articular); may cause adverse effects similar to systemic use because of absorption (topical).

CLINICAL IMPLICATIONS

General

- Determine why drug is being taken. Consider implications of condition on dental treatment.
- Be aware that signs of bacterial oral infection may be masked and anticipate oral candidiasis.

- *Osteoporosis:* Patient may be high-risk candidate for pathological fractures or jaw fractures during extractions.
- Place patient on frequent maintenance schedule to avoid periodontal inflammation.
- Anticipate Addisonian or cushingoid complications affecting the head and neck area (tablet).
- Despite the anticipated perioperative physiological stress (i.e., minor surgical stress), patients undergoing dental care under local anesthesia should take only their usual daily glucocorticoid dose before dental intervention. No supplementation is justified.
- Chronic dry mouth is possible; anticipate increased caries and candidiasis (inhalation).

When used or prescribed by DDS:
- *Lactation:* Undetermined.
- *Children:* Children may be more susceptible to adverse effects from topical use.
- *Hypersensitivity:* Reactions, including anaphylaxis, may occur.
- *Overdosage:* Moon face, central obesity, striae, hirsutism, acne, ecchymoses, hypertension, osteoporosis, myopathy, sexual dysfunction, hyperglycemia, hyperlipidemia, peptic ulcer, electrolyte and fluid imbalance (excessive or long-term use).

Pregnancy Risk Category: Category C (oral inhalation/nasal/topical).

Oral Health Education
- Teach patient to rinse mouth and gargle vigorously with water after inhaled steroid use to minimize the potential for candidiasis (inhalation).

When used or prescribed by DDS:
- Explain name, dose, action, and potential side effects of drug.
- Advise patient to read the *Patient Information* leaflet before starting therapy and again with each refill.
- Advise patient to continue taking other medications for same condition as prescribed by health care provider.
- Explain that effects of drug are not immediate. Benefit requires daily use as instructed and usually begins to occur within 1 or 2 days, but full benefit may take 1 to 2 wk, depending on the condition being treated and the dose and route of administration of medication being used.
- Caution patient not to decrease the dose or stop using the drug unless advised by health care provider.
- Caution patient not to increase dose but to inform health care provider if symptoms do not seem to be improving or are worsening.
- Advise women to notify health care provider if pregnant, planning to become pregnant, or breast feeding.
- Caution patient not to take any prescription or OTC medications, dietary supplements, or herbal preparations unless advised by health care provider.
- Advise patient that follow-up visits may be required to monitor therapy and to keep appointments.
- *Dental paste:* Teach patient proper technique for applying the paste: press a small dab (about 1/4 in) on the lesion until a thin film develops. Caution patient not to rub the paste into the lesion.
- Advise patient to apply at bedtime if being used once a day and after meals if being used more than once a day.
- Advise patient to stop using and inform health care provider if any of the following local reactions occur: burning, itching, new blistering or peeling, irritation, new sores.

---

triamcinolone acetonide — see triamcinolone

triamcinolone diacetate — see triamcinolone

triamcinolone hexacetonide — see triamcinolone

Triaminic AM Decongestant Formula — see pseudoephedrine

Triaminic Infant Oral Decongestant Drops — see pseudoephedrine

Triaminic Pediatric — see pseudoephedrine

Triaminic Thin Strips Cough and Runny Nose — see
diphenhydramine HCl

Triamsicort — see triamcinolone

triamterene (try-AM-tur-een)

Dyrenium

Drug Class: Diuretic, potassium-sparing

PHARMACOLOGY

Action

Interferes with sodium reabsorption at distal renal tubule, resulting in increased excretion of sodium and water and decreased excretion of potassium.

Uses

Treatment of edema associated with CHF, hepatic cirrhosis, and nephrotic syndrome; treatment of steroid-induced edema, idiopathic edema, and edema caused by secary hyperaldosteronism; management of hypertension in patient with diuretic-induced hypokalemia or at risk of hypokalemia.

➡◀ DRUG INTERACTIONS RELATED TO DENTAL THERAPEUTICS

No documented drug-drug interactions. The absence of evidence is not evidence of safety.

ADVERSE EFFECTS

⚠ **ORAL:** Dry mouth.

CNS: Weakness; fatigue; dizziness; headache.

GI: Diarrhea; nausea; vomiting.

MISC: Anaphylaxis; muscle cramps; photosensitivity; thrombocytopenia; megaloblastic anemia.

CLINICAL IMPLICATIONS

General

- Determine why drug is being taken. Consider implications of condition on dental treatment.
- Monitor vital signs (e.g., BP, pulse pressure, rate, and rhythm) at each appointment to assess disease control. Do not provide elective dental treatment when BP is ≥180/110 or in the presence of other high-risk CV conditions. Refer to the section entitled "The Patient Taking Cardiovascular Drugs" in Chapter 6: *Clinical Medicine.*
- Use local anesthetic agents with vasoconstrictor with caution based on functional capacity of the patient and use aspirating technique to prevent intravascular injection.
- Determine ability to adapt to stress of dental treatment. Consider short appointments.
- Monitor pulse rhythm to assess for electrolyte imbalance.
- Chronic dry mouth is possible; anticipate increased caries activity, candidiasis, and lichenoid mucositis.
- Blood dyscrasias rarely reported; anticipate increased bleeding, infection, and poor healing.
- Place patient on frequent maintenance schedule to avoid periodontal inflammation.

Oral Health Education

- Encourage daily plaque control procedures for effective self-care in patient at risk for CV disease.
- If chronic dry mouth occurs, recommend home fluoride therapy and use of nonalcoholic oral health care products.

Triatec-30 — see acetaminophen/codeine phosphate

triazolam (try-AZE-oh-lam)

Halcion

■✲■ Alti-Triazolam, APO-Triazo, Gen-Triazolam

Drug Class: Sedative and hypnotic, benzodiazepine
DEA Schedule: Schedule IV (Canada: Schedule F)

PHARMACOLOGY

Action
Potentiates action of GABA (gamma-aminobutyric acid), an inhibitory neurotransmitter, resulting in increased neuronal inhibition and CNS depression, especially in limbic system and reticular formation.

Uses
Treatment of insomnia.

➜◀ DRUG INTERACTIONS RELATED TO DENTAL THERAPEUTICS

Clarithromycin: Possible triazolam toxicity (decreased metabolism)
- Avoid concurrent use.

ADVERSE EFFECTS

⚠ **ORAL:** Dry mouth; taste disturbance; stomatitis; glossitis.

CNS: Anterograde amnesia; headache; nervousness; drowsiness; confusion; talkativeness; apprehension; irritability; euphoria; weakness; tremor; incoordination; memory impairment; depression; ataxia; dizziness; dreaming/nightmares; hallucinations; paradoxical reactions (e.g., anger, hostility, mania, muscle spasms).

CVS: Palpitations, tachycardia.

GI: Heartburn; nausea; vomiting; diarrhea; constipation; anorexia.

MISC: Dependence/withdrawal syndrome (e.g., confusion, abnormal perception of movement, depersonalization, muscle twitching, psychosis, paranoid delusions, seizures). Rebound sleep disorder (recurrence of insomnia worse than before treatment) may occur during first 3 nights after abrupt discontinuation; leukopenia, granulocytopenia.

CLINICAL IMPLICATIONS

General
- Chronic dry mouth is possible; anticipate increased caries and candidiasis.
- Monitor vital signs.

Oral Health Education
- If chronic dry mouth occurs, recommend home fluoride therapy and use of nonalcoholic oral health care products.
- Encourage patient to follow daily plaque control procedures for effective self-care.

Tricor — see fenofibrate
Triderm — see triamcinolone
Tridesilon — see desonide

---

trifluoperazine HCl (try-flew-oh-PURR-uh-zeen HIGH-droe-KLOR-ide)

Trifluoperazine HCl

■✲■ Apo-Trifluoperazine

Drug Class: Antipsychotic, phenothiazine

PHARMACOLOGY

Action
Effects apparently related to dopamine receptor blocking in CNS.

Uses
Management of schizophrenia; short-term treatment (<12 wk) of nonpsychotic anxiety.

➡◀ DRUG INTERACTIONS RELATED TO DENTAL THERAPEUTICS
No documented drug-drug interactions. The absence of evidence is not evidence of safety.

ADVERSE EFFECTS
⚠ **ORAL:** Tardive dyskinesia; dry mouth; tongue protrusion.

CNS: Lightheadedness; faintness; headache; weakness; tremor; fatigue; slurring of speech; insomnia; sedation; vertigo; seizures; twitching; ataxia; drowsiness; lethargy; paradoxical excitement; pseudoparkinsonism; motor restlessness; oculogyric crises; opisthotonos; hyperreflexia; dizziness; dystonia.

CVS: Hypotension.

GI: Dyspepsia; constipation; adynamic ileus (may result in death); nausea; anorexia.

RESP: Laryngospasm; bronchospasm; shortness of breath.

MISC: Increases in appetite and weight; polydipsia; heat-related illness; neuroleptic malignant syndrome; elevated prolactin levels; blood dyscrasias (e.g., anemia, leukopenia, thrombocytopenia, others).

CLINICAL IMPLICATIONS

General
- Determine why drug is being taken. Consider implications of condition on dental treatment.
- Clients with psychological disease may present with behavior management problems.
- Extrapyramidal behaviors can complicate performance of oral procedures. If present, consult with MD to consider medication changes.
- Chronic dry mouth is possible; anticipate increased caries and candidiasis.
- Monitor vital signs.

Oral Health Education
- Evaluate manual dexterity; consider need for power toothbrush.
- Encourage patient to follow daily plaque control procedures for effective self-care.
- If chronic dry mouth occurs, recommend home fluoride therapy and use of nonalcoholic oral health care products.

Triglide — see fenofibrate

triiodothyronine — see liothyronine sodium

Tri-K — see potassium products

Trileptal — see oxcarbazepine

Trilone — see triamcinolone

---

trimethoprim/sulfamethoxazole (try-METH-oh-prim/suhl-fuh-meth-OX-uh-zole)

Synonyms: co-trimoxazole; sulfamethoxazole/trimethoprim; TMP-SMZ

Bactrim, Bactrim D.S., Bactrim IV, Bactrim Pediatric, Cotrim, Cotrim D.S., Cotrim Pediatric, Septra, Septra DS, Septra IV, Sulfatrim, Uroplus DS, Uroplus SS

■✦■ **Apo-Sulfatrim, Bactrim Roche, Novo-Trimel, Novo-Trimel D.S., Nu-Cotrimox, Septra Injection**

Drug Class: Anti-infective

PHARMACOLOGY

Action

Sulfamethoxazole (SMZ) inhibits bacterial synthesis of dihydrofolic acid by competing with PABA. Trimethoprim (TMP) blocks production of tetrahydrofolic acid by inhibiting the enzyme dihydrofolate reductase. This combination blocks two consecutive steps in bacterial biosynthesis of essential nucleic acids and proteins and is usually bactericidal.

Uses

PO/PARENTERAL: Treatment of UTIs caused by susceptible strains of bacteria, shigellosis enteritis, and *Pneumocystis carinii* pneumonitis.

PO: Treatment of acute otitis media and acute exacerbations of chronic bronchitis; treatment of traveler's diarrhea.

Unlabeled Uses

Treatment of cholera, salmonella-type infections, and nocardiosis; prevention of recurrent UTIs in women; prophylaxis of bacterial infections in susceptible patients; treatment of prostatitis; prophylaxis of *Pneumocystis carinii* pneumonitis.

➤◆ DRUG INTERACTIONS RELATED TO DENTAL THERAPEUTICS

No documented drug-drug interactions. The absence of evidence is not evidence of safety.

ADVERSE EFFECTS

⚠ ORAL: Glossitis; stomatitis.

CNS: Headache; mental depression; ataxia, tinnitus; vertigo.

GI: Nausea; vomiting; anorexia.

RESP: Pulmonary congestion.

MISC: Allergic skin reactions (e.g., rash, urticaria); arthralgia; myalgia; agranulocytosis; thrombocytopenia; leukopenia; hemolytic anemia; hyperkalemia.

CLINICAL IMPLICATIONS

General

- Determine why drug is being taken. Take precautions to avoid cross-contamination of microorganisms.
- If oral infection occurs that requires antibiotic therapy, select an appropriate product from a different class of anti-infectives.
- If GI side effects occur, consider semisupine chair position.
- Blood dyscrasias rarely reported; anticipate increased bleeding, infection, and poor healing.

Oral Health Education

- Encourage daily plaque control procedures for effective, nontraumatic self-care.

Trimox — see amoxicillin

Triostat — see liothyronine sodium

Triptone — see dimenhydrinate

Tristoject — see triamcinolone

Tritace — see ramipril

Trixilem — see methotrexate

Triyotex — see liothyronine sodium

Trizivir — see abacavir sulfate/lamivudine/zidovudine

Trocal — see dextromethorphan HBr
Tromigal — see erythromycin
Trompersantin — see dipyridamole

---

trovafloxacin mesylate/alatrofloxacin mesylate (TROE-vah-FLOX-ah-sin MEH-sih-LATE/al-at-row-FLOX-ah-sin)

Synonym: alatrofloxacin mesylate/trovafloxacin mesylate

Trovan

Drug Class: Antibiotic, fluoroquinolone

PHARMACOLOGY

Action

The intravenous (IV) form is rapidly converted to trovafloxacin, which interferes with microbial DNA synthesis.

Uses

Treatment of nosocomial pneumonia, community-acquired pneumonia, complicated intra-abdominal infections, complicated skin and skin structure infections, and gynecological and pelvic infections caused by susceptible organisms.

➡◀ DRUG INTERACTIONS RELATED TO DENTAL THERAPEUTICS

No documented drug-drug interactions. The absence of evidence is not evidence of safety.

ADVERSE EFFECTS

CNS: Headache; dizziness; lightheadedness.
GI: Nausea; diarrhea; vomiting; abdominal pain.
MISC: Application/injection/insertion site reaction (IV use).

CLINICAL IMPLICATIONS

General

- Determine why drug is being taken. Take precautions to avoid cross-contamination of microorganisms.
- If oral infection occurs that requires antibiotic therapy, select an appropriate product from a different class of anti-infectives.
- If prescribed by the DDS, ensure patient knows how to take the drug and how long it should be taken, and to immediately report adverse effects (e.g., rash, difficult breathing, diarrhea, GI upset). See Chapter 4: *Medical Management of Odontogenic Infections.*
- Antibiotic-associated diarrhea can occur. Have patient contact DDS immediately if signs develop.
- Prolonged use of antibiotics may result in bacterial or fungal overgrowth of nonsusceptible microorganisms; anticipate candidiasis.

Trovan — see trovafloxacin mesylate/alatrofloxacin mesylate
Truphylline — see aminophylline
Tryptanol — see amitriptyline HCl
T/Scalp — see hydrocortisone
Tukol — see guaifenesin
Tusibron — see guaifenesin
Tussin — see guaifenesin
Tusstat — see diphenhydramine HCl

Twilite — see diphenhydramine HCl
Twin-K — see potassium products
Tylenol Arthritis — see acetaminophen
Tylenol Caplets — see acetaminophen
Tylenol Elixir with Codeine — see acetaminophen/codeine phosphate
Tylenol Extended Relief — see acetaminophen
Tylenol Extra Strength — see acetaminophen
Tylenol Infants' Drops — see acetaminophen
Tylenol Junior Strength — see acetaminophen
Tylenol Regular Strength — see acetaminophen
Tylenol w/Codeine — see acetaminophen/codeine phosphate
Tylenol w/Codeine No. 2 — see acetaminophen/codeine phosphate
Tylenol w/Codeine No. 3 — see acetaminophen/codeine phosphate
Tylenol w/Codeine No. 4 — see acetaminophen/codeine phosphate
Tylex — see acetaminophen
Tylex 750 — see acetaminophen
Tylex CD — see acetaminophen/codeine phosphate
Tylox — see acetaminophen/oxycodone HCl
U-Cort — see hydrocortisone
Ulcedine — see cimetidine
Ulpax — see lansoprazole
Ulsen — see omeprazole
Ultracaine-DS — see articaine HCl
Ultracet — see acetaminophen/tramadol HCl
Ultradol — see etodolac
Ultram — see tramadol HCl
Ultravate — see halobetasol propionate
Uni-Ace — see acetaminophen
Unidet — see tolterodine tartrate
Uni-Dur — see theophylline
Uniphyl — see theophylline
Unisom Extra Strength — see diphenhydramine HCl
Unisom Extra Strength Sleepgels — see diphenhydramine HCl
Uni-tussin — see guaifenesin
Univasc — see moexipril HCl
Unizuric 300 — see allopurinol
Urecholine — see bethanechol chloride
Urispas — see flavoxate
Uromol HC — see hydrocortisone
Uroplus DS — see trimethoprim/sulfamethoxazole
Uroplus SS — see trimethoprim/sulfamethoxazole

Uroxatral — see alfuzosin HCl
Urozide — see hydrochlorothiazide
Uvega — see lidocaine HCl

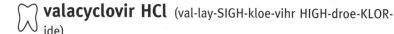 **valacyclovir HCl** (val-lay-SIGH-kloe-vihr HIGH-droe-KLOR-ide)

Valtrex: Tablets: 500 mg, 1 g

Drug Class: Anti-infective; Antiviral

PHARMACOLOGY

Action
Converted to acyclovir, which then inhibits viral DNA replication by interfering with viral DNA polymerase.

Uses
Treatment of herpes zoster (shingles); treatment or suppression of genital herpes; treatment of herpes labialis (cold sores).

Contraindications
Hypersensitivity or intolerance to valacyclovir, acyclovir, or any component of the formulation.

Usual Dosage
Herpes zoster
ADULTS: *PO:* 1 g tid for 7 days (initiate therapy within 48 hr of onset of rash).
HIV-infected patients
ADULTS: *PO:* 500 mg bid for HIV-infected patients with CD4 cell count of at least 100 cells/mm³ (efficacy beyond 6 mo of therapy has not been established).
Herpes labialis
ADULTS: *PO:* 2 g bid for 1 day approximately 12 hr apart, initiated at earliest symptoms of cold sore (e.g., tingling, burning, itching).

Pharmacokinetics
ABSORP: Rapidly absorbed from the GI tract. Bioavailability is about 55%. C_{max} is less than 0.5 mcg/mL.
DIST: Extensive tissue distribution.
METAB: Converted to acyclovir and L-valine by first-pass intestinal or hepatic metabolism.
EXCRET: About 46% is recovered in urine. About 47% is recovered in feces.
SPECIAL POP: *Renal failure:* Dose reduction is recommended.
Elderly: Dose modification may be necessary in geriatric patients with reduced renal function.

➡◀ DRUG INTERACTIONS

Ceftriaxone: Possible increased risk of renal toxicity (mechanism unknown)
 • Avoid concurrent use or monitor renal function.
Meperidine: Meperidine toxicity (decreased renal excretion)
 • Monitor clinical status.
Probenecid: Possible valacyclovir toxicity (decreased renal excretion)
 • Avoid concurrent use or monitor renal function.
Theophylline: Possible theophylline toxicity (decreased metabolism)
 • Avoid concurrent use or monitor theophylline concentration.

Zidovudine: Severe drowsiness and lethargy (mechanism unknown)
- Monitor clinical status.

ADVERSE EFFECTS

CVS: Hypertension; tachycardia.

CNS: Headache (38%); depression (7%); dizziness (4%); aggressive behavior; agitation; ataxia; coma; confusion; decreased consciousness; dysarthria; encephalopathy; mania; psychosis (including audio and visual hallucinations); seizures.

GI: Nausea (15%); abdominal pain (11%); vomiting (6%); diarrhea.

MISC: Arthralgia (6%); acute hypersensitivity reactions (e.g., anaphylaxis, angioedema, dyspnea, pruritus, rash, urticaria); facial edema; leukocytoclastic vasculitis; photosensitivity; leukopenia; thrombocytopenia.

CLINICAL IMPLICATIONS

General
- Determine why drug is being taken. Consider implications of condition on dental treatment.
- If GI side effects occur, consider semisupine chair position.
- Blood dyscrasias rarely reported; anticipate increased bleeding, infection, and poor healing.

When prescribed by DDS:
- Ensure patient knows how to take the drug, how long it should be taken, and to immediately report adverse effects (e.g., rash, difficult breathing, diarrhea, GI upset). See Chapter 4: *Medical Management of Odontogenic Infections.*
- *Lactation:* Undetermined.
- *Children:* Safety and efficacy not established.
- *Elderly:* Dosage reduction may be necessary, depending on underlying renal status.
- *Renal failure:* Dosage reduction is recommended; exercise caution when giving valacyclovir to patients with renal impairment or those receiving potentially nephrotoxic drugs.
- *Immunocompromised patients:* Valacyclovir is not indicated for use in immunocompromised patients.
- *Thrombotic thrombocytopenic purpura/hemolytic uremic syndrome:* May occur and has resulted in death in patients with advanced HIV disease and also in allergenic bone marrow and renal transplant recipients receiving 8 g/day of valacyclovir.
- *Overdosage:* Acute renal failure, anuria.

Pregnancy Risk Category: Category B.

Oral Health Education
- Advise patient to initiate treatment at the earliest sign of oral herpetic symptoms.
- Recommend that toothbrush be replaced following clearance of oral infection.

When used or prescribed by DDS:
- Explain name, dose, action, and potential side effects of drug.
- Review dose and appropriate dosing schedule depending on condition being treated (e.g., shingles, cold sores, or genital herpes). Instruct patient to take medication exactly as prescribed and not to stop taking or change the dose unless advised by health care provider.
- Advise patient that medication can be taken without regard to meals but to take with food if stomach upset occurs.
- Remind patient using medication for cold sores that it is not a cure and to initiate therapy at the first symptom of a cold sore (e.g., tingling, itching, burning). Remind patient that treatment should not exceed two doses taken about 12 hr apart.
- Advise patient to contact health care provider if medication does not seem to be controlling lesions and/or symptoms or if intolerable side effects develop.
- Caution patient to avoid unnecessary exposure to UV light (i.e., sunlight, tanning booths) and to use sunscreen and wear protective clothing until tolerance is determined.
- Advise women to contact health care provider if pregnant, planning to become pregnant, or breast feeding.

- Instruct patient not to take any prescription or OTC medications or dietary supplements unless advised by health care provider.
- Advise patient that follow-up visits may be necessary to monitor therapy and to keep appointments.

Valisone — see betamethasone
Valisone Scalp Lotion — see betamethasone
Valium — see diazepam
Valium Roche Oral — see diazepam

---

valproic acid and derivatives (VAL-pro-ik acid)
Synonyms: divalproex sodium; sodium valproate

Depacon, Depakene, Depakote, Depakote ER

■✦■ **Alti-Valproic, Apo-Divalproex, Apo-Valproic, Epiject, Gen-Valproic, Novo-Divalproex, Novo-Valproic, Nu-Divalproex, Nu-Valproic, PMS-Valproic Acid, ratio-Valproic, Rhoxal-valproic, Rhoxal-valproic EC**

■✦■ **Atemperator-S, Cryoval, Depakene, Epival, Leptilan, Valprosid**

Drug Class: Anticonvulsant

PHARMACOLOGY

Action
Believed to work by increasing brain levels of gamma-aminobutyric acid (GABA). It may also inhibit catabolism of GABA, potentiate postsynaptic GABA responses, and affect potassium channels or directly stabilize membranes.

Uses
Sole and adjunctive therapy in simple (petit mal) and complex absence seizures; adjunctive therapy in multiple seizure types, including absence seizures; monotherapy and adjunctive therapy in complex partial seizures that occur in isolation or with other seizure types; manic episodes associated with bipolar disorder (divalproex sodium delayed-release tablets); prophylaxis of migraine headaches (divalproex sodium delayed-release and extended-release [ER] tablets).

Unlabeled Uses
Treatment of atypical absence, myoclonic, and tonic-clonic (grand mal) seizures and atonic, elementary partial, and infantile spasm seizures; prevention of recurrent pediatric febrile seizures; intractable status epilepticus in patients who have not responded to other therapies; treatment of minor incontinence after ileoanal anastomosis (subchronic administration); management of anxiety disorders and panic attacks.

➡✦ DRUG INTERACTIONS RELATED TO DENTAL THERAPEUTICS

Aspirin: Possible valproate toxicity (displacement from protein binding)
- Avoid concurrent use.

Clonazepam: May precipitate absence status (mechanism unknown)
- Avoid concurrent use.

Diazepam or midazolam: Possible IV diazepam or midazolam toxicity (displacement from protein binding)
- Monitor clinical status.

ADVERSE EFFECTS

⚠ **ORAL:** Dry mouth, glossitis, periodontal abscess, stomatitis, tooth disorder, tardive dyskinesia (1% to 5%).

CNS: Tremor (57%); somnolence (30%); asthenia (21%); dizziness (18%); insomnia (15%); nervousness (11%); amnesia (7%); headache (5% or more); depression (5%); ataxia, emotional lability, abnormal thinking, paresthesia (1% to 5%); anxiety, confusion, abnormal gait, hypertonia, incoordination, abnormal dreams, personality disorder, agitation, catatonic reaction, dysarthria, hallucinations, hypokinesia, increased reflexes, speech disorder, vertigo (>1% but <5%).

GI: Nausea (34%); diarrhea, vomiting (23%); dyspepsia (13%); abdominal pain (12%); anorexia (11%); increased appetite (6%); constipation (1% to 5%); flatulence, hematemesis, eructation, fecal incontinence, gastroenteritis, GI disorder (>1% but <5%).

RESP: Infection (20%); flu-like syndrome (12%); rhinitis; dyspnea (1% to 5%); epistaxis, pneumonia, sinusitis, increased cough (>1% but <5%).

MISC: Infection (15%); back pain (8%); injection site pain (3%); injection site reaction (2%); fever, chest pain, vasodilation, peripheral edema, accidental injury, chills, face edema, viral infection (1% to 5%); malaise (>1% but <5%); lupus erythematosus; anaphylaxis.

CLINICAL IMPLICATIONS

General
- Determine why drug is being taken. Consider implications of condition on dental treatment.
- Determine ability to adapt to stress of dental treatment. Consider short appointments.
- Determine level of disease control, type, and frequency of seizure and compliance with medication regimen.
- Chronic dry mouth is possible; anticipate increased caries and candidiasis.
- Extrapyramidal behaviors can complicate performance of oral procedures. If present, consult with MD to consider medication changes.

Oral Health Education
- If chronic dry mouth occurs, recommend home fluoride therapy and use of nonalcoholic oral health care products.

Valprosid — see valproic acid and derivatives

---

valsartan (VAL-sahr-tan)

Diovan

Drug Class: Antihypertensive; Angiotensin II antagonist

PHARMACOLOGY

Action
Antagonizes the effects of angiotensin II (vasoconstriction and aldosterone secretion) by blocking the angiotensin II receptor (AT_1 receptor) in vascular smooth muscle and the adrenal gland, producing decreased BP.

Uses
Treatment of hypertension either alone or in combination with other antihypertensive drugs; heart failure.

➡️◀ DRUG INTERACTIONS RELATED TO DENTAL THERAPEUTICS
No documented drug-drug interactions. The absence of evidence is not evidence of safety.

ADVERSE EFFECTS
⚠ **ORAL:** Dry mouth (<1%).
CNS: Headache; dizziness; fatigue.
GI: Abdominal pain; diarrhea; nausea.
RESP: Cough (infrequent).
MISC: Fatigue; viral infection; edema; arthralgia.

CLINICAL IMPLICATIONS

General
- Monitor vital signs (e.g., BP, pulse pressure, rate, and rhythm) at each appointment to assess disease control. Do not provide elective dental treatment when BP is ≥180/110 or in the presence of other high-risk CV conditions. Refer to the section entitled "The Patient Taking Cardiovascular Drugs" in Chapter 6: *Clinical Medicine.*
- Use local anesthetic agents with vasoconstrictor with caution based on functional capacity of the patient and use aspirating technique to prevent intravascular injection.
- Determine ability to adapt to stress of dental treatment. Consider short appointments.
- Place patient on frequent maintenance schedule to avoid periodontal inflammation.

Oral Health Education
- Encourage daily plaque control procedures for effective self-care in patient at risk for CV disease.

---

valsartan/hydrochlorothiazide (VAL-sahr-tan/ HIGH-droe-klor-oh-THIGH-uh-zide)

Synonym: hydrochlorothiazide/valsartan

Diovan HCT

Drug Class: Antihypertensive combination

PHARMACOLOGY

Action
VALSARTAN: Antagonizes the effects of angiotensin II (vasoconstriction and aldosterone secretion) by blocking the angiotensin II receptor (AT_1 receptor) in vascular smooth muscle and the adrenal gland, producing decreased BP.

HYDROCHLOROTHIAZIDE (HCTZ): Increases chloride, sodium, and water excretion by interfering with transport of sodium ions across renal tubular epithelium.

Uses
Treatment of hypertension.

➤← DRUG INTERACTIONS RELATED TO DENTAL THERAPEUTICS

COX-1 inhibitors: Decreased antihypertensive effect (decreased prostaglandin synthesis)
- Monitor blood pressure.

ADVERSE EFFECTS

⚠ **ORAL:** Dry mouth.

CNS: Headache; fatigue; dizziness; increased appetite; anxiety; insomnia; decreased libido; paresthesia; somnolence; asthenia.

CVS: Postural hypotension.

GI: Diarrhea; constipation; dyspepsia; flatulence; nausea; abdominal pain; vomiting. HCTZ: Pancreatitis; sialadenitis; cramping; gastric irritation.

RESP: Cough; URI; dyspnea; epistaxis; bronchitis.

MISC: Viral infection; back pain; chest pain; allergic reaction; anaphylaxis; asthenia; dependent edema; arthralgia; muscle cramps; muscle weakness; arm pain; leg pain; angioedema. HCTZ: Hypersensitivity (e.g., purpura, photosensitivity, urticaria, necrotizing angiitis, fever, respiratory distress, anaphylactic reactions).

CLINICAL IMPLICATIONS

General
- Monitor vital signs (e.g., BP, pulse pressure, rate, and rhythm) at each appointment to assess disease control. Do not provide elective dental treatment when BP is ≥180/110 or in the presence of other high-risk CV conditions. Refer to the section entitled "The Patient Taking Cardiovascular Drugs" in Chapter 6: *Clinical Medicine.*

- Use local anesthetic agents with vasoconstrictor with caution based on functional capacity of the patient and use aspirating technique to prevent intravascular injection.
- Determine ability to adapt to stress of dental treatment. Consider short appointments.
- Monitor pulse rhythm to assess for electrolyte imbalance.
- Chronic dry mouth is possible; anticipate increased caries, candidiasis, and lichenoid mucositis.
- *Postural hypotension:* Monitor BP at the beginning and end of each appointment; anticipate syncope. Have patient sit upright for several min at the end of the dental appointment before dismissing.
- Place patient on frequent maintenance schedule to avoid periodontal inflammation.

Oral Health Education

- Encourage daily plaque control procedures for effective self-care in patient at risk for CV disease.
- If chronic dry mouth occurs, recommend home fluoride therapy and use of nonalcoholic oral health care products.

Valtrex — see valacyclovir HCl

Vancenase Pockethaler — see beclomethasone dipropionate

Vanceril — see beclomethasone dipropionate

Vancocin — see vancomycin

Vancoled — see vancomycin

---

vancomycin (van-koe-MY-sin)

Lyphocin, Vancocin, Vancoled

■◆■ **Balcoran, Vancocin, Vanmicina**

Drug Class: Anti-infective; Antibiotic

PHARMACOLOGY

Action

Inhibits bacterial cell wall synthesis and alters cell-membrane permeability and RNA synthesis.

Uses

PARENTERAL: Treatment of serious or severe infections due to susceptible bacteria not treatable with other antimicrobials (such as *Staphylococcus*).

ORAL: Treatment of pseudomembranous colitis caused by *Clostridium difficile*; treatment of staphylococcal enterocolitis.

Unlabeled Uses

IV prophylaxis against bacterial endocarditis in penicillin-allergic patients.

➔← DRUG INTERACTIONS RELATED TO DENTAL THERAPEUTICS

No documented drug-drug interactions. The absence of evidence is not evidence of safety.

ADVERSE EFFECTS

CVS: Hypotension (IV route).

GI: Nausea.

RESP: Wheezing; dyspnea.

MISC: Anaphylaxis; drug fever; chills; red person syndrome (hypotension with or without rash over face, neck, upper chest, and extremities – IV route); neutropenia, thrombocytopenia.

CLINICAL IMPLICATIONS

General

- Determine why drug is being taken. Take precautions to avoid cross-contamination of microorganisms.

- If oral infection occurs that requires antibiotic therapy, select an appropriate product from a different class of anti-infectives.
- Blood dyscrasias rarely reported; anticipate increased bleeding, infection, and poor healing.

Vanmicina — see vancomycin

Vanos — see fluocinonide

Vantin — see cefpodoxime proxetil

Vaponefrin — see epinephrine

---

vardenafil HCl (var-DEN-ah-fil HIGH-droe-KLOR-ide)
Levitra

Drug Class: Agent for impotence

PHARMACOLOGY
Action
Enhances the effect of nitric oxide at the nerve ending and endothelial cells in the corpus cavernosum by inhibiting phosphodiesterase type 5 in the corpus cavernosum of the penis. This results in vasodilation, increased inflow of blood into the corpora cavernosa, and ensuing penile erection upon sexual stimulation.

Uses
Treatment of erectile dysfunction.

➡◆ DRUG INTERACTIONS RELATED TO DENTAL THERAPEUTICS
Ketoconazole or itraconazole: Possible vardenafil toxicity (decreased metabolism)
- Avoid concurrent use.

ADVERSE EFFECTS
⚠ **ORAL:** Dry mouth; dysphagia; esophagitis.

CNS: Headache (15%); dizziness (2%); hypertonia, hypesthesia, insomnia, paresthesia, somnolence, vertigo (<2%).

GI: Dyspepsia (4%); nausea (2%); abdominal pain, diarrhea, gastritis, gastroesophageal reflux, vomiting, gamma-glutamyl-transpeptidase increase (<2%).

RESP: Dyspnea, epistaxis (<2%).

MISC: Flushing (11%); accidental injury, flu-like syndrome (3%); anaphylactic reactions, asthenia, face edema, pain; photosensitivity (<2%).

CLINICAL IMPLICATIONS
General
- Concurrent administration with nitroglycerin may lead to severe hypotension. Avoid concurrent use.
- Monitor vital signs because of potential CV effects.

Vasotec — see enalapril maleate

Vasotec IV — see enalapril maleate

Vatrix-S — see metronidazole

VaZol — see brompheniramine

Veetids — see penicillin V

Veetids '250' — see penicillin V

Velosef — see cephradine

Velosulin BR — see insulin
Velsay — see naproxen

---

venlafaxine (VEN-luh-fax-EEN)
Effexor, Effexor XR

■■■ Efexor

Drug Class: Antidepressant

PHARMACOLOGY
Action
Potentiates norepinephrine, serotonin, and dopamine neurotransmitter activity in CNS.

Uses
Treatment of depression; generalized anxiety disorder (Effexor XR).

➡◀ DRUG INTERACTIONS RELATED TO DENTAL THERAPEUTICS
Alprazolam: Possible decreased alprazolam effect (mechanism unknown)
 • Monitor clinical status.
Sympathomimetic amines: Possible increased risk of serotonin syndrome (additive)
 • Monitor clinical status.

ADVERSE EFFECTS
⚠ **ORAL:** Dry mouth (22%).
CNS: Headache (34%); nervousness (32%); somnolence (26%); dizziness (24%); insomnia (23%); asthenia (17%); anxiety (11%); tremor (10%); decreased libido (9%); abnormal dreams (7%); agitation (4%); depression, hypertonia, paresthesia (3%); twitching, abnormal thinking, confusion (2%); depersonalization (1%); migraine, trismus, vertigo, emotional lability, amnesia, hypesthesia ($\geq$1%); catatonia; delirium; extrapyramidal symptoms; neuroleptic malignant syndrome–like events; involuntary movements; serotonin syndrome; shock-like electrical sensations; panic.
CVS: Increased blood pressure.
GI: Nausea (58%); anorexia (20%); constipation (15%); diarrhea, vomiting, abdominal pain (8%); dyspepsia (7%); flatulence (3%).
RESP: Dyspnea ($\geq$1%).
MISC: Yawn (8%); chills (7%); infection, flu-like syndrome (6%); accidental injury (5%); chest pain, trauma (2%); arthralgia ($\geq$1%); congenital anomalies; night sweats; pancreatitis; hemorrhage; anaphylaxis; renal failure; rhabdomyolysis; pulmonary eosinophilia; increased prolactin.

CLINICAL IMPLICATIONS
General
 • Determine why drug is being taken. Consider implications of condition on dental treatment.
 • Depressed or anxious patients may neglect self-care. Monitor for plaque control effectiveness.
 • Determine ability to adapt to stress of dental treatment. Consider short appointments.
 • Monitor vital signs.
 • Chronic dry mouth is possible; anticipate increased caries and candidiasis.
 • Extrapyramidal behaviors can complicate performance of oral procedures. If present, consult with MD to consider medication changes.
 • Place on frequent maintenance schedule to avoid periodontal inflammation.

Oral Health Education
 • Evaluate manual dexterity; consider need for power toothbrush.
 • Encourage daily plaque control procedures for effective self-care.

Ventisol — see ketotifen fumarate
Ventodisk Disk — see albuterol
Ventolin — see albuterol
Ventolin Diskus — see albuterol
Ventolin Nebules — see albuterol
Ventolin Oral Liquid — see albuterol
Ventolin Rotacaps — see albuterol
Veraken — see verapamil HCl
Verapamil — see verapamil HCl

verapamil HCl (veh-RAP-uh-mill HIGH-droe-KLOR-ide)

Calan, Calan SR, Covera-HS, Isoptin, Isoptin SR, Verapamil, Verelan, Verelan PM

■✚■ **Alti-Verapamil, APO-Verap, Chronovera, Gen-Verapamil, Gen-Verapamil SR, Isoptin I.V., Novo-Veramil, Novo-Veramil SR, Nu-Verap**

■▨■ **Chronovera, Dilacoran, Veraken, Verdilac**

Drug Class: Calcium channel blocker

PHARMACOLOGY

Action

Inhibits movement of calcium ions across cell membrane resulting in depression of mechanical contraction of myocardial and vascular smooth muscle and depression of impulse formation (automaticity) and conduction velocity.

Uses

ORAL: Treatment of vasospastic (Prinzmetal variant), chronic stable (classic effort-associated), and unstable (crescendo, preinfarction) angina; adjunctive treatment with digitalis to control ventricular rate at rest and during stress in atrial flutter or fibrillation; prophylaxis of repetitive PSVT; management of essential hypertension.
SUSTAINED-RELEASE: Management of essential hypertension.
PARENTERAL: Rapid conversion of PSVTs to sinus rhythm; temporary control of rapid ventricular rate in atrial flutter or fibrillation.

Unlabeled Uses

Treatment of migraine and cluster headaches; treatment of hypertrophic cardiomyopathy.

➱◀ DRUG INTERACTIONS RELATED TO DENTAL THERAPEUTICS

Fluconazole, ketoconazole, or itraconazole: Possible verapamil toxicity (decreased metabolism)
 • Avoid concurrent use.
Aspirin: Increased antiplatelet effect (additive)
 • Avoid concurrent use.
Midazolam: Marked increased in midazolam effect (decreased metabolism)
 • Avoid concurrent use.
Bupivacaine: Severe hypotension and bradycardia (mechanism unknown)
 • Avoid concurrent use.
Clarithromycin: Cardiovascular toxicity (decreased metabolism)
 • Avoid concurrent use.

ADVERSE EFFECTS
⚠ **ORAL:** Dry mouth; gingival hyperplasia.
CNS: Dizziness; lightheadedness; headache; asthenia.
CVS: Hypotension (2.5%).
MISC: Increased bleeding (antiplatelet effect).
GI: Nausea; constipation.
RESP: Shortness of breath; dyspnea; wheezing.

CLINICAL IMPLICATIONS
General
- Determine why drug is being taken. Consider implications of condition on dental treatment.
- Monitor vital signs (e.g., BP, pulse pressure, rate, and rhythm) at each appointment to assess disease control. Do not provide elective dental treatment when BP is ≥180/110 or in the presence of other high-risk CV conditions. Refer to the section entitled "The Patient Taking Cardiovascular Drugs" in Chapter 6: *Clinical Medicine*.
- Use local anesthetic agents with vasoconstrictor with caution based on functional capacity of the patient and use aspirating technique to prevent intravascular injection.
- Determine ability to adapt to stress of dental treatment. Consider short appointments.
- Chronic dry mouth is possible; anticipate increased caries and candidiasis.
- Anticipate increased bleeding during procedures that result in bleeding.
- Anticipate gingival hyperplasia; consider MD consult to recommend different drug regimen if periodontal health is compromised.
- Place on frequent maintenance schedule to avoid periodontal inflammation.

Oral Health Education
- Encourage daily plaque control procedures for effective self-care in patient at risk for CV disease.

Verdilac — see verapamil HCl

Verelan — see verapamil HCl

Verelan PM — see verapamil HCl

Vergon — see meclizine

Versed — see midazolam HCl

Vertisal — see metronidazole

Vesanoid — see tretinoin

Vfend — see voriconazole

Viagra — see sildenafil citrate

Vibramicina — see doxycycline hyclate

Vibramycin — see doxycycline hyclate

Vibra-Tabs — see doxycycline hyclate

Vicks Dry Hacking Cough — see dextromethorphan HBr

Vicodin — see acetaminophen/hydrocodone bitartrate

Vicodin ES — see acetaminophen/hydrocodone bitartrate

Vicodin HP — see acetaminophen/hydrocodone bitartrate

Vicoprofen — see ibuprofen/hydrocodone bitartrate

Vigamox — see moxifloxacin HCl

Vilona — see ribavirin

Vilona Pediatrica — see ribavirin
Viracept — see nelfinavir mesylate
Viramune — see nevirapine
Virazide — see ribavirin
Virazole — see ribavirin
Viread — see tenofovir disoproxil fumarate
Virlix — see cetirizine
Visken — see pindolol
Vistaril — see hydroxyzine
vitamin A acid — see tretinoin
vitamin B2 — see riboflavin

---

vitamin E

Synonyms: d-alpha tocopherol; d-alpha tocopheryl acetate

Aquavit E, Dry E 400, Vitaplus E, d'ALPHA E Softgels, Vitamin E

Drug Class: Vitamin supplement

PHARMACOLOGY

Action

Assists in digestion and metabolism of polyunsaturated fats; reduces platelet aggregation to decrease blood clot formation.

Uses

Vitamin E deficiency; hemolytic anemia in premature neonates.

➔← DRUG INTERACTIONS RELATED TO DENTAL THERAPEUTICS

No documented drug-drug interactions. The absence of evidence is not evidence of safety.

ADVERSE EFFECTS

⚠ **ORAL:** Increased bleeding (doses higher than 3000 international units).

CLINICAL IMPLICATIONS

General

- Inquire about daily doses that have been consumed to determine potential risks of bleeding and possible CV effects.

Oral Health Education

- High doses of vitamin E have not been shown to protect against CVD. Evidence suggests high doses may precipitate CV events.

Vitaplus E — see vitamin E
Vitron-C — see ferrous salts
Vivelle — see estradiol
Vivelle-Dot — see estradiol
Volfenac Gel — see diclofenac
Volfenac Retard — see diclofenac
Volmax — see albuterol
Voltaren — see diclofenac

Voltaren Ophtha — see diclofenac
Voltaren Rapide — see diclofenac
Voltaren-XR — see diclofenac
Vomisin — see dimenhydrinate

---

voriconazole (vore-ih-KOE-nuh-zole)
Vfend

Drug Class: Anti-infective; Antifungal

PHARMACOLOGY

Action
Inhibition of fungal cytochrome P450—mediated 14 alpha-lanosterol demethylation, an essential step in fungal ergosterol biosynthesis.

Uses
Treatment of invasive aspergillosis; treatment of *Scedosporium apiospermum* and *Fusarium* spp., including *F. solani*, in patients intolerant of or refractory to other therapy; treatment of esophageal candidiasis.

➡◄ DRUG INTERACTIONS RELATED TO DENTAL THERAPEUTICS
No documented drug-drug interactions. The absence of evidence is not evidence of safety.

ADVERSE EFFECTS
⚠ ORAL: Dry mouth (2%).
CNS: Hallucinations (5%); headache (4%); dizziness (3%).
GI: Nausea (7%); vomiting (6%); diarrhea (2%).
MISC: Fever (6%); chills (4%); abdominal pain (3%); chest pain (2%); photosensitivity.

CLINICAL IMPLICATIONS

General
• Determine why drug is being taken. Take precautions to avoid cross-contamination of microorganisms.
• Monitor body temperature to determine disease control.
• This drug is used relatively short term; therefore, oral side effects generally do not contribute to oral disease.

---

warfarin (WORE-fuh-rin)
Coumadin

▮✦▮ **Apo-Warfarin, Gen-Warfarin, Taro-Warfarin**

▮✦▮ **Dimantil**

Drug Class: Anticoagulant

PHARMACOLOGY

Action
Interferes with hepatic synthesis of vitamin K—dependent clotting factors, causing in vivo depletion of clotting factors II, VII, IX, and X.

Uses
Prophylaxis and treatment of venous thrombosis and its extension; prophylaxis and treatment of atrial fibrillation with embolization; prophylaxis and treatment of pulmonary embolism; adjunct in prophylaxis of systemic embolism after MI.

Unlabeled Uses

Prevention of recurrent transient ischemic attacks and reduction of risk of recurrent MI; adjunctive treatment of small cell carcinoma of lung.

➟➟ DRUG INTERACTIONS RELATED TO DENTAL THERAPEUTICS

Acetaminophen: Increased dose-dependent anticoagulant effect (mechanism not established)
- Monitor clinical status.

COX-1 inhibitors: Increased bleeding (platelet inhibition)
- Avoid concurrent use.

Fluconazole or ketoconazole: Increased anticoagulant effect (decreased metabolism)
- Avoid concurrent use or monitor INR.

Clarithromycin: Increased anticoagulant effect (decreased metabolism)
- Avoid concurrent use.

Doxycycline: Increased anticoagulant effect (mechanism unknown)
- Avoid concurrent use.

Metronidazole: Increased anticoagulant effect (decreased metabolism)
- Avoid concurrent use.

ADVERSE EFFECTS

⚠ **ORAL:** Increased bleeding, difficulty swallowing; hemorrhage.
CNS: Dizziness; fatigue.
CVS: Hypotension, unexplained shock.
GI: Nausea; vomiting; diarrhea; paralytic ileus; intestinal obstruction; anorexia; abdominal cramps.
RESP: Shortness of breath.
MISC: Fever; cholesterol microembolization (purple toe syndrome); hypersensitivity.

CLINICAL IMPLICATIONS

General
- Determine why drug is being taken. Consider implications of condition on dental treatment.
- Determine prothrombin time or INR before completing procedures that may result in significant bleeding. Safe levels of INR for invasive dental procedures is 2–3. INR is calculated from PT.
- Monitor frequently to ensure adequate clotting during treatment that involves bleeding.

Oral Health Education
- Advise patient that gingival bleeding may be a sign of excessive dosage and M.D. should be consulted, as well as INR lab values considered.
- Encourage daily plaque control procedures for effective self-care in patient at risk for CV disease.

Welchol — see colesevelam HCl
Wellbutrin — see bupropion HCl
Wellbutrin SR — see bupropion HCl
Wellbutrin XL — see bupropion HCl
Westcort — see hydrocortisone
Winasorb — see acetaminophen
Wygesic — see acetaminophen/propoxyphene
Wytensin — see guanabenz acetate
Xalatan — see latanoprost
Xalyn-Or — see amoxicillin

Xanax — see alprazolam
Xanax TS — see alprazolam
Xanax XR — see alprazolam
Xeloda — see capecitabine
Xenical — see orlistat
Xolair — see omalizumab
Xopenex — see levalbuterol HCl
Xopenex HFA — see levalbuterol HCl
Xylocaina — see lidocaine HCl
Xylocaine — see lidocaine HCl
Xylocaine CO2 — see lidocaine HCl
Xylocaine Endotracheal — see lidocaine HCl
Xylocaine HCl — see lidocaine HCl
Xylocaine HCl IV for Cardiac Arrhythmias — see lidocaine HCl
Xylocaine MPF — see lidocaine HCl
Xylocaine Spinal 5% — see lidocaine HCl
Xylocaine 4% Sterile Solution — see lidocaine HCl
Xylocaine Viscous — see lidocaine HCl
Xylocard — see lidocaine HCl
Yodine — see povidone iodine
Zaditen — see ketotifen fumarate
Zaditor — see ketotifen fumarate
Zafimida — see furosemide

---

zafirlukast (zah-fur-LOO-cast)

Accolate

Drug Class: Leukotriene receptor antagonist

PHARMACOLOGY

Action
Inhibits three leukotriene receptor types. Leukotrienes have been associated with the longer inflammatory component of asthma.

Uses
Prophylaxis and chronic treatment of asthma in adults and children 5 yr of age and older.

➡️◆ DRUG INTERACTIONS RELATED TO DENTAL THERAPEUTICS

Aspirin: Possible zafirlukast toxicity with high doses of aspirin (decreased metabolism)
  • Avoid high doses of aspirin.

ADVERSE EFFECTS

CNS: Headache (13%); dizziness (2%).
GI: Nausea, diarrhea (3%); vomiting (2%); dyspepsia (1%).
MISC: Infection (4%); pain, asthenia, abdominal pain, accidental injury, fever, back pain (2%).

CLINICAL IMPLICATIONS

General

- Determine why drug is being taken. Consider implications of condition on dental treatment.
- Monitor vital signs (e.g., BP, pulse rate, respiratory rate and function); uncontrolled disease characterized by wheezing and coughing.
- Acute bronchoconstriction can occur during dental treatment; have bronchodilator inhaler available.
- Be aware that sulfites in local anesthetic with vasoconstrictor can precipitate acute asthma attack in susceptible individuals.
- Asthmatics often use a combination of inhalational drugs and orally administered drugs. Inhalation propellants may dry oral tissues when used chronically.

Oral Health Education

- If chronic dry mouth occurs, recommend home fluoride therapy and use of nonalcoholic oral health care products.
- Instruct patient to bring bronchodilator to each dental appointment.

Zagam — see sparfloxacin

zalcitabine (zal-SITE-uh-BEAN)

Synonyms: dideoxycytidine; ddC

Hivid

Drug Class: Antiretroviral, nucleoside reverse transcriptase inhibitor

PHARMACOLOGY

Action

Inhibits replication of DNA in HIV.

Uses

COMBINATION THERAPY: For the treatment of selected patients with advanced HIV infection.

➤◀ DRUG INTERACTIONS RELATED TO DENTAL THERAPEUTICS

No documented drug-drug interactions. The absence of evidence is not evidence of safety.

ADVERSE EFFECTS

⚠ **ORAL:** Dry mouth, glossitis, oral or esophageal ulceration.

CNS: Headache; dizziness; confusion; impaired concentration; peripheral neuropathy.

GI: Pancreatitis; nausea; dysphagia; anorexia; abdominal pain; vomiting; diarrhea; dyspepsia.

RESP: Nasal discharge; cough; respiratory distress.

MISC: Myalgia; arthralgia; foot pain; fatigue; anaphylactoid reaction; abnormal gamma glutamyl transferase (GGT).

CLINICAL IMPLICATIONS

General

- Determine why drug is being taken. Take precautions to avoid cross-contamination of microorganisms.
- Consider medical consult to determine disease control and influence on dental treatment.
- This drug is frequently prescribed in combination with one or more other antiviral agents. Side effects of all agents must be considered during the drug review process.
- Antibiotic prophylaxis should be considered when <500 PMN/mm^3 is reported; elective dental treatment should be delayed until blood values are above this level.
- Anticipate oral candidiasis when HIV disease is reported.

- Place on frequent maintenance schedule to avoid periodontal inflammation.
- Chronic dry mouth is possible; anticipate increased caries and candidiasis.
- If GI or respiratory side effects occur, consider semisupine chair position.

Oral Health Education
- Encourage daily plaque control procedures for effective self-care because HIV infection reduces host resistance.
- If chronic dry mouth occurs, recommend home fluoride therapy and use of nonalcoholic oral health care products.

Zamacort — see triamcinolone
Zamtirel — see salmeterol
Zanaflex — see tizanidine HCl

---

zanamivir (za-NA-mi-veer)

Relenza

Drug Class: Antiviral agent

PHARMACOLOGY

Action
Inhibition of influenza virus neuraminidase, with the possibility of alteration of virus particle aggregation and release.

Uses
Uncomplicated acute illness caused by influenza A and B virus in adults and pediatric patients at least 7 yr of age who have been symptomatic for no longer than 2 days.

➡️ DRUG INTERACTIONS RELATED TO DENTAL THERAPEUTICS
No documented drug-drug interactions. The absence of evidence is not evidence of safety.

ADVERSE EFFECTS
⚠ ORAL: Oropharyngeal edema (allergic manifestation).
CNS: Headache, dizziness (2%); seizures.
GI: Diarrhea, nausea (3%); vomiting (1%); abdominal pain (<1.5%).
RESP: Sinusitis (3%); bronchitis, cough (2%); bronchospasm; dyspnea.
MISC: Malaise, fatigue, fever (<1.5%); allergic or allergy-like reactions.

CLINICAL IMPLICATIONS

General
- Determine why drug is being taken. Take precautions to avoid cross-contamination of microorganisms.
- Monitor vital signs, including body temperature to assess disease control.

Zantac — see ranitidine HCl
Zantac 75 — see ranitidine HCl
Zantac EFFERdose — see ranitidine HCl
Zarontin — see ethosuximide
Zaroxolyn — see metolazone
Zebeta — see bisoprolol fumarate
Zegerid — see omeprazole
Zenapax — see daclizumab
Zerit — see stavudine

Zerit XR — see stavudine
Zestril — see lisinopril
Zetia — see ezetimibe
Ziac (with hydrochlorothiazide) — see bisoprolol fumarate
Ziagen — see abacavir sulfate

---

zidovudine (zid-OH-vue-deen)

Synonyms: azidothymidine; AZT; compound S

Retrovir

■✚■ APO-Zidovudine, Novo-AZT

■▨■ Dipedyne, Isadol, Kenamil, Retrovir AZT

Drug Class: Antiretroviral, nucleoside reverse transcriptase inhibitor

PHARMACOLOGY

Action

Inhibits replication of retroviruses including HIV.

Uses

In combination with other antiretroviral agents for the treatment of HIV infections; prevention of maternal-fetal HIV transmission.

➔← DRUG INTERACTIONS RELATED TO DENTAL THERAPEUTICS

Fluconazole: Possible zidovudine toxicity (decreased metabolism)
 • Avoid concurrent use.
Clarithromycin: Possible decreased zidovudine effect (mechanism unknown)
 • Avoid concurrent use.

ADVERSE EFFECTS

⚠ **ORAL:** Gingival bleeding; mouth ulceration; tongue or lip edema; dysphagia.

CNS: Headache; dizziness; insomnia; paresthesia; malaise; asthenia; decreased reflexes; nervousness or irritability.

GI: Anorexia; constipation; dyspepsia; nausea; vomiting; flatulence; rectal hemorrhage; eructation; abdominal pain.

RESP: Dyspnea; cough; epistaxis; pharyngitis; rhinitis; sinusitis; hoarseness.

MISC: Fever, diaphoresis; myalgia; arthralgia; muscle spasm; body odor; chills; flu-like syndrome; hyperalgesia; abdominal/back/chest pain; hypersensitivity reaction; anemia, neutropenia (infants).

CLINICAL IMPLICATIONS

General

• This drug is frequently prescribed in combination with one or more other antiviral agents. Side effects of all agents must be considered during the drug review process.
• Determine why drug is being taken. Consider implications of condition on dental treatment.
• Consider medical consult to determine disease control and influence on dental treatment.
• Antibiotic prophylaxis should be considered when <500 PMN/mm³ is reported; elective dental treatment should be delayed until blood values improve above this level.
• Anticipate oral candidiasis when HIV disease is reported.
• Blood dyscrasias rarely reported; anticipate increased bleeding, infection, and poor healing.
• Place patient on frequent maintenance schedule to avoid periodontal inflammation.

Oral Health Education
- Encourage daily plaque control procedures for effective self-care because HIV infection reduces host resistance.

---

zidovudine/lamivudine — see lamivudine/zidovudine

Zilactin-L — see lidocaine HCl

---

zileuton (zill-LOO-tuhn)
Zyflo

Drug Class: Leukotriene receptor antagonist

PHARMACOLOGY

Action
Attenuates bronchoconstriction by inhibiting leukotriene-dependent smooth muscle contractions.

Uses
Prophylaxis and chronic treatment of asthma.

➡️⬅ DRUG INTERACTIONS RELATED TO DENTAL THERAPEUTICS
No documented drug-drug interactions. The absence of evidence is not evidence of safety.

ADVERSE EFFECTS
CNS: Pain; dizziness; insomnia; somnolence; malaise; nervousness; hypertonia.
GI: Abdominal pain; dyspepsia; nausea; vomiting; constipation; flatulence.
MISC: Asthenia; myalgia; arthralgia; chest pain; fever; lymphadenopathy; muscle rigidity; pruritus.

CLINICAL IMPLICATIONS

General
- Monitor vital signs (e.g., BP, pulse rate, respiratory rate and function); uncontrolled disease characterized by wheezing and coughing.
- Acute bronchoconstriction can occur during dental treatment; have bronchodilator inhaler available.
- Be aware that sulfites in local anesthetic with vasoconstrictor can precipitate acute asthma attack in susceptible individuals.
- Asthmatics often use a combination of inhalational drugs and orally administered drugs. Inhalation propellants may dry oral tissues when used chronically.

Oral Health Education
- If chronic dry mouth occurs, recommend home fluoride therapy and use of nonalcoholic oral health care products.
- Instruct patient to bring bronchodilator to each dental appointment.

Zinacef — see cefuroxime

Zinnat — see cefuroxime

Zipra — see ciprofloxacin

---

ziprasidone (zi-PRAH-si-done)
Geodon

Drug Class: Atypical antipsychotic, benzisoxazole

PHARMACOLOGY

Action

Antipsychotic activity, apparently because of dopamine and serotonin receptor antagonism.

Uses

Treatment of schizophrenia; treatment of acute manic or mixed episodes associated with bipolar disorder; treatment of acute agitation in schizophrenic patients (injection only).

➤◀ DRUG INTERACTIONS RELATED TO DENTAL THERAPEUTICS

Ketoconazole: Possible ziprasidone toxicity (decreased metabolism)
  • Avoid concurrent use.

ADVERSE EFFECTS

⚠ **ORAL:** Dry mouth (5%); tongue edema (3%); increased salivation (dose related); tooth disorder (IM route).

CNS: Extrapyramidal symptoms, somnolence (31%); headache (18%); dizziness (16%); akathisia (10%); dystonia (4%); hypertonia (3%); speech disorder (2%); agitation, tremor, dyskinesia, hostility, paresthesia, confusion, vertigo, hypokinesia, hyperkinesias, abnormal gait, hypesthesia, ataxia, amnesia, cogwheel rigidity, delirium, hypotonia, akinesia, dysarthria, withdrawal syndrome, buccoglossal syndrome, choreoathetosis, incoordination, neuropathy (≥1%); anxiety, tremor (dose related); headache, insomnia, personality disorder, psychosis, speech disorder (IM).

GI: Nausea (10%); constipation (9%); dyspepsia (8%); diarrhea, anorexia (2%); vomiting (≥1%).

RESP: Respiratory disorder (e.g., cold symptoms, URI [8%]); increased cough (3%); dyspnea (≥1%).

MISC: Asthenia (6%); accidental injury (4%); myalgia (2%); abdominal pain, flu-like syndrome, fever, accidental fall, face edema, chills, photosensitivity reaction, flank pain, hypothermia, motor vehicle accident (≥1%); arthralgia (dose related); injection site pain, back pain (IM).

CLINICAL IMPLICATIONS

General

  • Determine why drug is being taken. Consider implications of condition on dental treatment.
  • Determine ability to adapt to stress of dental treatment. Consider short appointments.
  • Clients with psychological disease may present with behavior management problems.
  • Extrapyramidal behaviors can complicate performance of oral procedures. If present consult with MD to consider medication changes.
  • Chronic dry mouth is possible; anticipate increased caries and candidiasis.
  • If GI side effects occur, consider semisupine chair position.

Oral Health Education

  • Encourage daily plaque control procedures for effective self-care.
  • Evaluate manual dexterity; consider need for power toothbrush.

Zithromax — see azithromycin

Zmax — see azithromycin

Zocor — see simvastatin

Zofran — see ondansetron HCl

Zofran ODT — see ondansetron HCl

---

zoledronic acid (zoe-leh-DROE-nik AS-id)
Zometa
Drug Class: Bisphosphonate

PHARMACOLOGY

Action

Inhibition of bone resorption.

Uses

Treatment of hypercalcemia of malignancy; treatment of patients with multiple myeloma and bone metastases from solid tumors in conjunction with standard antineoplastic therapy.

➡◀ DRUG INTERACTIONS RELATED TO DENTAL THERAPEUTICS

No documented drug-drug interactions. The absence of evidence is not evidence of safety.

ADVERSE EFFECTS

⚠ **ORAL:** Sore throat; candidiasis; stomatitis; mucositis; dysphagia.

CNS: Agitation; anxiety; asthenia; confusion; decreased appetite; depression; dizziness; fatigue; headache; hypoesthesia; insomnia; paresthesia; somnolence.

GI: Abdominal pain; anorexia; constipation; diarrhea; dyspepsia; nausea; vomiting.

RESP: Coughing; dyspnea; pleural effusion; URI.

MISC: Aggravated malignant neoplasm; chest pain; chills; edema of lower limb; fever; flu-like syndrome; leg edema; metastases; nonspecific infection; progression of cancer; weakness.

CLINICAL IMPLICATIONS

General

- Determine why drug is being taken. Consider implications of condition on dental treatment.
- Patient may be high-risk candidates for pathological fractures or jaw fractures during extractions.
- Osteonecrosis of the jaw is reported; consider this adverse drug effect when osteolytic disease is suspected.
- Advise products for palliative relief of oral manifestations (e.g., stomatitis, mucositis, xerostomia).

Oral Health Education

- Encourage daily plaque control procedures for effective self-care.
- Consult with oncologist to determine whether alternative oral physiotherapy devices are appropriate to reduce risk of trauma to oral tissues.

Zolicef — see cefazolin sodium

---

zolmitriptan (ZOLE-mih-TRIP-tan)

Zomig, Zomig, Zomig ZMT

■✦■ **Zomig Rapimelt**

Drug Class: Analgesic; Migraine

PHARMACOLOGY

Action

Selective agonist for the vascular serotonin (5-HT) receptor subtype, causing vasoconstriction of cranial arteries and inhibition of pro-inflammatory neuropeptide release.

Uses

Short-term treatment of migraine attacks with or without aura.

➡◀ DRUG INTERACTIONS RELATED TO DENTAL THERAPEUTICS

No documented drug-drug interactions. The absence of evidence is not evidence of safety.

ADVERSE EFFECTS

⚠ **ORAL:** Taste disturbance (21% intranasal); dry mouth; dysphagia; throat and neck pain.
CNS: Paresthesia, dizziness, somnolence, vertigo, hyperesthesia (≥2%); headache.
CVS: Hypertensive crisis.
GI: Dyspepsia, nausea (≥2%); ischemic colitis; GI infarction or necrosis.
MISC: Asthenia, pain, chest pain, tightness, or heaviness, warm or cold sensations, sweating (≥ 2%).

CLINICAL IMPLICATIONS

General
- Determine why drug is being taken. Consider implications of condition on dental treatment.
- Monitor vital signs (e.g., BP and pulse). Drugs for prevention are sympatholytic; drugs for treatment of acute attack are sympathomimetic.
- Although this drug is used on a short-term basis, chronic dry mouth is possible; anticipate increased caries activity and candidiasis.

Oral Health Education
- If chronic dry mouth occurs, recommend home fluoride therapy and use of nonalcoholic oral health care products.

Zoloft — see sertraline HCl

---

zolpidem tartrate (ZOLE-pih-dem TAR-trayt)
Ambien

Drug Class: Sedative and hypnotic

DEA Schedule: Schedule IV

PHARMACOLOGY

Action
Mechanism is unknown but may involve subunit modulation of the gamma-aminobutyrate acid (GABA) receptor chloride channel macromolecular complex.

Uses
Short-term treatment of insomnia.

➨◀ DRUG INTERACTIONS RELATED TO DENTAL THERAPEUTICS

Ketoconazole: Possible zolpidem toxicity (decreased metabolism)
- Avoid concurrent use.

ADVERSE EFFECTS

⚠ **ORAL:** Dry mouth.
CNS: Amnesia; daytime drowsiness; dizziness; headache; lethargy; "drugged feelings," lightheadedness; depression; abnormal dreams; ataxia; confusion; euphoria; insomnia; vertigo.
GI: Diarrhea; constipation.
MISC: Allergy; back pain; flu-like symptoms; chest pain.

CLINICAL IMPLICATIONS

General
- Determine why drug is being taken. Consider implications of condition on dental treatment.
- Chronic dry mouth is possible; anticipate increased caries and candidiasis.
- Avoid prescribing opioids for dental pain.

Oral Health Education
- If chronic dry mouth occurs, recommend home fluoride therapy and use of nonalcoholic oral health care products.

Zometa — see zoledronic acid
Zomig — see zolmitriptan
Zomig Rapimelt — see zolmitriptan
Zomig ZMT — see zolmitriptan
Zonal — see fluconazole
Zonalon — see doxepin HCl
Zonegran — see zonisamide

zonisamide (zoe-NIS-ah-MIDE)

Zonegran

Drug Class: Anticonvulsant, sulfonamide

PHARMACOLOGY

Action
Unknown; however, may produce anticonvulsant effects through action at sodium and calcium channels.

Uses
Adjunctive therapy in the treatment of partial seizures in adult epileptic patients.

➡◆ DRUG INTERACTIONS RELATED TO DENTAL THERAPEUTICS
No documented drug-drug interactions. The absence of evidence is not evidence of safety.

ADVERSE EFFECTS
Because zonisamide is used as adjunctive therapy, figures obtained when zonisamide is added to concomitant antiepileptic drug therapy cannot be used to predict the frequency of adverse events in the course of usual medical practice. Except for potentially serious adverse effects (e.g., blood dyscrasias, CV events), which have been reported to occur in fewer than 1% of treated patients, the following adverse reactions have been reported in at least 1% of zonisamide-treated patients.

⚠ **ORAL:** Dry mouth; pharyngitis.

CNS: Somnolence; dizziness; headache; agitation; irritability; fatigue; tiredness; difficulty concentrating; memory difficulty; mental slowing; ataxia; paresthesia; confusion; depression; insomnia; anxiety; nervousness; schizophrenic/schizophreniform behavior; speech abnormalities; difficult verbal expression; tremor; convulsion; abnormal gait; hyperesthesia; incoordination.

GI: Nausea; anorexia; vomiting; abdominal pain; diarrhea; dyspepsia; constipation.

RESP: Rhinitis; pulmonary embolus; increased cough.

MISC: Flu-like syndrome; asthenia; accidental injury.

CLINICAL IMPLICATIONS

General
- Determine why drug is being taken. Consider implications of condition on dental treatment.
- Determine level of disease control, type and frequency of seizures, and compliance with medication regimen.
- Determine ability to adapt to stress of dental treatment. Consider short appointments.
- Place on frequent maintenance schedule to avoid periodontal inflammation.
- Chronic dry mouth is possible; anticipate increased caries and candidiasis.

Oral Health Education
- Evaluate manual dexterity; consider need for power toothbrush.
- If chronic dry mouth occurs, recommend home fluoride therapy and use of nonalcoholic oral health care products.

Zorbenal-G — see tetracycline HCl
Zorcaine 4% — see articaine HCl
ZORprin — see aspirin
Zostrix — see capsaicin
Zostrix-HP — see capsaicin
Zovirax — see acyclovir
Z-Pak — see azithromycin
Zurcal — see pantoprazole sodium
Zyban — see bupropion HCl
Zydone — see acetaminophen/hydrocodone bitartrate
Zyflo — see zileuton
Zyloprim — see allopurinol
Zymar — see gatifloxacin
Zymerol — see cimetidine
Zyprexa — see olanzapine
Zyprexa Intramuscular — see olanzapine
Zyprexa Zydis — see olanzapine
Zyrtec — see cetirizine
Zyrtec-D 12 Hour — see cetirizine HCl with pseudoephedrine HCl
Zyvox — see linezolid
Zyvoxam — see linezolid
Zyvoxam IV — see linezolid

Appendices

Appendix A

Drugs Listed by Therapeutic Category or Condition

ALZHEIMER DISEASE
donepezil (Aricept)
galantamine (Reminyl)
memantine (Namenda)
rivastigmine (Exelon)
tacrine (Cognex)

ANALGESICS
NONOPIOID
⟡acetaminophen (Tylenol)
NSAIDs
⟡aspirin
celecoxib (Celebrex)
diclofenac (Voltaren)
diflunisal (Dolobid)
etodolac (Lodine)
fenoprofen (Nalfon)
flurbiprofen (Ansaid)
⟡ibuprofen (Advil, Motrin, Nuprin)
indomethacin (Indocin)
ketoprofen (Orudis)
ketorolac (Toradol)
meclofenamate (Meclomen)
mefenamic acid (Ponstel)
meloxicam (Mobic)
nabumetone (Relafen)
⟡naproxen (Naprosyn, Anaprox)
oxaprozin (Daypro)
piroxicam (Feldene)
sulindac (Clinoril)
tolmetin (Tolectin)
OPIOIDS
buprenorphine (Buprenex)
codeine sulfate
⟡codeine phosphate/ acetaminophen (Tylenol #2, #3, #4)
fentanyl transdermal (Duragesic)
fentanyl transmucosal (Actiq)

⟡hydrocodone/acetaminophen (Lorcet, Vicodin)
⟡hydrocodone/ibuprofen (Vicoprofen)
hydromorphone HCl (Dilaudid)
meperidine (Demerol)
morphine sulfate (MS Contin)
oxycodone (OxyContin, Roxicodone)
⟡oxycodone/ASA (Percodan, Roxiprin)
⟡oxycodone/acetaminophen (Endocet, Percocet)
⟡oxycodone/ibuprofen (Combunox)
pentazocine (Talwin)
propoxyphene (Darvon)
propoxyphene/acetaminophen (Darvocet)
⟡tramadol (Ultram)
⟡tramadol/acetaminophen (Ultracet)

ANTACID
magaldrate (Riopan)
H₂ RECEPTOR ANTAGONISTS
cimetidine (Tagamet)
famotidine (Pepcid)
nizatidine (Axid)
ranitidine (Zantac)

ANTIANEMIC/IMMUNE BOOSTER
epoetin alfa (Procrit)

ANTIANGINALS
BETA-ADRENERGIC ANTAGONISTS
atenolol (Tenormin)
metoprolol (Lopressor)
nadolol (Corgard)
propranolol (Inderal)
CALCIUM CHANNEL ANTAGONISTS
amlodipine (Norvasc)

diltiazem (Cardizem, Cartia XT, Dilacor XR)
felodipine (Plendil)
nicardipine (Cardene)
nifedipine (Adalat, Procardia)
nisoldipine (Sular)
verapamil (Calan)

COMBINATION PRODUCTS
amlodipine/benazepril (Lotrel)
losartan/hydrochlorothiazide (Hyzaar)
valsartan/hydrochlorothiazide (Diovan HCT)

NITRATES
isosorbide dinitrate (Isordil)
isosorbide mononitrate (ISMO)
⋈nitroglycerin (Transderm-Nitro)

ANTIANXIETY/SEDATIVES
ANTIHISTAMINES
⋈diphenhydramine (Benadryl)
hydroxyzine (Atarax, Vistaril)
promethazine (Phenergan)

BARBITURATE
phenobarbital (Luminal)

BENZODIAZEPINES
⋈alprazolam (Xanax)
⋈chlordiazepoxide (Librium)
clorazepate (Tranxene)
⋈diazepam (Valium)
flurazepam (Dalmane)
⋈lorazepam (Ativan)
⋈midazolam (Versed)
oxazepam (Serax)
temazepam (Restoril)
triazolam (Halcion)

OTHERS
buspirone (BuSpar)
⋈chloral hydrate (Aquachloral)
eszopiclone (Lunesta)
doxepin (Sinequan)
zolpidem (Ambien)

ANTICOAGULANTS
COAGULATION FACTOR INHIBITOR
warfarin sodium (Coumadin)

LOW MOLECULAR WEIGHT HEPARIN
enoxaparin sodium (Lovenox)

PLATELET INHIBITORS
⋈aspirin
clopidogrel (Plavix)
dipyridamole (Persantine)
dipyridamole/ASA (Aggrenox)
ticlopidine (Ticlid)

ANTICONVULSANTS
carbamazepine (Tegretol)
⋈clonazepam (Klonopin)
diazepam (Valium)
divalproex (Depakote)
ethosuximide (Zarontin)
felbamate (Felbatol)
⋈gabapentin (Neurontin)
lamotrigine (Lamictal)
levetiracetam (Keppra)
mephobarbital (Mebaral)
oxcarbazepine (Trileptal)
phenobarbital (Luminal)
phenytoin sodium (Dilantin)
primidone (Mysoline)
tiagabine HCl (Gabitril)
topiramate (Topamax)
valproic acid (Depakene)
zonisamide (Zonegran)

ANTIDEPRESSANTS
ATYPICAL
bupropion HCl (Wellbutrin)
nefazodone HCl (Serzone)
trazodone HCl (Desyrel)
venlafaxine HCl (Effexor)

MONOAMINE OXIDASE INHIBITORS
phenelzine sulfate (Nardil)
tranylcypromine sulfate (Parnate)

SEROTONIN-SPECIFIC REUPTAKE INHIBITORS
citalopram HCl (Celexa)
escitalopram oxalate (Lexapro)
fluoxetine (Prozac)

fluvoxamine maleate (Luvox)
paroxetine (Paxil)
sertraline (Zoloft)

Tetracyclics
mirtazapine (Remeron)

Tricyclics
amitriptyline HCl (Elavil)
⚕desipramine HCl (Norpramin)
doxepin (Sinequan)
imipramine HCl (Tofranil)
nortriptyline HCl (Pamelor)

ANTIDIABETICS
Alpha Glucosidase Inhibitors
acarbose (Precose)
miglitol (Glyset)

Biguanide
metformin (Glucophage)

Combination Products
glipizide/metformin (Metaglip)
glyburide/metformin
(Glucovance)
rosiglitazone/metformin
(Avandamet)

Meglitinides
repaglinide (Prandin)

Sulfonylureas
acetohexamide (Dymelor)
chlorpropamide (Diabinese)
glipizide (Glucotrol XL)
glyburide (DiaBeta, Glynase,
Micronase)
glimepiride (Amaryl)

Thiazolidinediones
pioglitazone (Actos)
rosiglitazone (Avandia)

Others
insulins (see monograph for
proprietary brands)
nateglinide (Starlix)

ANTIEMETICS/VOMITING
chlorpromazine (Thorazine)
dimenhydrinate (Dramamine)
meclizine HCl (Bonine)

metoclopramide (Reglan)
promethazine (Phenergan)
scopolamine (Transderm-Scop)

ANTIHISTAMINES
azelastine HCl (Astelin, Optivar)
brompheniramine tannate
(BroveX)
cetirizine HCl (Zyrtec)
chlorpheniramine maleate
(Chlor-Trimeton)
clemastine fumarate (Tavist)
desloratadine (Clarinex)
dimenhydrinate (Dramamine)
⚕diphenhydramine (Benadryl)
fexofenadine HCl (Allegra)
hydroxyzine (Atarax, Vistaril)
ketotifen fumarate (Zaditor)
loratadine (Claritin)
meclizine (Bonine)
olopatadine HCl (Patanol)
promethazine (Phenergan)

ANTIHYPERTENSIVES
**Alpha-Adrenergic
Antagonists**
doxazosin mesylate (Cardura)
prazosin HCl (Minipress)
terazosin (Hytrin)

**Alpha/Beta Adrenergic
Antagonists**
carvedilol (Coreg)
labetalol (Normodyne)

**Angiotensin-Converting
Enzyme Inhibitor**
benazepril (Lotensin)
captopril (Capoten)
enalapril maleate (Vasotec)
fosinopril (Monopril)
lisinopril (Prinivil, Zestril)
moexipril HCl (Univasc)
perindopril erbumine (Aceon)
quinapril (Accupril)
ramipril (Altace)
trandolapril (Mavik)

ANGIOTENSIN II RECEPTOR ANTAGONIST
candesartan cilexetil (Atacand)
eprosartan (Teveten)
irbesartan (Avapro)
losartan (Cozaar)
olmesartan medoxomil (Benicar)
telmisartan (Micardis)
valsartan (Diovan)

BETA-ADRENERGIC ANTAGONIST
Cardioselective
atenolol (Tenormin)
betaxolol (Kerlone)
bisoprolol fumarate (Zebeta)
metoprolol tartrate (Lopressor)
nadolol (Corgard)
Noncardioselective
carteolol HCl (Cartrol)
penbutolol (Levatol)
pindolol (Visken)
propranolol HCl (Inderal)
timolol maleate (Blocadren)

CALCIUM CHANNEL ANTAGONIST
amlodipine besylate (Norvasc)
diltiazem (Cardizem)
felodipine (Plendil)
isradipine (DynaCirc)
nicardipine (Cardene)
nifedipine (Procardia XL)
nisoldipine (Sular)
verapamil (Calan)

CENTRALLY ACTING
clonidine (Catapres)
guanabenz acetate (Wytensin)
methyldopa (Aldomet)

COMBINATIONS
amlodipine/benazepril (Lotrel)
losartan/HCTZ (Hyzaar)

DIURETICS (SEE DIURETICS)

OTHER
guanadrel sulfate (Hylorel)
hydralazine (Apresoline)
minoxidil (Loniten)

ANTI-INFECTIVES

ANTIFUNGALS
⋈clotrimazole (Mycelex)
⋈fluconazole (Diflucan)
itraconazole (Sporanox)
⋈ketoconazole (Nizoral)
⋈nystatin (Mycostatin, Nilstat)
terbinafine HCl (Lamisil)

ANTIVIRALS
Hepatitis B
adefovir dipivoxil (Hepsera)
interferon alfa 2b (Intron A)
ribavirin (Copegus)
Herpes simplex
⋈acyclovir (Zovirax)
⋈docosanol (Abreva)
⋈penciclovir (Denavir)
⋈valacyclovir (Valtrex)
Herpes zoster
⋈famciclovir (Famvir)
valacyclovir (Valtrex)
Influenza
amantadine (Symmetrel)
oseltamivir (Tamiflu)
rimantadine (Flumadine)
zanamivir (Relenza)

CEPHALOSPORINS
cefaclor (Ceclor)
⋈cefadroxil (Duricef)
⋈cefazolin (Ancef)
cefdinir (Omnicef)
cefditoren pivoxil (Spectracef)
cefixime (Suprax)
cefpodoxime proxetil (Vantin)
cefprozil monohydrate (Cefzil)
ceftibuten (Cedax)
cefuroxime axetil
⋈cephalexin (Keflex)
⋈cephradine (Velosef)
loracarbef (Lorabid)

FLUOROQUINOLONES
ciprofloxacin (Cipro)
gatifloxacin (Tequin)

gemifloxacin (Factive)
levofloxacin (Levaquin)
lomefloxacin (Maxaquin)
moxifloxacin (Avelox)
norfloxacin (Noroxin)
ofloxacin (Floxin)
sparfloxacin (Zagam)
trovafloxacin (Trovan)

MACROLIDES

⬚azithromycin (Zithromax)
clarithromycin (Biaxin)
erythromycin (Erythrocin, Ery-Tab)

PENICILLINS

⬚amoxicillin (Amoxil)
⬚amoxicillin/clavulanate (Augmentin)
⬚ampicillin (Omnipen)
dicloxacillin sodium (Dynapen)
⬚penicillin V (Veetids, Penicillin VK)

TETRACYCLINES

⬚doxycycline calcium (Vibramycin)
⬚doxycycline hyclate, topical (Atridox)
⬚doxycycline hyclate, low dose (Periostat)
⬚minocycline HCl (Minocin)
⬚minocycline HCl, topical (Arestin)
tetracycline HCl (Achromycin)

OTHERS

⬚metronidazole (Flagyl)

ANTISIALAGOGUES (DRY MOUTH)

⬚atropine sulfate (Sal-Tropine)
propantheline bromide (Pro-Banthine)

ARTHRITIS/ANTI-INFLAMMATORY

allopurinol (Zyloprim)
⬚aspirin
auranofin gold (Ridaura)

celecoxib (Celebrex)
diflunisal (Dolobid)
etanercept (Enbrel)
etodolac (Lodine)
fenoprofen (Nalfon)
gold sodium thiomalate (Myochrysine)
⬚ibuprofen (Motrin)
indomethacin (Indocin)
infliximab (Remicade)
ketoprofen (Orudis)
leflunomide (Arava)
methotrexate (Rheumatrex)
nabumetone (Relafen)
⬚naproxen (Anaprox, Naprosyn)
oxaprozin (Daypro)
piroxicam (Feldene)
probenecid (Benemid)
sulindac (Clinoril)
tolmetin sodium (Tolectin)

ASTHMA/COPD

BRONCHODILATORS

⬚albuterol (Proventil)
albuterol/ipratropium Br (Combivent)
⬚epinephrine HCl (Primatene Mist)
ipratropium bromide (Atrovent)
levalbuterol HCl (Xopenex)
metaproterenol (Alupent)
pirbuterol (Maxair)
salmeterol (Serevent)
salmeterol/fluticasone (Advair Diskus)
terbutaline (Brethaire, Bricanyl Turbuhaler)

LEUKOTRIENE ANTAGONIST/INHIBITORS

montelukast (Singulair)
zafirlukast (Accolate)
zileuton (Zyflo)

MAST CELL STABILIZERS

cromolyn sodium (Intal)
nedocromil sodium (Tilade)

BIPOLAR DISORDER
lithium (Eskalith)
valproic acid (Depakene)

CANCER CHEMOTHERAPY
capecitabine (Xeloda)
fluorouracil (Efudex)
methotrexate (Rheumatrex)
tamoxifen (Nolvadex)

CHOLESTEROL REDUCTION
atorvastatin calcium (Lipitor)
cholestyramine (Questran)
colesevelam HCl (WelChol)
colestipol HCl (Colestid)
ezetimibe (Zetia)
fenofibrate (TriCor)
fluvastatin sodium (Lescol)
gemfibrozil (Lopid)
lovastatin (Mevacor)
niacin (Niaspan, Slo-Niacin)
niacin/lovastatin (Advicor)
pravastatin (Pravachol)
rosuvastatin (Crestor)
simvastatin (Zocor)

DECONGESTANT/ EXPECTORANT
guaifenesin (Mucinex)
pseudoephedrine (Neo-Synephrine)

DERMATOLOGICS
acitretin (Soriatane)
alefacept (Amevive)
alitretinoin (Panretin)
capsaicin (Zostrix)
doxepin (Zonalon)
isotretinoin (Accutane)
methotrexate (Folex)
minoxidil (Rogaine)
pimecrolimus (Elidel)
tacrolimus (Protopic)
tretinoin (Retin-A)

DIURETICS
LOOP
bumetanide (Bumex)
ethacrynic acid (Edecrin)
furosemide (Lasix)
torsemide (Demadex)
POTASSIUM SPARING
amiloride (Midamor)
spironolactone (Aldactone)
triamterene (Dyrenium)
THIAZIDE/THIAZIDE-LIKE
chlorothiazide (Diuril)
chlorthalidone (Hygroton)
hydrochlorothiazide (HydroDIURIL)
indapamide (Lozol)
metolazone (Zaroxolyn)

EMPHYSEMA
(see ASTHMA/COPD)

ERECTILE DYSFUNCTION
sildenafil (Viagra)
tadalafil (Cialis)
vardenafil (Levitra)

GERD
esomeprazole (Nexium)
lansoprazole (Prevacid)
omeprazole (Prilosec)
pantoprazole (Protonix)
rabeprazole (AcipHex)

GLAUCOMA
betaxolol (Betoptic)
carteolol (Ocupress)
latanoprost (Xalatan)
pilocarpine (Isopto Carpine)
timolol maleate (Timoptic)

GLUCOCORTICOIDS/ANTI-INFLAMMATORIES
INHALANTS
beclomethasone (Vanceril)
budesonide (Rhinocort)
flunisolide (AeroBid)

fluticasone (Flonase)
mometasone (Nasonex)
⚕triamcinolone (Azmacort)

SYSTEMIC

⚕betamethasone (Celestone)
cortisone acetate (Cortone)
⚕dexamethasone (Decadron)
fludrocortisone (Florinef)
hydrocortisone (Cortef)
methylprednisolone (Medrol)
prednisolone (Delta-Cortef)
⚕prednisone (Deltasone, Meticorten)
⚕triamcinolone (Aristocort)

TOPICALS

⚕betamethasone (Diprolene)
⚕clobetasol propionate (Olux, Temovate)
clocortolone pivalate (Cloderm)
desonide (DesOwen)
desoximetasone (Topicort)
⚕dexamethasone (Decaderm)
⚕diflorasone diacetate (Florone)
⚕fluocinonide (Lidex)
flurandrenolide (Cordran)
fluticasone propionate (Cutivate)
halcinonide (Halog)
halobetasol (Ultravate)
hydrocortisone (Allercort)
⚕triamcinolone (Kenalog, Kenalog with Orabase)

GOUT

probenecid (Benemid)

HEMOSTATICS

⚕absorbable gelatin sponge (Gelfoam)
⚕aminocaproic acid (Amicar)
⚕oxidized cellulose (Surgicel)
⚕tranexamic acid (Cyklokapron)

HIV DISEASE

NONNUCLEOSIDE ANALOGS

delavirdine mesylate (Rescriptor)
efavirenz (Sustiva)
nevirapine (Viramune)
tenofovir (Viread)

NUCLEOSIDE ANALOGS

abacavir sulfate (Ziagen)
emtricitabine (Emtriva)
lamivudine (3TC, Epivir)
stavudine (d4T, Zerit)
zalcitabine (Hivid)
zidovudine (AZT, Retrovir)

PROTEASE INHIBITORS

amprenavir (Agenerase)
atazanavir (Reyataz)
indinavir (Crixivan)
nelfinavir (Viracept)
ritonavir (Norvir)
saquinavir (Invirase, Fortovase)

COMBINATION PRODUCTS

abacavir, lamivudine, zidovudine (Trizivir)
lamivudine/zidovudine (Combivir)

OTHER

enfuvirtide (Fuzeon)

INCONTINENCE/ ANTICHOLINERGICS

oxybutynin Cl (Ditropan XL)
tolterodine (Detrol)

MANIA/ANTIPSYCHOTICS

PHENOTHIAZINES

chlorpromazine (Thorazine)
fluphenazine (Prolixin)
perphenazine (Trilafon)
thioridazine (Mellaril)
trifluoperazine (Stelazine)

OTHERS

aripiprazole (Abilify)
clozapine (Clozaril)

haloperidol (Haldol)
olanzapine (Zyprexa)
quetiapine (Seroquel)
risperidone (Risperdal)
thiothixene (Navane)
ziprasidone (Geodon)

MIGRAINE HEADACHE
almotriptan (Axert)
divalproex (Depakote)
eletriptan HBr (Replax)
frovatriptan (Frova)
propranolol (Inderal)
rizatriptan (Maxalt)
sumatriptan (Imitrex)
timolol (Blocadren)
zolmitriptan (Zomig)

OSTEOPOROSIS
alendronate sodium (Fosamax)
calcitonin-salmon (Calcimar)
ibandronate (Boniva) (see alendronate sodium)
raloxifene (Evista)
risedronate sodium (Actonel)
teriparatide acetate (Forteo)
zoledronic acid (Zometa)

PARKINSON DISEASE/ ANTICHOLINERGICS
amantadine (Symmetrel)
biperiden HCl (Akineton)
bromocriptine mesylate (Parlodel)
entacapone (Comtan)
levodopa/carbidopa (Sinemet)
pergolide mesylate (Permax)
pramipexole dihydrochloride (Mirapex)
ropinirole HCl (Requip)
selegiline HCl (Eldepryl)
tolcapone (Tasmar)

SKELETAL MUSCLE RELAXANT
carisoprodol (Soma)
cyclobenzaprine (Flexeril)
metaxalone (Skelaxin)
methocarbamol (Robaxin)

SMOKING CESSATION
bupropion (Zyban)
nicotine polacrilex (Nicorette)
nicotine transdermal (Habitrol, ProStep)

SUBSTANCE ABUSE
buprenorphine (Buprenex)
buprenorphine/naloxone (Suboxone)
disulfiram (Antabuse)
⊠flumazenil (Romazicon)
⊠naloxone (Narcan)
naltrexone (ReVia, Trexan)

THYROID DISEASE
HYPERTHYROIDISM
methimazole (Tapazole)
propylthiouracil (PTU)
HYPOTHYROIDISM
levothyroxine (Synthroid)
liothyronine (Cytomel)
liotrix (Euthroid)
thyroid (Armour Thyroid)

TUBERCULOSIS
aminosalicylic acid (Paser)
cycloserine (Seromycin)
ethambutol (Myambutol)
ethionamide (Trecator)
isoniazid (INH, Nydrazid)
pyrazinamide (generic only)
pyrazinamide/rifampin, INH (Rifater)
rifabutin (Mycobutin)
rifampin (Rifadin)
rifampin/isoniazid (Rifamate)
rifapentine (Priftin)

XEROSTOMIA/ CHOLINERGICS
⊠cevimeline (Evoxac)
⊠pilocarpine HCl (Salagen)

Appendix B

Abbreviations

A1C, Hg A1C	glycosylated hemoglobin lab test
ACE	angiotensin-converting enzyme
ADA	American Dental Association
ADHD	attention deficit hyperactivity disorder
apo B	apolipoprotein B
ASA	acetylsalicylic acid (aspirin)
AUC	area under the curve
AV	atriovenous
b.i.d., bid	twice a day [L. *bis in die*]
BP	blood pressure
BPH	benign prostate hypertrophy
BT	bleeding time
BUN	blood urea nitrogen
CAD	coronary artery disease
C_{cr}, Ccr	creatinine clearance
CHF	congestive heart failure
Cl_R	renal clearance
C_{max}	maximal drug concentration
CNS	central nervous system
COPD	chronic obstructive pulmonary disease
COX	cyclooxygenase
CV	cardiovascular
CVD	cardiovascular disease
DIC	disseminated intravascular coagulation
DDS	doctor of dental surgery
DM	diabetes mellitus

Abbreviations

DNA	deoxyribonucleic acid
DVT	deep vein thrombosis
GABA	gamma aminobutyric acid
GERD	gastroesophageal reflux disease
GI	gastrointestinal
GU	genitourinary
H_1	histamine 1 receptor
HBr	hydrobromide
HCl	hydrochloride
HDL	high-density lipoprotein
HIV	human immunodeficiency virus
HMG-CoA	3-hydroxy-3-methylglutaryl-coenzyme A reductase
hr	hour
5-HT	5-hydroxytryptamine
IL	interleukin
IM	intramuscular
INR	international normalized ratio
INX	interaction
IV	intravenous
JRA	juvenile rheumatoid arthritis
LDL	low-density lipoprotein
LFT	liver function test
MAO	monoamine oxidase
MD	medical doctor
MI	myocardial infarction
min	minute

Abbreviations

MISC	miscellaneous
mo	month
MTX	methotrexate
NSAID	nonsteroidal anti-inflammatory drug
OCD	obsessive-compulsive disorder
OTC	over the counter
PAF	paroxysmal atrial fibrillation
PE	pulmonary embolism
PMDD	premenstrual dysphoric disorder
PMN	polymorphonuclear leukocytes
p.o., PO	by mouth, orally [L. *per os*]
p.r., PR	by way of rectum [L. *per rectum*]
p.r.n., prn	as needed [L. *pro re nata*]
PSVT	paroxysmal supraventricular tachycardia
PT	prothrombin time
PTSD	posttraumatic stress disorder
PUD	peptic ulcer disease
PX	prevention
q.6h., q6h	every six hours
q.i.d., qid	four times a day [L. *quater in die*]
RCT	randomized controlled trial
RNA	ribonucleic acid
RSV	respiratory syncytial virus
SC	subcutaneous
SL	sublingual
SR	sustained release
SSRI	selective serotonin reuptake inhibitor

Abbreviations

$t_{1/2}$	elimination half life
t.i.d., tid	three times a day [L. *ter in die*]
TJR	total joint replacement
T_{max}	time to maximum blood level
TMJ	temporomandibular joint
TNF	tumor necrosis factor
TX	treatment
URI	upper respiratory tract infection
UTI	urinary tract infection
Vd	volume of distribution
VLDL	very low density lipoprotein
VT	ventricular tachycardia
WBC	white blood cell
wk	week
XR	extended release
yr	year

Appendix C

Herbal and Nutritional Supplements of Interest to Dentistry

The information in this section addresses only the clinical implications relevant to oral health care when clients are taking a supplement. The common supplement name is followed in brackets by other names used.

When conducting a review of the patient's health history, ask the following questions:

- Do you take any supplements or herbal products?
- What do you take?
- How much do you take and how often do you take it?
- Why are you taking this/these product(s)?
- Did you take any today?

Herbs with theoretical antiplatelet/anticoagulant potential because they contain coumarin, salicylate, or other antiplatelet constituents: angelica, anise, arnica, asafoetida, bogbean, boldo, capsicum, celery, chamomile, clove, cranberry, cucurbita, danshen, dong quai, fenugreek, feverfew, garlic, ginger, ginkgo biloba, (Siberian) ginseng, (Panax) ginseng, green tea, horse chestnut, horseradish, licorice, *Lycium barbarum,* mango, meadowsweet, prickly ash, onion, papain, passion flower, poplar, quassia, quilinggao, quinine, red clover, tumeric, vitamin E–containing herbs (sunflower seeds), wild carrot, wild lettuce, and willow.[C-1]

Herbs with theoretical additive sedation effects: calamus, calendula, California poppy, catnip, capsicum, celery, elecampane, (Siberian) ginseng, German chamomile, goldenseal, gotu kola, hops, Jamaican dogwood, kava, lemon balm, sage, St. John's wort, sassafras, skullcap, shepherd's purse, stinging nettle, valerian, wild carrot, wild lettuce, withania root, and yerba mansa.[C-1]

Herb or Supplement	Implications for Dentistry
aloe vera [burn plant, curacao aloe, Zanzibar aloe]	• Topical application of gel; oral liquid or juice is used to prevent periodontal disease; no randomized controlled trial evidence for support • Swallowing liquid aloe vera may inhibit absorption of oral drugs; allow 2 hr between doses • Overuse and subsequent K^+ loss may increase risks/side effects with corticosteroids • Hypoglycemic side effects: monitor client with diabetes

[C-1] Excerpted from Natural Medicines Comprehensive Database. www.naturaldatabase.com

Herb or Supplement	Implications for Dentistry
astragalus [milk vetch, huang chi]	• This herb has the potential to lower blood pressure; patient should be monitored for orthostatic hypotension • Monitor blood pressure in elderly, those with CVD, or clients fasting in preparation for surgery • May reduce effects of corticosteroids • Additive effects with benzodiazepines, CNS depressants, barbiturates, and opioids; monitor for orthostatic hypotension
bilberry fruit [blueberry, huckleberry, hurtleberry]	• Used as an astringent to relieve oral inflammation • At high doses, platelet aggregation may be inhibited, resulting in increased bleeding • Avoid use of NSAIDs for orodental pain
bistort [adderwort, dragonwort, snakeweed]	• Has been used as a mouthwash to treat periodontal disease, aphthous ulcers, and mouth ulcerations • Herb has no influence on dental treatment
black cohosh [black snakeroot, baneberry, squaw root, rattleroot]	• High doses can lead to hypotension, bradycardia, and gastric distress; monitor vital signs and use semisupine chair position • Contains salicylic acid; risk for toxicity when other salicylates are used • Additive hepatotoxicity: avoid use with acetaminophen, NSAIDs, macrolide antibiotics, azole antifungals, and dapsone • Hypotensive effects may be enhanced if used with anesthetics or sedatives
Boswellia [frankincense]	• In vitro studies have shown antiinflammatory effects • Herb has no influence on dental treatment; no drug interactions reported

Herb or Supplement	Implications for Dentistry
bromelain [bromelin, pineapple]	• Used for acute postoperative or posttrauma conditions of swelling, inhibition of blood platelet aggregation, and enhanced antibiotic absorption • Contains enzyme that may release kinin to stimulate prostaglandin E_1-like compounds • **Adverse effects:** GI disturbances, diarrhea • Has potential to increase bleeding time with NSAIDs, aspirin • Tetracyclines: increased plasma and urine levels of tetracyclines
butterbur [*Petasites*, blatterdock, butterfly dork]	• May have antiinflammatory, antispasmodic effects on smooth muscle; randomized controlled trials support use as antimigraine agent • Drug interaction: CYP3A4 inhibitors (erythromycin, azole antifungals) may increase hepatotoxicity of butterbur • Eugenol: May increase pyrrolizidine alkaloid toxicity
Calendula [marigold, holligold, marybud]	• Topical use to treat inflammation of oral mucosa, increase healing through anti-inflammatory and granulatory actions • Theoretical enhanced sedation and adverse effects with sedatives, drugs having CNS depressant properties
Capsicum [cayenne pepper, capsaicin, chili pepper]	• Used for toothache, pharyngitis, reducing muscle cramps, and joint pain • Topical OTC agent [Zostrix, others]; no drug interactions reported • **Oral use:** Platelet aggregation may be inhibited resulting in increased bleeding • Additive sedative and side effects with barbiturates and sedatives

Herb or Supplement	Implications for Dentistry
cat's claw [Una de Gato, Vine of Peru, Samento]	• Platelet aggregation may be inhibited resulting in increased bleeding • Avoid recommending aspirin, NSAIDs; additive bleeding effect • Advise to stop herb 2 wk before surgery • **Adverse effects:** diarrhea, hypotension, bleeding gums, bruising • Herb has potential to lower blood pressure; monitor for orthostatic hypotension • Theoretically may interfere with corticosteroid activity
chamomile [German chamomile]	• Used as mouthwash for aphthous ulcers, anti-inflammatory • Contains volatile oil and umbelliferone (coumarin-like ingredient) that may cause increased bleeding • **Oral use:** Enhanced sedation and adverse effects theoretically possible with CNS depressants, sedatives • Avoid recommending aspirin, NSAIDs; additive bleeding effect • Advise to stop herb 2 wk before surgery
chasteberry [chaste tree, hemp tree, monk's pepper]	• **Adverse effects:** dry mouth, tachycardia • Monitor pulse before treatment • If chronic dry mouth results, recommend home fluoride products for cariostatic effects • No dental drug interactions reported
chondroitin sulfate	• Used alone or in conjunction with glucosamine to relieve symptoms of osteoarthritis • Determine whether TMJ or fingers/wrist are affected and relation to oral hygiene effectiveness or ability to hold mouth open for dental treatment • No dental drug interactions reported, but be aware client may also be using salicylates (antiplatelet affect)

Herb or Supplement	Implications for Dentistry
clove [lavanga, caryophylli]	• Oil of cloves contains eugenol, used to relieve toothache and dry socket; component of temporary filling dental material; used as mouthwash and to relieve mouth and throat inflammation • Self-application of oil may result in gingival irritation and facial anesthesia • Platelet aggregation may be inhibited resulting in increased bleeding • Avoid recommending aspirin, NSAIDs; additive bleeding effect
coenzyme Q-10 [CoQ-10]	• Used to boost immune system; topically to treat periodontal disease; CHF, CVD, DM, and other reasons • Ask why supplement is used, consider effect of disease on dental treatment • Likely ineffective for periodontal treatment • No dental drug interactions reported
coleus forskohlii [forskolin, colforsin, borforsin]	• Additive effects with benzodiazepines, CNS depressants, barbiturates, opioids: herb has potential to lower blood pressure, monitor for orthostatic hypotension • Platelet aggregation may be inhibited resulting in increased bleeding • Avoid recommending aspirin, NSAIDs; additive bleeding effect
cordyceps	• Platelet aggregation may be inhibited resulting in increased bleeding • Avoid recommending aspirin, NSAIDs; additive bleeding effect • May decrease immunosuppressant effects of prednisone
cranberry [vaccinium vitis-ideae]	• Cranberry juice in large amounts can reduce urinary pH, theoretically causing increased excretion of opiates, antidepressants, some antibiotics
creatine	• Used in neuromuscular disorders to increase muscle mass • No dental drug interactions reported

Herb or Supplement	Implications for Dentistry
devil's claw [grapple plant, wood spider]	• Used topically as ointment for injuries; oral use: variety of uses • May cause loss of taste (8%) • **Oral use:** Claims of hypotensive effect; monitor blood pressure in elderly, those with CVD • May decrease blood glucose; monitor client with diabetes • Theoretically, because of increase in stomach acids, could enhance absorption of penicillin and doxycycline • Platelet aggregation may be inhibited resulting in increased bleeding • Avoid recommending aspirin, NSAIDs; additive bleeding effect
Dong quai [*Angelica sinensis*]	• Used in Chinese medicine for gynecological complaints • Additive effects with benzodiazepines, CNS depressants, barbiturates, opioids: herb has potential to lower blood pressure; monitor for orthostatic hypotension • Platelet aggregation may be inhibited resulting in increased bleeding • Avoid recommending aspirin, NSAIDs; additive bleeding effect • Tetracycline: photosensitization reactions possible • Enhanced sedation and hypotension theoretically possible with CNS depressants, sedatives

Herb or Supplement	Implications for Dentistry
Echinacea purpurea [purple coneflower, Kansas snakeroot]	• Used topically to treat mouth and pharyngeal inflammation • Daily use may depress immunity; anecdotal reports of oral candidiasis when used for more than 8 weeks • May interfere with corticosteroid action • Additive hepatotoxicity: avoid use with acetaminophen, NSAIDs, macrolide antibiotics, azole antifungals, and dapsone • Phenobarbital and other microsomal enzyme inducers may decrease the effects of echinacea • Discontinue echinacea before use of general anesthetics or 2 wk before surgery
Eleutherococcus [Siberian ginseng, devil's shrub, wild pepper, touch-me-not]	• Often contains ginsenosides with opposing effects: may cause either an increase or decrease in blood pressure or CNS stimulation or depression • **Adverse effects:** hypertension, tachycardia • Monitor blood pressure and pulse before dental treatment • Platelet aggregation may be inhibited, resulting in increased bleeding • Avoid recommending aspirin, NSAIDs; additive bleeding effect • Enhanced sedation and adverse effects theoretically possible with CNS depressants, sedatives • Use epinephrine with caution, in low doses • Siberian ginseng is different than Panax ginseng (American)
ephedra [ma huang]	• Sympathomimetic action: cardiovascular stimulation may cause fatal arrhythmia, myocardial infarction, stroke, hypertensive crisis • Action may be potentiated with propoxyphene • Use epinephrine with caution, low doses • Sale currently banned in United States

Herb or Supplement	Implications for Dentistry
essential oils	• Eugenol, thymol, carvacrol, menthol, eucalyptol, and oil of cloves are examples • Listerine contains menthol, thymol, eucalyptol, and methyl salicylate with alcohol • Antibacterial effect of combination product led to ADA approval as antigingivitis mouthrinse (not to be swallowed)
evening primrose [feverplant, night willow herb, scabish]	• Weak evidence supports use for periodontitis because of anti-inflammatory effects • Platelet aggregation may be inhibited resulting in increased bleeding • Avoid recommending aspirin, NSAIDs; theoretical additive bleeding effect • Monitor blood pressure because of potential hypotensive effect
feverfew [featherfew, midsummer daisy, *Tanacetum parthenium*]	• Primary use: migraine prophylaxis; used after tooth extraction as a mouthwash for anti-inflammatory and antiseptic properties • Chewing fresh leaves may cause mouth ulceration, loss of taste, and glossitis • Platelet aggregation may be inhibited resulting in increased bleeding • Avoid recommending aspirin, NSAIDs; additive bleeding effect—NSAIDs can theoretically decrease the effectiveness of feverfew

Herb or Supplement	Implications for Dentistry
garlic [*Allium sativum*, stinking rose]	• Determine why client is taking herb; often used to treat symptoms of CVD; consider effects of condition on dental treatment • Additive effects with benzodiazepines, CNS depressants, barbiturates, opioids: herb has potential to lower blood pressure; monitor for orthostatic hypotension • Monitor vital signs from cardiovascular effects • Platelet aggregation may be inhibited resulting in increased bleeding • Avoid recommending aspirin, NSAIDs; additive bleeding effect • Advise to stop herb 2 wk before surgery • Fresh garlic: Increased effects of triazolam because of inhibition of first-pass effect • Risk of hypoglycemia in client taking insulin or sulfonylureas
ginger [*Zingiber* rhizoma]	• Fresh ginger may be taken to reduce toothache • Additive effects with benzodiazepines, CNS depressants, barbiturates, opioids: herb has potential to lower blood pressure; monitor for orthostatic hypotension • Monitor vital signs from cardiovascular effects • Platelet aggregation may be inhibited resulting in increased bleeding • Avoid recommending aspirin, NSAIDs; additive bleeding effect • Risk of hypoglycemia in client taking insulin • May enhance barbiturate action
ginkgo biloba [maidenhair tree, kew tree]	• Determine why client is taking herb; often used to treat symptoms of CVD; consider effects of condition on dental treatment • Platelet aggregation may be inhibited resulting in increased bleeding • Avoid recommending aspirin, NSAIDs; additive bleeding effect • Advise to stop herb 2 wk before surgery

Herb or Supplement	Implications for Dentistry
ginseng, Panax [Asian, Chinese, Japanese or Korean ginseng, red ginseng, tartar root]	• Monitor vital signs due to cardiovascular effects • Additive effects with benzodiazepines, CNS depressants, barbiturates, opioids: herb has potential to lower blood pressure; monitor for orthostatic hypotension • Platelet aggregation may be inhibited resulting in increased bleeding • Avoid recommending aspirin, NSAIDs; additive bleeding effect • Advise to stop herb 2 wk before surgery • Risk of hypoglycemia in client taking insulin
glucosamine sulfate	• Used for joint dysfunction, osteoarthritis: question about use of aspirin, NSAIDs • No dental drug interactions reported
goldenseal [yellow root, *Hydrastis canadensis*]	• Used as mouthrinse to relieve gingival pain and herpes labialis • High doses have hypertensive effect: monitor blood pressure • Enhanced sedation and adverse effects theoretically possible with CNS depressants, sedatives • Additive photosensitization with tetracyclines
gotu kola [Centella, Indian pennywort]	• Used in oral rinse for anti-inflammatory effect, wound healing • High doses have hypertensive effect: monitor blood pressure • **Oral use:** Enhanced sedation and adverse effects theoretically possible with CNS depressants, sedatives
grape seed [*Vitis vinifera*]	• Determine why client is taking herb; often used to treat symptoms of CVD; consider effects of condition on dental treatment • No dental drug interactions reported

Herb or Supplement	Implications for Dentistry
green tea	• Tea bags can be used after tooth extraction for hemostasis • Caffeine component can decrease effectiveness of aspirin, APAP; also implicated in many drug interactions causing increased CNS stimulation and increased heart rate • Theoretically can reduce effects of benzodiazepines • Reduced metabolism of herb and increased CNS effects possible with fluconazole, CNS depressants
guar gum	• Decreased absorption of penicillin, aspirin; take 1 hr before or several hours after guar gum
guggul	• Used in Ayurvedic medicine for arthritis; in mouthrinse for anti-inflammatory effect and to promote healing • Question client about concurrent use of aspirin, NSAIDs • Platelet aggregation may be inhibited resulting in increased bleeding • May decrease absorption of many other drugs
hawthorn	• Determine why client is taking herb; often used to treat symptoms of CVD, hypertension; consider effects of condition on dental treatment • Monitor vital signs because of cardiovascular effects • Additive effects with benzodiazepines, CNS depressants, barbiturates, opioids: herb has potential to lower blood pressure; monitor for orthostatic hypotension
horse chestnut [buckeye]	• Platelet aggregation may be inhibited, resulting in increased bleeding • Avoid recommending aspirin, NSAIDs; additive bleeding effect • Advise to stop herb 2 wk before surgery • Theoretically, the saponin constituent of horse chestnut seed or extract might interfere with protein binding of oral drugs

Herb or Supplement	Implications for Dentistry
kava [kava kava, intoxicating pepper, kew]	• Chewing kava can cause intraoral numbness • Kava has analgesic properties not reversed by naloxone • Advise to stop herb 2 wk before surgery • Enhanced sedation and adverse effects theoretically possible with CNS depressants, sedatives • Additive hepatotoxicity: avoid use with acetaminophen, NSAIDs, macrolide antibiotics, azole antifungals, and dapsone • Long-term use may produce tolerance to benzodiazepines
lemon balm [honey plant, *Melissa*, dropsy plant]	• Topical use to reduce symptoms for herpes labialis • **Oral use:** Enhanced sedation and adverse effects theoretically possible with CNS depressants, sedatives • Theoretically, taking lemon balm with barbiturates can produce additive effects
licorice [*Glycyrrhiza*, sweet root]	• Ask why client is using herb: used for upper respiratory tract infections; monitor for infectious potential and disease transmission during dental treatment • Licorice candy does not contain the herb; it is flavored with anise • Overuse of licorice can produce cardiovascular toxicity, hypokalemia, increased blood pressure; monitor vital signs • Platelet aggregation may be inhibited resulting in increased bleeding • Avoid recommending aspirin, NSAIDs; additive bleeding effect. NSAIDS may also increase water retention • Increased activity of corticosteroids (oral and topical)

Herb or Supplement	Implications for Dentistry
lysine [L-Lysine, Lys]	• Used to reduce symptoms and healing time of herpes labialis • **Oral use:** 1,000 mg daily for 12 months and 1,000 mg three times a day for 6 months reported in clinical trials • No dental drug interactions reported
melatonin [pineal hormone, MLT]	• Melatonin can interfere with immunosuppressant drug action • Enhanced sedation and adverse effects theoretically possible with CNS depressants, sedatives
myrrh [*Commiphora molmol*]	• Resin used topically to reduce oral and pharyngeal inflammation, aphthous ulcers pain, and gingivitis • No dental drug interactions reported
nettle root [stinging nettle]	• Used to reduce symptoms of inflammation, osteoarthritis: may be taking aspirin, NSAIDs • **Adverse effects:** hypotension: monitor for orthostatic hypotension • Additive CNS depressant effects with CNS depressants
parsley	• Fresh parsley is chewed as a breath freshener • Herb has potential to lower blood pressure; monitor for orthostatic hypotension • No dental drug interactions reported
passion flower [maypop, passion vine]	• Platelet aggregation may be inhibited, resulting in increased bleeding • Avoid recommending aspirin, NSAIDs; additive bleeding effect • Enhanced sedation and adverse effects theoretically possible with CNS depressants, sedatives
peppermint oil	• Ask why client is using herb: used as inhalant to relieve upper respiratory tract congestion; determine risk for infectiousness • Primary constituent of the oil is menthol

Herb or Supplement	Implications for Dentistry
prickly ash [prickly yellowwood, toothache tree]	• Has been used to relieve toothache, ulcerations • Platelet aggregation may be inhibited, resulting in increased bleeding • Avoid recommending aspirin, NSAIDs; additive bleeding effect
probiotics [acidophilus]	• Product contains microorganisms to colonize GI flora while taking antibiotics • Determine why supplement is being taken; determine risk for infectiousness or relationship to dental treatment • Use of probiotics ½ hr before or 3 hr after taking antibiotics may prevent antibiotic-associated diarrhea
quercetin [meletin, sophretin]	• Determine why client is taking herb; often used to treat symptoms of CVD; consider effects of condition on dental treatment • Monitor vital signs because of potential cardiovascular effects • No dental drug interactions reported; may oppose effects of quinolone antibiotics
red clover [cow clover, beebread]	• Used to relieve symptoms of upper respiratory tract infection; determine risk for infectiousness during dental treatment • Coumarin constituents in red clover can result in increased bleeding • Avoid recommending aspirin, NSAIDs; additive bleeding effect
red yeast rice [monascus, ZhiTai]	• Determine why client is taking herb; often used to treat symptoms of CVD; consider effects of condition on dental treatment • Product contains lovastatin to block production of cholesterol in the liver • Additive hepatotoxicity: avoid use with acetaminophen, NSAIDs, macrolide antibiotics, azole antifungals, and dapsone • Azole antifungals, erythromycin: inhibits metabolism of red yeast rice; potential for toxicity

Herb or Supplement	Implications for Dentistry
rhatany [Krameria, mapato]	• Used topically for inflamed oral and pharyngeal mucosa, gingivitis, glossitis, stomatitis, and canker sores • No dental drug interactions reported
sage [*Salvia officinalis*]	• Used topically as a gargle for pharyngitis, stomatitis, gingivitis, or for oral injury • Sage and rhubarb mixed in cream used for herpes labialis • Additive effects with benzodiazepines, CNS depressants, barbiturates, opioids: herb has potential to lower blood pressure; monitor for orthostatic hypotension • **Adverse effects:** cheilitis, stomatitis, dry mouth • Enhanced sedation and adverse effects theoretically possible with CNS depressants, sedatives
SAMe [s-adenosylmethionine]	• Determine why client is taking supplement; consider relevance to dental treatment • Platelet aggregation may be inhibited resulting in increased bleeding • Avoid recommending aspirin, NSAIDs; additive bleeding effect • Theoretical concern that use with meperidine or tramadol may cause serotonin syndrome
saw palmetto [Serenoa repens]	• **Adverse effects:** GI complaints, nausea; determine whether semisupine chair position is desired • May enhance bleeding if aspirin, NSAIDS are taken

Herb or Supplement	Implications for Dentistry
St. John's wort [*Hypericum perforatum*]	• Determine why client is taking herb; consider relationship to ability to handle stress of dental treatment and motivation for self-care • Advise to stop herb 2 wk before surgery • Enhanced sedation and adverse effects theoretically possible with CNS depressants, sedatives • **Adverse effects:** GI complaints, photosensitivity • Interactions are possible with a variety of drugs, often leading to reduced drug action; potent CYP3A4 inhibitor • Increased risk for serotonin syndrome if used with tramadol or meperidine • Tetracyclines: increased potential for photosensitivity: advise to wear sunscreen if exposed to sunlight
stevia [sweetleaf, Yerba dulce]	• Cariostatic sweetener used in dental gels, mouthrinses • High doses can have hypotensive effect; monitor blood pressure • No dental drug interactions reported
tryptophans [L-tryptophan]	• Theoretical concern about serotonin syndrome with meperidine, tramadol • May cause dry mouth • Additive sedation with CNS depressants
turmeric [Curcuma, Indian saffron]	• Used for symptoms of dyspepsia, bloating: may need to use a semisupine chair position • Herb has potential to lower blood pressure; monitor for orthostatic hypotension • Platelet aggregation may be inhibited resulting in increased bleeding • Avoid recommending aspirin, NSAIDs; additive bleeding effect

Herb or Supplement	Implications for Dentistry
valerian [All heal; garden heliotrope, amantilla]	• Determine why client is using herb: used to promote sleep, relieve anxiety: determine relationship to ability to handle stress of dental treatment • Enhanced sedation and adverse effects theoretically possible with CNS depressants, sedatives • Avoid taking 2 weeks before surgery • May inhibit CYP3A4 isoenzymes
xylitol	• A cariostatic sweetener from birch tree bark in toothpaste, gum, or gels • No dental drug interactions reported
yohimbe	• Large doses: herb has potential to lower blood pressure; monitor for orthostatic hypotension • **Adverse effects:** salivation, tachycardia, hypertension • Monitor vital signs for cardiovascular effects • Use indirect-acting sympathomimetics with caution, in low doses, with aspirating syringe

BIBLIOGRAPHY

1. Agricultural Research Services. Dr. Duke's Phytochemical and Ethnobotanical Database. Available at: http://www.ars-grin.gov/duke/index.html.
2. Alternative Medicine Foundation. HerbMed database. Available at: http://www.herbmed.org.
3. American Botanical Council. Available at: http://www.herbalgram.org.
4. Gage T, Pickett F. Mosby's Dental Drug Reference [Appendix H]. St. Louis: Mosby, 2004.
5. Jacobsen P, Cohan R, Blumenthal M, Bruce G. Alternative Medicine in Dentistry. In: Yagiela JA, Dowd FJ, Neidle EA, eds. *Pharmacology and Therapeutics for Dentistry.* 5th ed. St. Louis: Mosby, 2004:880–889.
6. Jellin JM, Batz F, Hitchens, K. Pharmacist's Letter/Prescriber's Letter Natural Medicines Comprehensive Database. Stockton, CA: Therapeutic Research Faculty, 1999.
7. Jellin JM, Gregory PH, Batz F, Hitchens, K, et al. Pharmacist's Letter/Prescriber's Letter Natural Medicines Comprehensive Database. 7th ed. Stockton, CA: Therapeutic Research Faculty, 2005.
8. Little J. Complementary and alternative medicine: impact on dentistry. Oral Surg Oral Med Oral Pathol Oral Radiol Endod 2004;98:137–145.
9. National Cancer Institute. NCCAM Fact Sheets on Coenzyme Q10. Available at: http://cis.nci.nih.gov/fact/9_16.htm.
10. National Center for Complementary and Alternative Medicine. Available at: http://nccam.nih.gov/.
11. Therapeutic Research Faculty. Natural Medicines Comprehensive Database. Available at: http://www.naturaldatabase.com.
12. Touger-Decker R. Dietary Supplements and Oral Health: Should the dentist ask? Quintessence Intl 2005:36(4): 287–292.
13. U.S. Food and Drug Administration. FDA Office of Dietary Supplements. Available at: www.cfsan.fda.gov/~dms/supplmnt.html.
14. U.S. Food and Drug Administration. Food Health Claims. Available at: http://www.cfsan.fda.gov/~dms/flg-6c.html.

Appendix D

English/Spanish Dental Communication
Inglés/Español — Comunicación dental

From *Vamos al Dentista*, UTHSC, San Antonio, TX[D-1]

Basic Dental Terms	Términos dentales básicos
dental chair	la silla dental
dental floss	el hilo dental
dental office	consultorio dental
dentist	el dentista (male)/la dentista (female)
dentists	los dentistas
cavity	caries
a filling	un empaste un relleno
several fillings	unos empastes unos rellenos
tooth	diente
baby tooth	diente de leche
broken tooth	diente partido
gum (gingiva)	encía
abscess	absceso
the suture	la sutura
injection	inyección
toothbrush	el cepillo dental
toothpaste	la pasta de dientes
tongue	la lengua
lips	los labios
TMJ	la ATM articulación mandíbulo-temporal
Thank you.	gracias
You're welcome.	de nada

D-1 Adapted with permission from Glass BJ, Partida N, Rodriguez I, Arredondo DG. *Vamos al Dentista (Let's go to the Dentist): English to Spanish Translations of Commonly Used Terms and Phrases in the Dental Office.* UTHSCSA Dental School; 1999. To order the full booklet, please contact Becky Nixon, UTHSCSA Dental School, Office of Continuing Education, at (210) 567-3177 or by e-mail to Nixon@uthscsa.edu.

Basic Dental Phrases	Frases dentales básicas
I am the dentist.	Yo soy el (male)/la (female) dentista.
What is your problem?	¿Cuál es su problema?
How old are you?	¿Cuántos años tienes?
How are you?	¿Cómo está usted?
How long have you had the problem?	¿Por cuánto tiempo ha tenido este problema?
Did you brush your teeth?	¿Se cepilló los dientes?
I have to extract the molar.	Tengo que sacarle la muela.
We need to do an exam.	Tenemos que examinarlo (-a).
Are you in pain?	¿Tiene usted dolor?
Does this hurt?	¿Le duele esto?
Bite the gauze.	¡Muerde la gaza!
Use that towel.	¡Use esa toalla!
Drink the water!	¡Beba el agua!
Swish the water!	¡Enjuáguese con el agua!
Open your mouth!	¡Abra la boca!
Please say "ahh!"	¡Diga "ahh," por favor!
Please stick out your tongue.	Saque la lengua, por favor.
Lower/raise your chin.	¡Baje/suba la barba!
Breathe through your nose.	¡Respire por la nariz!
We are going to take some pictures of your teeth.	Vamos a tomarle unas fotografías de los dientes.
This lead apron is for your protection.	Este chaleco de plomo es para su protección.

General Office Terms	Expresiones comunes del consultorio
dental office	el consultorio dental
waiting room	la sala de espera
restroom	los servicios el baño
operatory	sala de operaciones
prescription	la receta la prescripción
dental instruments	los instrumentos dentales
suction	el succionador
x-ray machine	la máquina de rayos-x
x-ray film	la radiografía
receptionist	la recepcionista
dental assistant	la asistente dental
dental hygienist	la higienista dental
dental lab	el laboratorio dental
dental lab technician	el técnico (male)/la técnica (female)

Communication with the Receptionist	Comunicación con la recepcionista
What is your name?	¿Cómo se llama?
How are you, Mr./Mrs./Miss?	¿Cómo está, señor/señora/señorita?
Please sit down.	¡Siéntese, por favor!
The doctor will be with you in a moment.	El doctor/la doctora la verá en un momento.
Everything is going to be fine.	Todo va a estar bien.

FIRST DENTAL APPOINTMENT

PRIMERA CONSULTA DENTAL

Chief Complaint	Queja principal
What brought you here today?	¿Qué la trajo aquí hoy?
Are you in pain? Where?	¿Tiene dolor? ¿Dónde?
Where does it hurt the most?	¿Dónde le duele más?
Have you had a serious problem with previous dental work?	¿Ha tenido algún problema serio con previos trabajos dentales?
In case of an emergency, who should we call?	En caso de emergencia, ¿a quién llamamos?
We are going to take your medical history.	Vamos a preguntarle sobre su historia clínica.

Medical History	Historia clínica
Are you under the care of a physician?	¿Está consultando a un doctor?
When was the last time you visited a physician? Why?	¿Cuándo fue la ultima vez que visitó un médico? ¿Por qué?
Are you allergic to penicillin or other medicine?	¿Es alérgico (-a) a la penicilina, yodo o cualquier otro medicamento?
Have you ever had rheumatic fever, a heart murmur, heart surgery, or a joint replacement?	¿Ha tenido fiebre reumática, murmullo/soplo en el corazón, operación del corazón o le han reemplazado alguna articulación?
Are there recent dental x-rays of your teeth that we might borrow? If so, whom can we contact?	¿Le han tomado recientemente radiografías de sus dientes? ¿Podríamos pedirlas prestadas? ¿A quién podemos pedirlas?
Have you had a tumor or cancer? When?	¿Ha tenido un tumor o cáncer? ¿Cuándo?
Have you had a local anesthetic or general anesthetic?	¿Le han dado anestesia local o anestesia general alguna vez?
Have you had a reaction to an anesthetic?	¿Ha tenido reacción a alguna anestesia?
Do you have sinus trouble, asthma, hayfever, or severe headaches?	¿Tiene problemas de sinusitis, asma, alergias o severos dolores de cabeza?
Do you have high, low, or normal blood pressure?	¿Tiene la presión alta, baja o normal?

Medical History	Historia clínica
Have you had a heart attack or pains in your chest?	¿Tiene o ha tenido un ataque al corazón o dolor en el pecho?
Does mild exercise leave you short of breath?	¿Le falta la respiración cuando hace ejercicios ligeros?
Do you have heart problems?	¿Tiene problemas del corazón?
Have you had tuberculosis or another lung problem?	¿Ha tenido tuberculosis o algún otro problema con los pulmones?
Have you had a liver condition (hepatitis, jaundice, or cirrhosis)?	¿Ha tenido algún problema del hígado, (hepatitis, ictericia o cirrosis)?
Have you had sexually transmitted diseases?	¿Ha tenido enfermedades transmitidas sexualmente?
Have you had aphthous ulcers or cold sores?	¿Ha tenido úlceras, fuego o herpes labial?
Do you urinate frequently?	¿Orina frecuentemente?
How many times per night do you get up to urinate?	¿Cuántas veces se levanta por la noche para orinar?

Does anyone in your family have diabetes? Who?
    mother
    father
    brother
    sister
	¿Hay alguna persona en su familia que tenga diabetes? ¿Quién?
	    mamá
	    papá
	    hermano
	    hermana

Do you have diabetes?	¿Tiene diabetes?
Are you controlled by insulin? Diet? Medicine?	¿Está controlada con insulina? ¿Con una dieta? ¿Con medicamento?
Have you had seizures (such as epilepsy or fainting)?	¿Ha tenido ataques o convulsiones (como epilepsia o desmayos)?
Do you take medication for nervousness or depression?	¿Ha tomado medicinas para los nervios o depresión?
Do you have a tendency to bleed longer than normal?	¿Sangra mucho tiempo con cortadas pequeñas? ¿Tiene tendencia a sangrar más de lo normal?
Have you been hospitalized or received medical treatment within the past 5 years?	¿Ha estado en el hospital o ha recibido tratamiento en los últimos cinco años?

Medical History	Historia clínica

Have you taken any of these medications in the last 6 months?
   Cortisone or other steroids?
   Anticoagulants or blood thinners?
	¿Ha tomado alguna de las siguientes medicinas en los últimos seis meses?
	   ¿Cortisona o otros esteroides?
	   ¿Anticoagulantes o medicinas para la sangre?

Do you have any disease, condition, or problem not listed above? Any family or inherited diseases?	¿Tiene usted alguna enfermedad, o problemas de salud que no estén en este cuestionario? ¿Alguna enfermedad hereditaria?
Are you pregnant? Expected delivery date?	¿Está embarazada? ¿Fecha del parto?
Do you smoke or use tobacco? How many cigarettes per day?	¿Fuma o usa productos de tabaco? ¿Cuántos cigarrillos fuma usted al día?

Do you drink alcoholic beverages? What amount?
   rarely
   moderately
   heavily
   none
	¿Toma bebidas alcohólicas? ¿Cuánto?
	   raramente
	   moderadamente
	   mucho
	   nada

Are you taking medications?	¿Está tomando medicinas?
Which ones, please?	¿Cuáles, por favor?

Dental History	Historia dental
Have you been to a dentist before?	¿Ha consultado un dentista anteriormente?
Have you had an allergic reaction to dental anesthetic?	¿Ha tenido alguna reacción alérgica a la anestesia dental?
Where does it hurt?	¿Dónde le duele?
How long has it hurt?	¿Por cuánto tiempo le ha dolido?
Is it sensitive to cold or hot things?	¿Tiene sensitividad a cosas frías o calientes?
When was this tooth filled?	¿Cuándo le rellenaron este diente?
When was this tooth extracted?	¿Cuándo le sacaron ese diente?
Is the pain throbbing?	¿Es el dolor como una punzada?
Does anything make it feel better or worse?	¿Alguna cosa lo hace sentir mejor o peor?
Do you have a dry mouth?	¿Tiene la boca seca?

Dental Hygiene Appointment	Cita para la higiene dental
How often do you brush your teeth?	¿Cuántas veces se cepilla los dientes?
Do your gums bleed?	¿Sangran sus encías?
Do you use dental floss?	¿Usa seda o hilo dental?
I need to record what I find on your teeth.	Voy a documentar su salud dental.
You have plaque and calculus on your teeth.	Usted tiene placa bacteriana y sarro en sus dientes.
I am going to clean and polish your teeth.	Voy a limpiar y pulir sus dientes.
I am going to scale and debride your teeth.	Voy a hacerle un raspado radicular y alisado radicular en sus dientes.
I am going to give you a fluoride treatment.	Voy a darle un tratamiento de fluoruro.
I am going to place sealants over your molars.	Voy a poner unos sellantes sobre unas muelas.
Sealants protect teeth from decay.	Los selladores protegen sus dientes de picaduras (caries).
Please use a toothpaste with fluoride.	Por favor use una pasta dental que tenga fluoruro.
You have bone loss around your teeth.	Ha perdido hueso alrededor de los dientes.
Your gums bleed.	Sus encías sangran mucho.
You have gum recession.	Tiene retraídas las encías.
You will need surgical treatment of the gum disease to treat the gingiva and bone.	Necesitará cirugía de las encías y del hueso.

End of Appointment/Payment	Terminación de la cita/Pagos
Do you have dental insurance?	¿Tiene seguro dental?
We accept personal checks and credit cards.	Aceptamos cheques y tarjetas de crédito.
You can make payments.	Puede hacer pagos.
It will cost ＿＿＿ dollars and ＿＿＿ cents.	Le va a costar ＿＿＿ dólares y ＿＿＿ centavos.
We need to see you again. We will give you an appointment.	Necesitamos verla(-o) otra vez. Le vamos a dar una cita.
We want to see you in 6 months.	La(-o) queremos ver en seis meses.
Your next appointment is on (date) at (time).	Su próxima cita es ＿＿＿ a ＿＿＿.
Call us if you need to cancel the appointment.	Llámenos si necesita cancelar la cita.
Call us if you have a problem.	Llámenos si tiene problemas.
Our phone number is ＿＿＿.	Nuestro número de teléfono es ＿＿＿.

Appendix E

In-Office Preventive Products

FLUORIDE VARNISHES

Product	Manufacturer	Fluoride
AllSolutions	Dentsply 800-989-8825 www.professional.dentsply.com	5% sodium fluoride
CavityShield	Omnii Oral Pharmaceuticals 800-445-3386 www.omniipharma.com	5% sodium fluoride, pH 7.0; 0.25 ml (pediatric) & 0.40 ml (mixed dentition)
Duraflor	Medicom, Inc. 800-361-2862 www.medicom.ca	5% sodium fluoride, pH 7.0, xylitol as sweetener
Duraphat	Colgate Oral Pharmaceuticals 800-938-5388 www.colgateprofessional.com	5% sodium fluoride, pH 7.0
DuraShield	Sultan Dental Products 800-238-6739 www.sultandental.com	
Fluor Protector	Ivoclar Vivadent www.ivoclar.co.nz	
Fluoridex Lasting Defense	Discus Dental 800-422-9448 www.discusdental.com	
Varnish America	Medical Products Laboratories 800-523-0191 www.medicalproducts laboratories.com	

TOOTHPASTES WITHOUT SODIUM LAUREL SULFATE, CINNAMON, OR METHYLPARABEN

Product	Manufacturer
Advance Toothpaste for Sensitive Teeth	Arm & Hammer/Church & Dwight 800-524-1328
Biotene Dry Mouth Toothpaste	Laclede, Inc. 800-922-5856

Product	Manufacturer
Dental Care Baking Soda Tooth Powder	Arm & Hammer
Natural White with peroxide gel	
Pro_DenRx brush-on 1.1% neutral sodium dentifrice	Pro-Dentec 800-228-5595
Rembrandt Age-Defying Adult Toothpaste	Oral B/Rembrandt Products 800-268-5217 www.jnj.com
Rembrandt Naturals Toothpaste	Oral B/Rembrandt Products
Rembrandt Whitening Canker Sore Prevention Toothpaste	Oral B/Rembrandt Products
Rembrandt Whitening Natural Toothpaste	Oral B/Rembrandt Products
Revelation Toothpowder	Caswell-Massey 800-526-0500
Sensodyne Cool Gel	Sensodyne Products/ GlaxoSmithKline 866-844-2787
Sensodyne Tartar Control Toothpaste, Sensodyne (original) Toothpaste	Sensodyne Products
Slimer Gel	
Thermodent Toothpaste	Lee Pharmaceuticals 800-950-5337
Vince Tooth Powder	Lee Pharmaceuticals

XYLITOL PRODUCTS
Xylitol products with therapeutic dosage levels >1.55 g/serving

Product	Manufacturer
Beechies Xylitol gum	Richardson Brands www.richardsonbrands.com
Clen-Dent mints	Finnfoods, Finland 708-735-7819
Crest Multicare toothpaste	Procter and Gamble www.procterandgamble.com
Kloolerz gum	Hershey Foods Corp. 800-468-1714

Product	Manufacturer
Lotte XYLITOL gum	LotteUSA, Inc. www.lotteusainc.com 269-963-6664
Spry oral rinse, mints, gum, gel for infants	Xlear, Inc. www.sprydental.com
Squigle ADA Enamel Saver Toothpaste	Squigle, Inc. 610-605-5556
Starbucks — Peppermint & Cinnamon gum	Richardson Brands www.richardsonbrands.com
TheraGum, TheraMints, TheraSpray	Omnii Oral Pharmaceuticals 800-445-3386 www.omniipharma.com
V-6 Dental gum, mints	Scanlab, Sweden www.cadburyschweppes.com
Xylichew gum, mints	Naturemart, Finland www.naturemart.com
Xylifresh 100 Cinnamon	Leaf Mfg., Finland

Xylitol products not substantiated as efficacious xylitol content[E-1]

Product	Manufacturer
Advance Baking Soda Gum	Church & Dwight 800-523-1328
Altoids Chewing Gum	Callard & Bowser www.altoids.com
Biotene Mouthwash & Biotene Toothpaste	Laclede 800-922-5856
First Teeth Baby Gel	Laclede
Gerber Tooth & Gum Cleanser	Gerber Products www.gerber.com
Rembrandt Naturals Toothpaste	Oral B/Rembrandt Products 800-268-5217 www.jnj.com
Rembrandt Whitening Canker Sore Prevention Toothpaste	Oral B/Rembrandt Products
Rembrandt Whitening Natural Toothpaste	Oral B/Rembrandt Products

[E-1] Products contain xylitol at levels <1.0 g or unknown

Product	Manufacturer
SMINT Mints	Chupa Chups www.chupachupsgroup.com
Tom's of Maine Natural Mouthwash	Tom's of Maine, Inc. 207-985-2944, ext. 406 www.tomsofmaine.com
Tom's of Maine Toothpaste for Sensitive Teeth & Natural Toothpaste	Tom's of Maine, Inc.
Trident gum with xylitol	Cadbury Adams USA LLC 800-524-2854

ORAL RINSES WITHOUT ALCOHOL

Product	Manufacturer	Active Ingredients
BreathRx Anti-Bacterial Mouth Rinse	Discus Dental 800-422-9448 www.discusdental.com	Zinc, essential oils
Prevention Mouth Rinse – no alcohol	Prevention Products 800-473-1205 www.preventionmouthrinse.com	Zinc/hydrogen peroxide
Pro-Health Rinse	Crest www.dentalcare.com	7% cetylpyridinium Cl

Appendix F

Laboratory Values for Normal Limits

The full text for this appendix can be found on the *LWW's Dental Drug Reference with Clinical Implications* ✹ CD-ROM. The Table of Contents is included here for your reference.

Table of Contents

Cholesterol
Blood Urea Nitrogen
Uric Acid
Creatinine
Calcium
Phosphorus
Alkaline Phosphatase

BIBLIOGRAPHY